T0304751

E-HEALTH CARE INFORMATION SYSTEMS

E-HEALTH CARE INFORMATION SYSTEMS

An Introduction for Students and Professionals

Joseph Tan

Editor

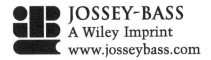

JOSSEY-BASS
A Wiley Imprint
www.josseybass.com

Published by Jossey-Bass
A Wiley Imprint
989 Market Street, San Francisco, CA 94103-1741   www.josseybass.com

Library of Congress Cataloging-in-Publication Data
E-health care information systems : an introduction for students
and professionals / Joseph Tan, editor.
      p. ; cm.
  Includes bibliographical references and indexes.
  ISBN-13 978-0-7879-6618-8 (alk. paper)
  ISBN-10 0-7879-6618-5 (alk. paper)
 1. Medical informatics. 2. Medical telematics. 3.
Public health—Information services. 4. Medicine—Communication
systems.
  [DNLM: 1. Delivery of Health Care—methods. 2.
Information Systems. 3. Computer Communications Networks. 4. Diagnosis, Computer-
Assisted. 5. Public Health Informatics. W 26.55.I4 E33 2005] I. Tan,
Joseph K. H.
  R858.E25 2005
  025.06'61—dc22

                                              2004022987

FIRST EDITION
HB Printing 10 9 8 7 6 5 4 3 2 1

CONTENTS

TABLES, FIGURES, and EXHIBITS

Tables

Figures

Exhibits

PREFACE

E-Health Care Information Systems: An Introduction for Students and Professionals is the latest in a series of works that I have published over the years, including *Health Management Information Systems* (first edition, 1995; second edition, 2001) and *Health Decision Support Systems* (1998). These works parallel the changes we have witnessed over the years in the evolution and development of health computing as a discipline. They also reflect the growth and maturation of my own reading and research in this intriguing and expanding field. Of course, this work represents the forefront of my research in the integration of information technology (IT), e-commerce, and health care.

Health Management Information Systems focused on the application of IT to replace manual clerical and information-processing tasks as well as to automate information flow models used to simulate well-structured (and not-so-well-structured) organizational and managerial activities in health care. The pieces of the health management information systems (HMIS) puzzle were put together to offer the reader a comprehensive view of how IT can be applied in health care organizations to facilitate efficient operational and tactical planning, administration, and evaluation. *Health Decision Support Systems* concentrated on the use of IT to extend the cognitive capacity and decisional expertise not only of health administrators and policymakers but also of clinicians, nurses, and other health professionals. Hence, health decision support systems (HDSS) moves one step forward from HMIS in applying the power of IT not just to achieve information-processing efficiencies but also to enhance decisional effectiveness on tasks that are mostly semi-structured and complex. Briefly, the purpose of

HDSS is to effectively enhance human thinking and extend human knowledge, to intelligently capture the interactions between end users and their health providers, and to creatively support organizational and clinical decision tasks.

E-health is next in line because the application of IT in health care is not confined to individual caregivers or even patients and should not be limited only to health organizations and urban communities. Indeed, if IT in health care is to flourish, its applications must be further enhanced with the potential for reaching the masses, especially those who are underserved, those who are elderly, and those who have no easy access to urban health care facilities. Accordingly, this publication was commissioned to remedy the lack of a comprehensive text on e-technologies in health care for students in all areas of medicine and health care, including population health and clinical epidemiology, nursing, pharmacy, occupational and environmental health, health administration, health policy and management, health education and health services research, and public and community health care programs. Such a work is especially needed in this era of explosive medical knowledge diffusion and rapidly advancing e-technologies, particularly the Internet. As we begin to see the pervasiveness of e-technologies in every aspect of health care and medicine, we will begin to understand why a course in e-health is logical for the health information systems curricula in medical schools as well as allied health, engineering, and business disciplines.

In light of these developments, we must understand the vision of future health in the context of evolving e-health systems and environments (Chapters One and Two). This book therefore offers the reader wide-ranging perspectives of e-health systems and environments (Chapter Three) and provides critical foundational knowledge of e-health in areas such as e-health records (Chapter Four), e-public health information systems (Chapter Five), and e-networks (Chapter Six). It surveys general and specific domains and applications of e-health, including e-rehabilitation (Chapter Seven), e-medicine (Chapter Eight), e-home care (Chapter Nine), e-diagnosis support systems (Chapter Ten), and e-health intelligence (Chapter Eleven). This book also provides information to increase the reader's understanding in key areas of e-health strategies (Chapter Twelve), e-health care technology management (Chapter Thirteen), e-security issues (Chapter Fourteen) and impacts of e-technologies (Chapter Fifteen). Finally, this work portrays the use of new and emerging e-technologies such as mobile health, virtual reality, and nanotechnology as well as how to go about harnessing the power of e-technologies for real-world applications (Chapter Sixteen).

The wide-ranging perspectives and interdisciplinary nature of e-health makes it impossible to expect any one individual to understand such an expansive field. Hence, the reader will soon discover, my collaborators are from diverse disciplines, including medicine, health sciences, engineering, business information systems, general science, and computing technology. Nonetheless, a single message has been conveyed throughout the text: the e-health paradigm shift is seen as a major transformation of our existing health care system and environment.

Instead of having to move patients to their caregivers, we are now going to be able to transmit medical information, knowledge, and relevant expertise to reach those who are in need of care, regardless of cultural, political, and geographical barriers as well as socioeconomic status. Even so, the future of e-health relates to further expansion of perspectives and clarity of the e-health vision (Parts One and Two of this text), new domains and emerging e-technology applications (Part Three), and new e-business strategies, management issues, and impacts (Part Four). All of these developments will ultimately lead to the blurring of corporate communities on one hand and user communities on the other hand. The defined roles of e-suppliers, e-providers, e-payers, and e-consumers are becoming less distinct. Therefore, it is still critical to come back, as we have done in the final part of this book (Part Five), to ask the questions "What is it that we want? How do we go about designing precisely what we want to achieve: the most accessible, available, affordable, and accountable medicine? How will such a system promote human health and well-being for the masses?"

Today, we stand at the crossroads where our current technology has the potential to be applied for the greatest good of many people, even entire populations, or to be used as a destructive weapon. The ongoing suffering in this world, the fighting over resources, the torturing of human beings, and the killing not only of animals but also of large numbers of human beings tell a story that must now be reversed. Technology can be a force for good only if humans know how to use it appropriately to better the lives of others. We have that power in our hands; its ultimate impact depends on how we go about using it. This, in essence, is the future of e-health care. The ideal and most significant paradigm shift will be the shift in human thinking—that is, applying new and emerging technologies not to destroy the human race but to create a peaceful and healthy world where illness is a thing of the past.

February 2005   Joseph Tan
Detroit, Michigan

ACKNOWLEDGMENTS

I am particularly indebted to my collaborators for their cooperative spirit and cheerful participation throughout this project. A listing of their names, official affiliations, and contact information is given elsewhere in the text. Here, I would like to note that I have taken an active role in many of these contributed works, presenting them to fellow colleagues at various universities and in major conferences, and have gained substantial feedback that has integrated the final versions of the contributed pieces.

Special thanks are also due to many others who have generously contributed to this project, including the reviewers, my colleagues, secretaries, students, and especially the academic and research assistants provided by the School of Business at Wayne State University. Naming each of these individuals runs the risk of missing someone important, but the abilities and selfless contributions of several individuals should be especially recognized: among my academic colleagues and peers from various universities: T. Butler, A. DePetro, W. Ragupathi, D. Matheson, M. Nies, R. Modrow, J. Gluesing, L. Weglicki, Y. Oscan, R. Lindstrom, L. Romilly, S. Satoglu, and W. Rogers; among the students at the British Columbia Institute of Technology, the University of British Columbia, and Wayne State University who either took courses from me or worked under me and provided me with pieces of related research information, A. Amnelahi, A. Arora, F. Barichello, S. Barr, Z. Bashir, A. Bhatnagar, J. Borsa, C. Buchner, T. Calice, Jr., R. Chernuka, R. Chun, K. Davis, L. Ebel-Wiebe, P. Erlendson, R. Habib, K. Hadad, J. Hanna, S. Hardiman, B. Harman, Z. Hirji, P Hutchison, S. Jafri, H. Javahery, M. Kassam, K. Kheirani, E. Kraus, A. Krystal,

J. Manton, F. McMahon, O. Mednik, J. Mills, M. Naidu, K. Narasimha, K. Nelson, C. Roach, K. Sarwal, H. Throng, J. Vadalabene, C. Xiao, and G. Yu; and my son, Josh Tan, who read and edited a number of the cases. He is growing up to be an avid reader and excellent writer on his own, and I am grateful that he shows an interest in my work. Without the help of all these special individuals, I am certain the work would not have been completed in a comprehensive and timely fashion.

I am also very grateful to the staff of Jossey-Bass: Gigi Mark (Jossey-Bass production editor), Susan Geraghty (freelance production editor), Carolyn Uno (freelance copyeditor), and David Horne (freelance cleanup editor). I appreciate their efforts and gratefully acknowledge all of the assistance, encouragement, and understanding I received during the various production stages, from beginning to the end.

Finally, one very special person has supported and encouraged me throughout the process of putting this book together. While I worked for long hours into the evening and sometimes past midnight over the last several months to bring all the materials together in a logical and meaningful fashion, editing various versions and rewriting many parts of chapters, my beloved wife, Leonie Tan, often woke up in the middle of the night to take care of my needs. She has been instrumental in ensuring that the manuscripts were generated on schedule and has provided me with warm and constant encouragement to keep my energy level sufficient to finish what I had set out to do. To her, I am and will ever be heavily indebted for any success.

Any errors and omissions within this text are my responsibility.

J.T.

THE EDITOR

Joseph Tan, Ph.D., currently on leave from the University of British Columbia, is professor and head of the Information System and Manufacturing Department at Wayne State University. He serves as guest editor and editorial board member for various journals and sits on key organizing committees for local, national, and international meetings and conferences. Tan's research—which has enjoyed significant support from local, national, and international funding agencies and other sources—has been widely cited and applied across a number of major disciplines, including health care informatics and clinical decision support, health technology management research, human processing of graphical representations, ergonomics, health administration education, telehealth, mobile health, and e-health promotion programming. He enjoys writing and editing books, book chapters, and journal articles; working on collaborative grant projects; engaging in philosophical discussions with colleagues and peers; and reading his son's work.

THE CONTRIBUTORS

Qiang Cheng, Ph.D., is an assistant professor in the Electrical and Computer Engineering Department at Wayne State University in Detroit, Michigan. He received B.S. and M.S. degrees from Peking University in China in 1994 and 1996, respectively, and his Ph.D. in electrical and computer engineering from the University of Illinois at Urbana-Champaign in 2002. He received the Invention Achievement Award from IBM's T. J. Watson Research Center in 2001. His research interests include multimedia computing and communications, watermarking, computer and communication security, human-computer interaction, and pattern recognition.

Tsang-Hsiang Cheng, Ph.D., is assistant professor in the Department of Business Administration at Southern Taiwan University of Technology in Taiwan. He received his Ph.D. in management information systems from the National Sun Yat-Sen University in Taiwan in 2003. His research interests include data mining, text mining, information retrieval, and schema integration.

Winnie Cheng, M.Sc., is a Ph.D. candidate in the Department of Electrical Engineering and Computer Science at the Massachusetts Institute of Technology. She received her M.S. in electrical engineering from Stanford University and her B.A.Sci in computer engineering from the University of British Columbia.

Avery Clouds holds an MBA and a doctorate in business administration. He has led the information management efforts at INTEGRIS Health, producing one of the most automated health systems in the country and winning the Most Wired award for four consecutive years. He is widely published and is a frequent speaker at academic and business meetings.

George Demiris, Ph.D., is assistant professor of health management and informatics and director of the health informatics graduate program at the University of Missouri–Columbia. He is also a member of the academic cabinet of the European Union Center and a member of the core faculty of the NLM informatics training grant at the University of Missouri. His research focuses on the use of telemedicine technologies in home care and the design and evaluation of smart home technologies.

George Eisler, Ph.D., is CEO of the British Columbia Academic Health Council. His career has taken him from polymer engineering and biomaterials research to bio-medical engineering, educational administration, and health care governance. Along the way, he earned an M.A.Sc. from the University of Waterloo, an M.B.A. from S.F.U., and a Ph.D. from the University of British Columbia. His research has focused on management of technology in health care. Eisler established and led one of the first clinical engineering departments in British Columbia. He has been dean of the School of Health Sciences at British Columbia Institute of Technology and served on the board of Vancouver Hospital and Health Sciences Centre. He has been asked to lead a council of senior health care and educational administrators in the further integration of health research, education, and practice in British Columbia.

Weiguo Fan, Ph.D., is assistant professor in information systems and computer science at Virginia Tech in Blacksburg, Virginia. He obtained his Ph.D. from the University of Michigan Business School in 2002. His research interests include knowledge management, information retrieval, text mining, and Web computing.

Pam Forducey, Ph.D., is a rehabilitation psychologist who has worked in rehabilitation for the past fifteen years. She is director of clinical research and development for the INTEGRIS Jim Thorpe Rehabilitation Center. Prior to that, she served as the clinical director for the INTEGRIS Rural Telemedicine Program. She received her doctorate from the University of Oklahoma.

Penny Grubb, Ph.D., is a founding member of the Yorkshire Institute for Clinical and Health Informatics and a lecturer at Hull University. During the 1990s, she headed one of the United Kingdom's first health informatics research groups, which became a world leader in the field.

Bob Hodge is manager of the local and wide area network for over seventy locations and oversees network specifications, installation, and maintenance for the INTEGRIS Health system. He was part of the planning team for the Rural Telemedicine project.

C. Ed Hsu, Ph.D., is assistant professor of health management and policy at the University of North Texas School of Public Health. He teaches health information systems and coordinates the Master of Public Health in Health Informatics program. Hsu has published in the area of spatial analysis of health and income disparities and is currently working on two projects that apply geographical information systems (GIS) in bioterrorism needs assessment training. He served as a programmer for a GIS-enabled community health information system to support his doctoral training. He received his Ph.D., (management and policy sciences), M.S. (health informatics) and M.P.H. (health services organization) from the University of Texas Health Science Center at Houston.

Paul Jen-Hwa Hu, Ph.D., is associate professor at the David Eccles School of Business, University of Utah. He received his Ph.D. in management information systems from the University of Arizona. His research interests include information technology applications and management in health care, management of system implementations, electronic commerce, digital government, and human-computer interaction. He has published articles in the *Journal of Management Information Systems*, *Decision Sciences*, the *Journal of the American Society for Information Science and Technology*, and other publications.

Patrick Hung, Ph.D., is assistant professor at the Faculty of Business and Information Technology in the University of Ontario Institute of Technology. Before that, he was visiting assistant professor at the Department of Computer Science in the Hong Kong University of Science and Technology and also a research scientist with Commonwealth Scientific and Industrial Research Organization in Australia. He has industrial experience in e-business projects in North America and Hong Kong. He serves as a panelist of the Small Business Innovation Research and Small Business Technology Transfer programs of the National Science Foundation. He is an executive committee member of the newly formed IEEE Technical Community of Services Computing , a W3C member, and also an editorial board member in several international journals. Further, he has published a number of technical papers in journals and conferences, and also has delivered many seminars at different institutions and research labs around the world. In addition, he has been a visiting Ph.D. student at RSA Laboratories West at San Mateo, California. His recent research interests include Service Computing, Web Services Security and Privacy, e-Business Process Integration, and Electronic Negotiation and Agreement.

Lee Kallenbach, Ph.D., is an epidemiologist in the Department of Community Medicine at Wayne State University in Detroit, Michigan. His career has spanned the public, private, and academic sectors. His research interest is in the measurement of improvement in community health as a shared responsibility of community partners.

Kawaljeet Kaur, M.D., M.Sc., completed medical school in India and received a Master of Science degree in health informatics from the University of Alabama at Birmingham. She is a Cisco Certified Network Associate. She worked at INTEGRIS Jim Thorpe Rehabilitation Center as a clinical development specialist and is currently pursuing her residency in medicine at the Medical College of Wisconsin.

Mengistu Kifle is a doctoral student in computer and system sciences at Stockholm University. The research for his dissertation is on the diffusion of e-medicine in Ethiopia. He has worked extensively in the field of health informatics in sub-Saharan Africa.

Liang-Ming Kung is a marketing engineer at IBM Taiwan Corporation. He received a B.S. degree from Soochow University in Taiwan in 1996 and an M.B.A. in management information systems from National Sun Yat-sen University in Taiwan in 1998. His research interests include data mining and electronic commerce.

Binshan Lin, Ph.D., is professor of operations and information management at Louisiana State University in Shreveport (LSUS). He is a six-time recipient of the Outstanding Faculty Award at LSUS and has published numerous articles in refereed journals and conference proceedings since 1988. He serves as editor-in-chief of *Industrial Management and Data Systems*, the *International Journal of Mobile Communications*, the *International Journal of Innovation and Learning*, the *International Journal of Management and Enterprise Development*, *Electronic Government*, and the *International Journal of Electronic Healthcare*. He is president-elect of Southwest Decision Sciences Institute (2003-2004), president of the Association for Chinese Management Educators (2003-2004), program chair of the Louisiana Information Technology Research Association 2003 meeting, and an active member of the International Association for Computer Information Systems. His research interests involve e-commerce, information technology management, quality management, and health care management.

Lin Lin has a Ph.D. in management information systems from the University of Arizona. His research interests include the application of machine learning and data mining algorithms in health care, system development, electronic commerce, and Internet marketing.

Barry P. Markovitz, M.D., is associate professor of anesthesiology and pediatrics, practicing pediatric critical care and anesthesiology at St. Louis Children's Hospital. He earned his medical degree at the University of Pennsylvania, completed a pediatric residency at Children's Memorial Hospital in Chicago, a residency in anesthesiology at the Hospital of the University of Pennsylvania, and a fellowship in pediatric anesthesiology and critical care medicine at the Children's Hospital of Philadelphia. He is chair of the ethics committee and medical director of respiratory care at St. Louis Children's Hospital. He has a strong interest in medical informatics and has been the Webmaster and principal editor of PedsCCM, The Pediatric Critical Care Website (http://PedsCCM.org) since its inception in 1995. He has served as chair of the medical records subcommittee of the St. Louis Children's Hospital medical staff and has played an important role in the ongoing development of electronic medical records at the hospital. His interest in evidence-based medicine and clinical epidemiology has involved him in co-editing the Evidence-Based Journal Club on the PedsCCM Web site, co-directing the journal clubs for pediatric and anesthesiology residents at Washington University School of Medicine, and teaching medical students and completing a Masters in Public Health degree at St. Louis University School of Public Health.

Sharline Martin works at an information technology company. She received an M.B.A. with a concentration in management information systems in 2000. Her research interests include the Internet, Web analysis and design, and electronic commerce.

Victor Mbarika, Ph.D., is assistant professor of information systems and decision sciences at Louisiana State University. He holds a Ph.D. in management information systems from Auburn University. His research interests focus on multimedia learning and the transfer of information technology to developing countries. He has written one book, *Africa's Least Developed Countries' Teledensity Problems and Strategies: Telecommunications Stakeholders Speak*, and numerous book chapters, journal papers, and conference papers.

Chitu Okoli, Ph.D., is assistant professor of management information systems at Concordia University. He received his Ph.D. in ISDS from Louisiana State University in 2003. He researches applications of the Internet in developing countries, strategic use of the Internet for competitive advantage, and remote electronic voting systems.

David Prouty is a network architect for INTEGRIS Health and played an important role in design, management, testing, and resolution of integration issues related to the Rural Telemedicine project.

Huyu Qu received a B.S. degree from the China Institute of Metrology in 1993 and an M.S. degree from the Department of Electrical and Computer Engineering at Wayne State University in 2003. He joined the technology department at China Telecom in 1993, mostly working with wired and wireless telecommunication network optimization. He is currently a Ph.D. student at Wayne State University in Detroit, Michigan. His research interests include wireless communication, network security, and telemedicine.

Anne F. Rutkowski, Ph.D., is assistant professor of information systems at Tilburg University in Tilburg, the Netherlands.. She received her Ph.D. in cognitive and social psychology. Since 1994, she has been involved in education and research activities in fundamental psychology. Her research interests and publications are oriented toward group decision making, problem solving, virtual and multicultural collaboration, and e-learning.

Cynthia Scheideman-Miller, M.H.S.A., advocates for legislative and third-party reimbursement changes to facilitate telehealth initiatives and improve the telehealth industry. She served as program director of the INTEGRIS Rural Telemedicine Grant from 1998 to 2003, and she holds a master's degree in health service administration from the University of Kansas.

Olivia R. Liu Sheng, Ph.D., is Presidential Professor and Emma Eccles Jones Presidential Chair of Information Systems at the David Eccles School of Business, University of Utah. Her research focuses on global knowledge management, including knowledge fusion and knowledge-refreshing technologies for portal management, biomedical, electronic commerce, digital government, risk management, telemedicine, telework, and distributed learning applications. She received a B.S. degree from the National Chiao Tung University in Taiwan and a master's degree and a Ph.D., both in computers and information systems, from the University of Rochester. She joined the management information systems faculty at the University of Arizona in 1985 and was department head from 1997 to 2002. She has also been a visiting faculty member at Hong Kong University of Science and Technology and at Tokyo Institute of Technology.

Sam Sheps, M.D., M.Sc., F.R.C.P., Pediatrics, is a Robert Wood Johnson Clinical Scholar and research fellow in the Department of Social Medicine and Administration at the London School of Economics. He is also professor in the Department of Health Care and Epidemiology at the University of British Columbia in Vancouver and director of the university's Western Regional Training Center for Health Services Research. He is a member of the college of reviewers for the Canadian Research Chair Program and a frequent journal reviewer. Sheps assisted in the development of the British Columbia Linked Database with colleagues from the Center for Health Services and Policy Research, where he is a core faculty member. He is a member of a national team that researches adverse medical events. His other research interests include waiting lists and wait times for surgical and other health services; high users of health services in British Columbia; and utilization of home care services. He has published on acute care utilization and the impact of hospital downsizing.

Mason Shieh is vice president and chief engineer of Pacific Meditech Inc., a medical application software company that specializes in picture archiving and communication systems (PACS), teleradiology, and system integration. He has extensive experience in implementation and maintenance of secure teleradiology operations through virtual private networks, broadband wireless networking, and other Internet-empowered technologies.

Yao Y. Shieh, Ph.D., is a clinical professor at the University of California Irvine Medical Center. His research interests include computer-aided diagnosis, medical image processing, and medical informatics. His research has been published in the *Journal of Digital Imaging,* the *International Journal of Healthcare Technology Management,* and *ACME Transactions,* among others.

Jung P. Shim, Ph.D., is professor of management information systems at Mississippi State University and has taught at Georgia State University, New York University, and the Chinese University of Hong Kong while on sabbatical. He has published numerous journal articles on the subject of management information systems. He is a seven-time recipient of outstanding faculty awards, including the John Grisham Faculty Excellence Award.

Sharon S. Smeltzer, M.S., CCC-SLP, is administrative director of the INTEGRIS Jim Thorpe Rehabilitation Hospital, a hundred-bed rehabilitation facility that is the largest in the state of Oklahoma and that includes several rural satellite clinics.

William E. Sorrells is a health care administrator and a captain in the United States Air Force. He served as secretary for the New Mexico Health Care Managers Forum, is a member of the Health Information Management and Systems Society and the American College of Healthcare Executives, and was the 2002 Air Force Materiel Command Medical Information Systems Officer of the Year.

Francisco G. Soto Mas, M.D., Ph.D., has a medical and public health background and extensive experience in disease prevention and health promotion. He received his medical degree in 1984 and worked as general practitioner for several years in his home country, Spain. Soto Mas completed two postgraduate degrees in sports medicine and nutrition and received his master's degree in public health from the University of Arizona in 1994 and his Ph.D. in health education from the University of New Mexico in 2002. For more than fifteen years, Soto Mas has been involved in academic and research activities related to social and behavioral sciences, including the development of theory-based health education programs. He is assistant professor in the Department of Social and Behavioral Sciences in the School of Public Health at the University of North Texas Health Science Center at Fort Worth.

Ronald Spanjers, M.Sc., started in 1992 as a financial consultant at the Jeroen Bosch Hospital in Den Bosch. From 1998 to 2002, he was managing director of the Division of

Perinatology and Gynecology at the University Medical Centre Utrecht. Currently, he is chief financial and information officer at Catharina Hospital in Eindhoven, the Netherlands. In addition, he is working on his Ph.D. in the Department of Information Systems and Management at Tilburg University.

Joshia Tan, currently a sophomore at Andover High School in Bloomfield Hills, Michigan, has excelled in every subject, maintaining a grade point average of 4.0. His hobbies include playing and listening to music, reading and composing works of literature, designing computer programs, and playing basketball.

Pency Tsai, M.B.A., is a translator and interpreter for Abcare Interpreter Service in Southfield, Michigan, providing interpreting and translating services to clients in various languages. She has worked as a market research analyst for Alliance Technology Inc. in Troy, Michigan, and received her M.B.A. from Wayne State University in 2004.

Yingge Wang received her B.S. degree from Peking University in China and an M.S. from the University of Illinois at Urbana-Champaign. She worked for CH2MHILL Inc. for two years. She was awarded the First Class University Award at Peking University, 1993–1994, the Huikai Academic Excellence Award at Peking University, 1994–1995, and the Contribution Award at CH2MHILL Inc. in 2002. Her research interests include signal processing, sensor technology, and biomedical sciences.

Chih-Ping Wei, Ph.D., is professor in the Department of Information Management at National Sun Yat-Sen University in Taiwan. He received his Ph.D. in management information systems from the University of Arizona. His papers have appeared in *IEEE Transactions on Information Technology in Biomedicine* and the *European Journal of Information Systems,* among others. His research interests include knowledge discovery and data mining; text mining and information retrieval; knowledge management; and multidatabase management and integration.

H. Joseph Wen, Ph.D., is associate professor of management information systems and chair of the Department of Accounting and Management Information Systems at Donald L. Harrison College of Business at Southeast Missouri State University. He holds a Ph.D. from Virginia Commonwealth University. He has published over ninety-five papers in academic refereed journals, book chapters, encyclopedias, and national conference proceedings. He has received over $6 million in research grants from state and federal funding sources. His areas of expertise are Internet research, electronic commerce, transportation information systems, and software development.

Harris Wu is a Ph.D. candidate at the University of Michigan Business School. He has had over ten publications in journals such as *Journal of the American Society for Information Science and Technology* and *Decision Support Systems*, at conferences such as CHI, Hypertext, ICIS and WWW, and in edited books.

David C. Yen, Ph.D., is professor of management information systems and chair of the Department of Decision Sciences and Management Information Systems at Miami University. He received a Ph.D. in management information systems and an M.S. in computer science from the University of Nebraska. He is active in research and has published three books and over one hundred articles. He was also a co-recipient of grants from the Cleveland Foundation (1987–1988), GE Foundation (1989), and Microsoft Foundation (1996–1997).

E-HEALTH CARE
INFORMATION
SYSTEMS

PART ONE

E-HEALTH OVERVIEW

If there were one phrase that could be used to describe the current status of e-health care system evolution, it would be *e-health paradigm shift*. Hospitals have been downsizing, reducing staff and closing hospital beds. Fiscal economics is playing a key role as governments scrutinize funding for health care services and delivery. New forms of alliances among health providers have also emerged, and new modalities of health service delivery have proliferated. The Internet has played an important role in many of these changes. Patients are becoming empowered e-consumers, demanding greater responsibility and accountability from their health care professionals. Health providers are challenged to go on-line. Even attitudes and views of health are changing, recognizing the value of e-health business alternatives and possibilities in terms of healing modalities, e-medicine, e-preventive care, e-health promotion, e-home care, and e-holistic medicine. Thus the evolving e-health care system is a dynamic entity that is being continually shaped by economic, political, technological, and social forces. In this book, the topic of e-health is not seen to exist in a vacuum but framed within this dynamic e-health paradigm shift. This part of the book unfolds the story line of the e-health paradigm shift as an outcome of changing e-consumer demands and increasing third-party payer expectations for more available, accessible, affordable, and accountable health care.

CHAPTER ONE

E-HEALTH

The Next Health Care Frontier

Joseph Tan

Learning Objectives

1. Articulate the emergence of revolutionary thinking in the e-health paradigm, business models, and practices
2. Identify basic components of an e-health care system
3. Recognize the underlying value propositions of an e-health care system
4. Understand the history of computing in health care and recognize how this process relates to the evolution of the e-health paradigm
5. Organize the range of current and emerging e-health care applications according to whether they require a high degree of internal integration or a high degree of external integration
6. Understand the scope of e-health care strategies and impacts

Introduction

The application and use of machines and computer-based technologies in health care have undergone an evolutionary process. Advances in information, telecommunication, and network technologies have led to the emergence of a revolutionary new paradigm for health care that some refer to as *e-health*. New experience and knowledge that crosses traditional disciplinary boundaries—particularly cross-disciplinary and multidisciplinary research in the fields of information technology and health care, along with emerging knowledge to promote evidence-based medicine (evidence-based medicine is discussed in the Case section of Chapter Thirteen), e-medicine, and remote e-health services—are causing not just episodic but systemic transformation of traditional health care systems and environments. Applications of electronic commerce (e-commerce) and electronic business (e-business) concepts to health care have resulted in efforts to use the availability of low-cost, high-speed Internet-related or wireless technology to revolutionize the health care business.

Health care administrators, clinicians, researchers, vendors, purchasers, and other health practitioners are facing increasing pressure to adapt to growing expectations for accountability from both the public and the private sector (see Chapter Sixteen). Major sources of this pressure include decreased government and third-party funding; increased patient education, participation, and expectations; and new and emerging forms of health organization reporting structures as well as breakthroughs in telecommunication and networking technologies. The simultaneous need for and technological opportunity to create more efficient, effective, secure, and economical health data sharing; large-scale health information processing; better and more effective communications; and seamlessly coordinated health knowledge management, data mining, and evidence-based health decision making demands a concerted effort to harness the power of e-technologies in the service of health care.

Those who understand electronic health (e-health) perspectives, domains, and challenges, as well as the potential benefits of e-health applications will be better prepared to work collaboratively through the use of computer-based groupware, virtual networks, and Internet appliances. E-health understanding will increase health awareness, improve decision-making effectiveness, cultivate more positive consumer-provider relationships, and enhance the partnership of e-health care product and service delivery networks. In addition, rapid shifts in the e-health market and environment also dictate a growing need for improved ergonomics and more intelligent interfaces in e-public health data systems and e-decision support applications and implementations.

E-health can be viewed as an integrated, multidisciplinary field, bridging the following key areas:

- Strategic health systems planning and e-marketing concepts
- Specialized e-record keeping and e-business operational analysis
- All forms of e-medicine linking health professionals to individuals
- Corporate and enterprisewide health technology management

E-technologies encompass the following:

- Complex information technology network design and methodologies for consumer-oriented system development
- E-health informatics (information sciences and methodologies)
- Wireless communications and emerging technological applications
- Web services implementation
- Ongoing evaluation of automated security of Web-based health information exchange
- Clinical monitoring and management systems

Three general topics characterize the eclectic field of e-health: (1) e-health foundations and benefits; (2) e-health domains and applications; and (3) e-health strategies and impacts.

Before discussing the e-health foundations and benefits, I will first attempt to answer a very basic question: "Can e-health help solve North America's health care crisis, particularly in terms of key challenges such as escalating health care costs, access for the underserved, and improving (or even maintaining) the quality of current health care service delivery?" Answers to parts of this question have remained unclear; e-health has sometimes been described as hype that may not make any appreciable difference in resolving current challenges. Thus, continuing investments and efforts that encourage investors, vendors, and purchasers to pursue e-health initiatives may well be limited by the lack of coordinated effort to unlock the potential benefits and powerful promise of the e-health paradigm shift (e-health paradigm shift is more fully explored in the beginning of Chapter Two). Essentially, the underlying argument is such that if we cannot diffuse medical and health care data, information, knowledge, and expertise from the e-providers and experts to the e-consumers so that we empower them to new heights of health and well-being rather than perpetuate their relentless dependence on care providers to cure their everyday problems, e-health investment will be fruitless. Until a few years ago, the thought of e-consumer empowerment from health information therapies was still a remote, far-fetched possibility. How could consumers have more current and detailed medical information on hand about their own illness or predicaments than their family physicians? Perhaps our question should be "Has the time come for us to move e-health knowledge and practice from being largely hype to being a new and respectable field?"

Understanding the values and benefits of investing in the e-health field is therefore critical to the future success of e-health initiatives. In the next section, we discuss e-health perspectives, infrastructures, components, and services and relate these concepts to core e-health value propositions by focusing on how core e-health values can benefit e-health's investors as well as its users, enhancing or supporting complex e-health technologies and applications.

Later, we survey and highlight major aspects of e-health domains and applications. Specifically, we review e-health history to show how emerging domains of e-health applications are derived from our understanding of health management information systems (HMIS), health decision support systems (HDSS), health informatics, and e-medicine (also called *telemedicine*). Following this, we organize e-health application clusters, dividing domains and applications that provide seamless internal system process integration from domains and applications that provide external linkages with e-stakeholders and the public. Finally, we shift the discussion to the significance of e-health strategies and impacts and conclude the chapter by examining how these various topics can be combined to achieve an effective understanding of the e-health field and provide the basis for considering how e-health practices in the coming era may be affected by changing e-consumer needs, trends, and expectations.

FOUNDATIONS AND BENEFITS OF E-HEALTH

To grasp the fundamentals of e-health technology, it is necessary to recognize its diverse perspectives, as well as its basic infrastructures and components. Part Two of this book is devoted to the details of the foundations of e-health and covers various theoretical perspectives of the e-health paradigm as well as concentrates on the different network infrastructures that make e-health care delivery systems possible. In this chapter, we emphasize basic e-health components, including the core value propositions and the basic characteristics of the e-commerce services as applied to e-health care (for example, business-to-consumer [B2C] and business-to-business [B2B] e-health models), the e-stakeholders, and future e-health impacts. Without these basic components, the e-health paradigm shift would never have been possible and patients would always have to travel to their doctors instead of having the best health care information sources transported to their fingertips.

In fact, the e-health paradigm shift did not begin with the linking of e-consumers to the e-care providers; instead, its current success has been largely the result of linking one health care business to another, increasing efficiencies and eliminating the need for manual administrative information exchange and off-line business transactions. We therefore begin by discussing electronic data interchange (EDI) methods used in typical B2B e-commerce applications in health care and then move to examine the design of Web sites using HTML versus XML standards to provide e-consumers with specific or specialized health information and dynamic electronic data interchange capabilities.

Since the advent of e-commerce, EDI has offered companies a largely automated way to conduct business transactions. Business processes that once required significant human intervention are now being done efficiently and effortlessly with little or no human interaction required. EDI, the standard method for conducting B2B e-commerce applications, is therefore considered the traditional basic infrastructure for electronic data sharing and transaction activities among e-stakeholders—for example, between a health provider and a payer. The best way to understand EDI processing is to divide the flow of data into several phases in the context of a provider-payer transaction, as depicted in Figure 1.1.

As shown, the provider sends data about services and care rendered to a selected clearinghouse by either using a value-added network (VAN) as an intermediary or using point-to-point (P2P) connectivity.

FIGURE 1.1. ELECTRONIC DATA INTERCHANGE TECHNOLOGY

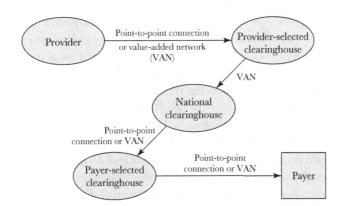

A VAN essentially functions as a post office for EDI transactions. Users are assigned "mailboxes" that store their data. Each mailbox is given a unique identity (ID) or communication code, accompanied by a qualifier. Together, the ID and qualifier serve as an address to which data can be mapped. Once the data arrive at the clearinghouse, they are translated and reformatted to the payer's specifications. Many clearinghouses make it possible to check the validity and completeness of the document. From the provider's clearinghouse, data are then sent to the national clearinghouse via VAN. In essence, a clearinghouse provides connectivity between health care providers (physicians, hospitals, pharmacies, and clinics) and payers (health maintenance organizations, insurers, and government entities such as Medicare). Clearinghouses take claims, eligibility requests, claim status checks, and other information from providers in various formats, translate and reformat them according to the prespecified or standardized formats demanded by payers, and transmit the reformatted versions to their destination. As an additional service, the clearinghouses may perform editing functions that check the claims.

At the national clearinghouse, data are further cleansed, and precautions are taken to ensure that the security, privacy, and confidentiality of the data set are kept intact. The data are then received at the payer-selected clearinghouse via a VAN or P2P connection. Then, data are again translated and reformatted before being sent to the payer via a P2P connection or VAN. With P2P connection, all of the data interchange and formatting activities discussed with the use of a VAN are preplanned and data transmission is performed through a secured channel.

If the data exchange process simply provides static health information from health information systems and legacy databases, then the information dissemination process is straightforward. In this case, the Internet and the typical HTML (Hypertext Markup Language) offer a convenient platform via which the information can be predesigned, validated, and captured or presented as a user-friendly multimedia document as with a P2P connection. To improve the data's timeliness, validity, and integrity, the preferred data collection method is automated and direct data input at the source—for example, using predesigned documents stored in organizational intranets or extranets, then warehousing the completed documents either centrally or via on-line distributed network technology. Data direct entry requires that the acquired data be converted into easily readable and appealing user-oriented information.

While most current documents on the Web are stored and transmitted in HTML because it is easy to use and generate, the need for dynamic and interactive Web interfaces as opposed to static ones resulted in the World Wide Web Consortium's introduction of a new standard known as XML (eXtensible Markup Language). With XML, data or even documents can be simultaneously transformed into useful, meaningful, and interactive information in a format that is readily retrievable, comparable and transactional, where data can be used for exchanging dialogues and executing monetary payments. The data transfer and data distribution functions (that is, data retrieval and transmission activities) become integrated with those of presentation, exchange, and use. A key problem with HTML data display is its inability to provide information by transaction and querying capability for users as well as its inability to convert e-commerce data into e-business information that can be further used in transactions. In contrast, XML technology allows the creation of multimedia and intelligent graphical Web interfaces and thus has the ability to compact large amounts of information conveniently. The information can be further packaged to support individual users by filtering out information that may not be needed for a particular application or for a particular data exchange transaction. For example, on an HTML Web site where an e-consumer may be looking for a quick answer to a question about the extent of her individual health insurance coverage, the presented information may only be tabulated. However, with an XML Web site, the e-consumer can ask the question via e-mail in an open format (that is, no special format is needed for the query to be understood and processed) and receive a direct answer within twenty-four hours through the secured Web site. On the same site, a direct transaction may be executed within a short processing time. Quality displays and functionality of Web-based e-health services are important because e-consumers are more likely to visit and use a Web site if it is dynamic rather than static.

Three common forms of data management technology can support Web-based information processing and management for data-centered and, to a lesser degree, for document-centered Web sites.

- Database management technology
- Model-base management technology
- Knowledge-base management technology

Database management enhances data collection and data storage activities, improves data integrity, reduces data update anomalies to ensure data consistency (see Tan, 2001), and promotes preservation and structuring of data for efficient data processing and effective data retrieval activities. *Model-base management* constructs, stores, manages, and interrelates models that may be needed by the user to make sense of the data being linked, analyzed, or computed. In fact, not all data collected are directly useful in the e-health care delivery or e-health information dissemination process. Some e-health information (including data elements and models) is collected merely to assist in the organization and generation of comparative data and statistics or simply for research purposes such as adding to the collection of data models and extending their applications.

More intelligent e-health data systems can assist e-health care providers and e-consumers in making complex decisions that may require provider-consumer interactions or teleconsultation (or e-consultation) in specialty areas. In this case, apart from the use of database and model-base management technologies, knowledge-base management systems come into play. *Knowledge-base management* assembles, stores, accesses, updates, and disseminates knowledge elements that may enhance specialized decisional processes. Regardless of the way e-health-related data are gathered, encoded, and entered as data or documents into a Web-based system, the information captured should be cleaned and meticulously verified for accuracy and validity. Put simply, bad data yield bad results, regardless of the sophistication of the systems that process them.

Basic Components of an E-Health System

The basic function of an e-health system is to gather and exchange appropriate and accurate data from various sources to satisfy the administrative, clinical, and transactional needs of e-health providers, payers, and users. Proposing an e-health business is not exactly the same as proposing a brick-and-mortar health business, and it is vital to understand the factors and barriers that determine e-health business success or failure. The fundamental components of an e-health system include

- Its core value propositions
- The characteristics of the e-health service model
- The community of e-stakeholders involved
- The potential to process a critical mass of transactions, to ensure enough revenue for sustainability and e-commercialization, that is, the potential for e-business ideas and models to thrive in a free online market system.
- The potential to accommodate future features such as product or service expansion, profitability, growth, and global development

First, understanding an e-health system's current value propositions is critical. *Value propositions* are the added values or quantifiable cost savings, efficiencies, or intangible benefits that can be achieved through implementation of a system. To evaluate these propositions, the observer needs to know the *characteristics* of the e-health service model—for example, whether the e-health business is to be set up as a completely virtual B2C or B2B enterprise or a more complex hybrid of brick-and-mortar and point-and-click models (called a *brick-and-point model*) in which the consumer can choose whether to get the service on-line or physically go to a designated service facility.

The *community of e-stakeholders* comprises the e-providers, e-payers, e-consumers, e-vendors, and e-purchasers connected to the system. It is important to know what each of these players see as the values that the e-health service model provides for them; all stakeholder groups will play by different rules.

The potential for a *critical mass of transactions* to be processed is significant because the number of transactions determines the amount of capital investment needed to implement the model and sustainability of the e-business model. The central business proposition boils down to the anticipated amount of dollar transactions generated from e-consumers or between the trading partners in a day versus the daily costs of maintaining the service. If there is no critical mass of transactions, there is no profit leading to e-commercialization.

Finally, the *business potential to accommodate future features* indicates potential future investment returns such as the potential for spin-off businesses that can take advantage of the operation of the current system. For example, a model that mimics Amazon.com or eBay by selling medical devices on the Web could have expansionary possibilities such as collaboration with other health equipment suppliers to resell used medical devices or recycling of expensive hospital-based medical technologies such as CT (computed tomography) scan and MRI (magnetic resonance imaging) equipment.

Careful consideration of each of these components is particularly important when proposing a new e-health business model. For instance, an e-health Web site that provides very specialized information on a specific illness such as ADD (attention deficit disorder) would not be likely to last very long. In fact, such a proposal could be very costly because it would most likely have only a limited number of users; the Web site might be completely static, with no interactive querying capacity; and more than a few hundred, even thousands, of competing Web sites might provide the same or better information, along with other valuable and useful functions. Many contemporary e-health Web sites allow the user to link to authoritative e-health providers or are supported by a major brick-and-mortar pharmaceutical chain and/or are sometimes endorsed by well-known professional associations. Successful Web sites will offer a unique mix of services and attract hundreds or even thousands of visitors daily.

E-Health Core Value Propositions

Both the United States and Canada face rapidly increasing health care costs. Health care expenditures in the United States now exceed 14 percent of the country's gross national product (GNP), which implies that Americans spend roughly $2 billion a day on health care products and services. Yet despite these large expenditures on health care, millions of Americans are denied access to medical care because they lack medical insurance coverage. In Canada, where the majority of health care funding comes from the government, citizens and residents are experiencing long waits and bed closures due to shortages of nurses, family physicians, and various health specialists.

Fortunately, the e-health paradigm shift has been supported by core value propositions that can help alleviate some of these problems by reducing costs and increasing efficiencies of processes in several areas. For example, e-health database management and on-line submission and processing of medical claims can vastly re-duce the need for clerical personnel. In addition, on-line processing will eliminate many unnecessary clerical errors due to faulty transcription; the need to satisfy repeated requests on status of claim processing; and submissions of identical patient informa-tion for different interventions, as well as the failure to simultaneously update redun-dantly maintained patient records in various physical files located in different places (update anomalies).

Virtual patient records (VPR) is an integrated health database processing engine that links the accurate and rapid collection of various patient-related information and knowledge elements to generate an aggregated, well-classified, and organized set of administrative and clinical information and knowledge that e-health providers (pri-marily nurses and clinicians) can retrieve, exchange, and disseminate as needed for e-clinical decision making, e-control, analysis, e-diagnosis, e-treatment planning and evaluation, and many other e-health-related cognitive activities.

Another core value proposition of most e-health domains and applications is improving two-way or multiple-party communications, thereby significantly improving access to e-health care, especially for those located in rural or remote areas. For exam-ple, technologies such as e-mail, Blackberries (wireless devices with organizer features providing access to email, corporate data, phone, and the Web), secured Internet Web sites, personal data assistants (PDAs), virtual private networks (VPNs) and wireless cellular phones can enhance long-distance communications among e-health professionals or be-tween e-health professionals and e-patients in different sectors, including communica-tions between e-physicians and e-patients, laboratory test clinics and doctors, e-consumers and e-home care workers, e-physicians and e-pharmacists for verification of on-line prescription orders, and e-generalists and e-specialists for e-consultations on various subjects.

An additional core value proposition often cited as a rationale for adopting an e-health paradigm is user empowerment through tele-education and e-learning. Video-conferencing and on-line health learning and Web-based educational technologies, for instance, may assist long-distance medical training and permit tele-educational and multimedia educational dialogues among doctors, nurses, mental health and other spe-cialists, and residents. The same videoconferencing and associated Web-based Inter-net training technology may be used for long-distance radiological consultations, remote medical consultations among doctors and specialists, and e-consultations by qualified doctors on emergency treatments that must be carried out by paramedics. Other e-health initiatives for tele-education and e-learning include on-line kiosks to provide software games and instructional materials for consumer education. Such e-health preventive initiatives, promoted to an entire population, can lead to huge cost savings in health care in the long run.

Benefits from the use of e-technologies in health care services should not be lim-ited to direct patient care; in fact, use of these emerging technologies to improve health care communications and reduce costs may also result in greater user satisfaction. New approaches to the same old routines may improve the quality of health care services, while unnecessary inefficiencies and undesired bottlenecks in the traditional system are eliminated or minimized. Clinicians and doctors, for example, may find it more convenient to receive clinical test results on-line or via EDI, appropriately filed into the respective e-patient records. E-consumers or e-patients may be delighted to be able to connect directly with doctors, nurses, or other health professionals without having to travel a long distance, only to be told, perhaps, that their test results have yet to be received or validated. Both providers and consumers will also benefit from having the confidence that insurers are efficiently reimbursing co-payments or services that they have claimed on-line. The reimbursements can easily be posted directly into recipients' bank accounts rather than delayed for reasons ranging from missing information on physical claim forms to postal strikes.

Aside from e-data management capabilities, improved communications, and tele-education, other core e-health value propositions include knowledge dissemination, intelligent support, better health decision making, and improved personal and community well-being. The use of the Internet, as well as intranets and extranets, to promote community learning and e-learning communities (e-communities), to increase virtual interactions between e-health experts and non-experts within a virtual health network environment, and to build partnerships among community and health care leaders can improve health service delivery. In addition, more effective implementations and uses of emerging e-technologies such as specialized Web services for intelligent health decision analysis and support—for example, helping an employer or employee choose among competing insurers and health maintenance organizations (HMOs)—can be of great benefit.

Evidently, the core value propositions underlying e-health can make critical and significant contributions to reduced health care costs, improved access to health care, and even enhanced quality of the health care workplace and environment. Thus, e-health domains and applications, properly structured, can greatly benefit individuals, groups, organizations, communities, societies, and populations. Still, the question remains as to what the best next steps are and who should lead the effort to mobilize human and other resources to transform e-health from hype or a concept found only in textbooks and conference papers into a set of successful real-world e-business practices and documented cases.

E-Health Domains and Applications

Everyone interested in e-health should study the historical evolution and knowledge development not just of e-health domains and applications but also of the general computing, health informatics, and telemedicine revolutions that preceded the e-health revolution.

E-Health History

The genesis of health care computing can be traced as far back as the early 1950s, when only mainframes were available and only the major hospitals of G7 countries could afford to house and use these machines. In that period, even the processing of a routine batch of health-related information took a considerable amount of coordinated effort among various health professionals and computer experts. Despite the demand on expertise, the end results were mostly fraught with mechanical and programming errors. The failures of this first era of computing in health care were due mainly to the lack of active support from hospital administrators and top management, the lack of continuing funding, and the lack of knowledge and skill in the design and use of automated systems.

From the early 1960s through the 1970s, a new era of computing in health care emerged. A growing group of hospitals, including Akron Children's, Baptist, Charlotte Memorial, Deaconess, El Camino, Henry Ford, Latter Day Saints, Mary's Help, Monmouth Medical Center, St. Francis, Washington Veteran's Administration, and others throughout the United States, as well as Sweden's Danderyd Hospital and Karolinska Hospital, England's London Hospital and Kings Hospital, Germany's Hanover Hospital, and others in Europe began to agree on the need to advance a patient information management system prototype. Despite the risk of major system failures, these pioneering hospitals invested large amounts of money, time, and effort to move toward computerization. Seeing the sudden surge of interest among these hospitals and the potential market opportunities, large computer vendors such as Burroughs, Control Data, Honeywell, IBM, and NCR joined in an effort to support patient information systems. Lockheed Information Systems Division, McDonnell-Douglas, General Electric (GE), Technicon Corporation, and several other companies with a reputation for effective management of complex systems also collaborated. Nonetheless, many of the early projects were almost complete failures: the complexity of the information requirements of a patient management system was gravely underestimated. Companies such as GE and Lockheed had to withdraw their participation due to a lack of continuing funding, interest, and management support. Many pioneering hospitals also had to fall back on their manual systems to keep their facility operating smoothly, and several of the hospital administrators had to make the difficult choice to abandon their hospital information systems project at a huge loss.

The Technicon system was the light that was eventually found at the end of the long tunnel of hospital-based patient information system failures. This particular system, initiated by Lockheed for El Camino Hospital in Mountain View, California, and later acquired and improved by Technicon Corporation under the leadership of Edwin Whitehead, became the successful prototype that laid the foundation for all future hospital patient information management systems throughout North America and Europe. The major lessons learned in the El Camino project were the importance of focusing on user information needs and the need to change user attitudes, particularly to overcome resistance from physicians and nurses. Owing to the success of this project, large-scale data processing applications in medicine and health record systems also began to take hold during the early and mid-1970s as the use of computers began to result in continuing gains in productivity and evidence of increased efficiency.

Nonetheless, these early successes were achieved at very high costs. Johns Hopkins Oncology Center, for example, acquired their first computer system in 1976 for a quarter million dollars; its processing power was only a fraction of today's desktop computers. Other successful early patient record systems include the Computer Stored Ambulatory Record System (COSTAR), the Regenstrief Medical Record System (RMRS) and The Medical Record (TMR). COSTAR, a patient record system developed at Massachusetts General Hospital by Octo Barnett in the 1960s, was later extended to record patient data relating to different types of ailments (for example, multiple sclerosis [MS-COSTAR]) and is used even today in several teaching hospitals and research universities across the globe. RMRS was a physician-designed integrated inpatient and outpatient information system implemented in 1972, and TMR is an evolving medical record system that was developed in the mid-1970s at Duke University Medical Center. Together with the success of the Technicon system, the efficiencies of these automated record systems soon provided considerable motivation for the integration of computing into health care systems.

As soon as health administrators and practitioners began to realize the efficiency and data processing power of computers, which increased when minicomputers were introduced during the late 1970s and early 1980s, computerization began to be seen as a magic bullet for controlling and managing the large and increasing volumes of medical and other administrative data processed on a daily basis. Medical data range from demographics of patients to clinical and health services data to epidemiological and health population statistics, such as the prevalence and incidence of tuberculosis (TB) along with statistics on TB morbidity and mortality. Health administrative data encompass health administrative and patient financial data and inventories of drugs and medical equipment, as well as routine transactional data, including the management of patient billing, insurance co-payments, accounts receivable and payable and general ledgers. By the early 1980s, computer miniaturization and cost reduction simultaneous with increases in processing power resulted in a dramatic move away from massive health data processing using mainframe or minicomputers to new and more efficient forms of health management information system (HMIS), office automation (OA), and networking technologies.

Whereas HMIS automates routine management reporting to support administrative and patient care applications, OA designs health office systems and processes to reduce time and effort expenditure on the part of health knowledge workers such as doctors, pharmacists and nurses. Networking technology is a relatively new aspect of computing and refers simply to the electronic transmission of data, text, or voice information from one computer (source) to another (destination). Each of these "islands" of health computing technologies comprise hardware and software components interacting with humans to provide a catalyst for change—in particular, a move toward greater ease in managing information flow between or among health care stakeholders. Early experiences led to awareness that integrating HMIS, OA, and networks would change how work processes needed to be "informated" in the different areas of health service delivery. Users at all levels also realized that the key to unlocking the usefulness of these technologies rested in successful design of the human-computer interface—that is, the information display interface that the users see as the computer.

Health networking and telecommunications were soon discovered to be the most powerful pieces in the puzzle of an integrated health care information system, bringing together the different technological islands. The focus on these two technologies opened up interest in e-clinical decision support and e-medicine applications in the early 1990s. E-medicine was first tried in the 1970s via low-cost telephone technology, but interest in this area dwindled quickly due to lack of funding. In the mid-1990s, however, advances in health computing and networking technologies rekindled interest in e-medicine and other areas of e-health administrative, clinical, and financial applications, including e-commerce applications, e-clinical decision support and expert systems, e-nursing support systems, and other e-health applications such as e-home care systems. Intelligent medical information systems and health decision support systems (HDSS), it was thought, should be able to mimic the thinking processes of clinicians. Researchers have always wanted to add intelligence to computer systems, and the extension to remote medical diagnostic systems was soon considered a valuable and noteworthy medical computing application domain, foreshadowing the e-health era.

In light of new technologies and the massive infusion of investment money provided by corporate businesses and venture capitalists in the late 1990s and also in the process of protecting health care assets from the Y2K threat, researchers, businesses, and end users all began to shift attention to Internet connectivity. Whereas Internet use had previously limited to academics, its sudden widespread diffusion and the discovery of e-mail as a convenient technology among end users led to the dissemination of e-commerce and e-business concepts among young entrepreneurs.

E-consumers and young risk-taking entrepreneurs began using current and emerging Internet technologies, giving rise to extended e-technologies and applications, including intranets, extranets, virtual public and private networks, e-business networks, Web-based businesses, community networks and learning communities, and Web development and maintenance services, all of which ultimately blossomed and extended into various e-health perspectives, domains, technologies, and applications.

While e-health constitutes only a tiny part of the lengthy history of the life and medical sciences, which, according to Jordan (2002), date back as far as 3,000 B.C., the wave of interest in and consumer-driven requests for e-health services on employers, clinicians, doctors and pharmacists in just the last several years is mind-boggling. In the context of the e-business revolution, e-health is seen as a paradigm shift from a physician-centered care system to a consumer-driven care system (see Chapter Sixteen). In other words, e-health systems place the e-consumers rather than the caregivers at the center. As one example, these systems are used primarily by e-patients to connect with member physicians when they want and wherever they want; patients are no longer limited by time and space. Further, if the quality of services or products or the level of health knowledge provided by a certain e-care provider or HMO does not meet the e-consumer's expectations, he or she has a convenient means of switching e-care providers. More significantly, the flow of e-health data, information, knowledge, and even wisdom will eventually empower e-consumers to take on new roles, not just seeking alternative care services from the best available and accessible sources but also educating themselves in evidence-based medical practices, in integrative (holistic) and gene-based medicine, in alternative and complementary clinical modalities, and in health-promoting lifestyles, activities, and behaviors. Eventually, these actions and changes in e-consumer health and lifestyle behaviors will result in new and creative forms of consumer-driven health information therapies.

Since we are now more aware of the numerous possibilities and channels through which e-health can be intelligently applied and practiced, we can turn our attention to the e-health application clusters that have been or can be implemented.

Domains of E-Health Applications

In general, e-health domains and applications can be divided into two primary clusters based on two key dimensions of systems integration characteristics (Raghupathi and Tan, 2002).

On one hand, systems that are characterized by a high degree of internal integration include applications such as the following:

- Virtual patient records (VPR)
- Document management (DM)
- Geographical information systems (GIS)
- Group health decision support systems (group HDSS)
- Executive information systems (EIS)
- Data warehouses (DW)
- Data mining

We define *internal integration* as the degree to which systems and technologies are integrated with one another within an organization.

On the other hand, systems that are characterized by a high degree of external integration include the following:

- Telecommunications, wireless and digital networks such as asynchronous transfer mode (ATM) networks
- Community health information networks (CHIN)
- The Internet
- Intranets and extranets
- Health informatics
- Telemedicine or e-medicine

External integration is defined as the degree to which systems and technologies interface with outside organizations and agency computer systems.

VPR technology houses uniquely identifiable information about an individual patient from various isolated sources. Accordingly, diversified data coded in different formats for use with different platforms can be converted for use with a common virtual platform. This is not just the creation of a massive traditional database but the design and development of a common network via a system which permits various components to interact and operate together (an open system) for the conversion and transmission of media-rich medical data from multiple distributed sources to support multiple users. TeleMed, a collaborative VPR prototype project created by researchers at Los Alamos National Laboratory and physicians from the National Jewish Medical and Research Center in Denver, supports real-time interactive uses of media-rich graphical patient records among multiple users at multiple sites. VPR technology is ideal for telemedicine practitioners.

Document management technology aims to put clinical and financial data online. DM applications can include document imaging, workflow optimization, electronic form processing, mass data storage and computer output to laser disk, among other possibilities. Many hospitals and health organizations use DM technology to handle the otherwise paper-intensive process of collecting and filing patient information. For example, notebook computers and customized software can allow busy nurses to rapidly and accurately update all patient and insurance records electronically instead of handwriting and later transcribing many documents and forms between their regular visits to patients. This technology frees up time for nurses to focus on patient care.

A geographical information system (GIS) is a powerful tool for collecting, recording, storing, manipulating, and displaying spatial data sets. A GIS uses spatial data such as digitized maps and can represent a combination of text, graphics, icons, and symbols on two-dimensional and three-dimensional maps. GIS technology might be used for digital mapping of a certain epidemic—for example, HIV infection among a subpopulation across various counties in a province or state. This knowledge can then be used to effectively target interventions for specific population groups.

A group health decision support system combines analytic modeling, network communications, and decision technology to support group decision-making processes such as group strategic thinking, problem formulation, and generation of goal-seeking solutions. Use of a group HDSS can reduce not only the cognitive burden but also the mental effort associated with group meetings. This technology also has the potential to increase the efficiency, effectiveness, and productivity of group interactions through asynchronous board meetings, on-line forums, or special group meetings in which board members and executives can network and share information with one another without being completely constrained by separation in time and geographical distance.

In the context of an e-health provider organization, an executive information system (EIS) collects, filters, and extracts a broad range of current and historical e-health-related information from multiple applications and across multiple data sources, both external and internal. This provides the organization's executives and other key stakeholders with the necessary information to identify key problems and strategic opportunities. A common EIS application entails an HMO executive using it in long-distance strategic planning sessions to determine the challenges and potentials of various business strategies. One popular feature is the ability of an EIS to narrow or expand information from one level to another, enabling executives to conveniently retrieve answers to special or ad hoc queries. For example, a DSS that allows a health manager to know who and why a group of people are "frequent" users of the organization's emergency services let the organization implement appropriate policies to prevent resource abuse or misuse. Another important feature is the ease with which EIS technology can be integrated with related technologies such as a geographical information system, an expert system (ES), an HDSS, or a group HDSS.

Data warehousing architecture for integrated information management simply provides an integrated source of aggregated, organized, and formatted data. The data in a DW are designed to support management decision making and strategic planning. Accordingly, these data may sometimes be stratified (categorized in various forms), and most likely have already been aggregated and filtered after coming from legacy systems. Again, a DW can be combined with an EIS, an ES, an HDSS, a group HDSS, or a GIS not only to increase data analytic and processing power but also to develop new and complex forms of e-health technologies.

Today, the most prominent use of a DW in e-health care is the automated collection of massive amounts of linked data from diverse sources for use in data mining (sometimes referred to as *data dipping*) techniques. Data mining techniques explore the data for hidden trends and patterns. Data mining tools include artificial neural networks, case-based (analogical) reasoning, statistical methods, genetic algorithms, and explanation-based reasoning. The opportunity for an HMO to explore and discover best practices by comparing and contrasting physician practice patterns for different treatment protocols corresponding to groups with specific case mixes is one benefit of applying DW and data mining technologies. The unraveling of the human genome to provide treatments for various challenging ailments is another noble example of DW and data mining technology applications.

Turning now to e-health systems and applications characterized by a high degree of external integration, we will start with e-health networking technologies. These essentially are applications that speed up large-scale movement and exchange of media-rich health information from one point of a network to another. The architecture of such a network may be a hub-and-wheel communication configuration; an open system configuration, including the use of the Internet, electronic data interchange (EDI), and extranet; a groupware application; or an intranet configuration (see Tan, 2001).

A community health information network (CHIN) may be conceived as a network that links health care stakeholders throughout a community or region. Such an integrated collection of telecommunication and networking capabilities can facilitate communications with patients as well as the exchange of clinical and financial information among multiple providers, payers, employers, pharmacies, and related health care entities within a targeted geographical area. Central to a CHIN's success is the practical implementation of a computerized patient record system at the community or regional level. Figure 1.2 shows the Wisconsin Health Information Network, an example of a participating CHIN. In this figure, WHIN connect software provides various business task applications to participating users. Whereas WHIN switch controls the mode and rate of access among the various users, WHIN processing ensures that data input provided by the users are cumulated to generate the required output (reports).

CHIN technology has become an important interactive research and communication tool, aiding both medical professionals and health consumers in search of health-related information and knowledge.

Intranets and extranets extend the concept of the Internet as a complex web of networks. Intranets and extranets use the same hardware and software as the Internet to build, manage, and view Web sites. Unlike the Internet, however, these virtual networks are private; they are protected by security software known as "firewalls" to keep unauthorized users from gaining access. An intranet supports Internet-based services only for organization members, whereas an extranet extends network access privileges to certain partners, giving them access to selected areas inside the private virtual network, thereby creating a secure customer or vendor network. A simple example of integrated Internet, intranet, and extranet use in health care is providing users such as e-patients, e-physicians, and other e-providers with access to on-line insurance service data. Electronic filing of insurance benefits and claims via an extranet

FIGURE 1.2. WISCONSIN HEALTH
INFORMATION NETWORK (WHIN)

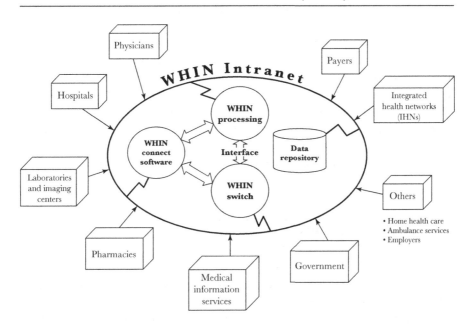

dramatically cuts agency and other labor costs while increasing the accessibility of the information for both patients and providers as well as providing administrative insights into health care trends and medical best practices. The use of intranets and extranets ensure the security and the accuracy of these transactions as the information is encrypted and transmitted over secure lines to ensure confidentiality. Whereas the intranet are used to share the internal data of an organization, the Internet and the extranet connect users from outside the organization primarily to information that may be released to the public.

The chief emphasis of health informatics and telemedicine is clinical and biomedical applications of e-health technologies. At the clinical level, e-health decision support systems (e-HDSS), e-clinical decision support systems (e-CDSS), and e-expert decision support systems (e-EDSS) are being developed to assist physicians and other medical specialists in diagnosis and treatment. An example of an e-CDSS is an interactive videodisk system that helps a client enter personal health data in order to weigh the pros and cons of surgery. HDSS is a generic term used among the administration staff whereas e-CDSS denote a clinical focus and are systems used by health providers. In contrast, e-EDSS are domain specific systems used amongst specialists (see Tan and Sheps, 1998). Other examples include systems that monitor heart rates and alert care providers if they are abnormal, that guide prescribing pharmacists to potential adverse drug interactions, and that educate patients on preventive health care and health-promoting activities.

Finally, e-medicine, which is a more generic term, unlike traditional "telemedicine" thinking, is the use of digital networks to perform virtual diagnosis of disease and disorders. In teleradiology, among the first successful applications of e-medicine, X-rays or scanned images of patients are digitized and stored electronically so that they can be shared among multiple health providers at geographically distant sites. Other e-medicine applications include teleconsultation—for example, in teledermatology and telepathology; telesurgery, including telegastroscopy (see Chapter Ten); robotics and virtual reality (see Chapter Sixteen); telelearning—for example, using videoconferencing or on-line medical education; and telecare (see Chapter Nine).

E-HEALTH STRATEGIES AND IMPACTS

Among the most critical aspects of e-health systems are planning e-health business strategies, e-health care technology management and diffusion, e-health system implementation and evaluation, and envisioning and monitoring the impacts of e-health technology.

The planning aspect involves building a strategic vision to align the goals of senior management with the changing needs of the e-health marketplace. Technology management and system implementation relate to managing the diffusion of e-health innovations, redesigning work practices so that both workers and users can work virtually (e-work), and addressing issues of user acceptance or failure arising from the implementation and evaluation of an e-health system. Not only is it important to focus on the impacts of e-health systems on individuals, groups, communities, and societies, but it is also critical to realize how the implementation of an e-health system may ultimately affect the larger context of our health care delivery system both nationally and globally.

Planning E-Health Strategies

Planning e-health strategies includes identifying e-consumer needs and business requirements, applying systems theory and decision theory, materializing telemarketing and virtual network management concepts, planning e-data warehouse mining and e-technology strategies, and championing sound methodologies for growing new and complex e-health applications. Most important, the mission of the system analyst group should reflect the vision of the system creator and should serve as a thematic rationale for integrating individuals and virtual group teams toward the achievement of planned goals and objectives.

A major trend in planning e-health strategies is shifting responsibilities and power from traditional health providers and health system analysts to e-consumers, the people who ultimately determine the survival, use, and growth of the e-health business ventures. Traditional approaches have concentrated on satisfying business needs with little attention paid to e-consumers. The decisions of leaders and system analyst groups should echo and reflect more appropriately the active participation, expressed needs and recorded feedback of e-consumers. This trend reflects growing acceptance of the notion that e-health data, information, and knowledge are shared resources and that the acceptance of any e-health business model and the accompanying interface design requires a consensus of e-health providers, payers, and consumers. Given the rapid shifts in the e-technology marketplace and the lengthy delays often experienced between the vision of a new e-health system and its realization, it is generally wise to revisit the decisions made during planning sessions and to conduct intensive market research and prototyping before implementing an actual e-health system.

More recent approaches call for shorter gaps between system strategic planning sessions and more attention given to the changing marketplace (see Chapter Twelve). In addition, an environmental assessment must always be conducted before formulating a strategic plan. Scenario planning is one approach to system strategic planning. Here, competing futures are envisioned, and strategies are developed and tested against these possible futures. The e-technology vision is then determined on the basis of the scenario results, taking into account current technological and system capabilities. For example, if the e-technology vision calls for handheld devices to be employed by all the e-health home care workers, who currently use only cell phones, then the transition to the new e-technology will call not only for changes in work practices and habits but also for finding new ways for patients to connect with workers, examining how workers monitor their patients remotely, and determining how workers are to be monitored and managed virtually (see Chapter Nine).

Successful e-health system planning also requires effective e-health care technology management (e-HCTM). Briefly, e-HCTM is management of the entire e-health technological infrastructure and the information processing capacity of the virtual business system. Top management must work to ensure that information resources and e-technology are best adapted to meet the needs of the marketplace. In many cases, the necessary work process restructuring for efficient e-health information processing and effective decision making will not happen without significant leadership at the executive level, including extracting past experiences and expertise within the e-business community (see Chapter Thirteen). Moreover, the increased complexity of the e-health care environment and the rapid rate of change in technological capabilities make the process of e-HCTM increasingly complex and difficult.

E-Health Implementation and Evaluation Issues

E-health system implementation and evaluation include responsibility for overseeing the integration of e-technologies, the incorporation of e-health transactional activities into the virtual e-health system, the incorporation of security and privacy mechanisms to ensure user acceptance and satisfaction, and the training and education of users migrating from legacy systems to the e-health system. Not only should e-technologies be integrated with old and new equipment within the existing virtual network configuration, but system transactional procedures must also be integrated into existing administrative procedures. Administrative issues may also include the privacy, security, and confidentiality of virtual patient and e-patient records; legal and ethical considerations regarding data collected, analyzed, and distributed electronically; and policies regarding security and network standards (see Chapter Fourteen). Among other important goals and objectives of e-health system implementation and evaluation are the following:

- To achieve significant operational cost savings
- To generate revenues without sacrificing quality patient care
- To project an improved professional image by relieving health care workers of tedious physical reporting activities so that they can concentrate on patient care
- To achieve user satisfaction, especially for e-consumers who will be relieved of travel costs and other inconveniences

One significant goal of e-health system implementation and evaluation strategy for a virtual system is to ensure that top management gives adequate attention to ensuring a smooth interface between the technological and human elements. Such interfaces occur at two levels: first, the human-computer interface (HCI) between the individual users and software applications, and second, the system technology interface (STI) between the various users and organization technologies as a whole, including human considerations involved in work processes and transactions, and the e-technology. STI focuses on the overall alignment of technology and human resources in pursuit of the overarching business goals, while HCI emphasizes building applications to augment specific functions for users. Many problems faced in system implementation and evaluation have to do with inadequate HCI design or poor STI configuration. The significance of these interfaces cannot be overemphasized, because the users, whether e-workers or e-consumers, do not have face-to-face interactions but conduct their businesses completely through these interfaces.

The challenges of e-health system implementation and evaluation are therefore interwoven with many other factors, including the integration of quality planning, quality control, and quality improvement processes to evolve a secure, well-managed, and quality-focused e-health care environment and the integration of network technology management, organization technology management, and user-interface technology management to build efficient, enterprisewide system infrastructure and interfaces. Integrating electronically gathered data, model, and knowledge elements to design effective applications is key to sharing these resources. Together, these challenges point to the need to integrate environmental, technological, and administrative components in order to successfully drive and direct the implementation and evaluation of various e-technologies and applications within the larger context of Web services and the Internet, intranets, and extranets.

Finally, any e-health system implementation and evaluation will lead to suggested system modifications and changes—for example, to the e-networking infrastructure; to the level of computing competence required of current and future e-workers; in the information flow processes and business processes; and in the belief systems, ethics, lifestyles, and behaviors of e-workers and users. To ensure that these workers and users will have the critical knowledge, skills, and attitudes to address concerns arising from these changes, the system should also address staffing, training, and education issues. For example, attracting and retaining valuable technical staff calls for aggressive recruitment and telemarketing programs, new opportunities for staff training and development, and the employment of e-learning strategies for sharing knowledge among workers.

E-Health Impacts

E-health will have an impact on the individual user, the workgroup, and the forms of emerging health systems—for example, virtual alliances, virtual work management, virtual group interactions and networking capability, collaborative decision-making effectiveness, and shared intelligence and expertise. Aside from the government and venture capitalists, several other major e-stakeholder groups are involved in e-health care systems: e-consumers, e-providers, e-employers, e-vendors, and e-insurers. Each of these groups has a set of interrelated needs and desires that are not being met by the traditional health care information and network infrastructure.

At the individual level, for instance, users want to know if the introduction of an e-health system will result in better productivity and decision-making effectiveness for them. For example, a traveling health manager equipped with a personal data assistant (PDA) that acts both as a cellular phone with an automated directory and an Internet appliance with the ability to access e-mails and Web sites will probably be able to better perform his or her duties irrespective of his or her whereabouts.

At the workgroup level, e-health will affect the ability of group members to share data, to coordinate activities, and to network effectively. A virtual health record system used by multiple care providers, for example, will integrate all the information from different care providers regarding a single patient.

At the system level, we have noted that e-health will create change on many fronts—for example, system structure and culture. E-health will improve managerial productivity, increase control of information flow, flatten reporting hierarchies, increase the power of decentralized units, change the power and status of individual workers, and open up possibilities for new units and services. E-health systems will result in new cultural expectations for system behavior. In keeping with the e-health diffusion phenomenon, for example, automated intelligence, on-line training capabilities, and virtual networking may completely change the way a given system performs health care services.

The impacts that e-health systems have at the level of a single isolated system may be extended to the entire health care delivery system at a societal level. For example, the use of the Internet to transfer massive amounts of media-rich patient data and the availability of knowledge systems such as robots and automated intelligent systems may engender legal and ethical questions about privacy, security, and individual and institutional property rights. One such question that is frequently asked is "Who owns all the different pieces of stored medical information about a particular patient?" Other questions may be "What information should or should not be kept on-line about an individual, and who has priority access to the information?" Follow-up questions to those could be "How accurate and secure is the information being stored, and what prevents the on-line information from being misused?" Other societal impacts of advances in e-technology include the following:

- Changes in employment levels for mainstream health workers and how their work may be performed (for example, telecommuting)
- Changes in the role of disabled, women, and minority workers in the health workplace
- New opportunities for cybercrime and misuse of power
- New ways for e-consumers to purchase health care products and services
- New ways to prevent injuries from work in hazardous environments
- New gadgets and automated devices to help seniors and the disabled
- New modalities and ways of reaching distant consumers and the underserved
- Improvements in e-medicine and e-home care services, societal well-being, and the quality of life in general

Conclusion

By the last half of this new millennium, hospitals and other health service organizations will face increasing pressures to move toward an e-health model, due to changing demographics, changing governments, a changing e-technology marketplace, and changing health care environments. We have already seen how a young discipline such as the e-health field can grow and expand quickly to affect every aspect of daily health care—particularly our acute care systems and our public health systems.

Chapter Questions

1. Do you feel that e-health phenomenon is a temporary fad or that it will become a permanent reality? Why?
2. What is the significance of understanding the basic components of e-health? Why is it important to understand the major themes of the e-health field?
3. Compare and contrast the e-health system with the mainstream health care system. What key factors distinguish e-health care from conventional health care?
4. Imagine that you're living in the age of mobile health where wireless connections prevail. How might you choose among a list of available mobile physicians? What criteria will you use? Cost? Response time? Other measures? How would you go about determining and measuring these criteria?

References

Jordan, T. J. (2002). *Understanding medical information: A user's guide to informatics and decision making.* New York: McGraw-Hill, 2002.

Raghupathi, W., & Tan, J. (2002). Strategic IT applications in health care. *CACM, 45*(12), 56–61.

Tan, J. (2001). *Health management information systems: Methods and practical applications* (2nd ed.). Sudbury, MA: Jones & Bartlett.

Tan, J., with Sheps, S. (1998). *Health decision support systems.* Sudbury, MA: Jones & Bartlett.

The Telebaby® Case

Ronald Spanjers, Anne F. Rutkowski

New information technologies can be efficiently used to fill the human need for communication during the difficult time when a family member is hospitalized. The Telebaby® project, designed and supported by the University Medical Centre Utrecht, links parents at home to their newborn receiving intensive, high, or medium care. Telebaby is simple enough to be easily adopted by parents; however, implementing Telebaby in a hospital environment proved to be a real challenge.

Background

The concept of attachment is central to most discussions of parenting. The purpose of bonding may sound paradoxical: the natural phenomenon of bonding enables a child to develop feelings of security in strange environments and later to separate from the main caregiver (Bowlby, 1969, 1988). If skin-to-skin contacts are recognized as primordial in the development of healthy premature newborns, any separation of a mother and her child affects not only the child but also the mother (Klaus and Kennel, 1976, 1985). Attachment is gradual, not automatic, immediate, or to be instantly expected of the mother; however, caregivers often experience traumatic stress and anxiety when separated from their newborn.

The idea of an Internet facility to link premature infants with their parents was conceived in order to support parents during the difficult period of separation. The researchers assumed that it would give caregivers a feeling of greater control of their relationship with their newborn and thus reduce their anxiety. Reviewing previous experiences in linking mothers with their hospitalized children encouraged the researchers to persevere (Bialoskurski, Cox, and Hayes, 1999; Lupton and Fenwick, 2001; Woollet and Phoenix, 1991).

Sponsorship by the "Friends of the Wilhelmina Children's Hospital" made it possible to implement a system that allows a mother to view her newborn on the intensive, high, or medium care unit from her hospital bed through an internal video circuit. Later, the concept of Telebaby originated from the idea that video images could be distributed over the Internet. Technology that provided a connection between the hospital and patients' homes was built: Telebaby was born. Parents were enthusiastic about using the Telebaby facility as a complement to their regular visits at the hospital. Telebaby was surely an appealing concept. More important, Telebaby contributed to the well-being of the caregivers and thus the health of their newborns.

This case study begins with a description of the project and the supporting technologies used. The results of monitoring parents' login activity and the preliminary results of a parent survey questionnaire are also presented. We then conclude by examining some research limitations and suggestions for future developments.

Project

The Perinatal Center of the University Medical Centre Utrecht consists of two wards, Obstetric Care and Neonatal Care. The center has four hundred employees and an annual budget of 20 million Euros. Obstetric Care handles 10,000 new cases per year, with 30,000 follow-up consults. Of 4,500 admissions, 2,500 are adults and 2,000 are newborns, of which 1,000 need low care, 500 medium care, and 500 intensive or high care. In total, the admissions and 600 short-stay days generate 30,000 nursing days in eighty to one hundred beds and cribs.

In the planning stages of Telebaby, several issues concerning privacy and safety were raised. Given their nature, only practice could prove the extent of their relevance. More practical issues such as costs and image quality were dealt with before the project started. One major concern was the "gimmick effect," the fear that the system, once developed, would have a short-term appeal for its concept and innovation but would not be appreciated for its contribution to the well-being of patients and families.

The Telebaby project started small and experimental. An exploratory team of three persons was formed, covering all necessary skills such as programming, financing, and understanding the medical and nursing activities of a perinatal center. Managers assigned a minimal and recoverable budget of 7,500 Euros. If the project had failed, most of the computer equipment could have been used elsewhere. The goal of the team was to test the concept and the technology. Within half a year, the team decoded and transmitted the signals required for transmission using standard Internet technology. Exhibit 1.1 presents a picture of a baby that was transmitted through the internal video circuit and that was used in a corporate campaign on innovation within the University Medical Centre Utrecht. Physicians, nurses and parents became curious.

EXHIBIT 1.1. VIDEO IMAGE OF A BABY AS TRANSMITTED THROUGH THE TELEBABY VIDEO CIRCUIT

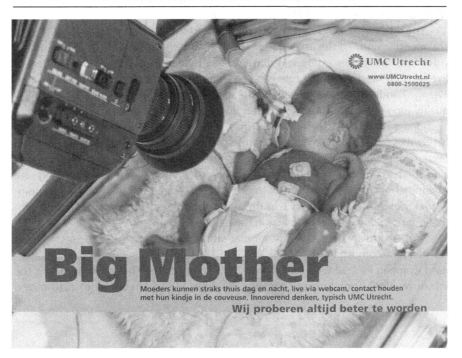

The hospital's automation department, working with Infoland, an Internet streaming company, ensured the stability of the technology. Providing maximal support to the users (parents and nurses) was recognized as the most important factor for success or failure (Oudshoorn, Brouns, and Van Oost, 2005). A budget of 75,000 Euros was acquired through the Friends of the Wilhelmina Children's Hospital. The largest part of the budget (55,000 Euros) was used for hardware and software, including the server, encoders, laptops, adaptation of the internal video circuit, and customized software. An estimated 400 hours were spent developing and implementing the concept (excluding software development by Infoland), for a total of 20,000 Euros in personnel costs.

Hardware and Software

The internal video circuit consisted of twenty analogue Panasonic cameras, mounted on a standard equipment rail on the crib with a fixed focus. They were connected to an internal coaxial network with an XLR plug that also provided power. Because the camera was located outside the crib, the image sometimes lost quality when the plastic top of a crib produced shimmering. The cameras were routed to the television in the mother's hospital room (or an Internet stream) using a patch bay that connects specific cribs with specific destinations inside and outside the hospital. This way, fifty cribs could be connected to fifty different beds.

The internal video circuit had to be adapted for Internet video streaming. An encoder transformed the analogue signal of the internal video circuit into a digital video stream. The encoding was done on-line in real time with a delay (buffer) of five seconds, and the frame rate was ten frames per second. A 56K modem on an average bandwidth network was able to adequately handle the data flow. A higher-quality modem did not provide a better image of the newborn, because the load of encoded data was relatively low: changes in light intensity were few, the newborn hardly moved, and movement around the crib was limited. Sound was not encoded because of privacy considerations rather than technical limitations; the microphone of a newborn in one crib could transmit speech from physicians or nurses providing care to another nearby newborn. Furthermore, it is was feared that parents might misinterpret sounds on the ward, such as the audio control signals from respiratory equipment, thus raising instead of lowering their anxiety.

The streams are offered to a server that distributes them to the viewers. The server is a standard Compaq PC (800 MHz, 16 GB, 522 MB). The four encoders are also standard Compaq PCs, all with four Osprey 200 Codec cards. The software used is the Windows 2000 operating system with Windows Media Encoder and customized

I-stream software from Infoland. Telebaby is accessible through a standard browser on the hospital's Web site. The login screen includes a "thank you" page that lists the sponsors and a disclaimer page that covers legal issues. The four types of users—the administrator, the automation department, the nurse, and the parent—have different menus. The administrator (supervisor) has access to all menus, including the system users menu (where types of users can be set), the camera control menu (which holds IP settings of the streams) and the general fields menu (where the patient data fields displayed along with the stream can be defined). The automation department and the nurses can access the menu where streams are assigned to patients and predefined patient data fields are filled in. The camera overview menu gives a thumbnail page of active streams (Exhibit 1.2). The parents (Exhibit 1.3) have access only to the parents' menu, which displays the stream of their newborn and some patient data fields such as name, unit, bed, the unit's telephone number, and the name of the primary nurse. No other menus were accessible from outside the hospital.

EXHIBIT 1.2. TELEBABY CAMERA OVERVIEW MENU

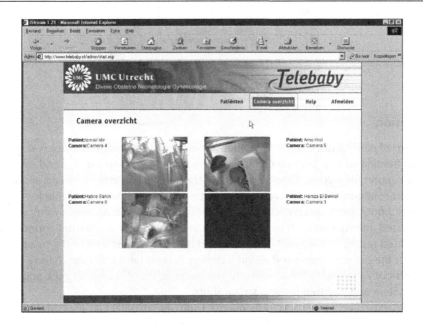

EXHIBIT 1.3. PARENTS AT HOME,
WITH ON-LINE TELEBABY CONNECTION

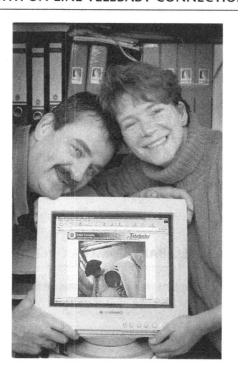

Implementation

A team of nine "Ambassadors of Telebaby" nurses was formed. This team was given extra training so that they could facilitate the implementation process and provide basic support for parents. Over 50 percent of the parents had Internet access at home. Five preconfigured laptops, each with an Internet account, were available for those who did not have a personal computer. Parents had to fill out an intake form, which requested information such as their address and which type of Internet connection they used (cable, phone, ISDN). Nurses used the intake sheet to add the newborn's data in the patients' menu and assign a stream. Parents (and other users) were given a hard-copy manual that was comprehensive in terms of navigating the software and system and had step-by-step screen shots.

An extensive, more technically oriented software manual was accessible via the Web site. Parents were asked to log in on a demonstration stream first, to reduce anxiety when logging in to see their newborn for the first time. Only after they had successfully logged in on the demonstration stream were parents given the login name and password for their child's video stream. More than one viewer can access the stream for a given infant at one time; parents were free to pass on the login name and password to relatives. Once parents could see the demonstration stream, almost no technical barriers could keep them from logging in to see their newborn. A blue or black stream indicated that the camera had been unplugged or covered at the unit; for example, parents who visit the unit will not need the camera, or the camera may be physically in the way when providing care to the newborn.

Implementing an externally oriented information system in a hospital triggers safety issues, particularly when this system crosses the boundaries of the hospital's networks. Hospitals have tight security policies. In this case, the streams were rerouted through the completely separate and more open network of the medical faculty. Acceptance of the system by physicians and nurses was obtained by relating it to the perinatal center's basic philosophy of keeping mother and child as close together as possible in a clinical setting. Telebaby extends this philosophy when the mother is discharged. Physicians and nurses had the basic right to switch the camera off when providing care to the newborns. However, it was stressed to parents that the quality of care was the same regardless of whether the camera was switched on. The twenty-four-hour nature of perinatal care, combined with the fact that some of the nurses only took night shifts, made the training difficult to plan and demanded a clear instruction manual.

Results

The login activity of the parents was closely monitored. The log file contains data such as duration and frequency of use (Exhibit 1.4) such as via a unique viewer identifier generated by the Windows Media Player. Usage was high between 11 A.M. and 3 P.M. A clear pattern of "anxiety visits" can be discerned. These short but frequent visits at 2 P.M. and 9 P.M. offer parents a feeling of control. They quickly see their newborn and log off, most likely after seeing the baby moving. At 10 P.M., the unit's lights dim and image quality drops, so usage is minimal after that hour.

System use over time varied and depended on the admission and discharge of patients and parents. Mothers who used the internal video circuit usually applied for the Internet streaming facility when they were discharged and their newborn stayed in the hospital. Average frequency of system use usually drops after the first few days and picks up shortly before the newborn is discharged, exceeding the initial use. System use on the weekends is low because parents visit the hospital more frequently on weekends. One important finding was that parents with access to the Telebaby system did not visit their newborn less frequently. Physical visits were always parents' first choice.

A questionnaire (n = 31) was distributed to parents after they had used the system. Parents were asked to rate the Telebaby system on a five-point Likert scale from –2 (not useful at all) to +2 (very useful). In preliminary results, parents rated the system very useful (M = 1.84, SD = 0.38). The parents were positive about the value that Telebaby added to the general level of health care provided to their newborns (M = 1.70, SD = 0.67). When using the system, parents worried less about their newborns (M = 1.26, SD = 0.82).

EXHIBIT 1.4. DURATION AND FREQUENCY OF TELEBABY USE

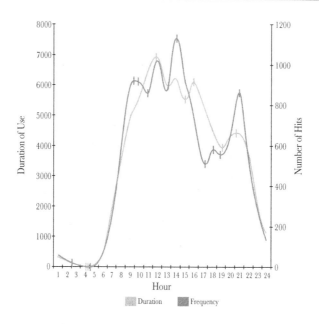

Parents were slightly less enthusiastic about the quality of the picture but generally satisfied (on a ten-point scale, with 10 as the maximum score, M = 6.35, SD = 1.10). Parents who used the hospital's internal video circuit found the streaming image quality less satisfactory, while parents who had never used the internal video circuit rated the overall image quality (both refresh rate and size) higher.

Conclusion and Limitations

Parents were enthusiastic about the possibility of using Telebaby as a complement to their regular hospital visits. The login activity of parents showed that using standard Internet technology to distribute multimedia images allowed parents to visit their newborn more often than they could have without the technology and markedly reduced the anxiety associated with the mother-child separation. The preliminary results of a questionnaire administered to parents (n = 27) indicated that Telebaby gives the parents a feeling of control in regard to knowing the state of their newborn. Parents of newborns are preoccupied; lack of a working system lowers their feeling of control over the state of their newborn and raises anxiety.

A system like Telebaby could become standard for perinatal centers. However, more investigations into experimental, ethical, legal, cultural, medical, and developmental issues should be conducted. For clear ethical reasons, we could not design a control group of parents who did not benefit from the Telebaby system. Monitoring of the login activity of parents revealed that the parents did share the password and login information to allow family members and friends to virtually visit their baby. If this trusting attitude toward such technology generalizes to other similar systems, ethical considerations of privacy and security should be given serious consideration. It would be interesting to see how people from different cultures react to such a project. Adding dynamic medical data such as saturation and heart rate could make the system more useful for physicians and nurses (Gray and others, 1998; Halamka, 2001). Because research suggests that the mother's voice plays an important role in the mother-child bonding, an auditory expansion to allow babies to hear their mother's voice would be worth investigating. Broadband Internet could make the transfer of sound from a parent's home to a hospitalized newborn more feasible (Dekkers and others, 2002).

In conclusion, valuable contributions to the quality of patient care can be made by applying standard information technology. While a system like Telebaby cannot replace the skin-to-skin contact of a baby with his or her caregivers, it nonetheless contributes to the relaxation of the parents. Spitz (1945) would surely agree that such a system can only be favorable for the hospitalized newborn's well-being. With health care moving toward a much more patient-orientated approach, we suggest that a relatively simple and low-cost application such as Telebaby can also contribute to the well-being of the caregivers and thus of their newborns.

Case Questions

1. How feasible would it be to apply the Telebaby system in your country or workplace?
2. Can you envisage improvements in the hardware and software integration of the Telebaby system?
3. If you were involved in implementing Telebaby, how would you ensure, evaluate, and even enhance its effects and effectiveness?
4. What are the psychosocial aspects and benefits of Telebaby? Can you identify any negative aspects? If so, how would you go above resolving these challenges?

References

Bialoskurski, M. Cox, M. C., & Hayes, J. (1999). The nature of attachment in a neonatal intensive care unit. *Journal of Perinatal and Neonatal Nursing, 13,* 66–77.

Bowlby, J. (1969). *Attachment and loss: Vol. 1. Attachment.* New York: Basic Books.

Bowlby, J. (1988). *A secure base: Parent-child attachment and healthy human development.* New York: Basic Books.

Dekkers, L., Dijkhuizen W. J., Van Geelen, N., Golder, T. J., Huizinga, H., & De Jager, M. (2002). Een Toekomst van Glas: Vooruitlopen op de Doorbraak van Breedband-technologie [A future of glass: Being ahead of the broadband breakthrough]. *Stichting Maatschappij en Onderneming* [small promotional book on broadband that uses Telebaby and similar applications as an example]. Den Haag.

Gray J., Pompilio-Weitzner, G., Jones, P. C., Wang, Q., Coriat, M., & Safran, C. (1998). Baby CareLink: Development and implementation of a WWW-based system for neonatal home telemedicine. *Proceedings of the AMIA Annual Symposium* (pp. 351–355).

Halamka, J. (2001). Inside a virtual nursery. *Health Management Technology, 6.* Retrieved from http://www.healthmgttech.com

Klaus, M., & Kennel, J. (1976). *Maternal-infant bonding.* St. Louis, MO: Mosby Press.

Klaus, M., & Kennel, J. (1985). *Parent-infant bonding.* St. Louis, MO: Mosby Press.

Lupton, D., & Fenwick, J. (2001). They've forgotten that I'm the mum: Constructing and practising motherhood in special care nurseries. *Social Science & Medicine, 53,* 1011–1021.

Oudshoorn, N., Brouns, M., & Van Oost, E. (2005). Diversity and distributed agency in the design and use of medical video-communication technologies. In H. Harbers (ed.), *Inside the Politics of Technology.* Amsterdam: Amsterdam University Press.

Spitz, R. (1945). Hospitalism: An inquiry into the genesis of psychiatric conditions in early childhood. In A. Freud (Eds.), *Psychoanalytic Study of the Child,* (Vol. 1, pp. 53–74). New York: International Universities Press.

Woollet, A., & Phoenix, A. (1991). Psychological views of mothering. In *Motherhood: Meanings, practices and ideologies* (pp. 28–46). London: Sage.

CHAPTER TWO

E-HEALTH VISION

Drivers of and Barriers to E-Health Care

Joseph Tan

Learning Objectives

1. Realize how the e-health paradigm shift has resulted in thinking, business models, and practices that differ from traditional health care
2. Conceptualize e-health in the context of other related health care systems and environments

3. Identify the primary goals and benefits of e-health systems
4. Articulate the range of potential barriers and challenges to implementing e-health applications

Introduction

Over the last several years, the belief that our current health care systems in the United States and Canada, as well as many other countries, need major restructuring has been strengthening in the minds of a growing number of Canadians and Americans, including the insured, the underserved, and the underinsured; unionized workers as well as nonunion workers; and employees of major corporations, universities, nonprofit organizations, and federal, state, and municipal governments. Seminars, forums, working groups, special task forces, and major conferences have been organized at local, regional, national, and international levels to discuss this topic. Most people are now convinced that something must be done quickly to stop the spiraling costs of health care. Given the wide availability of the Internet and the ubiquity of wireless technologies, one promising approach is to investigate how access to quality health care services and products can be achieved in a more economical and equitable fashion using e-health concepts, infrastructures, technologies, interfaces, and strategies.

Indeed, based on figures released by the National Science Foundation on survey data aggregated between 1985 and 1999 and reported in Blendon and others (2001), I assert that the United States has now passed the first major stage of a technological revolution that is transforming the lives of Americans. The percentage of Americans who use a computer at work or at home more than doubled over those years, growing from 30 percent in 1985 to 70 percent by the end of the last century. More striking is the increase in home computer ownership, which quadrupled from 15 percent to 60 percent of Americans between 1985 and 1999. During an approximately five-year span in the mid-1990s, the number of Americans who had used the Internet at some point in their lives jumped from fewer than one in 5 (18 percent) to almost two-thirds (64 percent) of those surveyed. Moreover, in 1995, only 14 percent of Americans sampled in the survey reported that they had gone on-line to send or receive e-mail or to access the Internet; by 1997, this figure had reached 36 percent and by 2001 had risen to 54 percent. In addition, 92 percent of those surveyed who reported having used a computer were younger than 60. Among those, 75 percent have used the Internet and 67 percent have sent an e-mail message. Finally, most Americans feel that the computer's impact on society has been largely positive. More than half surveyed indicated that the computer has given them greater control over their lives. Given these statistics, it is anticipated that the diffusion of e-health care is imminent.

In the previous chapter, we reviewed the three general themes encapsulating the evolution of the e-health field: foundations and benefits of e-health, domains and applications of e-health, and e-health strategies and impacts. We noted that new experience and knowledge are transcending the mainstream disciplinary boundaries of information technology (IT). Advances in information, telecommunication, and network technologies and their applications in e-commerce have led the way to new forms of health care delivery, specifically, e-health.

In contrast to traditional health care systems, e-health has developed to become a niche industry with the potential of providing, in one way or another, greater access to a growing range of health care products and services. Access can be increased in rural, inner-city, and remote areas; in underdeveloped as well as developing countries that lack the medical expertise or technology to protect and promote the health and well-being of their populations; and in areas that are difficult to reach, such as prisons, military bases, or aircraft, cruise ships, and space shuttles. As long as emerging e-technologies can be applied successfully, there is potential for e-health systems to evolve, survive, and thrive.

In this chapter, we conceptualize e-health as it relates to other existing health care systems and environments. Indeed, some health care hierarchies could be considered parents or grandparents or conversely, sons and daughters of the e-health care system. We need to recognize some of the interrelationships among these systems at different hierarchical levels. Our primary focus, therefore, will be to describe the overarching vision of the e-health paradigm shift, providing the reader with an understanding of the primary role of e-health systems, their goals and benefits, and why they should exist and be promoted in the face of increasing complexities and environmental uncertainties. We will look carefully at the drivers of and barriers to e-health systems— that is, (1) what drives the e-health revolution and (2) what challenges e-health systems must overcome in order to thrive and grow. As we lay down the tracks for the e-health train to move forward, we must ask ourselves what impediments we must be aware of and how we should respond to these impediments.

The E-Health Paradigm Shift

Many of us are familiar with the concept of a paradigm shift, a revolution of thoughts and actions that often results in a complete turnaround of earlier generational or traditional thinking and models in a field or even an era. For example, Einstein's theory of relativity was a paradigm shift in physics from Newton's law of gravity. Similarly, the industrial revolution, which began in England in the middle of the eighteenth century, was a paradigm shift, transforming society as machines began to replace animals and human workers.

In a similar vein, the technological revolution discussed at the beginning of this chapter is a paradigm shift that in turn is ushering in the e-health revolution that we are witnessing today. E-health can be conceived as a paradigm shift away from traditional approaches to health care and service delivery. In traditional health care systems, the focus is on caring for the sick rather than promoting wellness; in e-health systems, the focus is on preventive care and ubiquitous health care services. The traditional health care system transports the sick and those in need of treatment and healing to the doctors and specialists; the e-health care system moves or transmits key data, information, knowledge, and even products and services to the e-consumers and anyone who needs the data, information, knowledge, products, or services, including paramedics, nurses, and general practitioners.

In essence, transforming the way in which health care information, data, knowledge elements, products, or services are transmitted from a physical mode to a digital mode completely changes the way health care business can be conducted. At least in theory, e-consumers or their intermediaries (for example paramedics) will be able to access evidence-based medicine. Evidence-based medicine is the conscientious, explicit and judicious use of current best evidence in making decisions about the care of individual patients (see Case section of Chapter Fifteen). This will help seek out the best experts in any medical specialty field at the click of a mouse; specialists, doctors, psychologists, and nurses will be able to connect directly with e-patients and e-consumers or other intermediaries without being limited by time, space, or geographical location. And data could be shared among general physicians and specialists without face-to-face meetings.

Marvelous as this paradigm shift may sound, in order to realize its benefits, we must be able to articulate a clear vision of e-health that encompasses a comprehensive understanding of its general purpose, goals, and benefits.

Vision

From a practical perspective, the e-health vision must begin with a national strategy to create a common platform to do business. Extending this idea to a global perspective would translate into international agendas for (1) information and technological standards, (2) public health information infrastructures and highways, (3) electronic and digital networks to connect different health care professionals from all over the globe, and (4) a philosophy that good health care should be ubiquitous.

From an ideological perspective, e-health must go beyond the fear that universal health care may result in long waiting lines and a socialist or communist state paying for the poor and unproductive. It is argued that the vision of e-health is to promote general health care as a public good and to fight for greater public accountability on public investments in health care. It is a vision of more available, accessible, and affordable health care for everyone.

From a philosophical perspective, the e-health vision takes a positivist, evidence-based view, which leads to more secure and improved sharing of health care data and records for efficient and effective health care delivery and the promotion of citizens' well-being.

As we shall see, this vision applies to all areas of health care, including preventive health and health promotion, occupational and environmental health, population and public health, maternal and child health, emergency and non-emergency health care, and health education and training.

In the domain of preventive health and health promotion, e-health agendas could focus on smoking cessation, responsible driving, workplace accident prevention, healthy lifestyle behaviors, diet and nutrition, or walking and exercise. New opportunities could be created through the use of e-interventions and e-technologies. A network strategy, for example, could be employed to permit a sharable platform, perhaps using XML (see Chapter One) and on-line analytic processing (OLAP) to analyze and process data on a real-time basis. Initially, the network might serve a small number of connected, powerful servers, and the incoming data stream might be directed into a data warehouse for periodic cleaning, organizing, and mining. As the system grows, the network could be made accessible through the Internet, and data acquisition, cleaning, and analysis could be completed in real time. Such a system would provide the necessary infrastructure to support a national or even international information network that could track the health status of individuals, groups, communities, societies, and populations. Various data mining techniques could be applied, not just to monitor the effects of unhealthy behaviors or circumstances but also to track positive outcomes. The vision of such a system is to promote the health and well being of the population linked to this network. Indeed, such automated results of analysis might also prove useful for export to less developed nations (see Chapter Eight).

In the domain of public health care, for example, Yasnoff, Overhage, Humphreys, and LaVenture (2001), see a demand for a continual stream of information to be transmitted electronically "from a wide variety of sources regarding the health status of every community, to be collected, analyzed, and disseminated." Through the use of intelligent electronic health records, they argue, "automated reminders could be presented to clinicians for individually tailored preventive services, immediate feedback on community incidence of disease could be available, and public health officials could activate specific surveillance protocols on demand. Furthermore, customized, individualized prevention reminders could be delivered directly to the general public." Such a proposal could easily be extended to an international level, whether in public health or other areas, such as occupational and environmental health. Similarly, a surveillance system at a national level could be created to guard against major bioterrorism threats or pandemic and epidemic disasters caused by viruses such as HIV/AIDS, SARS, avian flu, West Nile virus, chicken pox, and monkey pox.

Applying this sort of thinking at an international level, therefore, our vision of e-health will specifically involve creating a real-time, on-line global disease surveillance network to maintain and promote the health of populations living in different communities across different countries, all of which would sponsor, support, or contribute data to this network. Any potentially threatening patterns of infectious diseases could be quickly detected and reported. The information could immediately be disseminated to all public health authorities and agencies subscribing to the global network. Such efficiency would be extremely beneficial because time is a vital factor in this kind of disease surveillance, monitoring, and prevention.

In the domain of maternal and child health, a similar national or international health information strategy could be instituted. Pregnant women could be tele-educated about (1) the positive effects of breast-feeding, proper diet and nutrition, and use of vitamins and supplements; (2) the negative effects of smoking, excessive drinking, and other behaviors; and (3) the identification of risk factors throughout the various stages of pregnancy and labor. Midwifery teletraining and education modules could also be developed to provide midwives with critical knowledge on how to prevent or overcome conditions that lead to maternal or child death or injury. Training modules on family planning, use of contraceptives, and the risks of sexually transmitted diseases could also be provided. Key to success is the will of the government and the people of a country to support the diffusion of e-technologies. Of course, strong leadership from the top is critical, especially in developing and less developed countries, to making the e-health vision a reality.

E-Health Versus E-Commerce, E-Marketing, E-Medicine, and E-Home Care

Conceptually, *e-health* is the umbrella term for applying existing and emerging e-technologies in combination with innovative or improved processes to transform mainstream health care business practices. Business processes require innovation and improvement because, in many instances, the delivery of e-health information, products, and services requires a different way of doing business. Whereas traditional health care information exchange, product retailing, and service delivery focus primarily on empowering health providers and professionals, the vision of e-health focuses on empowering users, typically laypersons or consumers, without limiting its potential to empower other stakeholders, including health professionals. Several key e-health domains have already diffused and are becoming popular and even profitable—for example, e-marketing (telemarketing), e-medicine (telemedicine), telehealth, and e-home care (telecare). (The term *e-marketing* is used here because *telemarketing* has been overused and connotes the use of telephones more than the use of the Internet or other digital media.)

E-health (sometimes referred to as *telehealth*) is one of the most broadly defined terms in this text (see Chapter Eight for more on definitions). It encompasses e-commerce and e-marketing and all forms of e-medicine (or telemedicine), decision support, e-business intelligence in health care, and e-home care applications. It can be defined as the use of existing and emerging e-technologies to provide and support health care delivery that transcends physical, temporal, social, political, cultural, and geographical boundaries. Examples of services include but are not limited to e-marketing, e-medicine, e-consulting, e-learning, e-diagnosis, e-imaging, e-home care and emergency support, and transactional transmissions.

E-commerce is another very comprehensive term referring generally to the application of e-technologies in order to realize business transactions. E-health includes e-commerce information exchange and transactional activities; in recent years, three important classes of e-commerce have grown in popularity. One of these is *business-to-business (B2B) transactions.* The business entities on either side of a B2B transaction can include e-vendors, e-caregivers, e-payers, and e-regulatory agencies. Another class of e-commerce is *business-to-consumer (B2C) transactions. Consumer-to-consumer (C2C) transactions,* a more recent development, contribute to the creation of virtual health networks and e-learning communities (e-communities). B2C applications are most closely related to our vision of e-health because they focus on delivery of data, information, knowledge, products, and services directly to e-consumers.

E-marketing (or *telemarketing*) systems are B2C applications, selling goods and services on-line to increase market share and profitability and also working to create a brand name over time. For example, www.WebMD.com offers Internet health care that connects e-physicians and e-consumers and allows e-consumers to choose physicians, schedule appointments, check claims' status, and view laboratory results. In addition, the site promotes a brand name (WebMD) to differentiate its e-physicians from mainstream physicians. ViagraPurchase (www.ViagraPurchase.com) offers on-line consultations for e-patients seeking Viagra through the Web, with guaranteed forty-eight-hour delivery of the Viagra. Brand names such as Johnson & Johnson skin care and baby products, OneTouch's ultrasoft automatic blood sampler and other medical devices and McNeil's Tylenol and other pharmaceutical products have all become known through traditional advertising and retailing. E-marketing promises to do the same for emerging Internet-based businesses, providing both retail potential and image advertising.

Many health insurers, HMOs, and e-health groups are also using e-marketing not only to create brand names but also to project a professional public image. The time may indeed have come for these entities to present themselves as being on the leading edge and fully able to deliver goods and services through the Internet, community health information networks, third-party portals and Web services, or the private networks of multinational health insurer and provider organizations. These systems are also used (1) to sell health information or provide e-consultation to e-consumers and e-providers on specific topics, (2) to fulfill e-prescription orders, and (3) to dispense over-the-counter health care products, medical devices, books, and associated services. For instance, MedSite (www.Medsite.com) e-markets products such as medical books and "doctor's bag" equipment from its on-line health care specialty store.

E-medicine (or *telemedicine*) is the deployment of information and telecommunication technologies to allow remote sharing of relevant information or medical expertise, regardless of the patient's location. Broadly speaking, e-medicine is a subclass of technological innovations that have been evolving to bring affordable medicine to the masses as well as to remote places. A key feature that distinguishes e-medicine applications from simple videoconferencing systems is the use of associated peripheral devices that enable e-clinicians to better approximate an on-site examination. These include electronic versions of standard examination tools, as well as other sensitive electronic instruments such as close-up cameras, microscopes, and dermascopes. These tools are not readily available at this point in time as they require large communication bandwidths, powerful servers and sophisticated AI-based systems. We expect most e-medicine applications to provide mostly e-monitoring of patients' vital signals through remotely controlled equipment.

E-home care (or *telecare*) is the application of e-technologies to assist patients who choose to be located at home rather than at a health care facility (see Chapter Nine). Many patients who have chronic illnesses such as diabetes; broken limbs; or mental illnesses are aided through electronic monitoring devices and other e-care services, such as e-transmission of blood test results picked up through sensors in the home. The latest developments in telecare have been moving toward integrating expertise from specialists such as psychologists, architects, computer scientists, clinicians and specialists, and builders and contractors trained in "smart homes" for the disabled, homebound patients, and seniors.

Figure 2.1 illustrates how various e-health care concepts relate to one another. The figure shows that the e-health care system is complex and its environment mutifaceted. This may partly explain why IT in health care tends to fall behind IT applications in business (as is discussed in the next section).

FIGURE 2.1. E-HEALTH CARE SYSTEMS AND SUBSYSTEMS

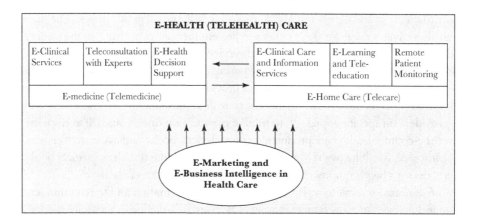

For many years, mainstream health care has been driven largely by primary health (acute) care needs, with attention shifting under special circumstances to secondary and tertiary care (referrals to rehabilitation and home care). While traditional health care provision may be the best form of acute and emergency care, most needs today have to do with non-emergency, secondary, or tertiary care areas—for example, chronic pain, management of cancer or heart problems, malnutrition, mental illness, excessive fatigue and stress, lifestyle and social behavioral problems, poor immune systems, and palliative care. E-health services are appropriate for these types of care. Hence, e-health care may be seen as a transforming health care agent because of its focus on preventive health and wellness, health promotion, non-emergency health care, self-care, health information therapy, and more directed self-care such as checking blood glucose and taking medications as prescribed.

We will now turn to the specific goals and benefits of e-health systems that will drive the future growth and development of e-health.

E-Health Drivers and Barriers

If the vision of the e-health system is to achieve better health and well-being for the general population through the application of e-technologies, the key goals must be to improve and enhance the efficiency and effectiveness of the existing system by making products and services more available, accessible, affordable, and accountable. We therefore begin by looking at system goals and benefits as underlying drivers for the paradigm shift. (See Chapter Twelve for more on challenges of e-health.)

System Goals and Benefits

As noted, the drivers of e-health are trends that should lead to achieving more comprehensive, reasonably inexpensive, and easy-to-access health care products and services for everyone. Yet the level or standard of e-health care in any given environment or system will likely be the minimum standard expected within that environment or system. Therefore, standards may vary significantly from one country or jurisdiction to another. For example, pursuing the goals and associated benefits of e-health care in the United States or most other developed countries could lead to expectations that all citizens could access health-promoting information, products, and services anywhere and anytime at a reasonably low cost, partly because of the huge amount of public investment that is made in health care on a yearly basis. If the same goals were pursued in developing areas such as sub-Saharan Africa (see Chapter Eight), the expectations would be vastly reduced because of the smaller economic means and lower health care standards there.

For these goals and benefits to be achievable, new legislation and policies will need to be implemented that are conducive to promoting e-health practices. Without supporting policies, all of the possibilities in this book will be totally theoretical, and we will be a long way from implementing and realizing e-health care.

As these policies and new legislations become implemented, e-health care can yield the following benefits:

- Availability and accessibility of health care knowledge and expertise, especially for the underserved and underinsured
- Availability and accessibility of quality health care on a more equitable basis to underserved rural and urban areas
- Comprehensive availability of e-clinical services, regardless of time, specialty, and geographical location
- Availability of e-health services for new and alternative (non-invasive) medical procedures
- Savings for e-providers and e-patients in procedural, travel, and claims processing costs
- Educational service networks for isolated health professionals, residents, and non-experts
- Empowerment of e-consumers and e-providers
- Reduced use of traditional emergency services
- Improved non-emergency services
- Decreased waiting time for non-emergency services
- Greater awareness of services among rural and remote residents and caregivers
- Availability and timely accessibility of critical information in the event of emergencies

If these benefits are to be realized, a gradual shifting from the traditional health care delivery system and environment to virtual forms of health care delivery systems and arrangements is needed. Thus, the evolution of e-health concepts, infrastructures, technologies, applications, interfaces, and strategies all contribute to the paradigm shift. For example, e-health concepts and strategies are vital for health care reform and new ways of thinking about health care delivery; e-health technologies and applications provide alternative means of delivering health care products and services; and e-health infrastructures and interfaces offer convenient mechanisms for transmitting medical and clinical knowledge to residents, non-experts, and health care workers. Moreover, e-health methods and strategies encourage innovations in non-invasive medical interventions, a focus on preventive measures, and greater emphasis on self-care and rural medicine.

In addition, e-health can aid in realizing rapid changes in a nation's health care infrastructures, financing, administration, management, and care delivery systems and procedures such as reduced administration costs and eliminating "inappropriate and unnecessary" emergency services. These goals and benefits, to the degree that they are realized, will further propel the growth and development of e-health in years to come.

Modern technologies are now pervasive in many societies. Citizens of developed countries, including the United States, Canada, and the United Kingdom, have significant access to consumer-oriented e-health information, albeit of variable quality. Entering a general word or phrase like *health care* into an Internet search engine will result in an overwhelming amount of information. Using the specific term *e-health* results in a number of relevant searches. This indicates a social trend in changing customer's attitudes toward e-health. More informed and better-educated consumers are also driving the e-health paradigm shift. Moreover, reduced administrative and medical costs due to more efficient information flow and more effective workflows will further reduce the cost of products and services, thereby adding to the growth of e-health. For instance, Web technology can replace fragmented paper trails and incomplete telephone messages with archived notes and electronically posted messages to coordinate time-consuming and complex communications between e-consumers and e-caregivers. Virtual private networks eliminate low quality, limited time-space connection while enabling secured transmission of large amounts of data among connected parties that are geographically apart. Costs associated with postage, paper, and long-distance phone calls can also be minimized.

Growing public awareness of the use of the Internet and its associated technologies and services also drive the growth and development of the e-health marketplace. E-consumers are able to search out relevant and useful information and work toward gaining continuing support from e-care professionals. Making information and tools available to e-consumers for planning their own treatment regimens and comparing notes with others will further enhance their trust in the e-health care system. It will also encourage them to share their many hidden concerns with e-caregivers, who can provide the virtual presence of someone who cares. People who suffer from chronic illnesses such as cancer, diabetes, fibromyalgia, and AIDS already draw support from other patients with similar challenges through Web chats, on-line support groups, e-mail messages, and newsgroups. (Trade-offs in regard to support groups will be pointed out later in this chapter.) Educating and empowering e-consumers on-line will enable them to become active participants in self-care, thus potentially resulting in greater satisfaction.

Today, when a patient walks into a physician's office, office personnel frequently use the phone to verify the scope of the patient's insurance. An e-health system can give physician's offices immediate access to such information. Once a service is rendered, on-line claims can be initiated and completed in just a few days, as opposed to the current weeks or even months it takes to get a reimbursement from an insurance company with manual form processing. Moreover, time and cost savings can quickly add up to hundreds of millions of dollars, including savings for the insured (who do not have to worry about a delay in verifying treatment eligibility or complete claim forms to find out that claims have been denied), the providers (who are spared delays in reimbursements and nonpayment for their services) and the insurers (who need less personnel for manual claims and experience fewer processing inefficiencies, such as keyboarding mistakes or illegible writing). The total savings on paper alone can sometimes be overwhelming: Hewlett Packard electronically stores ten terabytes of information per month, equivalent to a stack of paper three hundred miles high. Employees and consumers will also be able to access the information they desire precisely. This enhances the "pull" as opposed to "push" nature of the communication among insurers, providers, and patients. Global health corporations can facilitate instantaneous communication between e-providers and e-consumers, allowing them to have discussions that would not have previously been possible.

All of this has also created an expectation that future health services should eventually subscribe to the e-health vision. People, in general, expect the same level of services from an e-health care system as from the traditional health care system.

This brings us to a discussion of the barriers to reaching the e-health vision described in the beginning of this chapter.

E-Health Barriers and Challenges

Perhaps the most essential ingredient for vibrant e-health development is assurance for citizens and e-health care professionals that an e-health care system will in fact lead to improved health as opposed to fraud, medical misinformation, abuse of consumer data, marketing of products and services that are of little or questionable value, or e-care services that fail to satisfy their needs. In other words, evaluation of the existing e-health care system is important to ensure that the goals and benefits can be and are being achieved. Policies and mechanisms must be created to oversee the development and growth of e-health, including legislation against fraud and unethical practices and for protection of patient privacy and confidentiality of e-patient data.

Unfortunately, e-health is far less developed than traditional health care, which has been established over the last several centuries, or even e-business ventures, despite the similar transactional processes involved. Much skepticism has been expressed about the proliferation and diffusion of e-health, primarily because of fear of change, resistance from health care professionals, consumer concerns over privacy and security issues, competing interests among innovations for venture capitalists and funding sources, and continuing environmental and political uncertainties. Venture capitalists and investors are also wary of putting money into a health care system that is financially at risk, that lacks coherence and cost control, and that has byzantine requirements for computing costs and returns on investments. For example, even with state-of-the-art information systems in many health provider institutions, it is difficult, if not impossible, to give the precise cost of any specific medical procedure. For example, the cost of a hip replacement surgery depends on the condition of the patient, the seniority and prestige of the surgeon, the cost of the specific materials used, the length of the patient's stay, the facility in which the procedure is to be undertaken, and many other factors.

The lack of standards or at least a coalescing consensus on standards can be detrimental to building e-health infrastructures and highways for rapid transmission of e-health information, products, and services. System chaos can result when there are too many different platforms, software standards, security procedures, and programming languages, each attempting to stake out a niche in the billion-dollar e-health technology marketplace. The complexity of implementing common shareware without compatible standards creates undue or unnecessary delays in collaborative projects. Lack of standards also presents the risk of strengthened user resistance, especially from health professionals. Not only can the installation of a proper infrastructure assist in managing multiway communications among e-stakeholders, but it can also motivate e-workers to share information and participate in discussions as to best practices and evidence-based medicine. Of course, the federal government or a multinational corporation like IBM or Microsoft will be expected to provide the strong consensus-based leadership needed to champion and oversee the process of achieving standardization among major e-stakeholders.

Another area of challenge is e-work design. In many instances, consumers, providers, and insurers are not prepared for the changes in their respective information management roles. The transition to e-consumer empowerment means that e-provider corporations will become information disseminators rather than information gatekeepers. Recognizing this change in business functioning is critical to the success of e-health operations. Workers must be trained differently and companies must begin to learn how to manage e-work. Information system analysts and Web developers may also feel threatened as e-consumers and e-providers dictate specific information management functions and requirements instead of relying on the "experts." Poor and inadequate e-technologies and interfaces will not be tolerated and will fall by the wayside. All of these changes will lead to new work processes for everyone in the system. Trial and error is inevitable, but continual quality improvement and well-designed evaluations are equally important.

Data security and confidentiality of patient information are two of the most important concerns in the application of e-health technologies. Security access is a major concern as e-health technologies become available to a huge number of users spread across literally boundless geography. Appropriate firewall protection, data encryption, and password access can all be employed to manage security issues; however, computing viruses are getting more sophisticated as security technology increases.

The American Medical Association has developed stringent security procedures to prevent unauthorized access to computerized patient records, including an indication that individuals or agencies can only access confidential medical data with bona fide intent. In order to use e-technologies effectively, it is important to define to whom access will be granted and what level of patient data may be shared. At Beth Israel Deaconess Medical Center in Boston, the five-hospital patient record network has a 512-bit key encryption, a level of encryption that is standard in many contemporary e-business applications. This ensures a secure transaction which is capable of running on multiple platforms. Audit trails and separation of duties can also be used to beef up data security.

Here is a brief illustration of one e-health challenge. As many as 20 to 30 percent of the world's people may have literacy problems. In addition, many U.S. citizens are monolingual, and large numbers of European, Asian, African and Latin American people speak limited or no English. The variety of languages and cultural assumptions of potential e-health users present a natural barrier to sharing information. While automatic translators could conceivably be installed to reformat Web sites in English into other languages, and user responses in various languages could also be translated back to English, many medical terms are difficult to translate, and hidden connotations in one language may result in missed concepts or information when remarks are translated. In addition, use of certain symbols, colors, and layouts may convey different meanings to people of different cultures. For example, any attempt to teleconsult by e-providers who do not speak the same language will always be a challenge.

Medicolegal Considerations

Because the present technology appears to be capable of handling the demands of e-health care in most applications, the question arises as to why it is not used more often. Liability concerns are one major reason (Daley, 2000). According to Kleinke (2000), "IT executives have long blamed physicians" and their resistance to computers for the lack of widespread IT adoption in health care, while those same IT executives were perpetuating the real impediment. In the training manuals and other documentation of all health care IT products, one finds a vendor's legal disclaimer for any negative clinical consequences, typically on the very first page.

The liability issue is not new, nor is it unique to e-health care. The part that is unique is the need to determine laws and standards of care that govern e-health practice. It has been much debated whether a patient's location should govern the issue of liability, to prevent physicians from "forum shopping"—that is, practicing in states or countries with the most favorable liability laws. Presently, there is little legislation or judicial precedent regarding e-health care services. Physicians hesitate to get involved when there is not a well-defined legal framework or standard of care. Many e-health Web sites simply cater to whoever would like to purchase products and services, without carefully considering the medicolegal implications of the transactions.

Another major obstacle to the growth of e-health care is the problem of reimbursement for services. E-health products that are sold as business goods can use existing electronic payment systems, but a broad system for reimbursement for e-health care services is still unavailable. From April 1999 through December 2000, only 235 instances of telehealth services (valued at $15,082) were paid for under Medicare. During the same period, the total amount paid by Medicare was $4,030,103,894 (Wachter, 2000). It is also unclear whether e-health care is an eligible and legally insured service under federally funded capitated payment or health maintenance organization programs.

Another hindrance to the diffusion of e-health care is the fact that physicians and licensed practitioners are legally required to have separate medical licenses to practice in each state. E-health care allows health care services to cross state boundaries, but some states have laws designed to keep out health professionals who are not licensed in that state.

Before the practice of e-health can diffuse and become widely accepted in the United States and other developed countries, their respective governments must enact policies regarding the appropriate use of the Internet for direct patient-provider e-consultations, e-clinical care, and e-prescribing. Ideally, there would also be limitations on practitioners' liability as a result of providing e-health care services. For e-consumers, there must be assurance that privacy and confidentiality will be protected in the transmission of sensitive information and e-storage of their personal records. The next part of this book provides a brief glimpse of some potential developments and breakthroughs that are shaping the future of e-networking.

Conclusion

This section has attempted to demonstrate, despite a lack of both theoretical and empirical published research, that the implementation of e-health in hospitals and healthcare organizations is a challenge that has to be overcome from many angles if e-health is to succeed. As we have seen, one major hindrance in deploying e-health applications is the lack of a legal infrastructure that can administer and manage them. We believe that there is huge potential for e-health to improve human health services and to achieve the vision set out earlier in this chapter, if humans can make appropriate and ethical use of electronic technologies. E-health is beginning to permeate all aspects of the health care industry. Many of these technologies are no longer new, and it is up to humans to implement them now.

Chapter Questions

1. What is meant by the phrase *the e-health paradigm shift?* Provide some examples of trends toward this paradigm shift.
2. What do you envision as the purpose of the e-health care system? What is the significance of this vision in the development of global health care?
3. Who would be primarily responsible for successful implementation of the e-health care system? What challenges must be overcome for e-health to survive and thrive?

References

Blendon, R., Benson, J., Brodie, M., Altman, D., Rosenbaum, M., Flournoy, R., & Kim, M. (2001). Whom to protect and how? The public, the government, and the Internet revolution. In *The Brookings Review* (pp. 44–48). Washington, DC: Brookings Institution Press, Winter 2001, Vol. 19 No 1.

Daley, H. (2000). Telemedicine: The invisible legal barriers to the health care of the future. *Annual Health L., 9*, 73.

DICOM Standards Committee and Working Groups. (1998, December). *DICOM committee procedures.* Retrieved May 15, 2001, from Digital Imaging and Communications in Medicine Web site: http://medical.nema.org/dicom/wgs.html

Kleinke, J. (2000, November–December). Vaporware.com: The failed promise of the health care Internet; Why the Internet will be the next thing not to fix the U.S. health care system. *Health Affairs.*

Wachter, G. (2000, March 26). *Two years of Medicare reimbursement of telemedicine: A post-mortem.* Retrieved May 15, 2001, from http://tie.telemed.org/legal/issues/reimburse_summary.asp

Yasnoff, W., Overhage, J. M., Humphreys, B., & LaVenture, M. (2001). A national agenda for public health informatics: Summarized recommendations from the 2001 AMIA spring congress. *Journal of the American Medical Informatics Association,* 2001, *8*(6), 535–545.

Cyber-Angel: The E-Robin Hood Case

Joseph Tan, Joshia Tan

Cyber-Angel is an e-health system sponsored by a few local Detroit radio and television networks and partly funded by nonprofit organizations and foundations, including the Detroit FreeCare Enterprise, Total HealthCare Union, and Michael Livingston Foundation. Cyber-Angel was created by a group of volunteer social workers, e-physicians,

This case is hypothetical, to be used for discussion purposes only.

e-health practitioners, e-health care activists, and e-nurses. During a local e-health care conference, these volunteers decided to spearhead Cyber-Angel with the hope of providing long-lasting empowerment for the underserved and underinsured through low-cost e-health information and knowledge diffusion. In listening to a keynote speech, these volunteers were convinced of the inadequacy of the current U.S. health care system, especially in Detroit, to meet the needs of America's poorest and least educated people, some of whom were living in rural areas as well as in inner-city areas in cities like Detroit.

Cyber-Angel Operations

To make Cyber-Angel accessible, secured kiosks using touchscreen technology were installed in public places such as railway stations and group homes. Essentially, Cyber-Angel is an innovative Web site that allows needy e-consumers to obtain e-health services without having to pay regular insurance co-payments. In most cases, users only pay a quarter, which allows them to operate the system for about twenty minutes. About sixty kiosks have been installed throughout the inner city, and more are being planned. Plans have also been made to incorporate voice recognition technology in order to reach more people. In an attempt to reach out to the elderly, some volunteers are contemplating installing systems on desktops placed in seniors' homes and providing free access IDs and passwords. Presently, Cyber-Angel volunteers and donors can get free access to the Web site via the Internet through the use of their IDs and a secure password; other e-consumers who want to access Cyber-Angel must use one of the installed kiosks. The possibility of providing a subscription capability for registered users who want to pay a regular fee for the service has been discussed, but nothing concrete has been decided.

Friends of Cyber-Angel

Cyber-Angel acts like an E-Robin Hood, taking resources from those who are wealthy and able and giving them to the poor and needy. The Web site therefore invites donations from anyone who would like to contribute time, money, or effort to aid fellow Americans who carry no medical insurance coverage. Cyber-Angel has managed to attract a large network of volunteers, including lawyers, social workers, physicians, psychologists, nurses, and students. Each donor or volunteer is automatically assigned an ID and asked to select a secure password.

Here are several examples of how the volunteer system works: Mary is a trained nurse who registered to provide volunteer e-nursing service (providing nursing advice on an e-consultation basis) on two weekend night shifts from her home PC. Meanwhile, John raises funds for Cyber-Angel by e-mailing the list of potential donors from time to time, tracking and monitoring pledges and fulfillment on his desktop computer. Heidi is a well-trained medical resident with extensive training in naturopathy. She seeks to pass on some of her medical training and to share her knowledge of naturopathy. During her volunteer hours, Heidi contacted a number of clients through

Cyber-Angel, which she installed on her portable handheld. One such client, Steven, who now volunteers for Cyber-Angel, ceased smoking under Heidi's care and got in the habit of performing stretching exercises on a daily basis as directed by Heidi. Soon, Steven moved out of his group home, altering his diet and daily habits. He found a job at the local supermarket and told Heidi that he would volunteer his time to help others like himself benefit from Cyber-Angel. He was encouraged to register as a fundraising volunteer in order to keep Cyber-Angel active and to perform tasks similar to John's. Steven even became a health activist in his old neighborhood, raising awareness of the adverse effects of smoking among the smokers he had been living with at the group home.

Each year, the sponsoring radio and television networks run a joint campaign for fundraising, featuring Cyber-Angel in order to raise awareness among the Detroit public. These campaigns have generally been very successful, with the mayor of Detroit or the governor of Michigan present to kick off the events. Names of donors are automatically entered into Cyber-Angel's system and displayed in a section of the Web site, along with information on the level of donations and the types of volunteer services that the donors are supplying. Donors are automatically assigned an ID, then choose a password for Cyber-Angel and enter the amount they would like deducted from their bank account or credit card. In return, donors at all levels receive access to Cyber-Angel free of charge for their donation year. The average donor gives about $43 or an hour per month of their time, which is the recommended time commitment for volunteers.

Lessons from Cyber-Angel

Cyber-Angel's kiosks are currently available in three counties in and around Detroit, but more counties will soon have kiosks installed. E-health activists and professionals from other American cities are aware of this system. Some have traveled to Detroit to observe how the system works and have also initiated or welcomed similar concepts. Conferences are being planned to demonstrate some of these systems and to share information about the core value propositions, the infrastructure and e-technologies used, and the effects of these systems on users as well as on e-providers.

A recent analysis of Cyber-Angel reveals a number of core value propositions:

• Cyber-Angel is readily available and easy to operate, especially for those who need non-emergency health care services and cannot afford to see a doctor or a health practitioner. (Most users want to ask for medical advice and need someone to talk to about getting back their health and getting themselves out of their bad habits, services which do not require physical visits.)

• The system builds rapport between e-consumers and e-caregivers because Cyber-Angel services are not rendered based on monetary rewards for the caregivers but for the purpose of assisting users in need. Caregivers get satisfaction from resolving non-emergency health problems that could become serious if neglected. In addition, over time, e-caregivers get to know their clients, and e-consumers are welcome to e-mail their e-caregivers directly anytime. E-caregivers have the choice of replying to e-mails only at the times that they are scheduled to work.

• The Cyber-Angel system accumulates and houses important information in a data warehouse for future mining. Researchers are convinced that data analysis will unveil critical needs of the underserved, based on the types of questions and interactions that are being analyzed. Analysis of these data will almost certainly lead eventually to a better version of the Cyber-Angel software, as well as improved information for policy-making, particularly in the areas of public health and individual health care for the underserved and underinsured.

• Finally, the Cyber-Angel system promises to alleviate some of the demands on emergency care provided by local hospitals, because people, especially those who do not require immediate health care attention and cannot afford to pay, can be directed to use Cyber-Angel instead.

Conclusion

Despite its many advantages, Cyber-Angel faces many challenges and ethical questions. The City of Detroit recently ordered a review of the legality of the medical advice being provided. At the same time, some HMOs and other established insurers are threatening to place a court order to stop Cyber-Angel from further operation. The creators of Cyber-Angel have hired legal experts to look into the ethical and legal implications of its operations. The future of Cyber-Angel is now in question.

Case Questions

1. What features of Cyber-Angel distinguish it from traditional health care systems?
2. How would you envision the infrastructure that supports the functionality of Cyber-Angel? What types of e-health services are most likely to be appropriate for use in Cyber-Angel?
3. Do you agree that Cyber-Angel is an e-health system whose time has come? Why or why not?
4. Think about the ethical and legal issues of operating a program such as Cyber-Angel. What are the most significant challenges and barriers in operating Cyber-Angel?

PART TWO

E-HEALTH FOUNDATIONS

The history of computing in health care and its evolution in bringing about the e-health paradigm shift as described in Part One is just the beginning of a longer story. More specifically, the e-health paradigm shift is concerned with changes in and the integration of organizational structures and forms shaped by our evolving understanding of how to deliver goods and services that are needed to maintain the health and well-being of people around the world.

Part Two (Chapters Three through Six) continues to reflect the same concerns with a changed emphasis, offering a more in-depth understanding of various e-health perspectives (Chapter Three); e-health's conceptual foundations, including the significance of e-health records as the lifeblood of e-health (Chapter Four); the introduction of e-public health information systems as the most fundamental e-health applications (Chapter Five); and the complexity of e-networking as the skeleton structure for framing e-health in the past, present, and future (Chapter Six).

CHAPTER THREE

E-HEALTH PERSPECTIVES

General Systems Concepts, Chaos and String Theories, and Social Science Thinking

Joseph Tan

Learning Objectives

1. Relate general systems concepts to the e-health care system and environment
2. Apply systems thinking and analysis tools to understand the functioning of e-health systems
3. Conceptualize self-learning systems in the context of chaos theory and quantum mechanics
4. Articulate the concept of supersymmetry and its implications for changing the mind-set and redefining the role of e-health leaders
5. Apply virtual global team thinking in social science to address e-health system perspectives
6. Recognize how e-health systems can be conceived as evolving sociocultural entities

Introduction

This chapter allows the reader to take a closer look at the gradual breakdown of conventional thinking about organized health care delivery systems. Whereas in Part One this was done from the perspective of a historian, in this chapter it is done from the viewpoints of a systems philosopher, a physicist, and a social scientist. The reader may ask, "Why is it necessary to adopt such multiple views?" Perhaps the simplest answer is because e-health is a complex interdisciplinary field whose concepts, applications, methodologies, technologies, strategies, and impacts defy comprehension from a single perspective (see Part One). This chapter will provide a survey of theoretical perspectives applicable to e-health.

First, we review general systems concepts and discuss how these concepts relate to the e-health care system and environment. Next, we examine chaos theory and concepts of quantum mechanics, including a brief survey of different versions of string theories and an attempt to see how these theories may help transform our understanding of e-health. Following this, we examine emerging thinking in social sciences with respect to virtual global teams and relate this thinking to the development of e-health.

General Systems Concepts

General systems theory (GST) begins with the observation that what we see, hear, and interact with may be rationalized as a hierarchical network of systems and subsystems. In light of this, systems can be whole and be part of other systems (subsystems) at the same time. Examples of systems range from the galaxy to cells, organelles, and various submicroscopic and particulate systems to bed allocation systems, hospital information systems, the e-health care system, and the general health care system.

A system must have a purpose. In fact, a *system* may be defined simply as a set of interrelated parts that function together as a whole toward achieving a common purpose. Systems can also be characterized as being open or closed. For example, the U.S. health care system, which interacts actively with its environment on a minute-by-minute basis, is an open system, whereas a hospital room directory system, which is absolutely self-contained, is a closed system. The Canadian public health care system, for example, has the overarching goal of achieving excellence in public health and improving the quality of life and well-being for all Canadians. This purpose is expected to guide all subgoals of its embedded subsystems, including the bed allocation system, various health information systems, and various networks designed to support the main system. Systems can also range from simple (for example, a computerized payroll system) to very complex (for example, the computer network system for the New York Stock Exchange).

Open complex systems are characterized by input-process-output triads and feedback loops. GST easily describes the flow of appropriate and relevant information about sick patients (input), who are placed into the different subsystems of the acute health care system to be treated and cared for (process) until they are ready, perhaps, to be transferred to another subsystem such as a group home (intermediate output) before being discharged as healthy individuals who can continue to contribute to their work organizational systems (final output). Continual monitoring of the health status of these patients becomes the feedback loop in the system. These loops ensure the reliability and quality of health services provided, including those before and after the patients are discharged. A common example of an information system that controls this acute patient care process in a hospital setting is the admission-discharge-transfer (ADT) system.

In earlier works (Tan, 2001), the principles of GST concerning the behaviors of organizational systems and subsystems were used to think about the design of different classes of clinical and administrative health management information systems required to run hospitals and health provider organizations. To apply GST to the e-health care system and environment, the first step is to identify the various associated subsystems in terms of their inputs, processes, outputs and feedback loops. One subsystem that comes to mind is e-health records (EHRs), which will be discussed in detail in Chapter Four. In this system, the input consists of patient records stored in a data warehouse or a database. The processes are comprised in the management of those records, including automatic data gathering, cleaning and verifying, adding or deleting information, and retrieving or combining data to answer queries. The output of the system is the information or knowledge from the records that is displayed when queries from e-physicians or other e-caregivers are answered. Feedback loops in the system may include responses from e-patients on the information given to their e-physicians such as information on allergies and responses to queries for information from the EHRs that e-caregivers may make to ensure complete, correct information in the system.

While this description may appear unsophisticated and similar to the function of traditional health record systems, in part because EHRs are also used in traditional health care, in the e-health context, information sharing by the various e-stakeholders is far more complex. For example, information from police arrest documents may electronically follow the arrestee to the corrections facility. Understanding the types of data to be captured from e-stakeholders (multiple inputs) and the nature of the shared data flows (compound processes) needed to support the active exchange of information from EHRs (multiple intermediate and final outputs) in everyday activities can be challenging. Yet such understanding is needed to design relevant network infrastructures to support the many e-care delivery functions and continual data manipulation activities involved in the effective use of EHRs in e-health.

Systems Thinking and Analysis

Over the past fifty years, *systems thinking and analysis* have developed a body of knowledge and tools to make the complete patterns embedded in systems clearer and to help us see how to change them effectively. One such approach involves the execution of five learning disciplines: personal mastery, shared vision, mental models, team learning, and the overarching discipline of systems thinking (Senge, 1990). Systems thinking means seeing the connections among the processes of change, not just snapshots of changes; in other words, the focus should be on interrelationships rather than linear cause-effect chains. Owing to the prevailing focus on detail complexity at the expense of dynamic complexity, Senge notes that even elegant strategic planning fails, especially when the plan attempts to deal with too many variables and neglects dynamic cause and effect. Because dynamic complexity is subtle and does not necessarily happen at contiguous times, systems analysis efforts tend to focus on detail complexity. Unfortunately, the real leverage in most management situations lies in uncovering the underlying dynamic complexity.

In designing e-health care systems and networks, it is thus imperative to pay attention to the dynamic nature of e-health. In other words, not only should key factors and variables be tracked carefully, but moderating and intervening variables should also be monitored, to ensure more complete and intelligent management and decisions. For example, in developing an e-public health statistical system to examine and investigate the health of a population, key indicators such as average life expectancy (measured in number of years) and infant mortality (measured in infant deaths per 1,000 live births) must be tracked, and gender, age, race, and other moderating variables such as location and diet should also not be neglected. Ignoring intervening variables could result in an incomplete picture with too many unanswered questions. The power of e-technologies makes tracking all of these variables a less difficult task than it may seem.

Similarly, Capra (1996) identifies a number of key characteristics of systems thinking and analysis, including the shift from emphasizing the part to emphasizing the whole;

from viewing objects as of primary importance to viewing relationships as being of primary importance (also called *network thinking*); from paying attention to a single system level to moving between system levels; from using an analytic approach to promoting contextual thinking; and from employing objective analysis to applying epistemic science, in which the method of questioning is key to how scientific theories are understood.

In analyzing the data contained in an e-government refugee immigrant statistical system, for example, considerable attention should be paid to available support for lifestyle and cultural changes, community services, language education, on-the-job training, and location with a view to increasing the number of job opportunities for the refugees. Unfortunately, the analysis is often done in isolation and without adequate assessment of the impact of possible inadequate supporting infrastructures such as language education and on-the-job training, as well as possible failures of community services (for example, Australia sometimes only permits new immigrant refugees to settle in remote, underserved areas). If ongoing support for community services and language education as well as on-the-job training is inadequate, increasing the number of refugees every year may backfire: incoming refugee immigrants may just decide to go back to their own or on to other countries. Even worse, they may turn to crime or other destructive activities and become a burden to society.

Lindstrom, Matheson, and Tan (1998) note that in systems thinking and analysis, the need to distinguish fragmentation from wholeness in our tendency to lean toward analytic reductionism is an important step. They argue that there is often a propensity to think that having better and faster information at our disposal will lead naturally to better and faster decisions. Bohm (1980) indicates that this may not necessarily be true, because a fragmentary view may eventually lead to conflicting and confusing biases. In other words, if explanations of a system are a result of analyzing piecemeal and fragmented data, applying system methodology to understand the events that gave rise to the information in the first place will only result in a stovepiped mentality. If we extend this thinking to the e-government refugee immigrant statistical system, we might see a healthy and balanced rate of new job opportunities and be impressed by the comparative increase in number of employed refugee immigrants. In the real-world case from which this example is drawn, the data on the refugee population had an undiscovered trend of increasing job dissatisfaction and deteriorating working conditions. No account had been taken of the fact that many of these refugees were skilled professionals who were now limited to poorly paid unskilled labor. Hence, in analyzing systems, we must be sure to examine all the relevant pieces in order to get the whole picture.

Metaphors and Mental Models as Systems Analysis Tools

An important final point in the systems thinking and analysis approach to decision making is the development of *models* that are used to obtain valuable insights into the behavior of a system. For example, we often attempt to understand a system, such as the evolving e-health care system, by gathering and analyzing selected data and in-putting them into a model without due consideration for known intangible factors that affect the behavior of the system. Potential intangibles in e-health care include impacts from redesign of work practices, resistance from labor unions, and other sociopoliti-cal factors. Because many of these factors are too difficult or complex to simulate or model concretely, we try to piece together just the quantifiable parts to develop an ag-gregate. These quantifiable factors thus form the basis of our management or clinical decisions. Within the context of the e-health care system and its environment, vari-ables often are not easy to quantify; for example, consider the variables involved in ethical, legal, and privacy issues. Ultimately, improving e-health care and achieving better health status of e-patient populations depend largely on the extent to which we can accurately model the system and its inherent behaviors. Since e-health is complex and requires dynamic as opposed to static simulations, models can represent only the first cut at predicting complex system behaviors.

Notwithstanding, Lindstrom, Matheson, and Tan (1998) note that the use of metaphors and mental models in the application of systems theory to organizational studies and to studies of complex information and network systems in organizations is a particularly eye-opening and refreshing approach. Based on this perspective, a vir-tual health network may be conceptualized by using the analogy of a neural network. Basically a neural network (NN) may be conceived as a simplified emulation of the connections of the human brain. It is used here for depicting learning and self-organization within an artificial environment. Neural networks, with their remarkable ability to derive meaning from complicated or imprecise data, can be used to extract patterns and detect trends that are too complex to be noticed by either humans or simple mathematical and programming techniques. Just like an NN, an e-health organization is capable of adaptive learning, self-organization, and real-time opera-tion. This analogy will be relevant to our discussion of e-health network management.

Metaphorically, the memories, learning capacities, and mind-set of an organi-zational NN correspond to its enterprise-wide information, communications, and networked decision-making systems. Imagine John, the CEO of a major e-health care corporation, who is planning to retire. Before he steps down, he wants to ensure that critical pieces of information, communications, and decisions are captured in one form or another in a corporate enterprise resource planning (ERP) system. Perhaps this ERP system is a recently installed e-network, which is analogous to the NN. John's goal, then, is to make it possible for whoever succeeds him (he has his eye on his son, currently vice president of operations) to have access to the "neural network" capa-bilities and memories of the corporate culture now being captured virtually in the corporate ERP system. To the extent that this may be operative, John can have some assurance that the future administration of the corporation will have the benefits of his founding vision and his practices. Metaphorically, this implies that whoever takes over the corporation will understand John's history, strengths, culture, and orientation, and thus the corporation will continue to function and learn as if John were available to provide advice to his successors as needed. The ERP system or e-network thus projects a virtual mind-set and culture throughout the corporation.

How can the *metaphor* of the corporate neural network help us to understand the role of the e-health network infrastructure (enterprise system)? If system neural networks function in such a way as to pull together all of the necessary information and decision making processes of the organization, then we can argue that not only will these neural networks capture, store, process, and disseminate massive amounts of previously learned information, but they will also be able to coordinate and structure learning of new methods and better approaches among users so as to improve the management of the enterprise system (organization) over time. Morgan (1997) uses the term *network intelligence* to refer to this phenomenon. He believes that individuals, by accessing the "neural networks" from evolving knowledge networks and communication networks throughout an enterprise can become fully aware and participate in evolving networks of organizational memories and intelligence. System NNs create capacity for the evolution of a shared intelligence and memories. Going back to the example, John's intelligence and expertise, as well as his memories and learning during his leadership tenure, can now be easily and conveniently passed down to his son or whoever becomes the next CEO. Put simply, the NN metaphor implies that the communications among e-stakeholders within an e-health enterprise can be enhanced and enriched to a point where captured knowledge, key final decisions, and policies made by management can become easily accessible to those who need them.

To extend our NN metaphor and its implications for e-health networks and e-communities, evolving organizational knowledge and other enterprisewide networks could have major implications in altering or redirecting the bureaucratic principles of centralized control to a self-learning paradigm. The key here is to create a sharing network of interactions that can *self-learn*—that is, help generate further learning, shaped or driven by the intelligence of everyone involved in primary decision making throughout the virtual enterprise.

The "architecture of integration" articulated by Beckham (1993) is another interesting concept relevant to this metaphorical thinking. Integration in this sense is a process through which different parties (government, third-party insurers and payers, e-providers and e-vendors) can act as one mind within the system to serve e-consumers; that is, separate parties with individual minds can be meaningfully organized to act as if their minds were integrated. In many respects, the extent of integration can be used as an indicator of how well the networks support the infrastructure and functions of the virtual health care delivery system.

To determine the extent of virtual integration, especially in terms of network design and infrastructure, the following questions may be advanced:

- Are data collected electronically and directly from e-consumers? If so, how willing are e-consumers to provide the data? If not, why not?
- Do all e-providers have free virtual access to the same e-consumer records? If so, how is access authorization verified? Does the network provide the data unambiguously?
- Do the e-stakeholders operate as a well-coordinated virtual team in service delivery? If not, why not?
- Are e-consumer satisfaction and other measurable outcomes being tracked? If yes, how, and what other measurable outcomes are tracked? If not, why not?
- Does a single network serve the needs of e-stakeholders and decision makers at all levels? If not, why, and how can the challenges be overcome?

Mental models are also useful in systems thinking because they provide simplifications of complex e-health system structures. Networks can be designed using different mental models, depending on the perspectives of system users.

For B2C models, a service model perspective is most important because the availability of a convenient tool for e-transactions or e-purchases; on-line connection for inquiries to e-stakeholders, including e-providers, e-vendors, and e-insurers; and real-time access to relevant information resources are all key to meeting e-consumer needs.

For B2B models, the mental models reflect the views of the participating business entities. For instance, an e-vendor supplying prescription drugs wholesale to one or more retailers on-line will want to know the inventory status of the retailers, their account standing, and average monthly sales volume. An accounting model is therefore most relevant and appropriate.

Finally, for C2C models, active information exchange and potential for trading transactions lead to a model that balances the perspectives of the consumer-oriented service model and the transactional, accounting-oriented model; in other words, a hybrid model may be the best framework to pursue. In any case, mental models provide a starting point; system designers and leaders must interpret and determine what consumers and stakeholders expect and want from the system, since those consumers and stakeholders will eventually dictate the success of the new system.

The *rich picture approach* (Tan, 2001) is an especially powerful context-setting visual tool. It provides a powerful tool for mentally modeling any form of complex system as it allows various entities and relationships to be depicted in any ways that are meaningful to the users. Figure 3.1 depicts a rich picture of a multicommunity network designed to promote e-health activities among seniors interacting with high school students in a recently funded e-multicommunity health project, the Maria Madeline project (see the case discussion in this chapter), investigated by me and my colleagues

FIGURE 3.1. A RICH PICTURE OF AN E-MULTICOMMUNITY HEALTH PROMOTION PROJECT

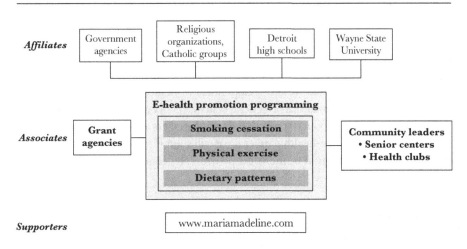

at Wayne State University School of Business. This is a "structural" depiction as opposed to a "pictorial" one. Typically, a rich picture allows the users to use any form of familiar symbols to depict ongoing activities and events or even conflicting views.

A convenient tool for documenting themes or issues for an ill-defined problem situation, the rich picture is especially suited to our mental modeling of soft and fuzzy issues such as conflicting views and attitudes among different stakeholders. In the case of this project, which focused on designing and offering Internet-based Web access primarily to underserved seniors living in inner-city Detroit, one such issue is the scope of computing training that may be needed by the seniors. Our project emphasized intergenerational programming by having high school students partner with seniors interested in learning to use the Internet. This instructional approach prepared the seniors to teach themselves to access available e-health services. The seniors first learn to extract data from the Internet via the Maria Madeline Web site (www.mariamadeline.com) and then via the World Wide Web, using various search engines. The rich picture we generated is only a simple first-cut mental modeling of the system based on one possible scenario of who would be these stakeholders in the system and what interactions will be expected among them.

Enriching this mental modeling process is the creation of *differing realities,* independent of the data observed. These differing realities can be initially investigated by using rich pictures to explore different scenarios to see how different designs of the community network would affect various e-stakeholders. These realities are imagined possibilities (idealized results), which are a combination of changing events, states of events and sequences of events. Further, when designing the network, exploring the relevance of different pieces of information (input or process variables) in the context of several metaphorical perspectives (which can be translated into different rich pictures) demonstrates that no given piece of information is of primary importance; instead, the entire metaphor or mental model is central to understanding the way the health care business should be changed, the way new e-health strategies should be implemented, and the way each of us read, understand, and shape our thinking and thereby our community, culture, and sociopolitical work life.

As we address the limitations of general systems theory and see how other frameworks can help us think about the role that decision makers and information will play in shaping the emerging e-health care era, we will soon discover new and emerging perspectives and conceptual frameworks provided by chaos theory, quantum mechanics, and string theories.

Chaos Theory and String Theories

The tools of systems thinking and systems analysis help us study and describe health care systems, including traditional hospital bed allocation systems; various administrative, financial, and clinical information systems; and even the traditional health care service delivery system (see Tan, 2001). Yet the application of these tools to self-learning systems, which are more dynamic in nature, is limited. Fortunately, recent developments in particle physics, chaos theory, quantum mechanics, and string theories together have unveiled further insights into the nature and characteristics of very complex systems.

Chaos Theory and Quantum Mechanics

Chaos theory, a mathematical science that has been examined subsequent to the era of computing and office automation, observes that extremely small changes, or perturbations, in the starting conditions of a set of equations or a mathematical model can lead to extremely different solutions. Nonetheless, solutions for any starting conditions derived by the mathematical model are always contained within a restricted set of solutions, commonly referred to as the *strange attractor*. Other aspects of chaos theory, such as the study of changing shapes and patterns known as fractals, are built on the idea of evolving complex structures that mimic natural biological systems. In fact, these complex structures behave like neural networks built on the successive "mutations" of simple equations. In other words, they reflect iterative applications of the initial equations, with each step depending on the results of previous steps. The methodology of neural networks is further described and illustrated in Hammad (1998).

Based on chaos theory, we can confidently infer that for any given set of constraints in an e-health system environment, small perturbations in a network can lead to major consequences. Moreover, this environment is not fixed in a set configuration but is dynamically changing. Just like any other organizational system, an e-health care system can be characterized as a living system thriving in an environment that has the potential for it to grow sensibly, creatively, and intelligently. It will be able to adapt to its changing environment and will seek order in order to maintain its meaning. An e-health system will naturally tend to organize itself, be it through a formal reporting structure or through informal structures such as virtual task groups and teams. Because the system is dynamic, its identity will continue to mutate, largely because of a changing infrastructure and evolving environment. In fact, there may be very little difference between the e-health system I am discussing here and the many social and political communities that we interact with in real life, except for the virtual aspect of the e-health care system.

Societal life is becoming more complex because of the increasing number of relationships being formed, the growing amount of information and knowledge that is available in each passing year, and turmoil in the daily sociopolitical environment. The interconnectedness and interdependence of these systems are reflected in the interconnectedness and interdependence of components within the e-health system. Such systems dictate new forms of behavior that may be difficult to predict intelligently. Attempts to decompose the systems into series of fragmentary parts without a clear understanding of the interfaces among the various parts will result in a limited worldview that also lacks understanding of the system dynamics. Thus, we have to go beyond the GST approach when studying nontrivial systems.

In quantum mechanics and physics, how we observe electrons determines whether a field of energy or a particle exists. Because electrons are known to have the capacity to be either energy waves or particles, fields can affect particles and particles can affect fields. Coupled with the observations of chaos theory, new discoveries in quantum physics tell us that the basis for the reordering and restructuring of elements and interactions (particles and fields) within systems is perturbation; in short, some uncertainties are inevitable because perturbation can be conceived as part of what creates the system, and such perturbations are needed if we want the system to yield responses that will in turn evolve toward order. As nature is inherently orderly or will be "attracted" to order, perturbation in the system will lead to balancing change occurring in a system until a steady state is achieved. Therefore, however small and subtle the perturbations may be, when they are introduced at the very beginning of a process, they will eventually lead to changes that may not always be small; indeed, even significant transformations can result from subtle movements. As we have learned, the evolution of e-health systems is an outcome of successive perturbations experienced and witnessed in traditional health care, caused by factors such as user dissatisfaction, governmental interventions, and changes in directions of health leadership. Moreover, we would expect the current e-health environment to change further via some form of evolutionary strategy rather than through an act of force.

Just like any living system, e-health networks cannot and therefore should not be forced to change to achieve particular results within a set time period. Accordingly, strategic planning is best achieved by means of the natural forces influencing change instead of imposed change. The emphasis should be on balancing between "forced" change that is drastic in nature and no change at all because it is not characteristic of living systems to behave in both these manners. In view of our current understanding of dynamic systems and particle physics, we foresee that the evolving networks in e-health enterprises will be best altered in subtle ways as self-learning occurs. Nevertheless, a sense of achievement may be realized at particular times, representing milestones in the history of the health enterprise computing.

Even so, solutions derived from a virtual collaboration among team members resulting in "change" will be very different from those imposed by an individual or even those arrived at during a face-to-face meeting, because the change process will be different. For example, some team members who shy away from participating in face-to-face meetings may be aggressive and vocal in on-line communications. Conversely, those who are usually active in physical meetings may not be as active on-line. Others, feeling the need to show that they are listening and paying attention, may contribute new insights to group thinking. With virtual networking, results achieved may be more likely to be seen as the decision of the entire group and not of any one particular individual, making any proposed changes much easier to implement and sustain over the longer term.

Lindstrom, Matheson, and Tan (1998) note that in quantum physics, a "field" governs the particles within itself and that "fields" themselves may be perceived as particles and hence be governed by a larger field. In an interconnected e-health system, fields are analogous to the visions, missions, values, and goals of subsystems embedded in larger fields with overarching visions, missions, values, and goals. The clarity of the overarching e-health vision and goals (see Chapter Two) will reflect the clarity of a still larger field and will dictate how its subsidiary particles (or embedded fields) will respond. To a large extent, this process will define the strange attractor that forms the set of solutions to any perturbations that may affect the entire system (Lindstrom, Matheson, and Tan, 1998). Put simply, the interconnectedness among elements in e-health networks constrains the emergent solution set. The fact that even a very small perturbation instituted at the beginning of the process can lead to a major change in the system leads to reflection on how we should encourage exchange of ideas, even disagreements, among affected stakeholders in order to arrive at a reasonably acceptable consensus. In this system, fields (representing vision, mission, values, and goals) guide outcomes, leading to suitable and acceptable solutions, but do not predict those outcomes. Conversely, lack of clarity in the fields or vision will lead to the risk of inappropriate and inadequate "solutions." In this view, the fact that the same values can be shared holistically among all e-stakeholders in an e-health network will naturally lead to self-learning and order, stabilizing the entire system.

Self-learning systems can therefore be defined as systems with "the ability of all living systems to organize themselves into patterns and structures without any externally imposed plan or directions" (Wheatley and Kellner-Rogers, 1995). In a self-learning system, change is not only inevitable but is a powerful, creative force resulting from earlier stages of system instability. Instability is sometimes desirable, even necessary. Purposeful (but subtle) perturbations can, if appropriately encouraged and balanced, lead to a desirable order for the system. If a system has always been stable, no change is ever warranted and no new learning can be achieved. For example, if the traditional health care systems were sufficient and there had been no technological advances, economic pressures, or breakthroughs in system thinking, health care would never have evolved into the e-health era.

Left alone, self-learning systems would improve over time on their own because they are preprogrammed to learn and adapt to changing environments. In our e-health network example, clarifying any ambiguity in the vision and values over time, welcoming contributions from team members and letting go of those who may hinder organizational productivity, as well as providing a means for everyone in the network to stay interconnected, will eventually result in a network that achieves the continuous improvements in availability, accessibility, affordability, and accountability that were discussed in Part One of this text.

Supersymmetrical Thinking

According to Lindstrom, Matheson, and Tan (1998), the principles of chaos theory and quantum mechanics offer insights into how to characterize the evolution of knowledge about complex structures and systems. It is suggested here that because complex structures and systems are mostly organic and dynamic with characteristics of self-learning, predicting the behavior of these systems therefore requires application of conceptual frameworks that may themselves be complex, that is evolving over time given the many interacting components that are to be modeled. The science of particle physics has been undergoing a revolution, and its theoretical development has provided new insights into how the properties of particles can be transformed. This is where string theories come in. Although there are many string theories, here we will examine only the underlying concept of supersymmetry.

Physicists can now safely infer that all known particles can be classified either as bosons or as fermions. *Bosons* are particles that transmit forces and can occupy more than one state at the same time—for example, energy and light—whereas *fermions* are particles that make up matter and can occupy only a single state at a given time—for example, the components of tables and chairs. In other words, fermions are physically visible and space-occupying objects, while bosons are, in a practical sense, energy forms of particles that can be digitally (or electrically) transmitted from one point to another and be in both places at the same time.

Both human beings and walls are made up of fermions. Since fermions can be in only a single state at any one time; that is, we cannot walk through walls without hurting ourselves. In particle physics, this idea is referred to as *the exclusion principle*.

The properties of bosons—for example, in light—are just the opposite. If we flash the beams of two flashlights at each other, we see that the two beams appear to pass right through each other without any interference. This is because bosons can occupy more than one state at the same time, allowing them to occupy the same space at the same time. Thus, the beams can overlap each other and still be part of both each other and themselves. In contrast, if we overlap two streams of voice—say, one coming from a radio and another from a television—what do we expect? Although these voices may appear to overlap, they will also appear scattered or disintegrated. This scattering is mostly electrical because the voices could have been electrically streamlined into one voice, given some transformational processes and time such as synchronizing the different analog sound waves into a single digital voice stream with equal speed and similar signal sequence intensity. This is just an analogy from which we can see that different signals appear to have produced the "scattering" that is felt. Hence, you can still hear two separate voices, when in fact, both voices are of the same form of energy.

Jim Gates, one of the foremost scientists in string theory, uses the example of connecting two streams of water from separate hoses into one. Because water may be transformed into a form of electrical energy, according to Gates, even if you could turn off the electrical charges from the separate hoses where the two streams hit each other and merge into one, the exclusion principle would still apply; hence, the water streams behave as if composed of fermions, although as a form of energy in transmission, they are essentially bosons. This phenomenon is known as supersymmetry and this same phenomenon applies to information, as will be demonstrated later. Here, our purpose is to provide counter examples of fermions and bosons behaving supersymmetrically.

As indicated, the world we see, hear, touch, smell, and taste comprises an apparent separation of fermions and bosons. The moment we question why we should limit our thinking to this apparent dichotomy, we begin to move towards a skepticism known as *supersymmetry thinking*, which is the core dilemma in string theories. Indeed, would not the world be or become more symmetrical (supersymmetrical) if some forms of matter could pass right through one another, just as energy and light do, and if some forms of energy could scatter one another just as "physical matter" such as water does? To take another example, is information all bosons? It can be digitized and passed through electrical cables to our television screens or fax machines; however, if this information is displayed as physical words or images occupying some space, and we need to erase and change the written words or graphic images for one reason or another, is it then fermions on the output medium (for example, television screen or fax paper) but bosons in the brain or cable?

The basic idea of *supersymmetry*, then, is that perhaps both matter and energy can be transformed into either fermions or bosons, bringing about some convergence of the properties inherent in the two classes of particles. Such a finding would be a scientific breakthrough (a significant paradigm shift) that would defy and transform our conventional thinking about nature. If that becomes a possibility, we will soon arrive at supersymmetrical thinking. In the world of particle physics, the idea of supersymmetry is to break away from the stereotypical thinking of fermions versus bosons to define the world we live in. Right now, this is purely hypothetical. Many scientists are hopeful that this idea will one day be verified, bringing together the different string theories and collapsing all of them into a single *M theory* (the "mother" of all string theories).

Applying supersymmetrical thinking to e-health networks and systems, we see that the key idea in moving toward an e-health paradigm is to provide ubiquitous access to e-health information. Instead of limiting knowledge and specialized medical information to just a few, those who need to be guided can now have access to specialized knowledge and information so as to capitalize on the transformational power of advanced networking infrastructure and technologies. In other words, doctors and specialists (fermions) will behave like complex information dispensing systems (bosons) and the media or digital devices can in term be used to dispense such e-health information (bosons) to those who may need it (fermions). Ultimately, this will result in producing a supersymmetrical world in which intelligent agents (including humans, information systems, and hybrid systems) will be able to combat many forms of diseases because of the ubiquity of e-health knowledge and information. Globalization, integration, and empowerment are all aspects of supersymmetrical thinking based on the foregoing reasoning of transforming human experts into intelligent agents and e-health information dispensing systems. Similarly, these e-health information dispensing systems can be engineered to produce intelligent human or hybrid agents interacting with each other via ubiquitous networks. Accordingly, the rapid exchange of specialized information via e-health networks will further promote globalization, integration, and consumer empowerment. In e-health networks, typically dependent consumers can become more central while the health providers who used to be independent controllers are now partners, essentially blurring the lines between specialists and generalists and between health providers and e-consumers that choose to self-care.

Globalization

For the purposes of this text, *globalization* refers to viewing the world as a single community for propagating the promotion of health and well-being through evolving virtual network and the sharing of e-health information and services. Owing to the many interacting components and agents within such a complex community as suggested by our understanding of "chaos theory," supersymmetrical thinking makes the transition to "globalization" possible because all of these agents can be "transformed" to behave like a common giant e-health knowledge and information dispensing and exchange system. The aim is to bridge social and cultural gaps by making health services affordable and conveniently available to anyone anytime, anyplace. Here, we are therefore using the word *globalization* differently from those in the antiglobalization movement, who are concerned about the exploitation of cheap labor forces and the export of jobs as well as the growth of multinational corporations.

Globalization of e-health care will require effective use of individual, group, community, organizational, and societal resources. With the implementation of global call centers and Internet-enabled transactional services, e-health purchasers and providers can significantly streamline many administrative and financial processes, promoting global exchange of data for scheduling, shipping, billing, ordering, and purchasing health care products and services.

Globalization of e-health services also has the potential to provide high-quality services to many underserved urban, rural, and remote areas. Another favorable outcome for e-consumers could be better morbidity and mortality rates, especially for e-consumers who choose e-home care and for those living in remote areas, including developing and underdeveloped countries. Another potential benefit not only for e-consumers but also for all participating e-stakeholders is learning from one another through shared responsibility, information exchange, and governance.

At the moment, only about 20 percent of the world's population receives 80 percent of the costly medical procedures and prescription drugs that advances in science and technology have made available. Globalization promises to close this gap and to extend these new discoveries to the underserved 80 percent. For e-consumers, global e-health networks can provide access to on-line consultations with qualified caregivers twenty-four hours a day, seven days a week; the potential for emergency assistance; and the portability of insurance coverage from one country to another. Other possibilities include e-prescription and e-claim services, instant messaging capabilities, real-time e-health information queries and retrievals, and on-line directory assistance.

Globalization also invokes the ideal of a universal e-health model rather than a competitive one. Currently, competition exists among major players, including venture capitalists, governmental bodies, nongovernmental organizations (NGOs) and multinational corporations. However, in order for the ideals of globalization to be realized, world leaders must be prepared to break down cultural gaps, conflicting views, and political differences among participating countries. Examples of health care initiatives that would be more effective should a global e-health infrastructure be put in place include the AIDS relief movements currently supported by the Gates Foundation, former U.S. president Bill Clinton, and former South African president Nelson Mandela.

Empowerment

Again, our supersymmetrical thinking of transforming the complex global community into one giant pool of an e-health knowledge and information dispensing system will lead to e-health consumer empowerment. *Empowerment* refers to providing on-line users of e-health systems, including e-consumers and other major e-stakeholders, with self-directed education, allowing them to participate actively in the decisions that affect them and their health. For example, an e-health service can permit prospective members to subscribe to information services; to check the scope of their insurance coverage; to change providers, choose options for coverage, and make premium payments; and to check out new products and services. Similarly, e-providers and e-caregivers can also be empowered via the use of e-health networks to exchange key patient data, to teleconsult, and to interact more frequently with clients, thus improving the quality of patient care.

Another aspect of empowerment is the ability of e-consumers to learn on their own or from one another, accessing current and relevant e-health information resources about treatments and medical procedures available for particular illnesses. Best practices can be easily shared. The increased ability of e-consumers to search, retrieve, store, learn about, and transmit specific health information regarding a certain disease group both for themselves and for others will make an appreciable difference in the management and control of these illnesses. Problems related to management of chronic ailments, such as diabetes and lower back pain, are especially amenable to this approach.

E-consumers can also benefit from being informed of breakthroughs in dealing with public health problems as well as potential symptoms arising from unknown exposures to hazardous bacteria, other dangerous biological agents, or threats due to bioterrorism (for example, anthrax). Medical problems that are on the minds of a growing number of both Americans and Canadians include AIDS/HIV, SARS, West Nile virus, mad cow disease, and avian flu. Many people turn to the Internet and other media for authoritative information about these life-threatening diseases. Knowing as much as possible about the vectors, symptoms, and treatment of these potentially threatening ailments is the best medicine; knowledge is power, and access to information may eventually offer some protection or, when no protection is available, at least the comfort of understanding the scope of the problem.

Integration

Finally, the supersymmetrical transformation will eventually lead to the creation of an integral e-health knowledge and dispensing system and an integration of intelligent agents among humans and machines. *Integration* is an ideal state, a longer-term goal to strive for as we make the e-health paradigm shift. Integration brings together various subcomponents of e-health care (stakeholders; hardware, software, and interface technology; and processes, tasks, and work designs) to create a practical solution that meets the needs of e-consumers. Integration needs to be achieved from several perspectives, including integration between or among e-stakeholders; integration of e-technologies; and integration of e-health processes and services.

Integration between and among e-stakeholders implies the clarification of their shared vision, mission, values, and goals. Without shared vision, mission, values, and goals, no e-health system or network will be profitable or even sustainable; strategies will be inadequately planned and poorly executed. Regardless of the amount of investment that has been sunk into e-health initiatives, the clarity of vision and goals must be the overriding concern. Achieving integration at the stakeholder level, though not an easy task, is nonetheless a necessary first step. Turf claims among competitors with conflicting visions and goals must be broken down. Turning those competitors into partners requires building trust among major e-stakeholders and nurturing their readiness to act as a unified entity. Integration among stakeholders represents a fusion of the vision, mission, values, and goals (reflecting the neural network metaphor and supersymmetrical thinking).

Integration of e-technologies is the ability to harness different e-technological developments, including network infrastructure, relevant hardware and software, and Web interface design, into a single, flexible, and integrated platform for the delivery of a seamless continuum of care. The Web development language chosen must be both flexible and functional in different computing systems, Web browsers, and search engines. As indicated in earlier chapters, the use of XML to support interactive functions and secured transactions on the Internet is one approach to a common and convenient interface. Other technologies that might be harnessed and integrated include an information grid to organize the piecemeal information captured throughout the Internet, with a language translator facility to extract information captured in different languages, and effective document management systems to ensure fast and effective delivery of information to e-consumers.

The integration of processes and services implies the ability to streamline, combine, and create new administrative, clinical, and financial processes from sometimes disjointed and poorly conceived procedures of legacy systems and to interconnect these functions within the e-health network. Integration also implies the use of advancing multimedia interface technologies so that health professionals can have access to integrated patient records and images, coordinate the scheduling and billing of on-line patient visits, monitor patient conditions intelligently on a remote basis, and provide e-consumers with integrated advising services.

Employing supersymmetrical thinking of ubiquitous exchange of e-health knowledge and information among e-stakeholders, then, our goal is that we should no longer be able to differentiate between e-consumer needs and e-stakeholder policies and procedures; between what customers expect and how providers offer what is expected;

and between integrated information flow and user satisfaction with transactional processing. Customer and provider requirements should be simply translated into integrated information flow, a flow that essentially reflects e-health products and services as they are demanded in the e-marketplace. Thus, integration of e-stakeholders, integration of e-technologies, and integration of processes and services ultimately lead to integrated information flow that satisfies joint e-stakeholder requirements. Thus, integration is a crucial component of e-health care leadership and management and essential to the success of the e-health care system model, which represents a transformation of the fragmentary and piecemeal approach inherent in traditionally managed organizations. This brings me to the next topic, sociocultural entities—a move from a hard science to a social science perspective.

Sociocultural Entities

A final framework for our thinking about currently evolving e-health groups and communities (e-communities) is the perspective of virtual global teams and learning communities. Understanding the characteristics of sociocultural entities will enable us to generate meaningful e-health solutions, notably in the context of interrelationships among users of e-groups and e-communities.

E-Communities as Sociocultural Entities

With e-businesses and multinational corporations actively competing on a global scale in today's e-marketplace, global virtual teams are being formed at an unprecedented pace. These teams typically include experts from various countries who meet via e-technologies for the purpose of designing innovative approaches to corporate challenges. Members of these groups may have very few opportunities to meet one another face to face. Cultural differences among them are a key barrier that must be broken down if they are to work together successfully. Moreover, some form of socialization must take place among members of these groups if they are to become productive work partners. Time is needed for group members to get to know one another. Virtual group leaders (leadership may be rotated among the members) must learn how to create reliable working relationships among members of the group. For example, leaders must design tasks and set conditions that are conducive to collaborative learning both before and after the formation of the group.

E-learning cannot be overemphasized on virtual teams. For team members to work collaboratively and learn within a virtual context, their working conditions must be conducive to nurturing critiques, comments, and feedback on one another's work, with guided directives and summaries of discussions from the leaders. When individuals who are not familiar with one another's work habits are placed in a vacuum, they will assume that everyone else has the same sociocultural, economic, and political background, when the opposite is true. Conflicts will abound as perspectives are shared. When virtual teams include people from different sociocultural backgrounds, the context for working together is invariably complex. Over time, as team members exchange views and freely engage in discussions until they feel comfortable with one another's beliefs, cultural viewpoints, and social status, some differences will disappear. In other words, a virtual community will have members from many distinct cultures. Initially, when a person does not know another person's culture, it will not be easy for the two of them to communicate. Nonetheless, the virtual group is able to communicate because all the participants have agreed to use the same language—for example, English—and they are focusing their energy on a common task. When this works, the virtual group will evolve a *sociocultural entity* of its own that will have a group-defined identity.

Community health information networks (CHINs) that have evolved in recent years parallel the concept of global virtual teams (or e-communities). CHINs are virtual teams that are community-based and involve participants and e-stakeholders within a well-defined geographical region. A CHIN therefore represents a community-based electronic organization: essentially, a regional ring to transmit clinical, financial, and insurance data among not only e-providers and e-payers but also e-claimers (consumers), e-business coalitions, and other e-stakeholders, in order to conduct business transactions or simply to share information. The complexity of the CHIN shadows precisely the complexity of the global virtual teams.

According to Julia Gluesing and Cristina Gibson (2003), the complexity that the global virtual team (or virtual community) faces in meeting its objective can be characterized along several dimensions: task, context, people, time, and technology. We have already noted that *time* is important in allowing team members to get to know each other and *technology* is the means by which virtual teams choose to meet and work collaboratively. Hence, the focus of the following discussion will be on task complexity, people, and context.

Task complexity comprises four elements: workflow interdependence, task environment, external coupling, and internal coupling. *Workflow interdependence* relates to how much the team members are independent of or dependent on one another in completing a certain task. *Task environment* can vary from static to dynamic; a static environment is easily predictable and stable, whereas a dynamic environment is shifting and uncertain. *External coupling* refers to how tightly a team is linked to or affected by what goes on in its task environment—that is, tight versus loose coupling. *Internal coupling* describes how crucial the relationships among team members are to the task at hand and can be described as weak or strong. Team members who are weakly coupled do not have to be integrated with one another in order to accomplish their tasks.

Virtual teams are composed of *people*. The extent to which people are motivated to participate in the team varies depending on their workload, the degree of organizational support they receive, the level of endorsement from other team members, their own personal interest in the assigned task, and the acceptance of their work from those with whom they are linked within their organization. In global virtual teams, members are often required to perform numerous tasks and take different roles. These multiple demands can create conflicting roles, ambiguous decision making or policy-making, and unclear responsibility.

Single Versus Multiple Contexts

In addition to task characteristics, contextual differences also determine the complexity of global teams. *Context* is defined as "the way of life and work within a specific geographic setting characterized by its own set of business conditions, cultural assumptions, and unique history." Essentially, work complexity is determined by the extent to which differences are represented on the team and the number of different contexts team members must negotiate in order to accomplish their tasks. Hence, when team members work in a common context, a single national culture frames their work and they share the same physical conditions, work environment, and sociopolitical framework.

In contrast, virtual global teamwork often must evolve across *multiple sociocultural contexts*. For this reason, virtual team members must be sensitive to how things appear in varying sociocultural contexts and thus must integrate differing sociocultural perspectives. If high-quality work is to be achieved within this multiplicity of sociocultural contexts, the team must address the following questions:

- Despite differences in opinions and sociocultural background, how can team members work together to make intelligent decisions?
- Which team members should be assigned to and be responsible for what part of the task, and why?
- How can information be integrated from all sources to help team members accomplish the task at hand?
- What would it take for individual team members to be able to see eye to eye with one another? If that is not possible, how can the concerns of team members be resolved?
- What and how can team members learn from one another, and what is the significance of this learning in the context of the task to be completed?
- How can learning from one another lead to a better understanding of the shared sociocultural contexts that will help in designing further tasks for virtual team members?

The world, and more specifically its e-health system, is often understood in terms of subsystem components that, when reconstituted and re-interpreted, give an illusory or mistaken view of the whole. Proliferation of virtual global teams that cut across sociocultural contexts has the potential to reduce or even eliminate this fragmentation.

What is important then, is not the differences in opinions among the virtual team members (which represent a fragmented view) but the emergent, acceptable view, the solution that integrates the differing views and perspectives.

Increasingly, we ignore contexts by unwittingly focusing too heavily on gathering data (creating fragmented views) to support individual and isolated arguments. In fact, some virtual team members will be preoccupied with large amounts of data (but perhaps too little information). Such preoccupation with supporting our own biases locks us into stereotyped learning. When we focus on a fragmented view in relation to a single context, we become blind to information shared by other team members who move in other contexts. Consequently, we lose an essential understanding of the whole system or even its parts. Invariably, much team conflict is due to some team members wanting to select and observe information from within a single sociocultural context. To be useful, emergent solutions must be relevant to the understanding of the whole.

Conclusion

Concepts of systems theory, systems thinking, and integration, combined with advances in mathematics and physics such as chaos theory, quantum physics, and string theories, as well as social sciences thinking, all provide us with useful frameworks for deciphering the meanings of e-health. Application of these principles can provide direction and guidance to students, practitioners, and proponents of e-health. The process of system evolution and creation is continual and is built on the ideas of globalization, empowerment of e-stakeholders, and integration of e-stakeholders, e-technologies, and e-processes.

Lindstrom, Matheson, and Tan (1998) argue that few of the health administrative skills we have valued in the past—for example, planning and controlling—will remain important. According to them, controllers, planners, and leaders have overplanned the world into forms that were thought to be wanted and required but that have not succeeded very well. What is needed is more participation and less planning in order to allow an emergent new world to appear.

Thus, transformational health care leadership begins with a transformation of one's thinking. An example of this possibility is an attempt to resolve the problems of AIDS and malnutrition on the African continent via some form of e-technology (see Chapter Eight). Lindstrom, Matheson, and Tan (1998) note that health care leaders and managers, including chief executive officers, chief operating officers, and chief information officers, are facing new challenges during these turbulent times. Indeed, for brick-and-mortar health care organizations to move successfully into the e-health care realm calls for a profound shift in the way health executives and administrators think and do business. Similarly, health care educators need to rethink the way they have been teaching health care concepts, strategies, and planning. I have argued that health care is shifting between two paradigms: from a huge, difficult-to-manage, and traditionally fragmented system to a more unified, holistic, and integrative system based on collaborative partnerships, virtual interactions, and active contributions to a common vision, mission, values, and goals.

In addition to the usual external environmental opportunities and threats (including sociopolitical, economic, cultural, technological, and demographic factors), three major trends will determine the growth and future development of e-health networks: globalization, empowerment, and integration. While this argument has been inferred from time to time throughout the chapter, it is at this point that we consider these issues more thoroughly.

In light of this observation, e-health leaders today should behave more like coaches, facilitators, and team leaders in a virtual global team context. They should break away from stereotyped thinking and learn to transcend disciplinary boundaries in clarifying and focusing the vision and values of the e-health system. They must be prepared to adopt supersymmetrical thinking in order to face more complexity, uncertainty, and ambiguity.

Finally, the dynamic functioning of e-health networks must be understood beyond the use of metaphors and mental models. Key to successful design and implementation of e-health systems will be recognition of the limitations of fragmentary thinking in a single sociocultural context and a correspondingly greater emphasis on the multiplicity of contexts and cultures within which emergent solutions can be achieved. Shifting from thinking and problem solving within a single sociocultural context to a network-based sharing of thoughts within multiple sociocultural contexts will be an ongoing challenge.

Chapter Questions

1. Explain why changes in mainstream health care have prompted new ways of thinking about planning and redefinition of business processes in the evolving e-health care system.
2. How does supersymmetrical thinking combine various aspects of e-health? What is the significance of supersymmetrical thinking in redefining the roles and responsibilities of e-consumers as opposed to other e-stakeholders?
3. Use the rich picture approach to portray an instance of a multiagency e-health system. What are the implications of globalization, empowerment, and integration for e-health systems?

4. How does the neural network metaphor apply to evolving sociocultural entities in an e-health system? Can it be applied to an e-community? What is the significance of viewing e-communities as evolving sociocultural entities?

5. Illustrate how an e-health system like the MMP project (see the case at the end of the chapter) can be conceived as an organic and self-learning system.

References

Beckham, J. (1993). The architecture of integration. *Healthcare Forum Journal 36*(5), 59.

Bohm, D. (1980). *Wholeness and the implicate order.* London: Routledge.

Capra, F. (1996). The web of life: A new scientific understanding of living systems. New York: Bantam Doubleday Dell.

Gluesing, J., & Gibson, C. (2003). Designing and forming global teams. In H. Lane, M. Maznevski, M. Mendenhall, & J. McNett (Eds.), *Handbook of global management: A guide to managing complexity*, forthcoming, Malden, MA: Blackwell.

Hammad, T. (1998). Computational intelligence: Neural networks methodology for health decision support. In J. Tan & S. Sheps, *Health decision support systems* (pp.). Sudbury, MA: Jones & Bartlett.

Lindstrom, R., Matheson D., & Tan, J. (1998). Organizational health decision support systems: The application of systems concepts, chaos theory, quantum mechanics, and self-organizing systems. In J. Tan & S. Sheps, *Health decision support systems* (pp.). Sudbury, MA: Jones & Bartlett.

Morgan, G. (1997). *Images of organization.* Thousand Oaks, CA: Sage.

Senge, P. (1990). *The fifth discipline: The art and practice of the learning organization.* New York: Doubleday.

Tan, J. (2001). *Health management information systems: Methods and practical applications* (2nd ed.). Sudbury, MA: Jones & Bartlett.

Wheatley, M., & Kellner-Rogers, M. (1995). "Self-organizing systems conference." Sundance, Utah.

Multicommunity E-Health Promotion Programming Case

Joseph Tan

In Detroit, the Maria-Madeline Project, Inc. (MMP) provides e-technology training for seniors: young adults teach seniors how to use computers in nursing homes, assisted living facilities, retirement communities, senior apartment complexes, and community

I acknowledge the contributions of my colleagues from the School of Nursing at Wayne State University, especially Mary Nies, Rosalind Peters, and Linda Weglicki for their input and feedback on the Green-Kreuter diagram discussed in this case as well as Tim Butler and Alexandra DePetro for their contributions to generating a survey instrument for use in this project.

centers. The goal of the MMP is to provide developmentally appropriate informational e-health interventions for urban, at-risk populations. To that end, the program staff plans to develop, implement, and evaluate interactive, Web-based informational and expert consultation sites.

The MMP can be viewed as a complex system composed of many interacting agents (for example, seniors, school children, stakeholders who fund the project, e-health care providers and on-line professional consultants, evaluators such as university professors, and others) with diverging perspectives and decisions. The resulting behavior of this complex system is difficult to predict; yet the social and cultural exchanges amongst these various parties follow predetermined or predictable patterns depending on the relationships and partnerships that are built over time. Where string theory and supersymmetrical thinking apply is the partnership among the seniors and school children in the use of advancing telecommunication and network technologies to allow these seniors to absorb the free-flowing e-health information and knowledge provided through the on-line consultations with the experts to the point that they become confident of their own use of this dispensed knowledge.

Background

The United States in general and cities such as Detroit in particular face a formidable challenge in delivering and promoting health services efficiently and equitably in the face of competing resource demands from sources that include bioterrorism and homeland security, natural calamities, environmental concerns and global warming effects, K–12 education and higher learning, and, on the federal level, international relations and foreign affairs. During this era of shrinking resources paired with information and knowledge explosion, several major federal and national initiatives indicate that government agencies, health care providers, and consumers expect information technology, particularly e-technology and Web-based services, to contribute to meeting this challenge. People are looking to information technology to facilitate increased clinical expert consultations, rapid health information access, equity in health care delivery, and increased comprehensiveness and accountability of health care services through security and policy regulations. One theme permeating many recent conferences sponsored by major health care agencies has been the development of an e-health technology infrastructure.

With continued and increasing use of on-line health services, the question arises as to whether the on-line environment will provide effective health care services to urban at-risk populations. One mental model of e-health programming suggests that the Internet can be a convenient environment for senior patients who wish to obtain health information. The MMP asks important questions of both students and seniors to yield insights into the truth of this model.

The Maria-Madeline Project, Inc. (www.mariamadeline.com) began in 1999 to serve nine facilities of the Archdiocese of Detroit. There are now a total of thirteen centers in metropolitan Detroit, plus a growing number of facilities in Texas and New York.

In addition, the MMP recently secured funding to work jointly with the Society of St. Vincent de Paul to further expand services. The MMP integrates technology into the lives of elementary and high school children and links them to senior citizens through a unique methodology called ExperienceSeniorPower®. Dell Computer Corporation is collaborating with the MMP, providing computers to all ExperienceSeniorPower locations at a significant discount. The MMP also works with Wayne State University School of Business researchers to better understand how seniors can be encouraged to change their health behaviors and lifestyles through the use of customized Web-based programming.

The Precede-Proceed Framework

We use the Green-Kreuter precede-proceed framework (Green and Kreuter, 1991) to guide our understanding in planning and evaluating this project. The overriding principle of this framework is that most enduring health behavior change is voluntary. This principle drives a systematic planning process that seeks to empower individuals with understanding, motivation, skills, and active engagement in community affairs. Thus, this model is applicable and practically helpful in the project planning, development, implementation, and evaluation stages of the MMP. These are nine phases of the precede-proceed model.

The first five phases of the precede-proceed model are diagnostic:

1. Social diagnosis of the self-determined needs, wants, resources, and barriers to fulfilling the needs and wants in the target community
2. Epidemiological diagnosis of the health problems
3. Behavioral and environmental diagnosis to determine specific behaviors and environmental factors for the program to address
4. Educational and organizational diagnosis of the predisposing, enabling, and reinforcing conditions that immediately affect behavior
5. Administrative and policy diagnosis of the resources needed and available in the organization, as well as the barriers and supports available in the organization and community

The left-to-right arrows indicate the impact that educational and environmental interventions can have on problem areas at each level. The process consists of systematic identification of health problems and their behavioral and environmental antecedents and the development of educational interventions aimed at those antecedents as well as at the problems themselves. The step-by-step process of the model, from the identification of social problems and their etiology to the implementation of appropriate community-based interventions, flows logically from the assessment findings and serves as a basis for community health promotion.

The four remaining phases relate to implementation and evaluation, with emphasis on using the latter to improve the former. Evaluation begins as soon as implementation does, in order to detect problems early so that they can be corrected. As implementation proceeds, the planner starts evaluating in the order in which program effects are expected. First, its immediate effects (impacts) are evaluated, in order to determine the extent to which the program needs modification. Finally, when enough time has passed, as specified in the objectives, the ultimate intended and actual effects on morbidity, mortality, and quality of life are assessed. This phased evaluation allows the project planners to see what works and what does not.

According to the precede-proceed model, Web-based informational programs to provide developmentally appropriate e-health-promoting interventions for urban, at-risk populations can only be effective if they also influence the precursors to behaviors (or the environments in which they occur), including (1) predisposing factors (factors that provide the motivation or reason behind a behavior—for example, knowledge, attitudes, cultural beliefs, and readiness to change); (2) enabling factors (factors that make it possible for a motivation to be realized—for example, available resources, supportive policies, assistance, and services); and (3) reinforcing factors (factors that come into play after a behavior has begun and that provide continuing rewards or incentives and contribute to repetition or persistence of behaviors—for example, social support, praise, reassurance, and symptom relief). Exhibit 3.1 shows our adaptation of the precede-proceed framework for the development of a state-of-the-art Web-based educational system for promoting changes in the healthy lifestyles of urban at-risk populations.

EXHIBIT 3.1. PRECEDE-PROCEED MODEL APPLIED TO E-HEALTH INTERVENTION

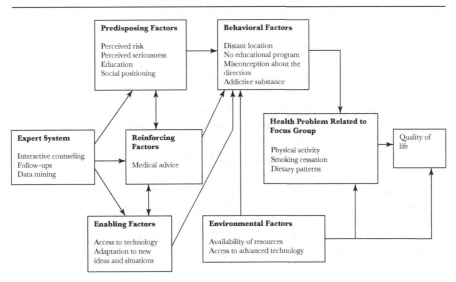

The precede-proceed framework is a comprehensive planning and evaluation system based on the needs of the people or community to be served. It starts with extensive research and analysis to assess those needs, then plans the steps that will meet them or eliminate them. It deals with the individuals to be served (in our case, the underserved seniors) and with others who have resources or influence on them, including intermediaries and partners such as community leaders, media decision makers, parents, peers, teachers, and health professionals.

Computers and Internet Use Among Seniors

Here, a key question is: "Does MMP promote better health because of access to computers?" To answer this question, we look at the literature regarding computer use and its impact on changing health behaviors. Bernard L. Bloom (1996) found that computer technology is playing an increasingly important role in personality and behavioral assessment, diagnostic interviewing and history taking, health education, mental health consultation, and clinical training. In these areas, the reliability, validity, and utility of computers compare favorably with those of clinicians. Evaluations of the computer use with psychiatric patients conclude that even those who are quite disturbed interact very successfully with computers, including many patients who are unable to interact with mental health personnel. Computer-assisted psychotherapy programs have been most successfully implemented in cognitive and behavioral psychotherapy. In the case of psychodynamic psychotherapy, computer programs appear to be limited by our failure to make fully explicit the rules governing therapist behavior and by the continuing inability of computers to comprehend natural language.

Once the initial cost and effort have been invested in their development, computerized teaching programs can be cost-efficient. Computer-mediated communications and computer-assisted instructional programs have been shown to "cost-effectively enhance patient outcomes, quality, satisfaction, [and] be used as part of large-scale prevention and educational efforts" (Budman, 2000). These tools can be easily accessible, time-efficient, and instructionally consistent, providing effective modes of instructional delivery (Peterson, 1996). Computer educational programs also help to increase users' attention to the material, perhaps because they are interactive in nature and people can remember better doing the interactions than just passively listening to a lecture. These programs allow users to progress at their own learning pace, maximizing the technology's potential as a self-help health education medium. Finally, they help users assume responsibility for their own learning (Paperny, 1997; Barber, 1990; Bixler and Askov, 1994).

Prochaska, DiClemente, Velicer, and Rossi (1993) used a computer program to individualize self-help materials for community-based adult smokers, although participants did not actually interact with a computer. A questionnaire was administered to determine subjects' readiness to change their smoking behavior, and then they were randomly assigned to one of four study groups. Compared with subjects in the group that received standardized manuals, subjects in the three other groups who were given various forms of summarized versus detailed computerized information and with or without repeated follow-up, regardless of their readiness to change, had significantly higher quit rates after six months and after twelve months. This indicates that detailed information and repeated follow-up was the most helpful in changing smoking behaviors. Schneider, Schwartz, and Fast (1995) developed a computerized, telephone-based, interactive smoking cessation program, using a toll-free call to activate the system. The system automatically composed messages to fit the needs, expectations, and progress of callers on a twenty-four-hour basis. Results indicate that 35.1 percent of users quit smoking while using the program and 14 percent were still not smoking six months after their first call. Of those who called five or more times, 68 percent reported quitting and 22 percent were abstinent six months after their first call.

McDaniel and others (2002) developed and conducted usability testing of an interactive computer program designed to promote smoking cessation in low-income women. Participants comprised one hundred women who received care at an inner-city community health center in Indianapolis. After baseline data were collected, the subjects completed the computer program in the clinic. Next, they completed a brief satisfaction instrument. Data indicated that satisfaction with the program was high (mean satisfaction score was 60.2 on a scale in which 70 indicated highest possible satisfaction). Average time required to complete the computer program was 13.6 minutes. In a follow-up survey, 79 percent of participants reported at least one behavioral change related to smoking. Results indicated that interactive computer technology might be useful for promoting smoking cessation in low-income women. Clearly, research is needed on the use of this mode of intervention not only for smoking cessation but also for other health-promoting activities.

MMP Evaluation Plan

The evaluation plan is the most important aspect of the MMP. The design of the project includes collection of data from participating seniors over a period of interactions. Data are collected both on their learning to use the Internet and on any self-directed attempts to extract resources from the MMP Web site. Although eating habits are an important aspect of the MMP, other e-health promotion activities and intervention developments are also being considered. In fact, the Web site currently allows seniors to ask questions of a nurse, a dietitian, and a dentist. The idea is to promote as many health-promoting behaviors as possible, including physical movement (such as walking), smoking cessation, and dental care. A questionnaire also obtains data directly from participating seniors on their training, satisfaction, and other impacts of the technology. The development of a questionnaire designed to extract these self-reported data for the purpose of determining the appropriate programming mix involves understanding different areas affecting the training process, the frequency of use of the MMP system for e-health purposes as opposed to other purposes, and how to define levels of satisfaction with the technology involved—that is, the Internet and Web browsers.

The data gleaned from this project are expected to be complex due to the varying e-health promotion activities involved (physical exercise, smoking cessation, dietary patterns, dental health, and so on). Efficient analysis, modeling, and evaluation of such a multidimensional data set in order to obtain useful, yet often subtle knowledge is a challenging task. Making health trend predictions is appealing but also challenging. Those involved in the project expect that analysis and assessment of the information will yield results that are particularly useful for promoting the health of urban, at-risk populations. We hope to find important yet somewhat latent factors associated with health risks and to evaluate lifestyles in order to accurately identify future health risks for individuals or groups. Based on such findings, we can alert these individuals (or groups) about unhealthy factors in their daily routines so that they will be better able to avoid risks.

Conclusion

The at-risk populations in the Detroit metropolitan area are multiethnic, multiracial, and multicultural. Each section of the city has different percentages of African Americans and whites represented in their respective populations. Arab Americans, Hispanic Americans, Asian Americans, and Native Americans make up a small percentage of the population in the metropolitan Detroit area.

The MMP project serves seniors from a variety of ethnic groups, all of low to middle socioeconomic status. This project may be conceived as the creation of a complex network that nurtures e-health promotional learning; the generation of a new sociocultural entity involving the interactions of students, seniors, and other key stakeholders; and the formation of an experimental learning community. Different e-stakeholders, including community leaders, grant agencies, government agencies, supporting religious organizations, children from the schools, and researchers from the university participate in this network. Central to this network are the participating seniors and students.

Key questions to be answered about the implementation and evaluation of the MMP include the following:

- What are the effective content themes for implementing an appropriate e-health promotion program such as the MMP?
- How effective is the use of an e-health promotional network for urban at-risk populations, specifically those served by the MMP, in terms of changes in healthy lifestyle awareness, attitudes, knowledge, and beliefs?
- What challenges are faced in diffusing the MMP, especially to seniors that live outside Detroit?
- How does MMP contribute to the globalization, integration and empowerment concepts discussed in the chapter?

While we expect results of the MMP evaluation to provide evidence that supports the use of the Internet and intergenerational programming in e-health initiatives, we may find that the seniors have not been empowered and have not benefited, perhaps due to inadequate planning, design, development, or even testing of the network. Moreover, the participants may not find e-learning an acceptable method of instruction. Conversely, we may find that the MMP brings about a positive relationship and a transformational perception among seniors and student groups. Also, other seniors may be brought into the learning community, so that learning among seniors comes not only from intergenerational programming but also from electronic connections with other seniors outside of Detroit. Awareness, attitudes, knowledge, and beliefs about e-health promotion activities may change due to new opportunities for the participants or the evolution of a strong learning community. In addition, the information resources accessible through the Web may empower seniors and further transform their lifestyles and daily routines. At this point, all of these outcomes are purely speculative. Hence, the emerging impacts of ongoing interactions between students and seniors, as well as among the seniors themselves, are worth examining. Moreover, the learning that emerges within the virtual senior group may be characterized by the sociocultural sharing of views. In the larger context of the e-health care system, we may expect this learning to be guided by the vision and values of the e-health network—that is, the vision as provided by the MMP.

Finally, the vision for the MMP project continues to evolve, expanding to include senior groups interacting with student groups across the nation. Current discussion includes ideas for generating an artificial intelligence–based programming prototype that would support e-health programming over the life span of the seniors being served. The activities to be facilitated can include physical exercise, management of common diseases such as diabetes, and pain management. If and when this happens, it will be interesting to mine the data on the use of new and powerful e-technologies to understand how an underserved population can truly be empowered to alter the quality of members' lives.

Case Questions

1. What aspects and features of the MMP qualify it as part of the e-health care system?
2. Why would the MMP appeal to seniors? What types of e-health services are most likely to appeal to seniors?
3. How would you go about determining the content for the e-health promotion programming in the MMP project?
4. Do you agree that students should be used to teach seniors how to use the Internet? Why or why not?
5. Think about the future growth and development of the MMP. What are the most significant next steps, challenges, and critical success factors in expanding the MMP within Detroit and Michigan? How does the MMP community mirror the social cultural entities as detailed in the chapter?

References

Barber, J. (1990). Computer-assisted drug prevention. *Journal of Substance Abuse Treatment, 7,* 125–131.

Bixler, B., & Askov, E. (1994). Characteristics of effective instructional technology. *Mosaic: Research Notes on Literacy, 4*(1), 7.

Bloom, B. L., & Berki, S. E. (eds.). (1996). *Cost benefit, cost effectiveness, and other decision-making techniques in health care resource allocation* (p. 87). New York: Biomedical Information.

Budman, S. (2000, November). Behavioral health care dot-com and beyond: Computer-mediated communications in mental health and substance abuse treatment. *American Pyschologist,* pp. 1290–1300.

Green, L. W., & Kreuter, M. W. (1991). *Health promotion planning: An educational and environmental approach* (2d ed.). Mountain View, CA: Mayfield Publishing.

McDaniel, A., Hutchison, S., Casper, G., Ford, R., Stratton, R., & Rembush, M. (2002). Usability testing and outcomes of an interactive computer program to promote smoking cessation in low income women. In *Proceedings of the AMIA Symposium* (pp. 509–513). American Medical Informatics Association, Washington, DC.

Paperny, D. (1997). Computerized health assessment and education for adolescent HIV and STD prevention in health care settings and schools. *Health Education and Behavior, 24*(1), 54–70.

Peterson, M. (1996). What are blood counts? A computer-assisted program for pediatric patients. *Pediatric Nursing, 22,* 21–27.

Prochaska, J., DiClemente, C., Velicer, W., & Rossi, J. (1993). Standardized, individualized, interactive, and personalized self-help programs for smoking cessation. *Health Psychology, 12*(5), 399–405.

Schneider, S., Schwartz, M., & Fast, J. (1995). Computerized, telephone-based health promotion: I. Smoking cessation program. *Computers in Human Behavior, 11*(1), 135–148.

CHAPTER FOUR

E-HEALTH RECORDS

The Lifeblood of E-Health Care

Joseph Tan

Learning Objectives

1. Understand the definition of e-health records (EHRs) in the context of e-health care system and environment

2. Review factors contributing to adoption of EHRs
3. Understand the purposes of EHRs
4. Identify the benefits and hurdles in implementing EHRs
5. Recognize privacy issues underlying the use of EHRs
6. Understand likely future issues in EHRs

Introduction

The health care industry is very data-intensive. This characteristic of the health care business will not change even if we move successfully from the era of traditional health care to the e-health care era. Among the key pieces of information in the health care system is the patient record. The patient record is central to the work of virtually everyone associated with planning, organizing, providing, directing, receiving, and reimbursing mainstream health care services.

E-health care services will only exacerbate the intricacy of managing the flow of consumer information and patient records. E-health activities demand even more speed from transactions between e-consumers and e-providers; are likely to generate large numbers of on-line information requests and query-related activities; and lead to a huge number of products and services that will be e-marketed, with a resulting quantity and variety of on-line clinical and administrative information that goes beyond just financial transaction figures. E-patient data gathering and e-consumer information retrieval and distribution activities will most likely define a large part of the functioning of an e-health system. Convenient interfaces and the potential for global connectivity will only add to the complexity of the e-health system and its need to store and manipulate consumer information and provide it to e-stakeholders in a timely and relevant manner that includes the management of e-patient records from a single, integrated source.

A key feature of e-health, which makes it more available, accessible, affordable, and accountable than traditional health care, is the shift in focus from the delivery of physical medicine (plagued by conflicting, fragmentary, and confusing patient data) to the delivery of timely, relevant, and integrated e-health information, specifically information that empowers e-consumers to make informed choices about their own health and well-being; information that assists e-providers in integrating business processes and administrative and clinical procedures in order to ease the delivery of health products and medical services on a real-time basis; information that can break down stereotyped thinking and long-standing barriers among and between various e-stakeholders; and information that cuts across economic, geographical, cultural, and sociopolitical differences among members of virtual communities to facilitate necessary therapies and treatments, especially for the underserved.

In this chapter, we examine more thoroughly the nature and characteristics of e-health information, particularly e-health records (EHRs). Despite more than half a century of exploratory work, millions of dollars in research, and the implementation of computerized patient records systems, efforts to automate the collection, storage, and management of the data in health records have not been very successful (Tan, 2001). This lack of success has limited opportunities for effective decision making from the bedside all the way to the formulation of national health care policy and the adoption of a global e-health strategy.

In an ideal EHRs system, identical electronic patient information will not be stored redundantly. Unfortunately, at the present time, the same patient information tends to exist in many different forms and in many different locations. For example, a physician may summarize a patient's complaints in a set of notes and enter them into the physician's handheld device. This information may then be downloaded into a larger electronic data collection and stored in a specific depository or database maintained by the health maintenance organization of which the physician is a member. The same data set could also be abstracted, reformatted, reorganized, and electronically recoded for placement in a data warehouse linked to a completely separate electronic health record system, then placed on another provider network that is accessible only to physicians who are members of that network and who are authorized to use this information when consulting with the patient. Indeed, if the accumulated data from all physician consultations is not rationally organized or appropriately merged with other data sets stored in separate databases to form a linked (integrated) EHRs system, imagine the consequences for future consultations with the patient. For example, when data on one patient can be found in several databases that are not centrally networked, it is possible for a physician to order a prescription that has an undesired interactive effect with another herb or drug that has already been prescribed.

In previous chapters, we have argued that the e-health care system will thrive only with support for its infrastructural and informational needs. EHRs (the central depository for patient information updates, further data analysis, and privacy controls) represent a major resource to fulfill these needs. Implementation of reliable EHRs will provide a convenient and easy way to access timely, relevant, and accurate information. As we shall see, transformation of the traditional health care system into e-health care relies on transformation of the management of health information and health information flow. E-patient records may thus be considered the lifeblood of e-health care.

In this chapter, we will first define EHRs based on perspectives from health authorities of three major developed countries: the United States, the United Kingdom, and Canada. Next, we will examine the trends influencing the movement toward EHRs technology and review the purposes of EHRs in the context of the evolving e-health system and environment. This is followed by an exploration of the benefits and hurdles in implementing EHRs. We then conclude with a look at the future of EHRs.

Definition of E-Health Records

Over the years, the concept of EHRs has become more transparent, although it has sometimes been confused or inappropriately interchanged with many other related terms such as *electronic patient records* (EPRs), *computer-based patient records* (CPRs), *automated or computerized clinical records, electronic incidental records,* and *electronic medical records.*

In 1997, the National Academy of Sciences' Institute of Medicine (IOM) conceptualized *computer-based patient records* and *electronic patient records* as a system specifically designed to support users by providing "accessibility to complete and accurate data, alerts, reminders, clinical decision support systems, links and guides to medical knowledge, and other aids" (Institute of Medicine, 1997). In other words, EPRs represent a data integration resource that functions as a supporting asset for health care providers. The U.S. Department of Veterans Affairs (1995), on the contrary, specifically defined *computer-based patient records* (CPRs) as records that are stored in "the Decentralized Hospital Computer Program" or any such electronically automated system—for example, an optical disk. Based on this observation, CPRs may be considered an institution-based system, whereas EPRs are an enterprisewide system.

In another attempt to clarify the emerging jungle of confusing terminologies, the United Kingdom's National Health Service (NHS) differentiated *electronic patient records* from *e-health records* according to the timeline and nature of the data recording for an individual's health care experience. According to the NHS, EPRs are institution-based, containing the periodic records of patient experience with a single provider organization, whereas EHRs are the records of longitudinal patient experiences from birth to death, including all encounters between a patient and a health care provider. Thus, EHRs would include data from the patient and family members; from community-based health centers; from public health agencies; from all of the patient's care providers, including physicians, nurses, and other health professionals and specialists; and from any other health-related organization or agency that may have collected data about the patient's health and health status.

More recently, in Canada, the Advisory Council on Health Infostructure (ACHI) and the Office of Health and the Information Highway (OHIH)—both part of Health Canada—provided further clarification on several terms (Advisory Council on Health Infostructure, 1999; Office of Health and the Information Highway, 2001). Through a series of public documents and Canadian governmental publications, the following terms were developed and defined in a successive fashion in order to better understand EHRs from a progressively inclusive perspective. *Incidental records* are records of selected data on a single patient for a specific incident or episode of care. If the data were gathered electronically, the records are referred to as *electronic incidental records.* In contrast, *patient records* are records of the accumulated incidents of a single patient, covering all encounters between a patient and a specific caregiver over time. If the data were gathered electronically, the records are called *electronic patient records*. Finally, *health records* are records of all encounters of all patients with all caregivers across all health provider institutions linked to the health records system, and if the data were gathered electronically, the records are called *electronic health records* (EHRs).

Interestingly, the ACHI-OHIH perspective echoes the IOM report in its contention that a number of core characteristics will help ensure EHRs' usability, functionality, and operability:

- List clearly a patient's clinical problems and associated current health status
- Support daily assessment of patient care outcomes through well-coordinated recordings of the patient's health status and functional level
- Provide a clinical rationale, documenting clinical decisions
- Link with local as well as remote databases and other patient or clinical records to provide a longitudinal care history
- Ensure patient confidentiality, privacy, and security of information collected, stored, manipulated, and disseminated
- Structure the stored data using a standardized or well-defined classification that supports direct data entry by health practitioners
- Guide the clinical problem-solving process through the use of decision support tools
- Assist in the management and evaluation of the quality and costs of care
- Permit timely access, selective retrieval and formatting, and flexibility for future expansion

For EHRs to fulfill these functions, Andrew and Dick (1995a, 1995b) note, five components are needed: a clinical data dictionary, a clinical data repository, flexible input capabilities, ergonomic data presentations, and automated decision support. A *clinical data dictionary* is a centralized repository of clinical information describing the content of the database, organized into files containing a range of clinical variables embedded and organized into predefined fields. A *clinical data repository* refers to the electronic database that holds the clinical data and the clinical data dictionary. *Flexible input capabilities* refers to the number of input devices and approaches that can be used to enter data. For example, data could be entered automatically via networked sources, directly by users, or indirectly through intermediaries such as third party agencies, including different clinicians and users. *Ergonomic data presentations* refers to user-friendly displays of output data, perhaps using multimedia or other graphical approaches. *Automated decision support* is the use of specialized decision-aiding software and tools to link necessary data and models in order to improve or expedite clinical, administrative, and managerial decisions.

Andrew and Dick (1995b) also argue that because it is more difficult to reach a consensus among care providers on issues relating to definition and policies, the development of the technical infrastructure of EHRs is not as challenging a problem as the ones resulting from sociocultural and political barriers. In any case, no existing system of EHRs contains all of the functions and characteristics identified by the IOM and ACHI-OHIH authoritative reports.

What is the significance of EHRs in e-health care? To address this question adequately, we must review the trends and purposes that drive the adoption and use of EHRs in the traditional health care era versus the coming e-health care era.

Trends in EHRs

Among the oldest surviving examples of medical data recording are papyri from ancient Egypt containing details of surgery and prescriptions. Those involved in the art and science of healing and treatment have always needed to pass on the details of successful procedures or medications either in writing or through an oral tradition. As medicine has evolved, this need has continued along two avenues: the need for structured data in order to derive conclusions (that is, use of objective measures and quantitative means) and the need for narrative data (that is, application of more interpretive and qualitative approaches). In *Doctors' Stories*, Kathryn Montgomery Hunter (1993) notes the need to value and listen to the patient's side of the story. She suggests that when physicians have a working knowledge of life histories and a sense of medical narrative that can accommodate the experience of illness, they are better able to provide good medical care, especially for those they cannot quickly cure. On the other hand, a structured approach such as the creation and use of EHRs can ensure that all the necessary information to arrive at sound medical decisions is at hand. Many factors influence the movement toward EHRs, including changes in the health care delivery system, sociocultural and political forces, and technological developments.

Increasing numbers of health care consumers are expressing a desire to play a more active role in the maintenance of their health. EHRs can potentially provide every individual with access to a comprehensive personal health profile. The shift toward providing more convenient, affordable, and comprehensive health services online has partly increased reliance on a wider range of health care professionals (for example, nurse practitioners, physiotherapists, and other alternative medical professionals) and locations (for example, hospitals and other acute care settings, outpatient clinics, ambulatory care settings, group residences, and other community-based care settings). EHRs provide a means of sharing information across this increasing range of practitioners and settings, thereby supporting the highest quality of care possible. In addition, increasing emphasis on public accountability and ethical practices will likely require EHRs to provide information in nonidentifiable or aggregate form for researchers, governments, administrators, investigators, and policymakers.

We have seen that the vision of the e-health care system of developed as well as developing countries is to provide borderless, seamless, accessible, and accurate health care that is free from red tape, redundancy, and duplication. Arguably, the union of technology and health will provide a transformational avenue to improve the quality, efficiency, accessibility, and effectiveness of health care delivery. As indicated at the beginning of this discussion, one means of accomplishing this is through universally accessible, lifelong EHRs that allow data to be shared among different health care providers in a safe, secure, and integrated fashion.

Put simply, EHRs should replace all other fragmentary data repositories found throughout our traditional health care system, in order to eliminate redundancies, anomalies, and errors in record updates. Another approach is the use of *virtual medical patient records,* in which data from all the different sources are merely linked electronically as and when needed. This would allow integration of patient information from all sources, including data from many ancillary health information systems used for enhancing patient care. In countries such as Canada and the United Kingdom, such an approach has already been accepted as a priority, as evidenced by the number of EHRs initiatives under way.

The lack of consensus on universal health care in the United States slows down progress toward EHRs. However, intensive efforts on the part of government research agencies such as the National Science Foundation, the National Institute of Health, and the Centers for Disease Control and Prevention; corporate and private funding agencies such as the Robert Wood Johnson Foundation and the Blue Cross Blue Shield Foundation; and many others—for example, the Institute of Medicine—have moved e-health care toward the development of standards, integrated network infrastructures, and linked databases to address some of the challenges with respect to implementing more accessible, affordable, and accountable health care. We can therefore expect that in the not-too-distant future, integrated EHRs or a hybrid form of EHRs with linked virtual patient record technology will become a reality.

Purposes of EHRs

EHRs technology serves many purposes. These include, for example, using EHRs as the basis to build a lifelong historical and legal account; to support medical education, clinical research, documentation, and communications; to enhance the efficiency and effectiveness of health professionals; to facilitate e-health work design and development; to describe and document preventive measures; to identify deviations from expected trends; and to anticipate future health problems and actions. In this section, we will focus on some of the more important uses of EHRs.

EHRs can serve to maintain an ongoing account of the e-clinical care provided by e-physicians. While the main part of their clinical use and value will be realized at the time of individual e-consultations (as part of building an ongoing patient-doctor relationship), EHRs will also aid e-clinicians to provide high-quality care over time, because they will contain prompts, reminders, and recognitions of uncertainties and dilemmas, as well as monitor objective measures such as height, weight, blood pressure, and sugar level. The retrospective data gathered in EHRs can also be transformed into review of past protocols to formulate future cases. Increasingly, e-clinicians need to study the factors influencing their clinical and management decisions and outcomes, to justify the use of e-technologies and e-health modalities. Because e-clinicians are seen as accountable both to e-patients and to the wider medical profession, the use of EHRs not only implies medicolegal responsibility but also the ethics of good e-clinical practice. Medical residents and students wanting to learn or teachers needing to assess student competence can make good use of EHRs in tele-education. The tools used for retrospective data collection in EHRs can be further enhanced, allowing the data to be used in e-clinical research.

Moreover, e-clinical care involves sharing responsibility among e-health care practitioners. Inevitably, parts of the EHRs must be shared. To do this effectively, EHRs must provide relevant views of patient data; in this way, overall quality of patient care is increased. The mobility of EHRs underscores the ways in which e-health can be portable and flexible; EHRs will move with e-patients to promote efficient, effective, and continuing care. On-line documentation of previous encounters will be easily available for e-consultations and reviews. Mainstream CPRs are often limited in availability because they are largely institution-based. Fortunately, EHRs can transcend CPRs, providing coordination among e-caregivers who practice in various locations at diverse brick-and-mortar institutions. The use of EHRs and e-medicine does not rule out the possibility of sending a patient to a physical facility for intensive care or treatment. With EHRs, however, a variety of e-caregivers, working within different professional contexts, can deal with a range of needs of the same patient (or different ones) at different times and places. Imagine, for instance, how a family in great distress feels when a family member is being cared for by over thirty social, medical, and other agencies, none of which have any formal means of communication with one another. This extreme example demonstrates not only the need for an integrated, well-ordered, and appropriately designed EHRs system but also the need to transform traditional health care services and delivery: the e-health paradigm shift.

In addition, many repetitive processes can be automated through the use of EHRs, including e-scheduling, e-prescription orders, e-billing, and e-claims, as well as automated analysis and reporting. Automating these processes will not only improve the efficiency of many related e-patient care processes and systems but also lead to more time for e-clinical services.

The ability to structure and view information and to locate and record such information at various levels of detail will mean that information can be retained in the record without overwhelming the e-clinician. For example, a blood test result that was scanned and evaluated as "normal" during a consultation may later need to be viewed in greater detail. The convenient interfaces supporting a common clinician or pharmacist patient data view in EHRs will lead to further reductions in medical procedural errors and medication errors. E-patients will also be able to view the data gathered in their EHRs and have some control over the release of any part of their records to specific clinicians.

Furthermore, effective EHRs could access individual values for the purpose of generating trends through a graphic display. Many serial measurements are made in all fields of medicine. Trends in serial measurements (for example, hourly blood gases, blood pressures, and hemoglobin levels) are difficult to ascertain without graphical representations. The ability to display serial measurements and relate them to normal or expected levels in a diagrammatic display is yet another advantage of EHRs. EHRs can also provide information to help e-managers allocate resources effectively, communicate with e-clinicians throughout the network system, share best practices and evidence-based medicine approaches, and minimize waste in the e-care system.

Moreover, it is anticipated that there is an increasing need to demonstrate e-clinical competence by drawing attention to preventive measures, possibly recording these items in a separate part of the EHRs system. Screening procedures are often performed because of an e-clinician's order rather than at the request of the e-patient. Prompting mechanisms from within the EHRs structure can greatly enhance the likelihood of these procedures being appropriately scheduled. The paper trail often used in mainstream health care systems has not been very successful, so EHRs can have a competitive advantage. As we have indicated, EHRs have the potential to reduce the risks of adverse medication interactions by capturing information on all current prescriptions and therapies, including data from complementary and alternative medical practitioners. EHRs will also aid in storing and retrieving data relating to future health care needs. Although local systems can anticipate future health requirements through improved structuring of past data entry, when physical medical files are transferred from one site to another, the urgent need to draw attention to medical actions that require monitoring at a future date often falls through the cracks. EHRs avoid this problem by storing all information virtually and ubiquitously.

E-Health Records: Benefits and Hurdles

Over the years, public and private hospitals as well as consolidated health provider institutions have invested millions of dollars in computerized health records systems that are mostly institution-based, automated, incidental, and clinical or a mix of clinical and administrative records. Largely due to increasing investments into vertically and horizontally integrated delivery systems (IDSs), we expect the market for EHRs to grow over time, not only for use in e-health systems but also to replace inadequate computerized patient record systems in traditional systems (Tan, 2001).

Benefits of EHRs

EHRs allow data to be used in many ways. As I have noted, EHRs can provide descriptive, graphical, and statistical analyses of e-clinical data through the use of standard statistical software packages. In addition, electronically stored data can be rearranged and sliced and diced in different ways to support ongoing quality assessment. This same information can also be used to provide e-physicians and e-patients with quantitative analyses of the risks of various conditions and suggested treatments. These are just a few of the many reasons that EHRs will proliferate as a technology, especially in the coming years with the advent of e-health.

Many patient records are still manually written on paper. EHRs will reduce the use of paper by combining records of e-clinical encounters and administrative records of the e-patient care process in a single integrated repository. In addition, EHRs will allow e-clinicians to conveniently access e-patient information anywhere and at any time. E-clinicians will not need to find a paper chart and will not be limited by geographical locations or time differences except when paper records are meant to serve as a backup system. Electronic retrieval of patient information is a central element of health care reform legislation and many reengineering efforts in the private sector. However, only a small percentage of physicians, hospitals, and even IDSs today have successfully implemented some form of EHRs, because of the complexity, costs, demand on administrative resources, and need for technical maintenance expertise. Nonetheless, the demand for electronic data by e-insurers, e-consumers, e-vendors, networked communities, and other e-stakeholders within the e-health care system will definitely grow over time. E-physicians and e-caregivers who make the changeover now will be ready and more able to serve e-consumers because they will be able to more easily measure outcomes, quality, and cost-effectiveness of future e-health services. Thus, switching to EHRs also provides a comparative advantage.

More significantly, EHRs also provide evidence that quality care and cost management need not be mutually exclusive. Networked electronic health records can be maintained at a fraction of the costs of manual record systems and can bring about a realization of the enormous value of shared protocols as quality tools and e-care drivers reduce time and increase processing efficiencies. Automated systems in conjunction with EHRs can help e-physicians investigate outliers in data or uncommon trends. Automated systems can be used to "flag" redundant testings and keep track of standard items relevant to a particular e-patient's condition. Alarms can also be set to alert the end user when two noncompatible drugs are prescribed. The IOM report indicates that, depending on the type and nature of data collected, electronic data system capabilities can facilitate both administrative and clinical decisions in numerous ways by organizing and ordering medical and patient records. Examples include rapid searching through single or multiple records; sorting information into one record or aggregating information across multiple records; organizing and aggregating information across patients by hospital, patient care unit, and department; and allowing easy abstraction of information throughout patient e-consultations or episodes of care.

In contrast to CPRs, users can expect EHRs to be more than just a place to store data. EHRs can provide at least five new kinds of tools: mechanisms for focusing attention, for patient-specific consultation, for information management, for data analysis, and for implementing quality assurance and cost management policies (see Barton and Schoenbaum, 1990; Tan and Bhatkhande, 2001). EHRs systems can also be a resource for guiding policies and practice by providing analysis of past e-clinical experience within an e-health provider setting. Furthermore, EHRs can help educate practitioners and keep them updated on new information by supplying easily accessible bibliographic information or other linked resources (for example, vendor information) relating to specific illnesses as needed.

Administratively, EHRs can assist in achieving higher-quality service at lower cost by providing improved access to necessary financial and e-clinical information. For any e-health care system, implementation of EHRs will be key and perhaps even mandatory because of the sheer number of e-care providers, e-patients, and other e-stakeholders that have a need for the information embedded in EHRs. Indeed, the larger the e-health network, the greater will be the impact of EHRs. If EHRs are used as an enterprisewide system to facilitate information flow between all e-health providers and e-consumers, their impact in areas such as reducing health care costs; decreasing misuse, abuse, and underuse of Medicaid and Medicare or national health services; and avoiding duplication, errors, and unnecessary repetition in data collection will contribute to a more available, accessible, equitable, affordable, and portable e-health care system. This is the unique vision and goals of an e-health care system supported with the appropriate EHRs and infrastructures: a system devoid of data redundancies and inconsistencies that can serve both the clinical and the administrative needs of connected e-stakeholders.

Hurdles in Implementing EHRs

A survey of 571 health care information managers on implementing electronic databases to house and manage patient information on-line revealed impediments to the diffusion of computer-based patient records (Bergman, 1993). Results of this survey are tabulated in Table 4.1. These hurdles would not be too different in an e-health care context.

As shown in Table 4.1, lack of funding; lack of technological know-how; lack of strong governmental leadership; lack of standards; resistance from health care practitioners (including physicians, nurses, and administrators); fear of breaches of security, violation of privacy, and compromised confidentiality of patient data; and lack of

TABLE 4.1. BARRIERS TO IMPLEMENTING ELECTRONIC DATABASES

Barrier	Percentage Agreeing That Barrier Exists
Hospitals lack funds and therefore are unable to make the first step in implementing an electronic patient record system.	23%
Technology is still lacking.	22%
Government has failed to set reporting standards, making installation of an electronic patient record system difficult and making it less usable.	20%
Clinicians are basically uninterested, and the reason for their resistance is usually that they are afraid to have their work documented for competitive reasons—that is, for fear of losing patients or clients.	13%
Hospitals are not committed, so hospital administrators choose to spend their time and focus on other projects or tasks.	10%
There are far too many regulations, either about security codes and passwords or about standardized vocabulary.	9%
Nonsupportive hospital policies—for instance, lack of policies on key issues such as privacy and medicolegal liability—make implementation of electronic records databases difficult.	4%

Source: Adapted from Bergman, 1993.

workable policies and procedures to protect patient data are among the key reasons underlying the lag in EHRs implementation. E-health executives and managers need to play an active and leading role in advocating for EHRs, while nurses and physicians need to be convinced that EHRs will not diminish their roles in the caregiving process. Support of e-stakeholders is key to success, including the government, e-vendors, e-purchasers, qualified and well-known physicians and other e-practitioners, as well as e-health consumer advocates and activists.

The one factor in Bergman's computer-based patient records survey that does not apply well in the evolving e-health era is technological lag. New advances in medical sciences and computing technologies have eliminated this deficiency. The mainstream health care system in general and the acute care or hospital system in particular have been very slow in applying new and emerging technologies to solve the problems of cost and quality of services. In contrast, many other industries and businesses (for example, the automobile industry or the banking industry) have been much more aggressive in transferring technological developments and applications from classrooms and research laboratories into the real world of practice. Given the enormous technological advances and developments since the time Bergman's survey was conducted, lack of adequate technology should not continue to be a major obstacle. Perhaps the greatest technological challenge is not the hardware or software, but the user interface. Effective interface design is critical to the acceptance of EHRs among health care professionals.

On the government side, the IOM report notes that some initial concrete steps should be considered at the national level, including the following:

- Development of national standards for documenting and sharing e-patient information
- Establishment of national standards for protecting the privacy and confidentiality of e-patient information
- Development of community health information networks
- Evaluation of the usefulness and cost-effectiveness of all requests for e-provider data by regulators and insurers

The development and establishment of national standards require the setting up of a high-level council of stakeholders from across all major e-health care sectors, including representation from government, universities, various e-practitioner groups, e-consumer groups, e-health insurers, and other e-stakeholders (for example, employers). A standards approval process should be put in place, with mechanisms to debate, approve, disseminate, and publicize the work of the council. The U.S. government, the largest employer and the highest payer for health care, is in the best position to play a leading role in championing the development and establishment of such standards. Initial costs of this sort of project, which must cut across institutional boundaries, break down sociopolitical and cultural differences, and inspire active participation from many e-stakeholders and third parties, will be immense, but the long-term benefits for many different users will more than offset the costs. The development and deployment of new and improved technologies for EHRs first require the generation and determination of standards for medical terms and data forms. A standard vocabulary, generally accepted coding for medical information, and consistent communication formats are all needed to advance the practice of e-medicine and e-health.

Privacy, confidentiality, security, and legal implications of the use of EHRs will continue to be a major hurdle in successful EHRs implementation. It has been argued that EHRs in fact offer more security than paper-based records because an audit trail can track who accesses electronically stored records and who makes changes, if any, to the stored data. Users of EHRs systems will presumably be required to use identity cards, keys, or passwords that are changed periodically in order to access any record.

For electronic patient records to be accepted by stakeholders, patient information must be protected so that people are not penalized or harmed because of their medical status. The establishment of privacy protection for patients and clinicians should be not only the responsibility of the government but also part of the culture and obligation of every e-health care provider. This will require formal sanctions for violation of confidentiality rules as well as informal sanctions in the form of consistent, meaningful disapproval of idle gossip or carelessness regarding patient information. All interested parties should be involved in deciding how information should be collected and disseminated so that privacy is preserved and protected. New technologies should continue to be explored in order to further enhance the security of information that has already been collected and stored electronically. In the long run, it may make sense for the government to transform itself to an e-government, providing the e-health industry with a model for maintaining consumer anonymity through coded unique identifiers in accumulating EHRs. However, some experts caution that too many security measures may become an unnecessary burden to users.

In an e-health care environment, there are several ways to address the confidentiality issue. One secure messaging and information storage company provides cryptographic solutions for securing corporate digital assets and protecting all forms of digital information, including e-mail, text, spreadsheets, audio, and video. Other options include secured identity verification, passwords, and more. These issues will be discussed in greater detail later in this book (Chapters Six and Fourteen).

Implementation of E-Health Records

The process of moving from a paper-based health record system to EHRs is multifaceted. The literature is packed with examples of the trials and tribulations of implementing health care information systems in countries such as the United Kingdom, Australia, Canada, and the United States. This section briefly covers the main concepts and issues involved in the creation and implementation of EHRs.

The development of EHRs can be divided into two major phases: (1) creation of electronic health records themselves, and (2) preparation of users and tools to allow convenient access to the records (Office of Health and the Information Highway, 2001). Figure 4.1 shows a model of EHRs that is advocated in the OHIH document. It portrays EHRs as comprising three components: interoperable databases, information access, and e-stakeholders.

The first component, *the interoperable databases*, consists of data about standards, procedures, and policies (data format, rules, and regulations); data about e-health care providers (data capture mechanisms); and linked databases that store data, including patient demographics, e-provider identifiers, clinical and administrative health information (data storage). The *information access* component refers to the user-friendly

FIGURE 4.1. CONCEPTUALIZATION OF
ELECTRONIC HEALTH RECORDS

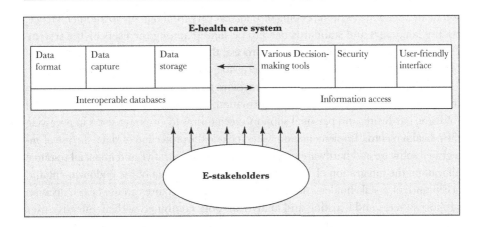

interface; the different tools available for making EHRs useful, such as decision support, analytical tools, and learning tools; and a security layer to ensure the protection
of the electronic health records. The *e-stakeholders* consist of e-patients or e-consumers;
the general public; e-health professionals, including e-health administrators and
e-caregivers; e-health policymakers and researchers; and third-party e-payers, including
employers and e-health insurers.

Much work and debate has been invested in the creation of EHRs. One challenge
is the data format of EHRs, which requires defining a standard set of codes to describe
medical concepts that can be shared by all e-stakeholders. Two examples of standardized sets of codes are the diagnostic related groups (DRGs) and the international classification of diseases (ICD-10).

Once a patient enters the e-health care system through contact with an e-care
provider, the desired information from all subsequent interactions should be identified or captured in some standardized way through direct entry, voice entry, or other
means, such as filling in on-line forms. Paper records used in the past have been portable,
easy to move physically from one location to another, and information—for example,
narrative clinical summaries—has been relatively unstructured. These paper records
are thus an informal medium, in which the few models used to interpret the information are within the knowledge base of most professional readers. Not only has the paper
chart been considered "the one place where everything can be found" (Tonnesen,
LeMaistre, and Tucker, 1999), but it has traditionally been the backup, especially in
health models of incremental EHRs implementation. In contrast, an electronic health
record should be structured and restricted to sets of codes. One commonly used standard of coding system is the ICD-9-CM (World Health Organization, 1977).

Once the codes are defined, classification hierarchies are needed to define more complex medical ideas or concepts. Often the translation from paper records to EHRs is a source of error, because interpretations of written data can differ from one person to another. Furthermore, coding of data can vary from one site to another. Hence, coding languages and standards need to be shared among the users of the system. Following the data capture and coding process, the collected information, with appropriate identifiers, needs to be stored in accessible data warehouses or databases.

The technology infrastructure (the provisions that allow e-stakeholders access within the e-health care network to stored information) refers generally to a combination of software, hardware, and personal support mechanisms to empower users in accessing the e-health records. Implementation issues include the protection of data, the use of integrated software and hardware support systems, administrative and financial resource allocation, the integration of interoperable systems, and finally, the endorsement and acceptance of e-stakeholders. As an example, an infrastructure can use health decision support systems and learning and analytical tools, combined with an effective user interface, to expand the uses of the stored data from routine administration and accounting to exploration and mining of epidemiological trends; trends in health care cost utilization; clinical guidelines and algorithms; interactive decision support areas useful for analyzing patient-specific data; medication tracking; patient history inquiries; and other investigative processes pertaining to shared or integrated care (Szende, 2001; Tan, 2001). As well, EHRs, if implemented appropriately, can permit analysis of e-health care system performance-based measures, including e-health system outcome, efficacy, and impact evaluation.

Because of its implications for all of the functions just described, it is evident that the effective design of the technology infrastructure for EHRs must involve all e-stakeholders, including e-health care providers, e-payers, e-vendors, and e-consumers: sharing ideas among all parties involved will determine what information is needed from the system, in what standardized format, and in what manner the information will be used (Tan with Sheps, 1998). As has been noted time and again, e-stakeholder endorsement and support is of paramount importance to the success of EHRs. Stakeholder buy-in can be facilitated by a user-friendly and flexible multimedia interface. Research in the design of automated computer systems that can interpret natural language in the complex domain of medicine is likely to enhance the capabilities of user interfaces with EHRs. Touchscreen paging technology currently allows users to read pages of documents displayed on computer screens as if they were reading a book. When this technology is applied to an EHRs system, e-caregivers will be able to read e-patient information without a keyboard. Advances in voice recognition software will permit speaking into the system rather than typing in commands or entering data via keyboards.

The actual implementation of EHRs requires clearly defined objectives; a responsive, logical technology infrastructure; and e-stakeholder participation and site testing. Methods of implementation are also an important consideration. Introduction of EHRs can be either "revolutionary" or "evolutionary" (Office of Health and the Information Highway, 2001; Tan with Sheps, 1998). *Revolutionary* approaches imply that system implementation occurs over a relatively short period of time, perhaps with the use of prototyping or rapid prototyping techniques. *Evolutionary* implementation involves incremental and systematic assimilation of various aspects of EHRs over time. The structured methods and traditional systems development life-cycle (SDLC) approaches underlie most of the evolutionary approaches (see Tan, 2001). In 1991, the Kaiser Permanente Rocky Mountain Division in Colorado envisioned and projected the full implementation of such a system in twenty-seven months; it actually took over five years. EHR system implementation is therefore not a trivial task to perform even for a large organization. The United Kingdom's National Health Service has adopted the incremental approach. Over a ten-year period, NHS's mandate is that "the implementation must proceed at a reasonable pace in relation to the flow of resources and the sheer scale and complexity of the technical, cultural and management challenges that will be faced" (Office of Health and the Information Highway, 2001).

In the revolutionary approach, it is possible to have an Internet-based EHR or a virtual integrated medical record system, discussed earlier, that could have been implemented within a relatively short period of time. In fact, several scientists believe that such an approach would be most logical as advancing technology allows data coded in different formats to be integrated virtually via a common platform just for retrieval and usage as per needed basis. Once the virtual system is logged out, these data are not stored or archived independently of the sources from which they were retrieved. In other words, issues of legality and privacy can be conveniently circumvented. While this approach has a lot of appeal and seems to overcome many of the shortcomings of the evolutionary approach, it nevertheless requires extensive collaboration among many stakeholders (federal, state, and local governments, HMOs, hospitals, third party payers such as insurance, employers and patients) which will be difficult, if not impossible, to achieve. However, several small-scale pilot projects that are community-based or hospital-based have been known to work quite amicably. We see this as another step towards future trends in e-health record keeping technology.

Implementation of EHRs can be bewilderingly complex. Managing the flow of information to and from EHRs is complex, particularly in the context of an evolving e-health care system, because of the frequency of information exchange and questions about who among the multitude of e-stakeholders has authority and priority to make changes to the stored information. With individual institutions, federal health agencies, statewide or provincial and regional governments, and private-sector organizations involved, custodianship of information, policing of information misuse, and linkage of separate databases will surely be problematic. Therefore, the initiative for EHRs should be coordinated at the national level, and the system should be standardized for common understanding among all stakeholders.

Finally, as I have already mentioned, strong support from e-stakeholders is key to the implementation success of EHRs. Large capital and resource investments are required, and without e-stakeholder endorsement, any development of EHRs will fail. E-stakeholders therefore must be convinced of the overall benefits of EHRs. Data sharing, e-provider liability, the growing numbers of medically informed e-patients through the Internet, and building the perception that EHRs are aimed at minimizing e-provider administrative chores, giving them more time to focus on patient care, are issues that need to be addressed. The public will need to see an improvement in patient care if EHRs, and more generally e-health care systems, are to thrive. Managers of virtual health networks, venture capitalists, and e-health investors will need to see cost-effectiveness and reasonable returns for such large investments. The full projected benefits of EHRs in terms of efficiency and cost-effectiveness have not yet been fully realized in any system thus far. Over time, with full implementation of EHRs, we can expect further innovations and advances in e-technologies to change the nature, scope, and usefulness of EHRs on a more global scale.

Privacy Considerations in Implementing EHRs

The improvement of public health and the quality of individuals' lives through the adoption of EHRs requires the acquisition, use, and storage of extensive health-related information over a long period of time. The electronic accumulation and exchange of personal data promises significant public health benefits but also entails significant issues of individual privacy. Breaches of privacy could lead to discrimination against individuals in employment, insurance, and government programs, as well as many other detrimental consequences, such as identity theft. A number of studies show that individuals concerned about privacy invasions may avoid clinical or public health tests, treatments, or research.

An e-health care environment has an even greater need than a traditional care environment to recognize the importance of establishing the appropriate balance between an individual's right to privacy and the many benefits of improved access to and use of health information by authorized e-health service providers. The stringent requirements for privacy in this environment are due to the massive amount of data that could be placed simultaneously in the wrong hands if access authorization becomes misused, and because of the ease with which the data are to be shared among multiple stakeholders, it would also not be easy sometimes to know precisely the source of initial or subsequent misuses. Regardless of the care environment, privacy requirements are among the most important factors that will influence or impede the pace at which EHRs will be implemented regionally, nationally, and globally. According to the Advisory Council on Health Infostructure of Health Canada, electronic health records, when implemented and used with particular care, can actually enhance privacy protection as well as improve patient care, enable tele–health care, empower citizens by allowing them greater control of their own health records, and serve as the foundation for an ever-improving information and evidence-based health system: "We believe that the level of privacy protection has the potential to be higher than today's paper-based world" (Advisory Council on Health Infostructure, 1999). Currently, the ACHI comprises a health information executive from each province—that is, someone who reports directly to the Minister of Health.

In both Canada and the United States, federal, provincial, and territorial jurisdictions each take different approaches to information privacy, and the level of information protection is not consistent throughout the country. Thus, a 1999 report by the ACHI called *Canadian Health Infoway: Paths to Better Health* recommended that federal, provincial, and territorial jurisdictions harmonize their legislation for privacy protection, taking into account international best practices (Advisory Council on Health Infostructure, 1999). In the United States, the Health Insurance Portability and Accountability Act of 1996, which will also be discussed in Chapters Eight and Fourteen, governs privacy protection for e-health records. Fair information practices and privacy-enhancing technologies must be implemented throughout the health sector. In addition to giving people control over their own health records, this would involve strict and explicit controls on access to health records, making these records available to e-health care professionals, researchers, and other e-stakeholders on a strictly need-to-know basis.

Some important questions on privacy issues related to EHRs are as follows:

- What information should be included in EHRs?
- Who should have authorized access to EHRs?
- Which information in EHRs should be shared with other providers, and under what circumstances?
- How would a patient be able to access his or her own data that are stored in EHRs?
- In what instances could the information in EHRs be used for secondary purposes (for example, research or administration)?
- When should consent from the patient be required for use of information in his or her EHR?

Privacy legislation and privacy codes are designed to provide individuals with the means to protect their personal information and control its use. Privacy legislation and codes provide individual control over the collection, use, disclosure, retention, and disposal of health information by collecting organizations. In Canada, the Privacy Act imposes restrictions on the collection, use, or disclosure of personal information by federal departments and specified federal agencies; protects the privacy of individuals with respect to personal information about themselves held by a government institution; and provides individuals with the right of access to that information. More specifically, the Canadian federal government adopted the Personal Information Protection and Electronic Documents Act (formerly known as Bill C-6) in order to initiate harmonized and consistent privacy policy and legislation among provinces and territories. This act establishes rules that govern the collection, use, and disclosure of personal information in a manner that recognizes the right of individuals to privacy and the need of organizations to collect, use, or disclose personal information for purposes that a reasonable person would consider appropriate.

Table 4.2 outlines the ten privacy principles identified by the Canadian Standards Association and Canadian legislation (the Personal Information Protection and Electronic Documents Act), providing comprehensive insight into the requirements that will be placed on EHRs.

TABLE 4.2. HEALTH INFORMATION PRIVACY PRINCIPLES

Principles	Implications	Requirements
Accountability	Organizations held responsible for personal information under custody or control; shall designate individual(s) to be accountable for compliance with privacy principles	Accountable person to manage personal information use/disclosure; verify adherence to principles; collect/monitor and report on status of controls; and assists in managing privacy issues
Identifying Purposes	Identify purposes for which personal information is collected at or before the time it is collected	Need to document purposes, track changes, support accountable person and document when and how individuals are notified of purpose and changes
Consent	Knowledge and consent of individuals required for collection, use, or disclosure of personal information	Document history of consent given and audit or review consent database

Principles	Implications	Requirements
Limiting Collection	Collect information by fair and lawful means; limiting the collection of personal information to that which is necessary for purposes identified	Document how each item supports purpose and how collection is made; review/audit collection; capture explanation of why and how data are collected; and collect information as per defined rules and definitions
Limiting Use, Disclosure, and Retention	Use or disclose personal information only for intended purposes, except with the individual's consent as required by law Retain personal information only as long as necessary for the fulfillment of those purposes as required by law	Document information use(s); authorize, manage and audit access and use; define roles; capture who can obtain access; log access requests; and report access requests outside of defined authorizations Deny use/access/receipt based on authorizations/permissions and exclusions; audit access/receipt; capture exclusions/permissions rules; and report access/receipt by excluded roles; track authorized disclosures/receipts Document rules for retention/information disposal; audit disposal of all information in a collection/destruction and verify, capture, hold, manage records for long retention periods; inventory all copies (backups, all subsets, all media); document/capture all steps in collection's life cycle
Accuracy	Personal information be accurate and current as necessary to fulfill purposes for which it is collected	Defined accuracy and maintenance checks; integrity designed into collection and retention mechanisms

TABLE 4.2. *Continued*

Principles	Implications	Requirements
Safeguards	Security safeguards to protect personal information against loss/theft, unauthorized access, disclosure, copying, use or modification, throughout its life cycle, regardless of the format in which it is held	Protect information with due diligence; security standards; high confidentiality and integrity objectives; limit right to access; safeguard selection based on requirements; standard approaches; specific data protection tools justified to meet objectives; for long-lived records, retrieval across generations of technology: software/hardware become part of the record so it can be read throughout its life
Openness	Specific information about policies and practices pertaining to management of personal information made readily available Inform individuals of the existence, use and disclosure of their personal information	Mechanism(s) for policy accessibility; for individual to receive/access status of information including use, disclosure (includes who has access to the information), disposal; and for tracking collection, use, disclosure, consents, disposal
Individual Access	Upon request, an individual shall have access to personal information. Exceptions to the right of access must be limited and specific An individual able to challenge accuracy and completeness of the information and have it amended as appropriate	Permit individual access to information; block exceptions (identification and authentication); record who requests, how, when; reliable change management process to record requests, action them, track changes and confirm to individual making the request; mechanism for propagating change across all copies of collections of individual's information
Challenging Compliance	An individual shall be able to address a challenge concerning compliance with privacy requirements to a designated individual or individuals	Audit compliance challenges and responses

Briefly, these principles include accountability, identifying purpose, consent, limiting collection, limiting use, disclosure, and retention, accuracy, safeguards, openness, individual access, and challenging compliance. This list indicates what will be required for the structuring of the information records generally and the protection of personal health information in EHRs specifically. For example, the principles of appropriate health record governance, the management of consent, use on a need-to-know basis, and individual access to the record will all require changes in the way business is currently conducted, especially if EHRs are to be shared among different e-stakeholders.

Thus, federal, provincial, and territorial governments in both the United States and Canada will need to develop consistent legislation and guidelines that will protect the personal health information of all individuals and that will prohibit all secondary commercial use of such information.

Moving Ahead

In order to move ahead with EHRs, top health leaders and executives in most developed countries agreed that instead of going for an integrated single EHRs system that would link a country from coast to coast, an incremental, evolutionary approach should be adopted. In this type of approach, the idea is to implement smaller shared systems such as e-laboratory systems (laboratory testing data are critical in supporting quality patient care). The next step could then be, for example, implementation of e-prescription systems, to ensure better pharmaceutical services for e-providers and e-consumers. After this, implementation could move on to e-radiological systems and EHRs.

Partnerships among key e-stakeholders (e-doctors, e-paramedics, governments, e-consumers, e-vendors, and corporate leaders) will provide the breakthroughs that result in successful EHRs implementation. As well, it will be important to get the information technology standards right so that compatibility problem are minimized.

The Institute of Medicine (1997) committee identifies five objectives for future health record systems. Extending these objectives to an e-health care environment, we note the following:

- EHRs must support e-patient care and improve its quality.
- EHRs must enhance the productivity of e-health care professionals and reduce the administrative burden and labor costs associated with e-health care delivery and financing.
- EHRs must support e-clinical and e-health services research.
- EHRs must be able to accommodate future developments in e-health care technology, policy, management, and finance.
- The importance of e-patient confidentiality must be emphasized, and confidentiality must be maintained while all the other objectives are being met.

In the future, EHRs will enable new functions through decision support tools, links to other databases, and reliable transmission of detailed information across substantial distances. To meet the needs of practitioners, EHRs will be linked to knowledge bases, clinical decision support systems, statistical software packages, and video or picture graphics. For example, in a virtual hospital setting, departments such as e-laboratory, e-nursing, and e-radiology will be able to automatically transfer data into centralized EHRs that are linked to national bibliographic resources such as MEDLINE to access digital radiological databases. In the larger e-health care environment, EHRs will be linked with e-networks of provider institutions, third-party payers, and other health care entities. All stakeholder needs should be taken into account, for if EHRs do not deliver an end product that the end users or e-stakeholders want, all of the investments—including money, the many personnel hours of technicians and programmers, and ongoing efforts to coordinate the project—will have gone to waste.

With new advances in technology, society has also become increasingly mobile. EHRs provide a means to keep track of medical histories regardless of location or modality of e-health service. As part of this technological evolution, interfaces between users and e-network systems are becoming more user-friendly through new concepts such as smart cards, smart cars, and smart houses. A smart card can retain a patient's vital medical information so that it can be easily retrieved by swiping the card through a reader after entering the necessary security information. The technology also permits mobile health care computing, so that products, medical treatments, or alternative medical therapies can be purchased wherever there is a card reader. Smart cars will direct their operators to the nearest emergency room or available clinician, using global positioning system technology and automated directories installed in the vehicles. Alternatively, a smart car could be designed to provide e-health services directly to the driver in an emergency or even for non-emergency needs. Smart houses allow monitoring of health variables (for example, blood pressure or sugar level) of homebound patients via remote sensors, satellite-operated cameras, or other smart e-technologies (for example, fiber optics wired into the house). A case illustration of a smart house for e-home care is provided in Chapter Nine.

Conclusion

Advances in information and communication technologies have the potential to transform the current health care system. EHRs are the lifeblood of e-health care and the key to promoting quality patient care and decision support. Although many barriers stand in the way of implementation of EHRs, including financial constraints; the complexity of the e-health system; resistance to change; and privacy, confidentiality, security, and access issues, EHRs are still the foundation of the future e-health care system.

Electronic patient record systems offer opportunities to improve patient care and reduce administrative and clinical costs by improving and streamlining the e-health care delivery process. Increasingly, e-stakeholders are realizing the potential of these systems and, as a result, are starting to voice their need for integrated EHRs. The extent to which e-health leaders, the government, and private investors will invest in EHRs, as well as which applications they will choose, will depend on the establishment of standardized vocabulary, availability of funds, improved e-security technologies, and other factors. Using EHRs means reengineering the work process—that is, changing the ways that e-clinicians process orders and test results and document patient care. It is hoped that the proliferation of EHRs will translate into healthier patients and more informed e-consumers.

Chapter Questions

1. Describe the benefits of EHRs. Suggest some steps toward building ideal EHRs as discussed in this chapter.
2. What do you envision in the future of EHRs? What do you think of virtual medical records as an alternative model?
3. Who would be primarily responsible for successful implementation of integrated EHRs in an e-health care system?
4. What are the major hurdles in implementing EHRs?
5. Imagine that integrated EHRs exist in a network from which you are able to access data that has been collected by e-practitioners about you. What would be your reaction if you discovered that not only were the data contained in the network plagued with errors, but also a good amount of the information provided about you in the network was sensitive and private? How would you go about ensuring that the information about you that was captured and stored in EHRs was reliably accurate and that the appropriate information was encrypted to protect your privacy and the confidentiality of your information?

References

Advisory Council on Health Infostructure. (1999). *Canadian health infoway: Paths to better health.* Final Report. Ottawa: Health Canada.

Andrew, W., & Dick, R. (1995a). Applied information technology. A clinical perspective feature focus: The computer-based patient record: Part 1. *Computers in Nursing,* 13(2), 80–84.

Andrew, W., & Dick, R. (1995b). Applied information technology. A clinical perspective feature focus: The computer-based patient record: Part 2. *Computers in Nursing,* 13(3), 118–122.

Barton, M., & Schoenbaum, S. (1990). Improving influenza vaccination performance in an HMO setting. *American Journal of Public Health, 80,* 534–536.

Bergman, R. (1993). The long march toward progress. *Journal of Hospitals and Health Networks, 67*(18), 42–46.

Hunter, K. M. (1993). *Doctors' stories: The narrative structure of medical knowledge.* Princeton, NJ: Princeton University Press.

Institute of Medicine. (1997). *Computer-based patient records.* Report no. 55. Washington, DC: National Academy Press.

Office of Health and the Information Highway. (2001). *Toward electronic health records.* Report no. 5-53. Ottawa: Health Canada.

Szende, A. (2001). A lifelong ehealth record. *Canadian Healthcare Manager, 55*(6).

Tan, J. (2001). *Health management information systems: Methods and practical applications.* (2nd ed.). Sudbury, MA: Jones & Bartlett.

Tan, J., & Bhatkhande, A. (2001). Evolving standards for integrating tomorrow's health care system: Toward a service process model. In J. Tan, *Health management information systems: Methods and practical applications.* (2nd ed., pp. 77–101). Sudbury, MA: Jones & Bartlett.

Tan, J., with Sheps, S. (1998). *Health decision support systems.* Sudbury, MA: Jones & Bartlett.

Tonnesen, A. S., LeMaistre, A., & Tucker, D. (1999). Electronic medical record implementation: Barriers encountered during implementation. *Proceedings of the AMIA Symposium* (pp. 624–626). Washington, DC: American Medical Informatics Association.

U.S. Department of Veterans Affairs. (1995, July). *Veterans Health Administration manual, M-I operations: Part 1. Medical administrative activities.* Publication 5.03. Washingon, DC: Author.

World Health Organization. (1977). *Manual of the international statistical classification of diseases, injuries and causes of death.* Publication ICD-9. Geneva, Switzerland: Author.

E-Primary Health Care and E-Health Records Cases

Penny Grubb

The primary care environment differs around the world. In some places, such as the United Kingdom, the general practitioner is the dedicated gatekeeper for all health services; other places, such as mainland Europe, offer comprehensive self-referral schemes. The means of funding, public or private, is one of the key drivers of how and where primary care is delivered. With new funding streams targeted at e-health initiatives, this in itself can make a difference. Thus, aspects of e-health provision can tip traditional balances, breaking barriers and initiating change in ways never before predicted.

A patient who directly pays a significant proportion of the cost of expensive treatment expects certain standards, including what might be termed frills: nicely appointed consulting rooms, hotel-standard service, no waiting time, and more. This reality drives health providers toward certain new technologies, placing a premium on being seen to be at the forefront, in order not to lose patients and therefore income. Wholly state-subsidized primary care, in which there are scant resources for frills, is at the other end of the scale. Patients have limited choice about where they go, and there is little direct financial motivation to please patients as though they were hotel guests. Thus, odd dichotomies come to light as the general context of health care changes. The extremes are very good and very bad: run-down public clinics at one end of the spectrum may provide state-of-the-art clinical expertise, while superbly appointed private clinics may keep costs down by skimping on specialist coverage. Both can lead to good and bad health care for different reasons.

In the United Kingdom, there is a push toward more integration of public and private health care at all levels, but many obstacles are being encountered. Partnerships are obstructed by the lack of quantitative data on comparative cost-effectiveness and on quality of care provided. In addition, cultural suspicion and even hostility between the sectors exist in many quarters.

In health care, not every eventuality can be predicted. This bedevils contracts between the public and private sector and can, for example, lead to clinical decision making on the basis of avoiding possible litigation rather than meeting genuine clinical needs. If the ultimate aim is good health care for all, there is room for all forms of primary care. The divisions that affect primary care are rooted in the history and traditions of the medical professions, as are the different types and contexts of care. E-technologies have a huge potential to smooth differences, to stretch resources, and to increase both effectiveness and efficiency. In doing so, they are likely to change the face of primary care.

Harnessing Information and Managing Knowledge

A great driver in any field is information, and the information explosion in health care has been as wide-ranging as in any context. However, information, by and in itself, is insufficient. Information overload can be as dangerous as information scarcity. Information must become knowledge, and it needs to be managed. Advances are continually made in both generalist and specialist medicine. As an illustration of the problem that this abundance of information creates, consider the following case: A primary health care clinician may justifiably wish to keep abreast of the latest developments in gastroenterology, given that roughly 15 percent of the patients he or she sees will have symptoms in this area. In a single year in the early 1990s, approximately 50,000 papers were published in this field. A clinician would need to read a paper every ten minutes or so, twenty-four hours a day, 365 days a year, to keep current. The technologies that facilitate such rapid advances must also allow the health care professional to access and harness the key research findings.

Gaps in knowledge are inevitable and still need to be addressed. All sorts of factors affect a primary health care clinician's knowledge and ability to provide effective care. For example, a study in Italy showed different levels of awareness relating to the age and experience of general practitioners (GPs). Younger GPs made greater use of scientific journals, while older GPs showed superior on-the-ground care skills, based on experience (Pavia, Foresta, Carbone, and Angelillo, 2003). One-size-fits-all knowledge management systems will not solve the problems.

Knowledge management skills have been essential in the changing face of primary care. No generalist can hold in his or her head sufficient knowledge to adequately service the diverse and shifting population that the twenty-first century lands on a provider's doorstep. In part as a response to this, primary care teams comprising doctors, nurses, and other appropriate therapists have developed. "The function of the team is to support and develop [the] therapeutic relationship between the patient and the professional" (Calman, 1994). This requires the development of new skills in teamwork and communication. Once again, the potential of the e-health context makes this possible.

The U.K. government has made it a statutory duty for primary health care groups to watch for ways to improve quality in their health care delivery (U.K. Secretary of State for Health, 1997), which means that they must keep current on research results. Keeping current would be impossible without the aid of e-systems such as regularly updated on-line research databases containing reviews and appraisals from trusted sources. In the United Kingdom, the National Institute for Clinical Excellence provides such a database.

Greater harnessing of information and knowledge within a team means that vastly greater amounts of sensitive medical data and information are available to many more people than were available a relatively short time ago. Thus, security and confidentiality are no longer as easy as remembering to lock the filing cabinet and keeping the key safe. E-technologies allow greater and more effective use but also potential for misuse of information, leading to the need for further technological aids to address information security and integrity requirements. The importance of continuing education both in monitoring and in improving skills and knowledge in the primary health care profession is well known. However, in some contexts, such as rural settings, literature is scarce and access to primary care may be difficult to come by. In these situations, caregivers rely even more on e-systems for access to up-to-date information (Murray, 1995). E-decision support systems, e-medicine, and e-home care become the obvious way forward (see Chapters Eight, Nine, and Ten).

A Greater Ability to Audit

Technology provides a means to harness information, analyze vast amounts of data with relative ease, and generate new knowledge. It permits ever more sophisticated audits of all areas of primary care. As in other areas of e-health, the potential for good is vast, and the ingenuity of people in contriving to get it wrong is impressive. Historically, audits of primary care in the United Kingdom were a financial necessity. A general practitioner was state-funded according to the number of patients on his or her books or the number attending routine clinics.

Now that information can be collected and analyzed quickly and accurately, there is a move to set targets and monitor progress toward their achievement. While this appears to be a force for good, it can lead to achievement of targets' taking precedence over patient care. For example, in the United Kingdom, the government set primary care teams the so-called 24/48 target: by 2004, all patients should be able to see a primary care professional (including nurses and other nonphysicians) within twenty-four hours, and a general practitioner physician within forty-eight hours. In setting the target, no allowance was made for the patients who, for a variety of reasons, book appointments in advance. This led to some primary care centers not allowing advance appointments, furthering their progress toward achieving the government target, and thus accessing funding, but causing great inconvenience to patients. No difference in the speed with which patients accessed primary care services resulted (McSmith, 2003).

Managing Chronic Disease in Primary Care

More appropriate audits could lead to more efficient and effective use of resources. Take diabetes care, for example. Primary care providers are often the routine caregivers for people with conditions such as diabetes. They run regular clinics and check patients' status and progress. A local clinic run by people the patients can get to know is more relaxing for the patients. Clinical tests are done in a more comfortable environment; patients are less likely to be stressed by unfamiliar surroundings, less likely to cheat on their tests, and more likely to attend. This leads to better overall health and management of the condition. Thus, resource use is more effective and overall expenditures are lower.

Still, if primary care practitioners in this local clinic have insufficient skill or knowledge, they may make inappropriate referrals to specialists: either too many routine cases referred, using scarce specialist resource unnecessarily, or cases not referred until too late to prevent serious problems—for example, amputation. Specialist clinics tend to insist on more referrals than necessary, on the assumption that it is better to be safe than sorry. Too few or too many referrals both lead to overload on specialist resources and thus lower standards of care.

Where E-Health Comes In

Using e-technologies, routine tests done in the primary care setting can be tracked automatically, both to see that these are being done and to track patient progress. The specialist can determine the template of care for the primary care team to follow. The primary care team's more intimate personal knowledge of patients can also be fed into the care templates.

Diabetes is a chronic condition that can be controlled but not cured. Good control is key in preventing serious complications such as blindness and amputation and in maintaining the patient's quality of life. Good control means maintaining blood sugar, blood pressure, and other relevant indicators at levels as near to normal as possible all the time. Maintaining normal levels on average is not enough. It is the peaks and troughs that cause the damage. The care of people with diabetes could be revolutionized by the use of e-primary care, as I will explain.

In the traditional primary care scenario, both routine testing and patient education are problem areas. Patients come to a primary care clinic every few weeks for tests. Satisfactory results may be recorded time after time, while a patient develops severe neurological complications and serious circulatory disorders. This may occur because the patient prepares for the clinic, consciously or subconsciously, by altering his or her diet for the preceding few days. This problem is also apparent when patients do home tests and bring their results to the clinic. They learn to massage the figures they write on the charts to give the doctor the "right" results.

The education problem is clear. People cheat on results to avoid a lecture on lifestyle, at the expense of their own long-term health. For years, patients have been given diet sheets and lifestyle advice, which have been improved over time. Tests now are far more sophisticated than they used to be. Despite this, the problem persists.

E-primary care in this context can both address the problem of misleading results and improve the efficacy of patient education. Home testing kits can gauge and store results electronically without the patient's intervention, and results can be sent electronically to the clinic. Automatic analysis of results provides a means to monitor the condition as changes occur rather than looking at what has already passed. Tests done in the home setting, when correctly recorded, give a more accurate reflection of the patient's health because they lack the element of "special occasion" that can have effects such as raising blood pressure.

The e-health context provides the means to obtain a far more complete and accurate picture of the progress of a patient's condition than that achieved through traditional means. E-health enables providers and patients to receive early warning of potential complications. Thus, intervention can be more timely, and advice on lifestyle can be more immediate and thus more effective. In this context, the barrier between primary and specialist clinics blurs as information and knowledge become ubiquitously available. The "virtual patient," in the guise of comprehensive and accurate test results, can be automatically transferred and analyzed.

Results, combinations of results, and specific vagaries of individual patients can potentially be tracked automatically. Automatic alerts can then be raised if a person needs specialist intervention or checking. The specialist clinic can take fewer routine cases with confidence, thus leaving specialist resources free for those genuinely in need. Automatic systems can learn from past situations as medical outcomes are fed back to them. This will spread in the future into home monitoring, in which automatic systems will check results and their integrity and thus ease the load on even the routine primary care clinics.

Early studies on e-home care for diabetics show encouraging results (Dansky, Bowles, and Palmer, 2003). However, for more sophisticated e-systems, the trust of primary health care professionals will be essential. A system that is not trusted will not be used, even when it has been shown to be clinically effective (Grubb and Takang, 2003).

The deployment of e-systems in the care of conditions like diabetes could lead to vast benefits. For example, a small percentage decrease in the number of amputations or the incidence of blindness translates into enormous quality of life benefits as well as huge cost savings. Even routine data exchange has been shown to make a difference (Grubb and Dixon, 1993). E-medicine and e-care systems such as those exchanging data between primary care and specialist clinics may have the potential to eventually bypass primary care altogether because specialists now can treat patients directly with or without the need of a referral. However, e-technologies are a long way from replacing the primary health care professional. Harnessing data and making them useful through information and knowledge management applied in teamwork and audit contexts may lead to better health care but cannot substitute for the relationship between a patient and a primary care provider. No e-medicine or robotic system will ever provide satisfactory service for the patient whose regular trip to the diabetes clinic is primarily for human contact.

The primary health care physician, faced with unusual symptoms and without recourse to the battery of tests and equipment of the specialist clinical setting, routinely makes difficult clinical decisions. We are a long way from technology that will bring the tests on-line to all primary care settings, let alone to the homes of individual patients; thus, the experience and expertise of primary care professionals remains essential.

Challenges in E-Health Records

The early days of primary care e-systems were as fraught with excitement and problems as the pioneering days of any other field. There were fully networked GP clinics in the early 1960s, but within a few years, they were struggling with hugely expensive maintenance charges, while newer systems were cheaper, faster, and more reliable and offered greater functionality. Moving decades' worth of stored medical information to take advantage of newer technologies was a costly business, often unreliable and sometimes impossible. Some practices, after making this costly leap, found themselves in the same position a decade further on. What was cutting edge when bought had become hopelessly slow and archaic, and swapping systems was costly and complex.

The 1990s saw the first serious investment in research on electronic medical records (Beale, 1994; Beale and Lloyd, 1995; Camplin, 1994; Ingram and others, 1995; Dixon, Grubb, and Lloyd, 2000a, 2000b)[1] and showed that the issue of fitting people inside their electronic health records was a far more complex business than it had first appeared to be. This issue accounted for many early failures. An interesting comparison is the computerization of people's tax records. This major task was relatively easy compared to electronic health records. Essentially, electronic records were created, and people's tax personas were fitted to them. The computerization of Inland Revenue records in the United Kingdom brought inconsistencies to light that led to changes in the tax laws. No such leeway is available to builders of medical records, since there is no law that can be changed in order to determine the way a person breaks a bone or develops a disease.

Many things had to be taken into account in the medical record, including, but by no means restricted to the following:

- *The need for the data to be kept, without loss of integrity, for long periods of time, maybe in excess of one hundred years.* We cannot envisage the technologies that will underpin twenty-second century e-health systems. Thus, trying to ensure long-term integrity of the information by requiring compatibility with a particular database or file format is inappropriate. It is not the format of the data (such as specifying alphanumeric characters to a maximum length) that is relevant, but the architecture of the record itself, including the type and characteristics of data entities and relationships to be captured.

- *The correct identification of a patient.* This issue has two sides. First, who is the patient? Second, which are the correct records? Unique patient identifiers have been proposed as a solution, but the area is fraught with technical, cultural, and political difficulties. Research suggests that patients in primary care see both the potential benefits and the pitfalls of unique patient identifiers (Bomba, 2003).

A young girl died in a London hospital in the 1990s as a direct result of reliance on name as the means of identifying the correct electronic record. On her second visit to the hospital, the record of her previous visit was not found, and ignorance of previously done tests led to misdiagnosis of what turned out to be fatal meningitis. The girl's name had been keyed in on one occasion with the middle initial and on the other without it. This case illustrates that the identification issue is not just an academic problem; lives may depend on solving it effectively.

In some cases when quick clinical decisions are needed—for example, when a patient is unconscious after an accident—the patient's name and other details may not be known. There have been many suggestions for solutions, including the following:

- *Smart cards.* Work has been done on the use of health care smart cards, but the issue of what information should be coded on the card remains a matter of contention. Such cards are also vulnerable to loss or misuse.
- *National and international identity databases.* On paper, such schemes may solve technical problems, but they are fraught with practical difficulties, including misuse. Any potential for medical data to fall into the wrong hands is problematic. There is already controversy over how much data should be accessible to insurance companies.
- *Retinal prints or fingerprints.* These can provide reliable identification, but only when matched against some central record; thus, they solve only the identity side of the equation, not the records side.
- *DNA.* In some circumstances—for example, following a serious accident—fingerprinting may not be possible. DNA will always be available. However, the problems of matching are the same as for fingerprints or retinal prints.

It may be that one day roadside testing of blood or DNA will provide emergency personnel with necessary medical information such as existing conditions, allergies, and drugs in the patient's system. If that becomes possible, identification of the patient will become clinically irrelevant, but it will still be an issue for other reasons—for example, determination of the patient's religious convictions or who pays for treatment. For now, medical record architecture needs to allow all forms of identification—name and demographics; fingerprints; retinal prints; photographs; and other key data—and must not preclude the addition of future means of identification that have not yet been conceived. Work done in the European Union–funded Electronic Healthcare Record

Support Action project led to the production of software that shows the depth to which the medical record architecture must be defined in order to provide long-term integrity, flexibility, and portability (Dixon, Grubb, Gosland, and Lloyd, 2000).

Impacts of E-Health on Primary Care

Primary care has always been the repository of large amounts of clinical data. Information is now becoming available in all sorts of new ways, bringing both problems and benefits. Trends and patterns can be identified through automatic analysis of primary care records. Screening becomes easier and more accurate, leading to better standards of care but also to concerns about overscreening, which can result in unnecessary worry and concern or even unnecessary surgery.

Primary care is not an exact science, but technological factors can sometimes make it appear so. For example,

- An e-system can give misleadingly authoritative results even if it has, among other possibilities, incorrectly set parameters.
- E-systems tend toward pseudoexactness and bald statements. There is a huge difference between "You might have cancer" and "The signs you are exhibiting are the same as those of a subpopulation, a small percentage of whom will go on to develop a condition that may lead, in a small percentage of cases, to cancer." A primary health care professional can select the right slant, based on knowledge of the patient. An e-system may give entirely the wrong signals because it cannot tailor the message.
- E-systems can give inappropriate weight to information. Inadequate lab procedures, for example, can lead to false positive or negative results, but these are nonetheless given a certain gravitas by appearing as a set of computerized results, the neatness of the printout somehow counteracting the careless technique of a lab technician having a bad day. As an illustration, a computer program will state an amount as 9.45678 mg. Impressive accuracy? Probably not. The program may be running on hardware incapable of accuracy beyond two decimal points.

The above illustrations of problems with e-health systems are, in our opinion, outweighed by the huge potential advantages. The problems can be serious because they affect people's health and well-being, but they are an indication of the immaturity of the health informatics and medical informatics fields and will inevitably be overcome.

Health Informatics and Medical Informatics

Early e-primary care systems were inadequate for several reasons:

- Neither hardware nor software was reliable enough.
- Systems built by information technology professionals did not meet clinical needs.
- Systems built by health care professionals did not have technical integrity.

These issues led eventually to the development of the new disciplines of health informatics and medical informatics, in which professionals with a foot in both the medical and the technical camps could build robust systems that met clinical needs.

E-Health Impacts on Traditional Primary Care Roles

An e-medicine project in the early 1990s required a nurse in a primary health care clinic to contact a specialist clinician via a teleconferencing link and to treat patients according to the specialist's advice. The aim was to see whether specific specialist referrals (with attendant problems, including waiting times) could be cut without compromising levels of care. The system was cumbersome and unreliable but was used for the duration of the project.

By the end of this project, the videoconferencing system was not used, but the nurses continued to consult the specialists in awkward cases by telephoning while the patient was with them. This direct contact, initiated at the nurse's convenience, would previously have been unheard of, but it benefited patients, nurses, and specialists. Neither nurses nor specialists had believed that frequent telephone conversations would be so useful. Without realizing it, they had been playing out their traditional roles, in which such informal contact was frowned on. Although the e-system itself was generally deemed worse than useless, the context of e-health broke down traditional barriers. The sophisticated teleconferencing system had empowered the nurse to use the old-fashioned telephone.

Roles and boundaries in different areas of health care have always been subject to debate, but the e-health context speeds things up and blurs boundaries in unpredictable ways. Traditional relationships between professions don't always hold when put under the e-health spotlight. This leads to differences in perception of primary care roles, among others. For example, primary care is taking a bigger role in public health issues, enabled by the extra functionality provided by new technologies that deliver better facilities and processes. Nonetheless, there are differences in perception between primary care staff based in the community and those based in clinics about what their role should actually be (Heller, Edwards, Patterson, and Elhassan, 2003). Where there was once a clearly defined line between medics and trained nonmedics, the e-health context seems to be blurring that line. Evidence from a Netherlands-based trial indicates that patient care support from trained nonmedics alters clinical decision making (Frijling and others, 2003).

Conclusion

E-health in the context of primary health care is at an early stage. Health informatics and medical informatics are new disciplines compared with medicine and even with information technology. Despite some serious challenges, the difficulties in the current e-health environment in primary care are essentially teething problems. Not only is e-primary health care bringing enormous improvements in the quality and effectiveness of care, but it is also a driving force behind what are likely to become fundamental shifts in the roles and responsibilities of different health care professionals.

Both hardware and software are now available at a cost and level of reliability that should allow primary health care to benefit far more than it has. One primary obstacle is the immaturity of health informatics and medical informatics as disciplines. We can send data around the world and book complex travel tickets in any downtown office, but we still don't have reliable linked primary health care systems that can guarantee data integrity, confidentiality, security, portability, and comprehensiveness. There are signs, however, of emerging solutions. Time, the traditional great healer, is an effective treatment for problems of immaturity.

Note

1. CEN TC251, the Technical Committee of the European Standards Organisation, is responsibility for developing standards that enable compatibility and interoperability between independent systems in health care. In 1996, its Project Team PT1–011 produced a preliminary standard, ENV 12265, for the Electronic Record Architecture (www.centc251.org). In 1998, CEN Project Teams 26, 27, 28, and 29 began working together to produce a four-part standard as an enhancement of ENV 12265. PT26 produced the Extended Architecture and Domain Model. PT27 produced the Domain Term List. PT28 produced the Distribution Rules. PT29 produced the Messages for the Exchange of Record Information (www.centc251.org).

   GEHR, the Good European Health Record project, an EU Framework III Telematics project, developed a comprehensive common data structure for using and sharing electronic health care records within Europe. Details are at http://www.chime.ucl.ac.uk/work-areas/ehrs/GEHR/.

References

Beale, T. (1994). *The GEHR systems architecture guide.* Retrieved from http://www.chime.ucl.ac.uk/work-areas/ehrs/GEHR/

Beale, T., & Lloyd, D. (1995). *The GEHR Object Model, Version 2.2.* Retrieved from http://www.chime.ucl.ac.uk/work-areas/ehrs/GEHR/, Good European Health Record Project

Bomba, T. (2003). A survey of patient attitudes towards the use of computerised medical records and unique identifiers in four Australian GP practices. *Journal on Information Technology in Health Care, 1*(1),35–45.

Calman, F. (1994). Working together, teamwork. *Journal of Interprofessional Care 8,* 95–101.

Camplin, D. (1994). *GEHR software tools and prototypes/application software integration.* GEHR Project Deliverable 16/17. Retrieved from http://www.chime.ucl.ac.uk/work-areas/ehrs/GEHR/

Dansky, K., Bowles, K., & Palmer, L. (2003). Clinical outcomes of telehomecare for diabetic patients. *Journal on Information Technology in Health Care, 1,* 61–74.

Dixon, R., Grubb, P., Gosland, J., & Lloyd, D. (2000, April). *Final illustrative demonstrations of EHCR (Electronic Health Care Record Support Action) architecture features using scenarios and worked examples.* Electronic Healthcare Record Support Action, an EU Framework IV Telematics project. Retrieved from http://www.chime.ucl.ac.uk/work-areas/ehrs/EHCR-SupA/

Dixon, R., Grubb, P., & Lloyd, D. (2000a, April). *Final recommendations to CEN for future work.* Electronic Healthcare Record Support Action, an EU Framework IV Telematics project. Retrieved from http://www.chime.ucl.ac.uk/work-areas/ehrs/EHCR-SupA/

Dixon, R., Grubb, P., & Lloyd, D. (2000b, April). *Guidelines on interpretation and implementation of CEN EHCRA.* Electronic Healthcare Record Support Action, an EU Framework IV Telematics project. Available at http://www.chime.ucl.ac.uk/work-areas/ehrs/EHCR-SupA/

Foy, R., & Warner, P. (2003). About time: Diagnostic guidelines that help clinicians. *Quality and Safety in Health Care, 12,* 205–209.

Frijling, B., Lobo, C., Hulscher, M., Akkermans, R., Drenth, B., Prins, A., Wouden, J., & Grol, R. (2003). Intensive support to improve clinical decision making in cardiovascular care: A randomized controlled trial in general practice. *Quality and Safety in Health Care, 12,* 181–187.

Glasziou, P., & Irwig, M. (2000). An evidence based approach to individualizing treatment. *British Medical Journal, 320,* 659–661.

Grubb, P., & Dixon, R. (1993, April). *The communication of diabetic patient information through IT.* Paper presented to the Royal Society of Medicine at the Forum on Computers in Medicine.

Grubb, P., & Takang, A. (2003). *Software maintenance: Concepts and practice* (2nd ed.) Hackensack, NJ: World Scientific Publishing Company.

Heller, R., Edwards, R., Patterson, L., & Elhassan, M. (2003). Public health in primary care trusts: A resource needs assessment. *Public Health, 117,* 157–164.

Ingram, D., Lloyd, D., Kalra, D., Beale, T., Heard, S., Grubb, P., Dixon, R., Camplin, D., Ellis, J., & Maskens, A. (1995, June 30). *GEHR Architecture, Version 1.0.* GEHR Deliverables 19, 20, and 24. Retrieved from http://www.chime.ucl.ac.uk/work-areas/ehrs/GEHR/

McSmith, A. (2003, June 29). Revealed: How GPs cheat on their patients. *The Independent on Sunday.* Report.

Murray, T. (1995). Education for rural primary health care workers. In *Rural general practice in the United Kingdom* (pp. 36–38). Royal College of General Practitioners, Occasional Paper 71.

Pavia, M., Foresta, M., Carbone, V., & Angelillo, I. (2003). Influenza and pneumococcal immunization in the elderly: Knowledge, attitudes, and practices among general practitioners in Italy. *Public Health, 117,* 202–207.

U.K. Secretary of State for Health. (1997). *A first class service: Quality in the new NHS.* London: Stationery Office.

CHAPTER FIVE

E-PUBLIC HEALTH INFORMATION SYSTEMS

E-Technologies for Public Health Preparedness and Surveillance

Joseph Tan, Francisco G. Soto Mas, C. Ed Hsu

Learning Objectives

1. Define public health and public health informatics in the context of the evolving e-health care system and environment
2. Understand the basic functions of e-public health information systems
3. Identify key features of e-public health information systems
4. Recognize the differences between legacy and e-public health technologies in practice
5. Understand the application of e-technologies such as geographical information systems (GIS), data warehousing, and data mining methodology in the context of public health preparedness and surveillance
6. Understand the application of GIS-based technology in public health surveillance and rapid epidemiological assessment

Introduction

In this era of knowledge diffusion, rapid advances in quantum sciences and developments in e-technologies promise to revamp every aspect of health and medicine. History documents that in 1793, over five thousand people in a Philadelphia neighborhood—about 10 percent of the city's population—lost their lives within just three months following an outbreak of yellow fever. Had computers been in place two centuries ago, the software would have been able to monitor population health, alert public health officials at an early stage to a possible outbreak, and permit epidemiologists to assess the event rapidly and respond by quarantining the ill, preventing the deaths of a significant number of people.

Present-day applications of information and communication technology (ICT), through the use of tools such as health decision support systems, geographical information systems, and data mining methodologies, can now automatically track and monitor significant health threats and other related events both locally and across the globe (Tan with Sheps, 1998). For example, one surveillance system used by Health Canada searches the Internet for information on potential outbreaks and epidemics. The information collected is then sent to the World Health Organization (WHO) for verification and analysis. This information, in turn, can be used to alert public health officials worldwide to take preventive measures. The WHO's ability to monitor and assist in controlling the spread of recent outbreaks of severe acute respiratory syndrome (SARS), avian flu, and other infectious diseases (for example, chicken pox and monkey pox) worldwide testify to the effectiveness of current public health information systems.

Access to well-documented, timely, and useful information is the key to preventing disease and promoting health. The collection, analysis, use, and communication of health-related information has been called a "quintessential public health service," because all public health work depends on the availability of accurate, comparable, relevant, and timely information (Seldon, Humphreys, Yasnoff, and Ryan, 2001–2002). Public health, then, is a natural venue for the use and application of advanced information technology. E-health technologies may be considered the hub of health care delivery at the macro level, because these technologies link communities to public health practitioners; provide government with information on population health status and changing statistics; allow greater quality improvement; enhance learning about effective methods for responding to outbreaks and other related threats; and channel epidemiologists and public health researchers to concentrate on the health and well-being of the population, on future public health care delivery, and on more effective decision making and policymaking at the community, public health, and governmental levels (Riegelman and Persily, 2001).

The ability to monitor, store, and track e-health information changes the way health care is provided. The preceding chapters discussed the vision and goals of e-health; in this chapter, we argue that the vision of e-health is to promote the health and well-being not only of individuals but also of groups, communities, and entire populations. Earlier chapters showed how e-technologies, in the form of e-health records and other e-technologies (for example, e-prescription systems, e-clinical care, and e-medicine), can assist in realizing such a vision and goals. This chapter focuses on the application of e-technologies in the field of public health—that is, e-health surveillance systems and geographical information systems (GIS).

We begin the chapter by defining *public health* and *e-public health informatics*. We then highlight the potential benefits of a convergence of public health and technology, discussing GIS, public health preparedness, and surveillance. We describe the basic terminology and examine how emerging e-technologies such as GIS, data warehousing, and data mining methodology can support public health readiness, response, and ongoing surveillance in relation to epidemiological and biodefense activities. Tan's model of health information processing functions (Tan, 1995) is adopted to illustrate the potential of various e-technologies and to show how technology such as GIS might enhance preparedness for bioterrorism. An application of GIS in epidemiological rapid assessment is used to illustrate how the scope of traditional public health surveillance can be extended by e-health applications.

The Field of Public Health

The term *public health* conveys different meanings to different people. For new parents, it might mean a vaccination shot to protect their child from Hepatitis B. For tourists in a foreign country, it might mean the comfort of knowing that the restaurants they will be dining in are regularly inspected. For public health students, residents, and practitioners, it might mean the investigation of food or waterborne epidemics in a community. But public health should not only mean preventing disease, injury, and disability. It should mean improving population health and health status and dealing with the most risky and prevailing health issues facing our society. In its early years, public health focused on preventing and dealing with infectious diseases such as yellow fever and tuberculosis. During the Industrial Revolution, public health shifted its attention to chronic disease management, focusing on diabetes, cancer, and heart disease. Today, new and more difficult challenges await us as we deal with newly emerged infections, bioterrorism, and antibiotic-resistant organisms (Yasnoff, Overhage, Humphreys, and LaVenture, 2001). Indeed, a key request expressed urgently by the U.S. government to scientists and researchers is for them to take up the challenge of preparing the nation against bioterrorism and biohazards.

Generally speaking, the science of public health studies the distribution and determinants of health-related states or events in a specific population and works to understand how the acquired information can be applied to control health problems. In differentiating between individual and public health, we may say that a clinician, whose focus is on individual health, will try to determine the disease that an individual has contracted, while a public health practitioner will try to identify the individuals most susceptible to a specific disease or condition. Koo, O'Carroll, and LaVenture (2001) suggest a four-step approach to public health problem solving:

1. Surveillance, or asking what the problem may be
2. Risk factor identification, or asking what the underlying cause of the problem may be
3. Intervention evaluation, or asking what works and what doesn't
4. Implementation, or asking how to go about applying what we have learned

They also propose that the three primary roles of public health practitioners are (1) assessing and monitoring the health of communities and populations at risk to identify health problems and priorities; (2) developing public policy designed to solve these identified health problems; and (3) ensuring that all populations have access to appropriate care, from health promotion to disease prevention services. In an e-public health environment, public health practitioners who can employ the most advanced information technologies will capture the most reliable and current information about disease trends and know the best practices and most effective methods for dealing with public health problems.

The players in the field of public health range from nurses, physicians, and epidemiologists to engineers, social workers, laboratory workers, sanitarians, lawyers, government legislators, and academics. Public health involves all these players because it covers wide-ranging issues from toxic waste disposal to water treatment, from school safety to promoting healthy lifestyles. The large number of players and the variety of issues make the adequate processing of information central to the core functions of public health programs. This leads us to ask, what is e-public health informatics?

E-Public Health Informatics

According to Yasnoff, Overhage, Humphreys, and LaVenture (2001), *public health informatics* may be conceived as "the systematic application of information and computer sciences to public health practice, research and learning. . . . The development of this field and dissemination of informatics knowledge and expertise to public health professionals is the key to unlocking the potential of information systems to improve the health of the nation" (p. 537). While this definition focuses on the role of ICT as a tool for public health professionals to engage individuals, groups, and communities in the process of behavioral and environmental change (Seldon, Humphreys, Yasnoff, and Ryan, 2001–2002), we surmise that in the context of the evolving e-health system and environment, the participation of all stakeholders—including public health professionals and workers, the public, the WHO, hospital physicians, clinicians, leaders in governmental and nongovernmental organizations, health authorities, first responders in emergencies (such as police and firefighters), policymakers, and academic researchers—is critical to the expanding field of e-public health informatics. Based on an expanded view of these earlier definitions, we therefore conceptualize *e-public health informatics* as networks of interconnected e-stakeholders working together through the systematic application of information and communication technologies and e-technologies to achieve timely, high-quality, and cost-effective public health surveillance, preparedness, and care services. E-public health informatics therefore integrates public health with ICT and e-health technologies. In other words, it is the systematic use and application of ICT and e-technologies as tools to support a large network of interconnected e-stakeholders, particularly e-public health professionals and the government, in their goal of protecting and promoting the health and well-being of the public. The discipline covers a gamut of specialties, from e-disease surveillance and e-disease registries to on-line injury and trauma tracking and occupational and environmental health risks monitoring. E-public health informatics also deals with the complicated relationships of ICT and e-technologies in community health services; population screening programs; immunization programs; emergency, disaster, and bioterrorism preparedness and response; and genetics programs. In fact, when e-public health informatics is used to its full advantage, e-public health systems can determine and describe the magnitude of health problems and their sources, analyze risk factors, identify community strengths and particular areas of weaknesses, continually evaluate, refine, and implement what works and promote the health and well-being of entire populations.

Because public health and e-health technologies seem so inextricably linked, it is easy to presume that e-public health informatics would be a well-defined and active discipline. However, just the opposite is true. While the public health community was among the very first in the health discipline to adopt computer technology, the technology was applied in pursuit of narrow, categorical applications rather than applications that would be easily integrated into functional systems for monitoring the health and well-being of communities. Until the last few years, there were only a very limited number of successful e-public health informatics applications. This is due, in part, to lack of resources, poor public health education, inadequate support for population-based public health programs, low-level use of advancing e-technologies and the complexity of e-public health information management problems. The basic computer and telecommunications infrastructure necessary for the implementation of effective e-public health information systems has been slow to develop, because data systems not only require a large front-end investment but are also difficult to change quickly in response to new decision-making trends.

Another problem that has hindered the development of e-public health ICT infrastructure is that public health officials typically do not have the training, necessary experience, or knowledge about the effective implementation of e-public health information systems to make strategic investment decisions about ICT. Although public health staff recognize the immense importance of integrated, computerized information systems as critical tools, the key components of public health ICT infrastructure have not historically been funded by large grants or endowments. This is true even in countries such as Canada and the United States that are known for heavy investment in health care research. For example, Koo, O'Carroll, and LaVenture (2001) state that the U.S. Congress will fund public health programs for disease prevention and control, but there is little or no incentive to fund program-specific ICT-related public health projects, such as development of integrated e-public health information systems that would benefit multiple community and public health programs. The result of this targeted funding approach is that local and state health departments in the United States use distinct, incompatible applications for the entry and analysis of public health data, resulting in data that cannot be easily exchanged, linked, or merged by different programs or used by public health personnel across geographical areas.

Nevertheless, in recent years, the field of e-public health informatics has exploded. The number of academic papers addressing the application of advanced ICT in public health has more than tripled, from only about twenty scientific papers between 1980 and 1984 to over nine hundred between 1996 and 2000 (Seldon, Humphreys, Yasnoff, and Ryan, 2001–2002). Recognition of this newly emerging field is also occurring in universities across the United States and Canada. Schools of public health and health informatics programs at North American universities are introducing new courses to teach the importance of health information systems to the success of public health programs. For instance, Dr. Richard Riegelman, a professor and administrator at the School of Public Health and Health Services at The George Washington University, insists that students of public health need core skills in health information systems, including basic concepts of information management in public health practice and the use of health data (Riegelman and Persily, 2001). E-public health information systems and health communications are the ties that bind the disciplines of public health, health services, and clinical medicine, and thus it is vital for public health practitioners to understand the applications of emerging e-public health technologies.

The linchpin of e-public health information systems is *electronic surveillance*, which is generally defined as automatic and systematic collection, analysis, and interpretation of health data for use in planning, implementing, and evaluating public health programs and practices. E-surveillance is a crucial element in the detection and description of emerging health problems. A critical point in e-public health informatics is that e-surveillance is not only intensively data-driven but also heavily resource-dependent. No single data source or system contains information for all diseases or conditions of interest. Therefore, an e-public health information system that coordinates the tracking and monitoring of all of these data would be an expensive solution. The data must be derived from various sources, including individual family physicians, laboratories, and birth and death certificates. Thus, e-public health informatics is frequently challenged to manage a variety of inconsistent data. A well-designed e-public health information system would create a networked system strong enough to reduce or eliminate these inconsistencies, translate the data into discernible trends and patterns, and discover or identify key population health problems before they become serious.

At this time, we turn to some specific examples and applications of legacy systems and e-public health information systems.

Legacy Health Systems Versus E-Public Health Information Systems

Several applications of legacy (traditional public health information and recording) systems and more current e-public health information systems have recently been put into practice with varying degrees of success. Given the complexity of these systems and the size of the public health field, it is no surprise that creating e-public health technology that catches, tracks, and appropriately assesses the necessary data to determine public health status is an extremely challenging task.

Emerging e-public health technologies include geographical information systems (GIS), data warehousing, and data mining methodology. These e-technologies, which have matured over the years, are now being applied to e-public health information

systems. Before focusing our discussion on specifics, we will survey the essential features of an e-public health information system and compare some legacy systems with
some Internet-based public health information systems.

Key Features of E-Public Health Information Systems

An e-public health information system must support the public health mandate of improving the health status of the community and the population at large. The information system must measure the health of the population against potential
determinants of health. Community health assessment, for example, requires the collection, analysis, interpretation, and communication of key health statistics, data, and
information.

Data-driven e-public health information systems must be comprehensive and take
a broad, strategic view of the community or population health status. These systems
should be feasible and sustainable. Data should come from existing available sources
and must have community-level granularity that can be aggregated to census tracts,
among other geographical identifiers, to address issues of regional variability. Data
from a variety of medical and nonmedical databases should be integrated to provide
the necessary information. Timely information is central to informed development of
public health policy. The output presentation should be easy to read and interpret so
that public health care workers and professionals can easily understand and use the
system.

Population health requires long-term strategies, so the indicators measured and
monitored should include both process (for example, number of hospital visits) and
outcome (for example, infant mortality) indicators. The tracked indicators must be integrated operationally and related to existing public health services. Quantitative indicators that form the community health profile must describe various
sociodemographic characteristics, health status, and quality of life such as morbidity
measures. Specifically, in developing an e-public health statistical system to measure
the health status of a region—say, metropolitan Detroit—we must be able to generally state the life expectancy (in number of years) and the infant mortality rates (infant
deaths per 1,000 live births), as moderated by such variables as gender, age, race,
and location, for residents of the city and its various suburbs.

It is important also to know where and how public health data are collected. Data
are collected in a variety of sites, including hospitals, laboratories, clinics, and workplaces. Several administrative jurisdictions influence the timing of data entry, which
is also influenced by workload and hardware and software access. For example, the
Centers for Disease Control and Prevention (CDC) mandate the registration of birth
in the United States for disease control purposes, but variations in this registration
process occur due to state regulatory requirements and individual hospital regulations.
The initial birth information is recorded locally within a week and sent to the state

department within one to four weeks. The information is then sent to the CDC, and it can take up to a full calendar year for the birth to be recorded in the national registry. In other words, there is a one-year time lag in national data resulting in delayed public health policy implementation and effective key decisions.

In practical terms, timely availability of information is required for effective public health policymaking and decision making; national and even international standards for the registration of information that is significant to population health are essential. Because different health care professionals will use the e-public health information system for different purposes, terminology must also be understandable across professions (Hardiker, Hoy, and Casey, 2000). Other areas of concerns include ease of data retrieval, quality of the data presentation interface, and data sharing among public health authorities and health care providers.

Data are filed by a variety of users, including police, doctors, community health nurses, and paramedics; not everyone who enters data will be aware of how the information is used for public health policy development. Although data from death certificates are used for morbidity and mortality statistics, physicians often complete death certificates quickly and inaccurately. The literature reports different levels of detail of information reported in active public health–initiated surveillance (for example, number of cases of influenza) and in passive surveillance (for example, number of flu shots administered). Other differences have also been found, especially when public health departments rely on different providers for data. Wide differences in terminology prevent the comparison and exchange of public health information. For effective data sharing and communications, efforts must be made to develop controlled vocabularies, classifications, nomenclatures, and thesauri. Ongoing national and international initiatives are striving to develop standard terminology (Hardiker, Hoy, and Casey, 2000).

Public health data about specific individuals must be accurately combined and aggregated at the population level. This information must also be provided to legislators, the community, and e-health care providers. Several nonmedical data sets can be used to monitor community health, including crime, housing, socioeconomic environment, lifestyle, transportation, education, and accidents, all of which should be monitored and reported. Much of this information is collected routinely and can be disaggregated to regional or community levels (Saunders, Mathers, Parry, and Stevens, 2001). Unique identifiers to link health outcomes with specific communities or areas are essential to the functioning of an e-public health information system.

More important, the information collected for public health is very personal, and the risk of harm to patients if information is incorrectly released is high. Safeguards must be implemented to protect the individual and ensure that the community has confidence in the data's security, privacy, and confidentiality.

The creation of a standardized vocabulary is necessary, but even a long-standing standardized classification system is not immune to interpretation errors. The international classification of diseases (ICD) was developed to allow international comparability of mortality and morbidity and has been in place for several decades. Nonetheless, current literature indicates problems with the accuracy of the system. Error rates appear to be related to medical complexity: a low error rate has been found in ophthalmology, and a high number of errors has been found in cardiovascular disease. Errors may also occur because coders, usually health records technicians, are not well trained. In addition, physicians may not specify the discharge diagnosis in the discharge report, or specialists may simply overlook the primary diagnosis.

Following are some specific examples of e-public health information systems that have been put into practice. We hope that the discussion of these examples will illustrate the need for further development of e-technologies for public health surveillance and preparedness.

CATCH

The Comprehensive Assessment for Tracking Community Health (CATCH) is a systematic framework that was developed in southern Florida by the Association of Schools of Public Health in collaboration with the CDC to measure community-level health status. CATCH links health status to resource allocation and policy formulation. CATCH is multidimensional and comprehensive and monitors over two hundred indicators organized into ten major categories, including socioeconomic status, maternal and child health, infectious diseases, and behavioral risk. These indicators are taken from multiple sources that are uniformly collected, available at a county level, and reside in an existing public database. Indicators reported are also comparable to state and national values.

CATCH allows communities to identify health needs of the community groups and to set priorities through the tracking of many indicators. Information collected over a five-year period also allows trend comparisons. CATCH supports displays of the aggregated information in numeric and graphical forms. County indicators that fall below average are listed and evaluated in terms of several key criteria, including the number of people affected, the economic impact, the availability of efficacious treatment or prevention strategies, the trend direction, and the magnitude of the difference between the county values and the average values. Results from using CATCH include achievement of a community focus on high-priority health problems and increased coordination across sectors and across the broad spectrum of community health partners.

CATCH can be considered a legacy public health information system because of the traditional ways in which data are collected within the program. Unfortunately, the program is labor-intensive, and information is collected via telephone, hard-copy documents, or faxes. Data collected must be verified; typically, the time lag between an event and registration of the information into CATCH is three to four months. This time-consuming labor, as well as delays, makes CATCH a very expensive tracking system. Studnicki et al. (2002) note that longitudinal trend analysis may not even be possible with CATCH. Hence, reengineering the data collection methods and building data warehouses to enhance CATCH may increase its process efficiency. The vision for the future is a state-of-the-art relational data warehouse, which must include the use of open network architecture, integrated and robust hardware, and an intelligent interface. Developing dataware to focus on capturing data from the various sources electronically, so that these data can be used to develop a set of CATCH indicators, is a critical next step. The intent is to use the information to establish and maintain a broad strategic view of the community's health status and the various factors that influence that status.

PAPNET

Cervical cytology has been advanced through the development of PAPNET, a computer-assisted screening program to assess cervical smears (PRISMATIC Project Management Team, 1999). The PAPNET system uses neural network–based artificial intelligence to present images of the cells that have the most abnormal appearance to public health screeners in a convenient and interactive fashion. PAPNET software has huge potential; the aim is to decrease screening errors and improve overall screening productivity. This is a clear example of how e-public health technologies can not only improve but also speed up needed interventions.

PAPNET is a health decision support system (Tan with Sheps, 1998) that moves away from legacy public health systems. Since the advent of mass screening programs in the 1960s, pap smear screening has remained unchanged. Screeners must examine countless normal smears just to identify a few abnormal ones. The use of microscopic slides makes the task an even more difficult, highly skilled, and time-consuming process, prone to both false negative and false positive results. The introduction of PAPNET changes the entire process. The system is first used as a primary screening method, in which the neural networks classify routine cervical smears either as negative or needing further screening. Human screeners can then focus on a much smaller set of smears to pick out the abnormal ones.

In a multicenter trial conducted in the United Kingdom to evaluate the screening of cervical smears on PAPNET compared with conventional primary screening, PAPNET-assisted screening showed significantly better specificity, identifying 77 percent of negative smears, while conventional screening identified 42 percent of negative smears. Not only was PAPNET more effective in identifying negative smears, but the system did so at almost three times the speed of conventional screening methods. Specifically, the study demonstrated that PAPNET's total mean time for screening and reporting was 3.9 minutes per smear, as opposed to 10.4 minutes per smear with conventional screening methods.

FluNet

Because our physical environments are constantly being attacked by an increasing number of hazardous and infectious viruses, it is important that we remain aware of virus activity in different parts of the world. FluNet, an Internet-based global surveillance system, is a critically valuable e-public health information system. The WHO developed the application to link its global network of influenza centers. The purpose of FluNet is to serve as an early alert system and to provide real-time epidemiological and virological information. Designated users enter data via secured access; the information is made available to the public through the Internet and thus must be easy to read and use. FluNet's displays are very flexible; information can be presented in a variety of formats, including graphs, maps, tables, and text. Information can also be downloaded and printed.

FluNet demonstrates the power of a global e-surveillance tool. Eighty-three countries work with the WHO through a network of over one hundred national influenza centers. to detect any new virus with pandemic potential—for example, the HIV/AIDS virus. Designated users can submit data, such as influenza activity and viral laboratory results, electronically via secured access; others can send information by e-mail or by fax to ensure up-to-date reporting from networks without FluNet access rights. FluNet then aggregates the data and provides summary statistics based on the analysis. Epidemiological activity and virological results are reported by geographical area for different periods of time. The information gathered by FluNet is also used to determine vaccine composition (Flahault and others, 1998).

Travelers moving from one major city to another may carry influenza viruses without knowing it—that is, even if they do not develop the familiar flu symptoms. Hence, it is easy for contagious viruses to spread from one country to another. It is obvious that FluNet cannot include data that are not available or simply not reported because the effects are not apparent until a breakout occurs. Thus, underreporting of influenza is a limitation of FluNet.

The FluNet system needs to establish some form of standard reporting of incidents and effects of contagious virus infections. Unfortunately, data are reported differently in North America than in Europe or Asia. There are no harmonizing links between the different systems, although FluNet's real-time feedback, which shows patterns of influenza, especially if it is linked with other information such as weather patterns, might provide researchers with clues to the mechanisms of outbreaks. To ensure the speed of reporting and access to FluNet, a mirror application duplicates all reported developments on a separate computer, which reduces waiting time during epidemics.

E-TECHNOLOGIES FOR PUBLIC HEALTH SURVEILLANCE AND PREPAREDNESS

In this section, we introduce the key e-technologies that are currently being applied to aid public health preparedness and surveillance.

GIS-Related Technologies

In recent years, *geographical information systems* (GIS) and associated technologies have been touted as transformational technologies that will facilitate beneficial changes in public health care and improve the speed, quality, cost, and accessibility of public health information and services. Like telemedicine, GIS-related technologies promise to conquer the challenges of space and place (Ricketts, 2003). These computer-based systems integrate and analyze geographically referenced data and comprise a set of tools that enable the collection, storage, manipulation, representation, and modeling of geographically referenced information (Cromley and McLafferty, 2002).

With GIS-related technologies, the physical locations of data items can be identified and presented in relation to various spatial references—for example, coordinates and elevation, geographical boundaries, or transportation arteries. GIS data sets can pertain to population health statistics and trends, community health immunization programs, and emergency or non-emergency health events or incidents. Coordinates (for example, longitude and latitude positioning) and elevation may be coded by means of geographical positioning technology via satellite or other means. Geographical boundaries may be defined by ZIP codes, school districts, census tracts, block groups, or counties, among others. Transportation arteries, of course, may be mapped by specific highways and roads. This mapping information will be crucial in readiness assessment, preparedness planning, and communication with the public.

Among the significant GIS-related technologies for public health preparedness and surveillance are data warehousing and data mining as they are computer-based and reference massive spatial data that need to manipulated, mined, and analyzed. A data warehouse can be of enormous benefit in clinical research, quality improvement, and decision support by enabling quick and efficient access to information from legacy systems and departmental databases. Covvey (2001) distinguishes an *administrative data warehouse* (ADW) from a *clinical data repository* (CDR) by the difference in the use of the two: the ADW is used for management decision making and the CDR for clinical decision making. While these systems both collect, retrieve, analyze, and present health data, the ADW may include clinical, operational, and financial data. Some authors and vendors use these terms interchangeably.

Education of public health students and researchers in e-technologies plays an important role, but other factors also lead to the successful implementation of a data warehouse system. Schubart and Einbinder (2000) specify what "successful usage" means, using concepts such as productivity, user acceptance, usability, and technical adequacy or system flexibility. Interviewing staff and end users, they found a difference between initial and continued use of the data warehouse. Initial use, as predicted, is affected by users' proficiency in computer applications, standard coding, and data retrieval, but continued use requires more: the availability of new information not available elsewhere. It is also important to distinguish between different types of users. For example, physicians and administrators may want and need different classes and types of information, while analysts, who might shape the question, retrieve the data, and clean them up or change the reporting format, may need a totally different set of data. Ultimately, an organizational culture must support the use of a data warehouse to make it effective at producing rich information for a wide variety of users.

Unfortunately, about 40 percent of e-health data warehouse implementation projects fail outright, and up to 85 percent fail to satisfy their owner's objectives. The underlying reason appears to be that data are often collected without a clear understanding of how they are to be applied. Prior to the data gathering and mining process, key questions to be answered include which population cohorts are to be studied, what the specific characteristics are of these cohorts, and what population-related analytic patterns are to be investigated. As well, many components are required, with specific interfaces needed for different queries; the questions that each user poses are varied and often complex. Covvey (2001) describes the creation of an ADW as a project to be approached "with some trepidation." He suggests two options for organizations planning to develop an ADW. One is to design their own components, starting by addressing the needs of the end user; primary considerations in the initial design would include indicators, processing and display of information, data organization, and how to get clean, consistent data from the feeder system. A second option is to acquire a preset, generic ADW and make customized modifications.

Data mining is the main reason for acquiring a data warehouse. *Data mining* involves identifying valid, novel, potentially useful, and ultimately understandable patterns in data; it is a knowledge discovery methodology for working with large databases. A variety of technologies, including neural networks, decision trees, and rule induction, are used to predict and to explain the rationale underlying unusual temporal patterns in the data. When the data are incomplete, imprecise, or redundant, they can be improved by using "rough set analysis" to find underlying relationships among data elements (Tan with Sheps, 1998).

Brossette and others (1998) report the use of data mining techniques to develop a public health surveillance system that was able to identify the occurrence of an infection and anti-microbial resistance in a hospital in Birmingham, Alabama. For instance, epidemiologists are often interested to find out if there may be some socioeconomic, cultural, or environmental factors affecting or causing the emergence of specific diseases in a particular neighborhood, such as a high rate of cancer due to poverty, unhealthy lifestyle practices such as smoking, or the presence of radioactive substances nearby. Such relationships are often hard to detect and require careful studies of correlations among massive amount of data and uncovering of interrelationships among seemingly unrelated variables. In many cases, such investigations could be performed efficiently using data mining techniques such as clustering methods to search for hidden patterns that are yet to be discovered. Epidemiologists may find this technique useful in identifying unusual disease clusters. The e-health records (EHRs) discussed in the previous chapter are an important component of data mining—for example, when integrated by a master patient index to allow record sharing across different settings or regions (Maheu, Whitten, and Allen, 2001). The applicability of data warehousing, EHRs, and data mining techniques to the field of public health lies in their combined ability to track the global spread of disease, to aid in the development of targeted prevention programs, and to examine the efficacy of ongoing public health research by exploring relationships among a large number of seemingly unrelated variables to discover hidden patterns and knowledge.

Figure 5.1 depicts a simplified model of the infrastructure of an e-public health information system.

FIGURE 5.1. MODEL OF AN E-PUBLIC HEALTH INFORMATION SYSTEM

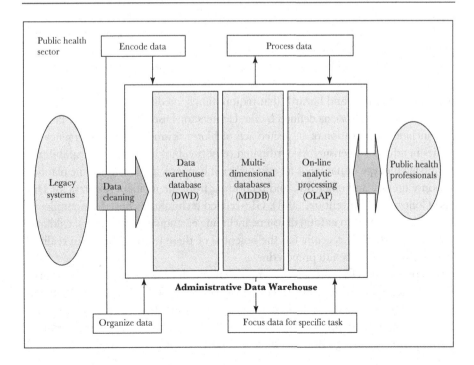

Figure 5.1 provides a model of an e-public health information system that combines the concepts of data warehousing, data mining, and on-line analytic processing (multidimensional data aggregation and data analysis for online queries) of the collected data into trends and patterns, information that is used to alert the public on epidemics or other threats. Data mining techniques have also been used to understand provider behavior, to explain why clinicians choose one treatment over another, and to uncover patient choice patterns related to compliance with medications. Pharmaceutical companies and other vendors also see data mining as a tool for marketing specialty products by detecting patterns of Web use behavior among online purchases and determining product mix.

Epidemiological Surveillance and Public Health Preparedness

Epidemiological surveillance is concerned with the determinants, distribution, and control of potential health hazards, while public health preparedness surveillance encompasses a series of biosecurity measures that can be taken before an emergency, and the subsequent routine collection of potential risk or hazard information. Biodefense efforts can be strengthened by the combined use of emerging GIS-related technologies and health resources repositories including various sources of health related databases (such as EMRs, MEDLINE, epidemiological databases) as well as those pertaining to health facilities and workforces. These e-technologies can also be used to plan and monitor ongoing syndromic or epidemiological surveillance. During biosecurity emergencies, prompt response and deployment of first responders including police, firemen, and public health providers are vital tasks. E-public health information systems that combine GIS-related and data management technologies can identify critical community assets, potential impacts that warrant heightened alert or evacuation, and risks and hazards that require timely mediation.

Preparedness activities, as defined by the Centers for Disease Control and Prevention, include identification of suspected acts of bioterrorism, planning emergency activities in advance to ensure a coordinated response, building response capabilities, identifying the type or nature of an event when it happens, implementing the planned response quickly and efficiently, and recovering from the incident (Centers for Disease Control and Prevention, 2001). GIS-related technologies have been employed for years in response to natural disasters, including earthquakes, tornadoes, wildfires, and hurricanes. Only recently has the potential of these technologies been realized in addressing public health preparedness.

In preparation for emergency response efforts, the federal government created the National Spatial Data Infrastructure by executive order in 1994, in order to encourage geospatial data acquisition and access. The initiative provides an unprecedented mechanism to support GIS-related applications in public health preparedness and response. Applying GIS-related technologies in biodefense may also help fulfill the CDC's objectives of upgrading state and local public health jurisdictions' preparedness for and response capabilities in case of bioterrorism, outbreaks of infectious disease, or other public health threats and emergencies. Use of GIS-related technologies will enable preparedness efforts in the CDC's "Healthy People 2010" priority areas, which focus on immunization and infectious diseases, environmental health, public health infrastructure, and surveillance and data systems (Centers for Disease Control and Prevention, 2001). Objective 23–3 of Healthy People 2010 seeks to increase the proportion of major national, state, and local health data systems that use geocoding. The current baseline indicates that in 2000, 45 percent of major national, state, and local health data operations had records geocoded to street address or latitude and longitude. The CDC set a target of 90 percent geocoded health data by 2010.

GIS-Related Technologies for Emergency Preparedness and Bioterrorism

Among university researchers, GIS-related technologies have been widely used for years in understanding disaster management. In two recent publications addressing the application of GIS-related technologies to preparedness for and responses to bioterrorism, a committee of the National Research Council advocated the integration of GIS into disaster preparedness infrastructure. The committee recommended further research into development of digital floor plans and maps of other physical structures (Science and Technology for Countering Terrorism: Panel on Information Technology, National Research Council, 2003). It was suggested that the resulting data could be stored in geospatial information systems, which would allow responders to focus on high-probability locations of missing people (such as lunchrooms) and avoid dangerous searches of low-probability locations (such as storage areas). The committee recommended research in wearable computers for search-and-rescue operations, so that responders could update GIS software in real time as they discovered victims and encountered structural damage (Committee on Science and Technology for Countering Terrorism, National Research Council, 2002). In practice, the past few years have also seen personal digital assistants and remote sensing technologies used in disaster relief.

Consider this example of how GIS-based equipment can help in an emergency. In the first four days of the rescue attempts in New York City after the World Trade Center attacks on September 11, 2001, no GIS equipment was available. Rescue workers had to create maps on cardboard or use shopping guides to draw maps of unstable buildings. Once GIS equipment and related software arrived, people from the Federal Emergency Management Agency were able to create maps of the World Trade Center site and lower Manhattan that ranged from simple maps showing locations of command posts, first aid centers, and food stations to others depicting hazards such as lingering fires and debris hanging from buildings ("Mapping the Hazards to Keep Rescuers Safe," 2001). GIS-related techniques that are usually used to determine structural soundness after earthquakes were applied to the World Trade Center area for rapid assessment of the surrounding structures (Nishenko, 2002). Having participated in the search and rescue effort in New York City, one specialist reported that GIS and location-based technologies were used extensively and proved extremely valuable (Kevany, 2003).

Both GIS-related technologies and public health surveillance are concerned with the spatial and temporal dimensions of public health problems. What is important is how human beings are represented in both dimensions when events unfold. Figure 5.2 illustrates these convergent interests. For example, in an event that raises biosecurity concerns, mission-critical challenges would be to identify the epicenter and boundaries of the event, understand the available resources, identify the affected populations and characteristics of the communities, and, of course, avoid potential hazards in a timely manner. Transportation intelligence, such as knowledge of major arteries and roads surrounding the event, would afford valuable information on how to reach vulnerable populations. Providing authorities with this critical information gives them the intelligent decision support they need in order to make informed actions and choices.

Although many recent experiences have indicated that GIS-related technologies will prove useful in disaster preparedness and relief, there is still a lack of literature examining their functional components and their application to public health surveillance and bioterrorism preparedness. The next sections show how GIS-related

FIGURE 5.2. THE CONVERGENCE OF GEOGRAPHICAL INFORMA-TION SYSTEMS, PUBLIC HEALTH PREPAREDNESS AND RESPONSE, AND EPIDEMIOLOGICAL SURVEILLANCE

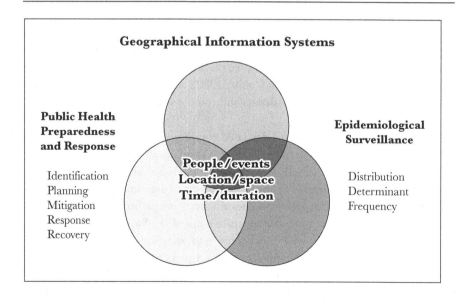

technologies can meet the needs of public health surveillance and illustrate how GIS-related technologies can be applied to support public health emergency preparedness, particularly biodefense preparedness efforts in specific targeted areas.

GIS-Related Data Management for Emergency Preparedness

According to an informatics model suggested in Tan (1995, p. 12), a basic health information processing system includes at least the following components: data acquisition and verification (data input); data storage, classification, computations, and update (data management); and data retrieval and presentation (data output). GIS-related technologies can meet these requirements and are well positioned to transform data into meaningfully stratified information, making the transition from aggregated information to valuable and strategically organized knowledge.

As part of an e-public health information system or application, GIS-related technologies can support direct or indirect (data extracted from available secondary sources) data input and verification from either a desktop computer or a Web-based browser that interfaces with a data storage system, which may be a data warehouse or a suite of databases. At least four data categories may warrant inclusion in a GIS-related application for use in biodefense preparedness.

- Assets data
- Data on hazard sites
- Data on transportation routes and utility networks
- Data on free space

Assets data are data groupings that identify priority areas to be protected or used—for example, population attributes, locations, repositories, facilities, and response teams. Some important population attributes include density of residents; subpopulations by age, race, and ethnicity; and vulnerable populations or their locations—for example, senior citizens, nursing homes, school districts, and non–English-speaking ethnic communities. Specific location data would include locations of health facilities, beds, and surge capacity; laboratories, pharmacies, and veterinarians; National Pharmaceutical Stockpile locations; emergency vaccine and drug administration locations; predesignated vaccine repositories; and waterways, including boundaries, flood plains, treatment plants, pumping stations, well locations, emergency water supplies, water towers, and reservoirs; public facilities; emergency management supplies; and community services and response teams, including fire departments and command centers. *Data on hazard sites* identify the priority areas to mediate or avoid, such as radiological sites. *Data on transportation routes and utility networks* can identify, for example, areas in service, restricted areas, or areas under construction. These data would be used for response actions, such as triage, relief, or evacuation. Finally, *free space data* would be critical in specifying locations for loading and unloading of emergency supplies, parking space, and temporary setup of safe and secured shelters.

For data management, GIS-related technologies will allow various users to manipulate data, perform data processing functions such as inserting data, updating entered data, appending new data to original data sets, or deleting stored data. Data mining methodology has powerful abilities to rotate, dice, and cluster "cleaned" data sets to reveal new knowledge, discover hidden patterns, or unveil general trends. Many sophisticated analytical methods and statistical techniques can be applied in data mining. As long as the captured data can be properly cleaned and verified, organized information can be managed and transformed into valuable knowledge for emergency response teams, including police, firefighters, and community leaders.

GIS output data can be aggregated, reformatted, mapped, and disseminated. The classes of output data specific to GIS-related representations and analysis include at least five major categories:

- Geocoded events
- Choropleth maps
- Buffer zones
- Network analysis
- Overlay analysis

Geocoded events refer to "pinned" maps (think of a map display with a pin indicating the location of each event) that indicate hot spots or display spatial patterns of affected areas or regions. This can be used to present thematic maps such as geo-coding the most intensely affected areas that describe a geographically referenced event. A *choropleth map* shows areas or regions that have the same characteristics, using color coding or shading to represent the magnitude of measures or indicators. Answers to spatial queries about specific affected locations, such as schools, nursing homes, and other public or community facilities, can be represented with spatially color coded or geographically referenced information. *Buffer zones* are represented by concentric circles or polygons that define the anticipated or actual scope of impact (exposure) and associated or corresponding response time. *Network analysis* can provide useful information to help determine travel time and the shortest routes available for rescue, evacuation, or other purposes. *Overlay analysis* can result in two forms of displays: *point-in-polygon maps*, which display whether data with specific attributes (such as incidence of a disease) fall within a certain circumference, and *polygon-overlaid maps*, which can be used to create a new map layer encompassing two or more existing layers.

Figure 5.3 presents an expanded GIS-enabled e-health technology framework, including data input, data management, and data output functions.

FIGURE 5.3. AN INTEGRATED GIS-BASED PUBLIC HEALTH PREPAREDNESS SYSTEM

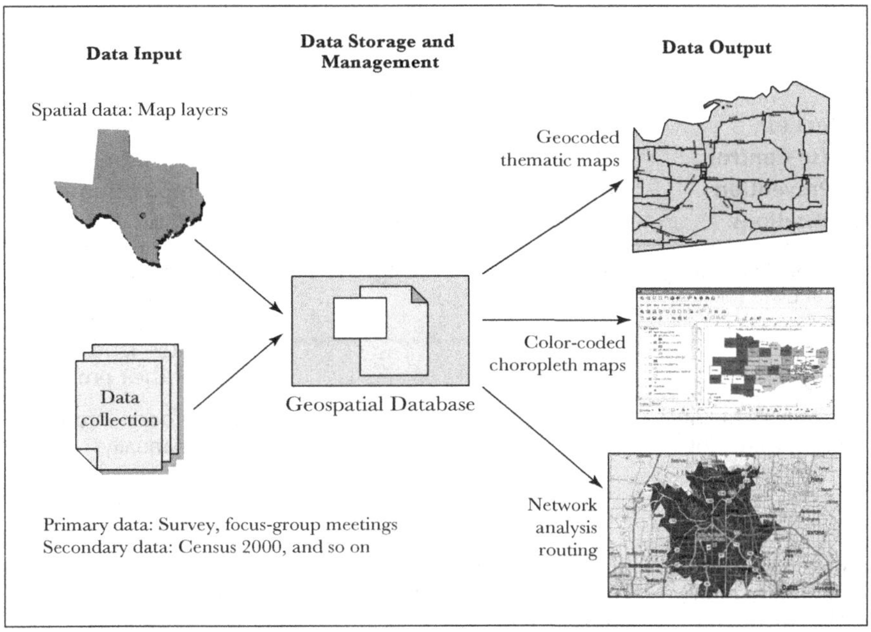

In generating guidelines for the application of ICT to biosecurity in 2001, the CDC produced a report describing the ICT functions and specifications for public health emergency preparedness and bioterrorism (Centers for Disease Control and Prevention, 2001). A GIS-enabled public health information system has substantial potential to fulfill all the functions and specifications provided by the CDC. For example, GIS-related technologies can use electronic clinical data for event detection, use data mining methodology to investigate possible hazard diffusion patterns, and manage and process electronic data from care systems at clinical care sites and laboratories.

For data analysis and visualization, GIS-related technologies can analyze, display, report, and map accumulated data from other public health partners and share data and technologies for analysis and visualization. A detailed list of GIS-related technology's ability to fulfill the CDC requirements is presented in Table 5.1.

The application of GIS-related technologies to public health preparedness is a classic example of how an e-public health information system could transform the future of public health preparedness and surveillance: in data acquisition, GIS-related technologies could enhance traditional data collection efforts, allowing rapid needs

TABLE 5.1. TAN'S HEALTH INFORMATION PROCESSING SYSTEM AND CDC-PROVIDED INFORMATION TECHNOLOGY SPECIFICA-TIONS FOR EMERGENCY AND BIOTERRORISM PREPAREDNESS

	Health Information Processing System (Tan, 1995)		
Centers for Disease Control and Prevention Specifications	Data Input • Acquisition • Verification	Data Management • Storage • Classification	Data Output • Retrieval • Presentation • Computation • Update
1. Use of Electronic Clinical Data for Event Detection	Receive,	manage,	and process electronic data from care systems at clinical care sites, laboratories, or their proxies
2. Manual Data Entry for Event Detection and Management	Accumulate,	manage,	and process information manually entered via a Web browser at a health agency or remote site
3. Specimen and Lab Result Information Management and Exchange	For laboratories involved in public health testing, receive laboratory requests, accept specimen and sample data,	manage these data,	and immediately report electronic results to public health partners
4. Management of Possible Case, Contacts, and Threat Data	Electronically accumulate,	manage, link	and process the different types of data (track possible cases detected, possible contacts, facility, lab results, prophylaxis or vaccination; monitor adverse events and follow-up)
5. Analysis and Visualization	Analyze, display, report, and map accumulated data, and share data and technologies for analysis and visualization with other public health partners		

Centers for Disease Control and Prevention Specifications	Data Input • Acquisition • Verification	Data Management • Storage • Classification	Data Output • Retrieval • Presentation • Computation • Update
6. Directories of Public Health and Clinical Personnel	Manually or automatically develop and	maintain directories of public health participants, including primary clinical personnel, participant roles, and contact information.	Geographically referenced information can be shown as a mouse rolls over its location on a map.
7. Public Health Information Dissemination and Alerting	Receive,	manage,	and disseminate alerts, protocols, procedures, and other information for public health workers, primary care providers, and public health partners in emergency response

Health Information Processing System (Tan, 1995)

Sources: Adapted from Centers for Disease Control and Prevention, 2001, and Tan, 1995.

assessment; in data storage and output, the use of a geospatial metadatabase will permit both primary data (such as needs assessment data collected from the field) and secondary data (such as census data) to be stored in a central relational database repository or, more likely, a data warehouse, either of which would allow the data to be mined and displayed in various ways.

A metadatabase (data about data), describes the content, quality, condition, and other characteristics of data. It refers to the federally mandated open geographical data structure that was approved by the Federal Geographic Data Committee. The open data warehouse structure will allow authorized agencies to query, present, and analyze the data for public health preparedness and response purposes.

A GIS-Enabled System for Health Surveillance and Epidemiological Rapid Assessment

Rapid public health assessment quickly determines public health needs in affected areas after disasters such as floods, bioterrorism, or toxic exposures. It can help determine the boundaries of affected areas; the duration and intensities of exposures; water and food supply disruptions; risks for various subpopulations; zoonotic disease risks; and the need for short-term health measures or quarantines. Rapid public health assessment can also be a point of departure for communicating public health advice and investigating longer-term health effects. A rapid assessment may be undertaken immediately after or even during an event, or it may be done as a preparedness or preventive measure. The assessment usually consists of identification of the area that is affected or could be affected, followed by a sampling scheme, and then the rapid assessment coordination. In this sense, GIS mapping technology can coordinate the communications among multiple first responders of where and how the affected area would be optimally secured for managing and containing the hazards.

GIS is central to providing maps of factors affecting the event area in response to emergencies. The CDC has identified seven key components, or focus areas, that are necessary for a comprehensive public health response:

- Focus Area A: Preparedness planning and readiness assessment
- Focus Area B: Surveillance and epidemiological capacity
- Focus Areas C and D: Laboratory capacity—specifically, biological and chemical agents
- Focus Areas E and F: Risk communication and health information dissemination
- Focus Area G: Training and education

How a GIS-enabled rapid assessment system can address CDC public health preparedness focus areas is discussed next.

A GIS-supported preparedness plan could assess preparedness by either geographical area or jurisdiction and provide logistical support for program planning, implementation, and quality assurance. As described earlier, GIS-related technologies can produce preparedness data inventories and thematic maps to assist in assessing the level of preparedness and offering strategic recommendations for coordination and resource allocation. The system can provide enhanced mapping and visualization of complex and changing data, coupled with spatial analysis that affords heads-up, next-step information for preparedness and response planning.

Obviously, such an e-public preparedness system can be used for ongoing surveillance of community health. The geographical characteristics of such data systems make it useful for

- Disease surveillance and reporting
- Sentinel measures: data from doctors, hospitals, pharmacies

- Early location of syndromes in space and time: detection of symptom and case clusters; identification of exposure sources; early detection of biological, chemical, or radioactive events
- Aiding issuance of health warnings and precautions
- Disease outbreak mapping; rapid assessment mapping
- Incidence and prevalence mapping in relation to health care locations or special populations; exposures and risk factors

In preparedness planning, GIS-related technologies can link databases containing updated data from various sources, as discussed previously. Having this repository of data at the preparedness stage makes a rapid assessment possible. In turn, this facilitates accurate forecasting of casualties and other public health needs for various scenarios. GIS-enabled activities can provide logistical support in reviewing surveillance systems, enhancing syndromic early alert capacity, contributing to regional efforts in training of health care providers and in developing an emergency decision support system (EDSS).

The EDSS can be supported by the GIS data collection and rapid assessment activities. Data collection includes geocoded, systematic syndromic surveillance data, which can be saved in GIS-compatible metadatabase format. Geographically coded metadata can be shared and used to conduct data analysis and produce maps across multiple platforms and agencies. In short, the health data saved in such a structure will be readable by most GIS software including the CDC's EpiInfo 2002 and EpiMap, the mapping component of EpiInfo 2002. Metadata products can include preparedness-related relational databases, thematic maps, and educational components for regional training activities.

Rapid assessment can be conducted by using geospatial analysis and epidemiological surveillance. Indeed, a rapid assessment may merely be an accelerated and focused step in routine disease surveillance. Using GIS in routine disease surveillance can facilitate the fine-tuning of geographical health analysis in an epidemiological surveillance activity. GIS-related technologies facilitate rapid identification of high-risk areas and populations; staff can develop expertise in this activity for risk identification and mitigation.

GIS-enabled activities can maintain geographically referenced databases of laboratories, including staffing personnel, capacity of internal and external proficiency testing, and other preparedness data. First, mapping changing capabilities and contact information will be extremely important to monitoring overall laboratory readiness. Second, in an emergency such as the anthrax attacks of 2001, a system that can locate where samples have been sent and where they are being processed will be extremely important. As well, GIS-related technologies can identify the populations in the catchment areas of hospitals, assessing the hospital's bioterrorism response capabilities (for example, isolation wards, decontamination units, personnel) and combining these data with information on the populations the hospital serves. GIS-related technologies work effectively in locating resources for use in cases of environmental exposure—for example, mapping where chemical assays are being conducted within the state and where advanced biomonitoring and testing can be obtained in a crisis. The databases will support health authorities in implementing triage procedures to prioritize intake and testing of specimens (samples) before analysis.

The combination of health information and geographical data in one analytical tool is still new for much of public health. In a public health emergency, geography assumes more importance because of limited mobility and the physical immediacy of health threats. The strength of GIS-related technologies in these situations is exemplified by rapid assessment—for example, determining which hospitals have both isolation units and certain kinds of laboratories, or determining from age distributions in census tracts the best school locations from which to administer vaccinations for vulnerable age groups. Where information is lacking on, for example, the prevalence of acute disease symptoms, GIS-facilitated rapid assessment can help professionals design a logical sampling scheme based on population density and proximity to an event.

In an emergency, risk communication is particularly important for communities with predominantly non–English-speaking populations. For this purpose, geographically referenced (mapped) information holds promise for helping to bridge language and semantic barriers in communications. Several schools of public health, the CDC, and large metropolitan areas and health departments have developed risk communication pre-messaging programs, in which messages in different languages are created in advance for use in case of emergency. As programs are developed, a repository can be created. A geographically referenced repository of risk communication tools will be critical to the preparedness effort. A GIS-enabled inventory can provide information on where these programs are and where they are needed and monitor the process of dissemination.

Finally training and education is critical if GIS-related technologies are to be used successfully. Currently, there is an apparent lack of expertise among organizational users including governmental agencies and first responders on the use and applications of GIS-related technologies to real world problem solving. These technologies provide useful insights into spatial data relationships and allow massive amount of data to be mined simultaneously. Many universities conduct courses and research in geographical information systems. Most of these courses are either offered by the geography department in collaboration with computer science, library science, or information systems. Public health scientists and professionals alike will therefore benefit significantly from acquiring expertise and skills in GIS-related technologies.

Conclusion

In a field exploding with possibilities, there are many challenges to conquer before the vision of an integrated, accessible, and accurate e-public health information system becomes a reality. Three areas represent major challenges to e-public health informatics: (1) developing coherent and integrated national and international e-public health information systems; (2) developing a closer integration of public health and clinical care; and (3) addressing pervasive concerns about the effects of information and communication technology on confidentiality and privacy, as discussed in Chapter Four. Beyond this, the hope is that we can apply e-technologies in unanticipated ways to remake public health and create new ways to protect and promote community health. In particular, aside from the promotion of health and the prevention of unnecessary disease, injury, and disability, there are unexplored and unimagined ways of harnessing the power of ICT to transform the way we as members of society take care of one another—for example, in public preparedness against bioterrorism and biohazards.

More than anything, the future of e-public health informatics is about globalization and a safer environment for all populations. The World Health Organization is committed to the measurement of health outcomes, using internationally agreed-on indicators at the level of populations (for example, community level), so comparisons of the value of specific strategies can be made. The U.S. government is focusing its public health efforts primarily on preparedness and surveillance for bioterrorism and other similar threats. Meeting the decentralized information needs of all stakeholders demands an excellent e-public health information system. Health needs, not the market, should drive the acquisition of technology. Given the difference in health care budgets among various stakeholders, collaboration among stakeholders is essential. As a group, they can take advantage of economies of scale to demand compatibility, open architecture, competitive prices, and pilot applications. The applications of e-public technologies may provide an interesting model for public health informaticians to watch and learn from in the future.

Chapter Questions

1. How can public health benefit from e-health informatics concepts? What are the barriers in introducing e-health informatics concepts in public health?
2. Differentiate legacy systems from e-public health information systems. Compare CATCH, PAPNET, and FluNet.
3. How can GIS technologies help with public health preparedness and surveillance?

4. Imagine that you are planning to visit a country that is experiencing an epidemic of avian flu. Travelers returning from affected countries are being screened, and you don't want to be stopped at customs or to be quarantined. What steps can you take to ensure that you are safe and that you will be able to get through customs quickly on your return trip? Where would you look for information?

References

Adams, M. (2000). Validity of birth certificate data for the outcome of the previous pregnancy, Georgia 1980–1995. *American Journal of Epidemiology*, 154(10), 883.

Brossette, S. E., Hardin, J. M., Jones, W. T., Moser, S. A., Sprague, A. P., & Waites, K. B. (1998). Association rules and data mining in hospital infection control and public health surveillance. *Journal of the American Informatics Association*, 5(4), 373.

Centers for Disease Control and Prevention, U.S. Department of Health and Human Services. (2001). *Public health response to biological and chemical terrorism*. Atlanta, GA.

Committee on Science and Technology for Countering Terrorism, National Research Council. (2002). *Making the nation safer: The role of science and technology in countering terrorism*. Retrieved from http://search.nap.edu/terror

Covvey, H. D. (2001). What's a data warehouse? *Health Care Information Management and Communication*, 15(3), 36.

Cromley, E. K., & McLafferty S. L. (2002). *Geographic information systems: GIS and public health*. New York: Guilford Press.

Flahault, A., Dias-Ferrao, V., Chaberty, P., Esteves, K., Valleron, A., & Lavanchy, D. (1998). FluNet as a tool for global monitoring of influenza on the Web. *Journal of the American Medical Association*, *280*, 1330–1332.

Hardiker, N., Hoy, D., & Casey, A. (2000). Standards for nursing terminology. *Journal of the American Medical Informatics Association*, 7(6), 523–528.

Kevany M. J. (2003). GIS in the World Trade Center attack: Trial by fire. *Computers, Environment and Urban Systems*, 27(6), 571–583.

Kirby, R. (2001). Using vital statistics databases for perinatal epidemiology: Does the quality go in before the name goes on? *American Journal of Epidemiology*, *154*(10) 889.

Koo, D., O'Carroll, P., & LaVenture, M. (2001). Public Health 101 for informaticians. *Journal of the American Medical Informatics Association*, 8(6), 585–597.

Maheu, M., Whitten, P., & Allen, A. (2001). *E-health, telehealth, and telemedicine: A guide to start-up and success*. San Francisco: Jossey-Bass.

Mapping the hazards to keep rescuers safe. (2001, October 4). *New York Times* Retrieved from http://www.nytimes.com/2001/10/04/technology/circuits/04MAPS.html?ex=100315>%201502&ei=1&en=204ee22d59ff49ea

Nishenko, S. (2002). *Critical infrastructure*. Presentation at the Natural Disasters Roundtable Forum on Countering Terrorism: Lessons Learned From Natural and Technological Disasters, Washington, DC.

Pinner, R. (1998, July–September). Public health surveillance and information technology. *Emerging Infectious Diseases*, *4*, 462–465.

PRISMATIC Project Management Team. (1999, April 24). Assessment of automated primary screening on PAPNET of cervical smears in the PRISMATIC trial. *Lancet*, *353*, 1381–1385.

Ricketts, T. C. (2003). Geographic information systems and public health. *Annual Review of Public Health, 24*, 1–6.

Riegelman, R., & Persily, N. (2001). Health information systems and health communications: Narrowband and broadband technologies as core public health competencies. *American Journal of Public Health, 91*(8), 1179–1183.

Saunders, P., Mathers, J., Parry, J., & Stevens, A. (2001). Identifying non-medial datasets to monitor community health and well-being. *Journal of Public Health Medicine, 23*, 103–108.

Schubart, J., and Einbinder, J. (2000). Evaluation of a data warehouse in an academic health sciences centre. *International Journal of Medical Informatics, 60*, 319.

Science and Technology for Countering Terrorism: Panel on Information Technology, National Research Council (2003). *Information technology for counterterrorism: Immediate actions and future possibilities.* Retrieved from http://www7.nationalacademies.org/cstb/project_counteringterrorism.html

Seldon, C., Humphreys, B., Yasnoff, W., & Ryan, M. (2001–2002). Public health informatics. *Current Bibliographies in Medicine, National Library of Medicine.*

Studnicki, J., Murphy, F., Malvey, D., Costello, R., et al. (2002, Winter). Toward a population health delivery system: First steps in performance measurement. *Health Care Management Review, 27*, 76–95.

Studnicki, J., Steverson, B., Myers, B., Hevner, A., & Berndt, D. (1997, September/October). Comprehensive assessment for tracking community health (CATCH). *Best Practices and Benchmarking in Healthcare, 2*, 197–207.

Tan, J. (1995). *Health management information systems: Theories, methods and applications.* (1st ed.). Sudbury, MA: Jones & Bartlett.

Tan, J., with Sheps, S. (1998). *Health decision support systems.* Sudbury, MA: Jones & Bartlett.

Yasnoff, W., Overhage, J. M., Humphreys, B., & LaVenture, M. (2001). A national agenda for public health informatics: Summarized recommendations from the 2001 AMIA spring congress. *Journal of the American Medical Informatics Association*, 8(6), 535–545.

E-Profiling of Community Health Performance Indicators Case

Lee Kallenbach, Joseph Tan

During times of increasing uncertainty, gathering massive amounts of data is insufficient without the ability to transform the data into critical information and organized knowledge to support intelligent decision making and policymaking at all levels. Information technology (IT) can play a significant role in that transformation. For example, a technologically driven program for public and community health that applies software tools and analytical methods such as intelligent software, data mining, expert systems which are domain-specific health decision support systems, complex simulation and mathematical models, and geographical information systems as well as Internet and wireless technologies can contribute significantly to individual and community health and performance as measured by specific indicators, promote community health and wellness such as healthy lifestyle and group behavioral patterns, and advance our understanding of critical steps needed to improve health for all.

The field of public and community health is growing and expanding. There is great potential to combine the fields of health and medical informatics, community health care, epidemiology, biostatistics, health management, and policy research. This confluence of disciplines could improve our understanding of how best to prepare the public, particularly at the community level, to deal with everyday threats, including HIV/AIDS, obesity, cancer, congestive heart failure, diabetes, and other chronic and infectious diseases, as well as potential threats from bioterrorism and other emerging challenges, including new or mutated contagious diseases. The first step is learning how to track and monitor community health performance data electronically, which is the focus of the case example discussed here.

The goal of the Community Health Institutes (CHI) at Wayne State University, in collaboration with the Detroit Medical Center, is to produce a set of indicators for community health performance monitoring (for example, health status) based on several key criteria. These include tracking data that have the following characteristics:

- Small geographic areas (smaller than counties)
- Annual measures
- Readily available indicators
- Data available for the entire tricounty Detroit area

Background on Community Health

In communities, health is a product of many factors, and many segments of the community can contribute to and share responsibility for health protection and improvement. Changes in public policy, in public-sector and private-sector roles and accountability in health and health care, and in public expectations present both opportunities and challenges.

Performance monitoring offers a tool to assess activities in the many sectors that can influence health and wellness at the community level. Assessing performance indicators at this level via the use of available and advancing e-technologies is also an effective means of promoting both collaboration and accountability among practitioners, researchers, and policymakers in working toward better health for the entire community, especially within the framework of a community-based health improvement process. Performance monitoring relies on selection of a set of meaningful and measurable indicators to determine community health.

As a starting point in measuring the health of its community, CHI has adopted the twenty-five indexes proposed by the Institute of Medicine (IOM) in their publication *Improving Health in the Community: A Role for Performance Monitoring* (1997). These twenty-five indexes (see Exhibit 5.1) represent six domains of health and community information: demographic characteristics (such as age, ethnicity, education, and employment status), health status (such as infant mortality and death rates), health risk behavior (such as prevalence of smoking and obesity), health care resource consumption (such as per capita Medicare spending), functional status (such as self-reported health status), and quality of life (such as satisfaction with existing health care systems).

EXHIBIT 5.1. INDEXES FOR COMMUNITY HEALTH PROFILE

#	Indicator Topic	4 Criteria*				CHI
	Sociodemographic	Zip	Annual	Available	Tri-county	Profile
1	Age and race/ethnicity	Yes	census	Yes	Yes	YES
2	Groups whose access to community services or resources may be limited	Yes	census	Consider	Yes	NO
3	Educational attainment (HS graduation)	Yes	census	Yes	Yes	YES
4	HS dropouts	No	Yes	Consider	Yes	NO
5	Household income (median)	Yes	census	Yes	Yes	YES
6	Children in poverty	Yes	census	Yes	Yes	Kids
7	Unemployment rate	Yes	census	Yes	Yes	YES
8	Single-parent families	Yes	census	Yes	Yes	YES
9	Persons without health insurance			No		NO
	Health Status					
10	Infant mortality	Yes	census	Yes	Yes	YES
11	Death rates, selected causes	Yes	census	Yes	Yes	YES
12	Incidence of communicable diseases	Yes	census	Consider	Yes	NO
13	Births to adolescents	Yes	census	Yes	Yes	YES
14	Child abuse and neglect	Yes	census	Consider	Yes	NO
	Health Risk Factors					
15	Preschool immunization	Yes	census	Yes	Yes	Kids
16	Older adult immunization	Yes	census	Consider	Yes	NO
17	Prevalence of smoking			No	Yes	NO
18	Prevalence of obesity			No	Yes	NO
19	Air quality	No			Yes	NO
20	Water quality (for recreational uses)	No			Yes	NO
	Health Care Resource Consumption					
21	Per capita Medicare spending	No	Yes	Consider	Yes	NO
	Functional Status					
22	Self-reported health status			No		NO
23	Recent poor health			No		NO
	Quality of Life					
24	Satisfaction with health care system			No		NO
25	Satisfaction with quality of life			No		NO

Available Data Source in Michigan (NOT in IOM)

	CHI Added Indicators	4 Criteria*				CHI
		Zip	Annual	Available	Tri-county	Profile
1	Preventable Hospitilizations (selected)	Yes	Yes	Yes	Yes	YES
2	Cancer Incidence (selected causes)	Yes	Yes	Yes	Yes	YES

Birth Indicators

	Kidscount Indicators	4 Criteria*				CHI
		Zip	Annual	Available	Tri-county	Profile
1	Percent of Teen Births	Yes	Yes	Yes	Yes	YES
2	Percent of Repeat Teen Births	Yes	Yes	Yes	Yes	YES
3	Percent of Births to Unmarried Women	Yes	Yes	Yes	Yes	YES
4	% to Mothers with <12 years of Education	Yes	Yes	Yes	Yes	YES
5	% of Births with Late or No Prenatal Care	Yes	Yes	Yes	Yes	YES
6	% of Births to Mothers Smoked During Pregnancy	Yes	Yes	Yes	Yes	YES
7	Percent of Low Birthweight Babies	Yes	Yes	Yes	Yes	YES
8	Percent of Preterm Babies	Yes	Yes	Yes	Yes	YES

* Status of availability

Source: Durch, Bailey, and Stoto, 1997.

The six domains were chosen to present a broad and inclusive picture of health and emphasize the context of community health improvement.

In addition, other available measures (for example, cancer incidence, birth indicators, and hospitalizations) were used as CHI community health profile indicators.

Community Diagnosis

Just as a physician or other health care practitioner makes a diagnosis based on an individual's signs and symptoms, so too can a community diagnose its own signs and symptoms. The community can make sense of the collected data, using information technology to transform the data into meaningful information in order to provide a diagnosis and develop a treatment plan involving interventions at the community level.

For example, we can track the life expectancy of various population samples in different counties, townships, or communities within metropolitan Detroit, gathering data on the various indicators to see how different counties or townships perform in terms of life expectancy, infant mortality, and other measures as moderated by the variables (for example, age, ethnicity). This information can be further analyzed and aggregated in different ways to provide us with a picture of the health status and the health needs of the different counties, townships, or communities. A plan for health intervention can then be developed to improve the health status (for example, life expectancy or infant mortality) of specific counties, townships, or communities.

Selection of Profile Indicators

The indicators reported in the CHI Profile include those recommended by the IOM based on data that are readily available for the tricounty metropolitan Detroit area from existing computerized data sources. The CHI Profile also includes detail related to births that is similar to that presented by kidscount.org, which is more detailed than the IOM recommendations. In addition, the CHI Profile includes a number of measures based on data available in Michigan (cancer incidence and hospitalizations) that are not part of the IOM recommendation. Many of the indicators recommended by the IOM depend on primary data collection through household survey. These types of data are not readily available, and so such indicators are not currently included in the CHI Profile.

Geographic Areas

The intention of CHI-Mart, as of any community database, is to be flexible and to provide information aggregated into a number of different geographic representations. This is best accomplished by building larger areas from information available for smaller areas, which serve as building blocks.

Generally, while we may not be interested in units as small as census tracts, we are interested in units that have been defined as aggregates of census tracts. Unfortunately, this means that the source information is coded to census tract, which requires street address–level information. Street address information, like names, is considered to be confidential because it can be used to identify individuals. Obtaining permission to acquire confidential data can be difficult without a specific research protocol.

The population that resides in each geographic area is related to the size of that area. The validity of the health indexes presented in the CHI Profile is affected by the number of events counted in relation to the size of the population in each geographic area. The discipline of epidemiology deals with the calculation of rates of disease or events in a population. Calculating a statistically stable rate requires a population of adequate size. For common events, this can be small, but when the event is rare, the population size required can become quite large. Counts of people or major events (such as births and deaths) can be presented for areas with small populations. However, when presenting numbers for detailed subgroups (white females aged 40–44) or when examining less common events (HIV infection), larger populations are desirable. Therefore, population size affects the determination of which geographic area is best for a particular information or data characterization purpose. For these reasons, we have initially chosen to aggregate information by zip codes or groups of zip codes with populations of at least 25,000. However, some of the indexes recommended by the IOM may not have information readily available for zip codes.

Timeliness

Timeliness refers to two aspects of data collection: frequency and time from collection to report. Some of the information required to develop the IOM indexes is collected yearly; some information is collected at longer intervals; and some information is not routinely collected at all. In addition, while some information may be collected on an ongoing basis, reporting of the information might be done a number of years later. This raises issues of how meaningful the information may be, which in turn affects the value of the reporting.

Data collected every year and reported before the end of the following year are considered to be very timely. Timeliness coupled with a need for geographic specificity presents a further challenge to producing a profile that contains useful information for real-time program planning and evaluation.

Exhibit 5.2 illustrates the community health data profiling for a single geographic area covered by the CHI Profile.

The CHI Profile was produced to provide members of a community and those that offer service to a community with information to help them improve their community's health. The CHI Profile can be used by many individuals, groups, and organizations to learn something new, make decisions, or solve problems related to their community's health. Thus, there will be many different uses of "report cards," a

EXHIBIT 5.2. COMMUNITY HEALTH PROFILE

CHI District Profile - 48227/Peer Area - Detroit

Population Description (2000)			Tri-County Area Detroit, Michigan
Total Population	**61,118**	**Rank**	
By Age Group	**N**	**(%)**	
0-17	19,783	32.37	
18-44	23,499	38.45	
45-64	13,045	21.34	
65+	4,791	7.84	
By Race/Ethnicity	**N**	**(%)**	
One Race Alone	60,336	98.72	
Black	58,764	96.15	
White	1,276	2.09	
Other	296	0.48	
Two or More Races	782	1.28	
Hispanic Origin	391	0.64	
Sociodemographic (2000)	**(%)**	**Rank**	
Single Parent Families	34.35	12/21	
High School Graduates	74.86	16/20	
Unemployment	12.20	15/21	
Median Household Income	$31,760	14/21	
Public Assistance Income	12.28	10/21	
Poverty Status	24.29	15/21	

CHI District
Peer Area

Peer Area Detroit **Total Population** 983,937
Black 80.54% **White** 12.92% **Other** 4.01%
0-17 31.01% **18-44** 39.23%
45-64 19.25% **65+** 10.51%

U.S. Census Bureau SF1, SF3, (2000)

Health Status/Health Resource Indicators
Characteristics of selected CHI District compared to all CHI Districts that make up the Peer area

Mortality (1995-98, N=2,131)			Cancer Incidents (1993-97, N=994)		
Selected Causes of Death	**Proportion**	**Rank**	**Selected Cancer Types**	**Proportion**	**Rank**
Heart disease	29.85	20/21	Prostate Cancer	19.12	14/21
All cancers	16.85	7/21	Lung and Bronchus	17.94	7/21
Homicide	5.87	3/21	Breast Cancer	13.77	3/21
Suicide	0.89	11/21	Colon Cancer	8.50	7/21
HIV/AIDS	2.53	3/21	Cervical Cancer	1.57	10/21
Diabetes Mellitus	2.67	10/21	**Infant Mortality (1997-99, N=61)**	**Rate**	**Rank**
Motor vehicle accidents	2.35	2/21	Infant Deaths/1000 Births	19.47	2/21
Hospitalizations (2000, N=9,285)			**Birth Characteristics (1999, N=968)**		
Selected Hospitalizations	**Proportion**	**Rank**	**Selected Birth Characteristics**	**(%)**	**Rank**
Congestive Heart Failure	3.73	8/21	Births to Teens	16.12	15/21
Bacterial Pneumonia	3.13	18/21	Repeat Births to Teens	26.28	12/21
Asthma	2.63	14/21	Births to Unmarried Women	76.96	7/21
Chronic Obstructive Pulmonary Disease	1.12	17/21	Births <12 Years Education	24.28	17/21
Diabetes Mellitus	2.26	9/21	Births Late/No Prenatal Care	7.23	15/21
Hypertension	1.93	14/21	Births Smoked in Pregnancy	12.50	17/21
			Low-Birthweight Babies	14.88	12/21
			Preterm Babies	18.49	7/21

Data Sources: MI Dept. of Community Health: Death Records, Live Birth Records,
State Cancer Registry, MI Hospital Assoc. - MI Inpatient Database

Source: Copyright © 2004 by Lee Kallenbach.

concept analogous to that of scoreboards. Likely users of the CHI Profile include the following:

- Community members or consumers of health care: individuals, families, and representatives of neighborhoods and of larger geographical areas
- Professionals in public health, clinical care, and social services
- Professionals in fields other than health: clergy, educators, attorneys, business professionals, press and media representatives
- Community advocates and organizers

The CHI Profile provides users with measures presented as both numbers and rankings, which can aid in understanding potential problems and associations in a particular community or set of communities. The numbers and rankings presented in the CHI Profile can be used in several ways:

- To determine the health level in the area—for example, by examining beneficial social qualities and characteristics or significant diseases, injuries, disabilities, and causes of death
- To discover health strengths, problems, or needs that were not previously understood or fully appreciated, including identification of populations at risk for adverse health effects, detection of an unexpected problem or health need, and identification of unforeseen determinants of health problems
- To make comparisons, for example, among zip code areas, with the state or nation, or with an objective standard
- To establish priorities among health problems or interventions
- To bring community members together to explore, investigate, discuss, or take action on issues of interest; to build coalitions; to empower users to resolve or improve the health of individuals or the community; or to educate the community
- To influence public or private policy

Conclusion

Based on the foregoing analysis, e-profiling community health indicators can yield significant benefits to the community, although key challenges must be overcome. Stakeholders in community health profiles can make more informed choices as to health interventions needed at the community level, deciding where community resources should best be applied to significantly improve community health services, as well as uncovering particular strengths or weaknesses in order to prepare the community as a whole for potential future hazards. Timeliness of data is an issue, along with security, privacy, and confidentiality of data. Availability, accessibility, reliability, and integrity of the data to be gathered, as well as validity and meaningfulness of our reported aggregates are all challenges that continually need to be addressed. While advances in information technology promise to make data gathering and analysis less error-prone and somewhat quicker, as well as make data easier to interpret and easier to access with emerging multimedia interface technologies, ultimately, the support and acceptance and leadership of community leaders and users will be needed to move e-profiling of community health care indicators forward.

Case Questions

1. What is meant by public and community health care?
2. Why is e-profiling community performance indicators analogous to the concept of the scoreboards?
3. What are the benefits and challenges of e-profiling community performance indicators?

4. Imagine that you are asked to e-profile indicators relating to the health status and preparedness of your community for future hazards. Where and how would you begin? What criteria and indexes would you use to move the project forward?

Reference

Durch, J. S., Bailey, L. A., & Stoto, M. A. (eds.). (1997). *Improving health in the community: A role for performance monitoring.* Washington, DC: Institute of Medicine.

CHAPTER SIX

E-NETWORKING

The Backbone of E-Health Care

Joseph Tan, Winnie Cheng

The authors would like to acknowledge the contributions of William J. Rogers, a graduate student in electrical engineering who was previously at Stanford University in Stanford, California.

Learning Objectives

1. Realize the e-networking requirements for the major classes of e-health applications: e-consumer health informatics, e-clinical care, and biomedical research
2. Identify e-networking standards for various components, including e-network infrastructure support, digital data formats and storage, and e-security
3. Conceptualize the open systems interconnect model and its significance for e-networking in health care
4. Differentiate between ISDN and mobile e-network infrastructures and among various satellite configurations for deploying e-health care applications
5. Understand medicolegal considerations in e-networking

Introduction

Traditionally, health care information systems have been deployed to provide rapid administration of patient data to support either mostly clinical or mostly administrative and financial services. These systems are highly autonomous, not designed to share information among administrators and caregivers working from various sites. Naturally, given the autonomous working environments, differing organizational cultures, and distinctive work ethics found in these settings, the information relating to a specific patient is typically captured in widely varying formats, impeding integration of information from different sources. Details of the patient's progress and treatment are often not included with the electronic patient records, even if these records were available, because isolated legacy systems using different coding standards are employed to capture and house that information. As a result, inefficiencies abound, leading to poor coordination and discontinuities in the care process among caregivers.

This lack of integration among legacy systems quickly spirals into unnecessary delays and poor-quality health care. In an emergency, for example, the patient's medical history is often not readily available to assist in diagnosis. Delays in treatment occur when requested copies of diagnostic results or images cannot be delivered quickly to the hospital or clinic. Information collated from the separate legacy systems is often time-consuming to locate, leading to further dissatisfaction with the quality of health care. Patients often complain about having to repeat the same information or, even worse, having to undergo a similar test procedure because results of the previous test were unavailable. Fortunately, rapid advances in computer memory and storage capacity, improved managed care processes, and recent consolidations among health provider organizations and health maintenance organizations into integrated delivery systems have all led to aggressive efforts by care providers to eliminate much of the inefficiency in health data processing and to provide greater accountability for health care services, gradually ushering in a new era of health care delivery, the e-health care era.

With the advent of e-health care, a wide range of technologies can now be applied to provide medical care products and services. In earlier chapters, it was noted that these technologies are the result of new advances in information and communication technologies, including the Internet and other advanced telecommunication and interactive network technology such as videoconferencing and wireless services. The use of e-technologies implies not only the ability to integrate information from many different sources but also the ability to practice medicine across long distances. Accordingly, e-health practices promise rapid access to shared, integrated administrative, financial, and even medical information and expertise regardless of the whereabouts of the patients as well as the caregivers.

Given these advances, the range of e-health care services can vary from on-line appointments to remote surgical procedures, including services directed by surgeons. Remote assessment of patient problems, on-line diagnoses, e-consultations between physicians and specialists, virtual consultations among patients and providers, massive digital data transfer, teleradiological transmissions of X-rays and magnetic resonance imaging archives, and interactive education and training sessions are all examples of emerging e-health care services and e-clinical applications. To understand the needs of the evolving e-health care system, this chapter provides a continuation and integration of the discussions of previous chapters by focusing on e-network infrastructures and configurations. Without e-networking, the backbone of all these emerging e-technological applications, limitations of time, space, location, and facility resources will restrict the provision of up-to-the-minute health care services.

E-networking is the term we will use to refer to the connectivity among various networks and their communication devices, such as servers, routers, and personal computers. Tan and Hanna (1994) argue for a three-tier implementation of e-network connectivity standards for health care applications: physical, systems, and applications connectivity. *Physical connectivity* has to do with promoting hardware compatibility, effecting teleprocessing, and administering network management. *Systems connectivity* refers to the use of flexible systems to interconnect platforms, and the concept of an open systems interconnect (OSI) model. *Applications connectivity* is concerned with software standards, as in the application of eXtensible Markup Language (XML), and user training. Together, these elements of network integration, which we refer to as *e-networking*, will result in the appropriate design and deployment of functional network infrastructures and configurations to link traditional health care networks and systems. E-networking will accomplish this integration not only by cutting across geographical and organizational boundaries but also by breaking down long-standing barriers to effective and productive exchange of key patient information.

This chapter first examines the e-networking requirements of three major categories of e-health applications: e-consumer health informatics, e-clinical care, and biomedical research. Next, we survey the e-networking standards for different components that support e-health networks and applications. Against this backdrop, we discuss the range of solutions offered by existing e-network technologies and, where applicable, the technical advances needed to solve these problems. We then review e-network infrastructures and configurations that have been tried for some e-health applications, highlighting broadly the issues that challenge the adequacy of these configurations. Equally important to the success of e-network technology are medicolegal infrastructures, which we explore briefly. Finally, we conclude the chapter with a look at the future growth and development of e-networks.

E-Networking Requirements

The evolution of e-health care services demands a wide range of applications with different e-networking requirements. In this chapter, we divide our discussion of e-health applications into three somewhat discrete categories—e-consumer health informatics, e-clinical care, and biomedical research—for the purpose of studying their varying e-networking needs. The e-networking requirements for each of these application categories are analyzed by examining their bandwidth, latency, security, and accessibility needs. Latency refers to the time delay prior to the transfer of data just after an instruction for its transfer has been received or provided (that is, from a storage device).

E-Consumer Health Informatics

E-consumer health informatics is probably the area in which e-health care products and services are most visible. Today, e-health care vendors and providers are recognizing the importance of engaging their clients and patients in order to provide more meaningful and effective e-health care information on products and services. More significantly, there is a global trend toward emphasizing preventive care and endorsing the general concept of self-care by empowering e-consumers with accurate and reliable information and knowledge. Promoting healthy lifestyles through systematic health education and changes in everyday routines and even through transforming current unhealthy behaviors (such as quitting smoking, becoming less sedentary by participating actively in walking and stretching exercises, and paying attention to eating disorders and poor eating habits) has caught on with younger people, who are often also well versed in the use of the Internet and other technologies. The e-consumers of tomorrow want accurate and reliable medical and other health-promoting information. E-consumer health applications include consumer-oriented Web sites, chat sessions, newsgroups, e-mail exchanges with medical experts, wireless and digital broadcasts, and other compilations of on-line resources.

The number of e-consumers searching for health information on the Internet seems to have been steadily increasing over the years. By 1999, just a few years following the initial diffusion of this e-technology into popular use, this number was already estimated to have reached a staggering 30 million at least (National Research Council Committee, 2000). It is believed that e-consumer health informatics will soon become the primary means of providing laypersons and nonprofessionals with health information.

As shown in Figure 6.1, e-consumer health informatics assumes a bidirectional information flow between the health care provider community and the general public. Notwithstanding, many health administrators and providers feel somewhat frustrated and helpless in trying to ensure that the health information and knowledge that e-consumers glean via the Internet or otherwise is authoritative or definitive. For example, e-consumers are constantly faced with uncertainties about the safety and effectiveness of particular health care products and services advertised on the Internet. Perhaps a clearinghouse to validate many such claims is badly needed. More and more private and governmental Internet sites and on-line surveys collect and disseminate demographic, accident, and work injury statistics to help promote preventive health and encourage the growth of e-consumer health informatics. However, such epidemiological data and biostatistics cannot be easily collected without a secured, publicly accessible infrastructure and platform. E-consumers are also demanding that the scientific accuracy of medical information or findings that are presented or released be verifiable and that potential biases be disclosed.

FIGURE 6.1. E-NETWORKING FOR E-CONSUMER INFORMATICS

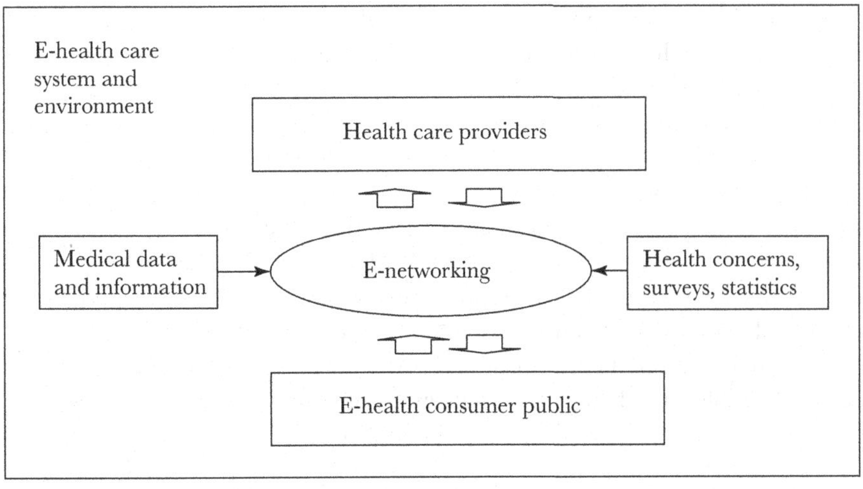

One approach to e-consumer health informatics is the community health information network (CHIN). Basically, a CHIN may be understood as a regional ring that links health care stakeholders throughout a community (see Chapter Three). Essentially, a CHIN refers to an integrated collection of telecommunication and e-networking capabilities that facilitate communications among patients and clinicians, as well as transfer financial information among multiple providers, payers, employers, pharmacies, and related health care entities, all within a specified geographical region. CHINs are further discussed in Tarn, Wen, and Tan (2001), who also provide several examples of how these networks can improve e-consumer informatics.

The bandwidth required by e-consumer informatics varies depending on the type of information to be transferred and on the number of users who will be accessing the information at any one time. For example, Web sites that provide a database of health risks and pharmaceutical products are usually adequately served by the access network (that is, a base station providing connection to associated networks that eventually lead to information site to be retrieved) capabilities offered by current Internet service providers (ISPs). On the Web server side, the bandwidth demand is driven largely by the volume of requests to be serviced. In most cases, e-consumer health informatics can accommodate interactivity that is characterized by a higher latency, except in such applications as on-line medical training courses where low latency interactivity is desired. While the networking requirements for e-consumer health informatics are not very stringent, architecture improvements are still necessary for the field to advance because of greater rising e-consumer expectations.

Of great importance to e-consumer health applications are issues relating to the accessibility, reliability, security, and legal aspects of e-health computing and networking. Some of these topics will be discussed in other parts of this chapter and this text. Here, we emphasize two general issues that need to be addressed. First, e-consumer health applications should be highly accessible, in order to serve the general public. To this end, the Internet plays a significant role in the dissemination of e-health information. However, with each passing day, the volume of information on the Internet is surpassing the ability of existing search tools. Search capabilities need to be further enhanced to allow the growing number of users to locate more precisely the information they are looking for. Moreover, people who are clearly underserved or disadvantaged due to the "digital divide"—for example, seniors, people living in poverty or in underdeveloped countries, and many others—still lack the knowledge of or training in how to get connected, how to extract relevant information, and how best to interpret the information gathered.

Second, health care policymakers and e-network designers can and should work together to institute mechanisms for providing e-consumers with accurate medical information. For example, policies can and should be established to identify sites that provide erroneous or misleading information. Authentication technologies may be applied to ensure that e-consumers are receiving information from approved sources. Also, e-consumer health applications require on-line anonymity and security because searching for information can reveal e-consumers' identities or health concerns about AIDS, sexual dysfunction, or other illnesses that may carry a public stigma. Appropriate infrastructures must be put in place to allow legitimate users to access accurate health information anonymously.

E-Clinical Care

E-clinical care involves the use of virtual clinics and medical services across distances. Virtual clinics are extending health care and clinical care services to a more geographically dispersed population than is possible with traditional care, including people in rural areas and in restricted places such as military bases, war zones, and planes and ships. In such instances, e-health care providers and e-patients typically do not meet physically; hence, medical specialists often interact with these patients via teleconsultation.

The success of e-clinical care today depends on the integration of four key application domains:

- Teleconsultation (or e-consultation)
- Digital medical imaging
- Remote patient monitoring
- Electronic health records

Teleconsultation (e-consultation) is a cost-effective alternative to staffing multiple clinics with the same set of specialists (Elsner, Kottkamp, and Hindricks, 2000). This e-technology allows rural areas, underserved urban areas, prisons, and other areas to receive medical services that may otherwise be unavailable (Kontaxakis, Walter, and Sakas, 2000). The bandwidth requirement for successful e-consultation varies depending on the types of data that are being transferred.

Table 6.1 specifies the bandwidth demands for five common categories of e-consultation interactions. As shown, the bandwidth demands for e-consultation can be quite significant for certain application categories. Current access networks for the Internet are based on an asymmetric upstream-downstream model in that downstream is much faster than upstream (Prior, 1996) and are not yet cost-effective enough to provide enough bandwidth to satisfy the demands of e-consultations. Latency guarantees are also necessary for e-consultation because this is a real-time, interactive application. As a result, dedicated networks are often needed.

Table 6.1. NOMINAL BANDWIDTH REQUIREMENTS FOR DIFFERENT TELEMEDICINE APPLICATIONS

Type of Consultation	Needed Bandwidth	Examples
High resolution, no motion	Store-and-forward	Radiology, dermatology, pathology
Medium resolution, low motion	128 kbps	Stethoscope, visual exams, psychiatric consultations, gastroenterology
Medium resolution, high motion	384 kbps	Cardiology, neurology, and emergency room consultations
High resolution, high motion	768 kbps	Cineo-angiography and echocardiograms
Very high resolution, High motion	Up to 2.5 Mbps	Gait analysis

Source: David Balch, East Carolina University, personal communication, Feb. 2, 1999.

Another aspect of e-clinical care that is closely related to e-consultation is sharing *digital medical imaging* information. This capability enables e-care providers to transfer medical information among specialists for interpretation as needed (Zhang and others, 2000). An on-line repository for medical images is commonly referred to as a *picture archiving and communications system* (PACS). The size of medical images varies: uncompressed radiographic images may range from several kilobytes to tens of megabytes. Table 6.2 summarizes the amount of medical imaging information that is typically transferred for the different image types. Up to hundreds of megabytes may be needed—for example, to store nuclear medicine images.

The bandwidth required to support digital image transfer applications depends on two factors: the amount of time in which the image must be transmitted and the degree of compression that can be employed. In many teleradiological applications, medical images may be sent as e-mail attachments with an interpretation or diagnosis turnaround time of one to two days. However, a busy mammography center may perform eighty to one hundred examinations per day. To transmit all of the results would require an average sustained throughput of approximately 1 megabyte per second without compression and a throughput of almost 100 kilobytes per second with 10:1 compression. Of course, any compression used must not degrade the image to the extent of possibly impairing interpretation. There are two types of compressions: lossless and lossy. *Lossless* compression emphasizes a coding technique that captures all information in a smaller number of bits. It allows a file size reduction by a factor of three or four. *Lossy* compression can typically provide a reduction by a factor of between ten and twenty without sacrificing diagnostic quality (Pradhan, 2001). Lossy compression uses a number of compression techniques that allow loss of information, for example scalar and vector quarantization, which are outside the scope

TABLE 6.2. NOMINAL FILE SIZES OF COMMON MEDICAL IMAGES

Image Type	Image Size (bits)	Images per Exam	Size of One Exam (megabytes)
Nuclear medicine	128 x 128 x 16	30-60	1-2
Magnetic resonance imaging	256 x 256 x 12	60	6
Ultrasound (color)	512 x 512 x 24	20-230	16-180
Digital angiography	512 x 512 x 8	15-40	4-10
Digitized electron microscopy	512 x 512 x 8	1	0.26
Digitized color microscopy	512 x 512 x 24	1	0.79
Computed tomography	512 x 512 x 12	40	20
Computed radiograph	2048 x 2048 x 12	2	16
Digitized X-rays	2048 x 2048 x 12	2	16
Digitized mammogram	4096 x 5625 x 16	4	184

Source: Huang, 1999.

of this discussion (for more info see Case section in latter part of this chapter). Further compression can be employed, depending on the application domain and the intended users. For example, a specialist reviewing a radiograph requires much higher resolution than a primary care physician looking at the same file. For some applications, such as mammography, how much the images can be compressed without significantly impairing their interpretation is a matter of some controversy. Techniques such as the use of intelligent systems to preprocess medical images may further reduce the bandwidth requirements. In general, medical imaging can benefit from faster e-networks with shorter turnaround time and greater access to the repositories.

A third domain of e-clinical care is *remote patient monitoring*. Remote patient monitoring provides a different interaction between the e-care provider and the patient. During an e-consultation session, it may be necessary for the provider to take vital signs and other measurements. In addition, some patients may require ongoing treatment and monitoring. Deployment of remote monitoring requires specific network infrastructure to be in place. Home networking is leading the way in the area of remote patient monitoring; for example, devices may be interconnected in a home using a local area network, with a central gateway governing the information access, processing, and control of these devices. Advances in micro-electromechanical systems are also enabling the control of microscopic mechanical devices such as pacemakers and sugar-level monitors via electrical signals. The amount of information communicated is usually small so that it is unlikely that high-bandwidth connections will be required. However, the aggregation of these devices may require careful management of e-network resources. In other words, latency and bandwidth control may be critical for some applications—for example, monitoring many patients simultaneously. The e-care provider should be able to handle an aggregate load of information from different remote devices and respond to critical situations in a timely manner. This type of monitoring also requires an e-network of high reliability.

Security and network availability are crucial to the success of remote patient monitoring. Data must not be altered while in transit through the network. In addition, the privacy of patient information must be protected. E-network downtime must also be within reasonable bounds and be as short as possible. The accessibility requirements for remote monitoring are analogous to those of emergency phone line support. Imagine the difficulties and confusions that accessibility problems would cause in dealing with patients undergoing e-clinical care. What if a particular instance of e-clinical care were a result of a bioterrorist attack that had caused the treatment location to be physically inaccessible to caregivers because of road closures and other transportation barriers?

Finally, *electronic health records* (EHRs) represent a critical component of e-clinical care. EHRs consist of a centralized on-line repository that enables authorized access to medical records (see Chapter Four). EHRs can house comprehensive records of patient information gathered from different sources over an extended period of time. Bandwidth demands for these on-line patient records vary depending on the type and nature of information stored. Web-based storage of medical records can provide needed accessibility; however, security measures should be implemented to protect patient privacy and guard against any inappropriate disclosure of highly confidential and sensitive data.

Biomedical Research

An important aspect of any e-health care system is preventing and controlling the spread of disease, injury, and disability. Chapter Five shows how Internet-based information exchange allows the timely dissemination of information and collection of data so that public health concerns and trends can be analyzed. Information and statistics are compiled on individual health, personal risk factors, and medical treatments. Data on potential sources of diseases and injury in the environment and resources that can be used to take effective action against such threats can be made available to the public, thus providing better prevention and control of epidemics and other disease outbreaks.

The Internet has demonstrated its power in promoting collaborative research. With rapid advances in communications, the biomedical field can benefit from the ability to quickly disseminate information. Not only can researchers share large databases, but they can also participate in linked simulations to exploit the power of distributed computing. Improvements in e-networking technologies will enable remote control of experimental apparatus, virtual reality training, and even remote surgery.

Again, in collecting biostatistics and epidemiological data, e-networks must provide mechanisms to protect patient privacy and confidentiality. Schemes and policies must be in place to ensure anonymity. Accessibility to patient information is also very important, as the information is relevant to the public and the individuals. The bandwidth and latency requirements are less stringent because most of the data transferred will be of manageable size. E-public health information systems should be supported by a network infrastructure that can accommodate a variety of bandwidths, allowing users connected to different networks to access the information.

Biomedical databases will differ from e-public health information databases in size and bandwidth requirements. Some biomedical databases shared among research projects cover DNA sequences, protein sequences, and human genetic diseases. A typical search retrieves a large amount of data; therefore, the demand on bandwidth may be high. To support a distributed computing environment in which linked simulations can occur among various high-end computing nodes, the network must provide enough bandwidth to allow results from one simulation to be fed to another simulation residing elsewhere in the network. Linked simulations impose both high bandwidth and stringent latency requirements on the e-network. However, in many cases, high-end machines are connected through private networks, so these requirements can be met through cost-effective sharing of these expensive computing workstations or servers.

Costly experimental equipment and apparatus such as electron microscopes, DNA sequencing facilities, and nuclear magnetic resonance spectrometers may also be shared. The ability to remotely control experimental equipment opens up resources to a broader research community and enables collaboration on the analysis of experimental results. A researcher from afar may send samples of interest to device operators, then run experiments remotely, specifying the desired magnification, controlling the focus and field of view, and retrieving images as desired. The researcher may also request another authorized researcher or expert to examine the image. Trainees can connect to video-streaming servers for on-line training classes or to simulation servers in order to participate in a virtual operation. Advances in robotics coupled with those in networking can bring virtual training as far as the performance of remote surgery in hard-to-reach areas (see Chapter Sixteen).

In most cases, biomedical research applications involve control data that must be transferred reliably and in sequence. The bandwidth requirements of these applications may vary. Because they are interactive applications, they require systems that meet latency specifications in order to be effective. Global accessibility is rarely necessary and in most cases is undesirable. Rather, only authorized researchers can have access to such costly and powerful equipment. Once again, authentication, encryption, and other standard security measures that ensure privacy and confidentiality are crucial to success.

E-Networking Standards

Having reviewed the e-networking requirements for major classes of e-health applications, we now move to discussing e-networking standards. More specifically, we will focus on standards that align technical advances in the various e-health component areas to support the development of e-health care applications, including e-network infrastructure support, digital data and image representation and storage, and e-security.

E-Network Infrastructure Support

E-network infrastructure support is concerned with achieving accessibility, bandwidth, and latency requirements. As we saw earlier, demands on the e-network infrastructure vary for different e-health applications. Low-quality networks may be adequate for some simple applications such as the transmission of on-line clinical reports. At the higher end of the spectrum, complex e-health transactions require sophisticated e-networks; one such application is the transmission of teleradiographic images and exchange of multimedia information for e-consultation and e-clinical services among networks connected via servers.

In real-time interactive e-health applications such as e-consultation, low latency and adequate bandwidth guarantees are required to sustain a session. These applications also demand symmetric link speeds, dictating an equal upstream-downstream data transmission rate that is not common in today's access networks. Medical information may contain high-resolution imaging data that are susceptible to data loss. E-health-related applications may involve critical functions that require fast and reliable information delivery. Hence, the field of e-networking faces many challenges. Recent deployments of faster networks that offer increased bandwidth have provided better resolution of images and some relief from network congestion. The predominant Internet Protocol (IP) networks currently operate on a best-effort assumption—an assumption that the best route will be traversed to satisfy requests; however, the need for quality of service (QoS) standards in the future is evident.

In recent years, considerable attention has been given to the need for QoS standards in e-networking. QoS parameters are used to distinguish traffic with different transfer requirements. For example, the audio stream of an e-consultation session requires much lower latency than e-mail traffic that may be competing for bandwidth simultaneously on a network. The transmission control protocol (TCP), which was developed a decade ago to ensure reliability in data transfer, has become the de facto standard, but it has many undesirable characteristics. First, it attempts to eliminate network congestion by pushing network utilization to its maximum until a retransmission caused by lack of capacity triggers it to backtrack. Moreover, the latency caused by retransmission may be unacceptable for real-time applications. Applications in e-health may also require the frequent exchange of multimedia information. Because multimedia traffic is likely to be carried over the same IP-based network as data traffic that typically uses TCP, this poses significant challenges. Unlike data traffic, multimedia traffic requires a minimum bandwidth to function. In order to guarantee multimedia services, the aggressiveness of TCP applications must be controlled to reserve at least the minimum bandwidth for multimedia traffic. Therefore, it is essential to employ e-networks with guaranteed QoS for more complex e-health applications in domains such as specialty e-consultations, real-time e-clinical care, and biomedical research such as a real-time, on-line clinical trial network for new drugs being tested on a global scale.

Two types of standardized QoS schemes have been discussed in the literature:

- Integrated services (IntServ)
- Differentiated services (DiffServ)

In addition to basic best-effort service, the IntServ model proposes two service classes—one that guarantees service and one that guarantees controlled load service, that is, it will be able to service all of the requests over time (Wachter, 2000). The precedence bits of the type of service (ToS) field in the IP packet header determine the packets relating to each service class (Skolnick, 1998). The IntServ model requires a telecommunications signaling protocol such as the Resource ReSerVation Protocol (RSVP). RSVP is therefore a policy-based network scheme that reserves paths on the Internet for transmitting video and other high-bandwidth messages. The IntServ model is characterized by the ability to reserve resource per-flow (in other words, a scheme to denote network resource reserved in a specific transmission) and, hence, provides end-to-end QoS guarantees. However, per-flow information must be stored and processed at each intermediate node in a network. This places high processing requirements on routers and inhibits scalability.

The DiffServ model alleviates the scalability problems encountered by IntServ. It aims to shift the processing to the edge of the networks by classifying and conditioning traffic at the boundaries before it enters the DiffServ domain (Woodward, Istepanian, and Richards, 2001). Core routers within the DiffServ domain can then provide fast switching. DiffServ supports a wider range of classes by replacing the To S field in the IP header with a new field, the differentiated services (DS) field. Per-class (that is, a scheme to specify the class of network resource to be reserved and used in a transmission) rather than per-flow information is then processed. A service-level agreement (SLA) may also need to be specified between the user and the network provider. SLAs may be negotiated statically or dynamically through the use of a signaling protocol such as RSVP (Clarke, Fragos, Jones, and Lioupis, 2000). In the absence of significant overprovisioning and explicit signaling to reserve resources, research has shown that simple DiffServ mechanisms can provide a high probability of meeting users' QoS requests for point-to-point communications. However, deployment of DiffServ is difficult over networks owned by different ISPs. Thus, end-to-end QoS will remain a challenge until new standards can be developed and agreed on by the various ISPs.

A QoS solution that can harness the advantages of both IntServ and DiffServ, overcoming scalability issues while providing end-to-end QoS guarantees is the Internet Engineering Task Force's (IETF's) Integrated Services over Specific Link Layers, which combines the end-to-end service definitions and signaling of IntServ with the scalable queuing and classification techniques of DiffServ. Another approach is the use of virtual overlay networks (VONs) (Tyrer, 2000). This technique aims to virtually divide the Internet into isolated networks such that different QoS and security requirements can be serviced independently. Packet flows belonging to different VONs are tagged with flow identifiers. For example, if a hospital creates multiple VONs to serve different applications, each network could connect to different end points and offer different levels of service. Routers would then determine how packets with different flow identifiers should be treated.

When bandwidth of a particular link is fixed, priority is often given to some packets at the expense of others in order to meet QoS demands. Ideally, all users would like their packets routed with the highest priority, but for some applications, average priority may be acceptable, while others may require a minimum guarantee at all times—for example, when transporting health-critical information in remote monitoring applications. Along with technology to support packet routing of different QoS classes, policies are needed to determine the priority of the traffic and hence the class to which each data packet should be assigned. RSVP is a flexible signaling mechanism that can allow some policy-related data to be exchanged. The Common Open Policy Service protocol has been defined to enable routers processing RSVP requests to exchange policy data with policy servers. These servers store policy information, such as types of requests allowed from a certain institution and the preemption priority of certain applications. Policy decisions are complex and require the agreement of the health care community as a whole.

Today, the predominant IP networks operate on a best-effort assumption in which packets are dropped when the network is close to saturation. Many health-related applications have critical functions requiring that information be delivered not only quickly but also reliably. Hence, networking faces many challenges in delivering the infrastructure needed to support these applications. Not surprisingly, despite ongoing research (for example, Tan and Hanna, 1994; Clarke, Fragos, Jones, and Lioupis, 2000), more studies in the area of health e-networks, particularly on data compression techniques for reduced bandwidth requirements, standardized QoS schemes, faster and more acceptable data and image transmission priority schemes, and ISP policy issues are still needed.

Data, Image, and Video Representation and Storage

We now turn to data format standards, particularly some commonly used standards in image and video compression techniques. For example, for the storage of medical information, systems known as *picture archiving communication systems* (PACS) have been developed to address some of the accessibility issues and e-networking requirements for the exchange of medical imaging data. Essentially, PACS are systems for storage of massive digital images. These systems also support simultaneous access to digital imaging data from various connected terminals, systems, and networks. E-health applications require storage and retrieval of images that can vary from 40 to 300 megabytes in size, with an average expected access time of 2 seconds or less. High compression ratios may cause important details that are crucial for proper diagnosis to be lost; hence, a high bandwidth requirement is often necessary (Sarek, 1997). To overcome these challenges, Stentor Inc. has proposed an innovative approach to lighten the load on e-networks. In this scheme, images are encoded using wavelet transformations (numerical techniques), thereby requiring only small chunks of data of 4 to 32 kilobytes to be exchanged at any one time and eliminating the need for dedicated links to support high bandwidth requirements. Moreover, instead of transmitting an entire medical study in one transfer, users can be presented with several low-resolution images that can then be separately "zoomed" to the image sizes with higher resolution needed at later points.

Other emerging standards for image and video compression have been applied to enhance the integration of multimedia applications with software and networks. The Joint Photographic Experts Group (JPEG) compression standard has been commonly used to compress both gray-scale and photographic-quality color images, but this compression technique is "lossy." The Moving Pictures Expert Group (MPEG) standards (MPEG-1, MPEG-2, MPEG-4, MPEG-7, and MPEG-21) can transmit different types of frames from a video clip. These techniques essentially compress the video clips into different types of frames, including intrapicture frames (I-frames), predicted frames (P-frames), and bidirectional frames (B-frames). Typically, I-frame is used as a reference for the B-frames and P-frames, which only record changes from the I-frames and thus use the I-frames to fill in the picture.

E-networking data format standards have been established among different e-stakeholders. Among these, Digital Imaging and Communications in Medicine (DICOM) and Health Level Seven (HL7) standards have aimed to specify the various hospital computer system interfaces DICOM provides guidelines on interfacing medical imaging devices, whereas HL7 comprises a set of data models that define data structure and transactions for communicating patient information and other financial and administrative data. HL7 is an organization accredited by the American National Standards Institute that is developing standards for representing and communicating data related to health care. The e-health care environment focuses on e-clinical and e-patient data such as EHRs (see Chapter Four). HL7 specifies a set of data models and transactions that have been adopted as the data interchange standard in many traditional as well as e-health applications. The HL7 data model has been implemented as a message-based format, as a relational data model, and as an object-oriented model. It has been extended to interoperate with eXtensible Markup Language (XML), which is becoming increasingly popular in implementation of e-health applications on the Internet.

The DICOM Standards Committee created a detailed specification that describes a means of formatting and exchanging images and associated information, particularly in a PACS environment for the storage and transmission of digital teleradiological images (DICOM Standards Committee and Working Groups, 1998; Rickards, 1996). DICOM guidelines apply to the operation of the interface used to transfer data in and out of an imaging device. The DICOM guidelines are a widely adopted standard for device interoperability in teleradiology, and it is probably at least partly a result of having such well-defined standards that teleradiology was one of the first forms of telemedicine to receive full reimbursement under Medicare and is among the most widely used forms of e-health services in the United States and worldwide. With standards in place, it can be determined whether an e-physician followed the standard of care.

E-Security

E-health applications frequently involve the exchange of sensitive information and knowledge. E-security opens doors to public acceptance of e-health care services by providing authentication of the identities of authorized users and ensuring patient anonymity in sensitive research, public health, and quality assurance applications. E-security features may be needed to authenticate parties before the exchange of confidential patient information (McDermott and others, 1999).

A common approach to ensuring e-security is the use of encryption technologies, which fall into two broad classes:

- Symmetric private key cryptography
- Asymmetric public key cryptography

Symmetric encryption uses the same key for data encryption and decryption. With this technique, distribution of keys is a major problem because security may be compromised.

Thus, in many cases, *asymmetric encryption* using two different keys (a private key and a public key) is preferred. When data and knowledge elements are encrypted using the private key, they can only be decrypted using the public key, and elements encrypted with the public key can only be decrypted with the private key. Authentication is accomplished when the sender encrypts a message with its private key and the recipient decrypts it by using the sender's public key. Privacy is protected in the reverse scenario, in which the sender encrypts the message with the recipient's public key and the recipient decrypts it with its private key. This method permits "strangers" to share information and knowledge, with both authentication and privacy. It is especially useful, for example, when two unaffiliated organizational entities need to share patient records.

Asymmetric encryption typically requires more bits than symmetric encryption in order to achieve the same level of security. In addition, the management and distribution of public keys in asymmetric encryption poses challenges. A user who wishes to use a certain public key for either authentication or privacy protection needs to know for certain that the key belongs to the appropriate entity. This problem is usually handled through digitally signed documents distributed by a certificate authority or through certificates that accurately specify public-key-to-entity relationships. Difficulty arises because of the large number of certificates that need to be given to all potential participants in a variety of simultaneous transactions. One proposed solution that would improve scalability is to arrange certificate authorities in a hierarchical fashion for improved security management, but this solution raises many other issues that are outside the scope of this discussion. *Public key infrastructure* (**PKI**) refers to the class of problems that deal with the distribution of keys and certificates.

Another important e-security feature is the revocation of certificates. Mechanisms are often needed to invalidate a public-private key pair and to disseminate this updated information. A downside to the current certificate authority models is the way they bind public keys to a particular organization or individual, which can significantly compromise privacy. A working group of the IETF (the Simple PKI working group) is developing an Internet standard that addresses these issues. Several techniques have been developed to provide user authentication and protection of messaging traffic. Early protocols were aimed at providing link-level security, whereas today security is enforced across a range of different layers to provide greater flexibility and reassurance. Internet Protocol Security (IPSec), Transport Layer Security (TLS) and Pretty Good Privacy (PGP) operate respectively at the network, transport, and application layers.

IPSec is an architecture and set of standards at the network layer that provides a variety of services, such as the encryption and authentication of IP packets. It was devised by the IETF to provide a general framework rather than a complete set of functionality and encryption algorithms. Thus, it allows a pair of communicating entities to use whichever algorithms are adequate for the application. For example, an application that employs IPSec can choose whether to use an authentication facility that validates the sender or an encryption facility that also ensures the confidentiality of the payload (McWherter, Sevy, and Regli, 2000). The security may also be asymmetric, with authentication applied in one direction only. IPSec can protect traffic across any local area network (LAN) or wide area network (WAN). Traffic can also be terminated at end systems or at gateways, with encryption and decryption applied at the two endpoints.

IPSec technology was first used in virtual private networks (VPNs) to secure messages exchanged via an encrypted tunnel. For example, it has been used for exchange of information between health care providers and the Health Care Financing Administration in processing on-line Medicare claims. VPNs have several limitations; the tunneling scheme does not scale well, and VPNs often require prior knowledge of where connectivity will be required.

TLS is commonly used on the Internet in the form of the Secure Socket Layer (SSL) system (National Research Council Committee, 2000). TLS uses asymmetric encryption to authenticate the server (and sometimes the client) and symmetric encryption to secure information exchange between the end user and the server. It is widely used by financial institutions in electronic commerce and therefore can be used similarly in e-health applications to capture sensitive information such as credit card numbers. SSL can support encryption in both directions between the server and the client; however, it normally provides authentication of the host organization's Web site. Support of bidirectional encryption requires certificates to be assigned to both the client and the server. This may be needed in many e-health applications in which the authentication of the user and the e-health care provider are equally important. This requirement imposes constraints on the deployment of e-health applications because it entails careful assignment and distribution of certificates to the communicating parties.

Several initiatives are under way to set up certificate authorities for future e-health applications. Recently, Intel has announced a joint effort with the American Medical Association to provide digital certificates that will enable doctors to transmit information such as test results to patients and other e-health care professionals (Kontaxakis, Walter, and Sakas, 2000). In e-consumer health informatics, WebMD has agreed to provide a similar service to physicians. WellMed and Franklin Health also have plans in place to enhance e-consumer informatics. A $2.5 million grant has been awarded for a five-state Health Key research initiative on facilitating electronic exchanges of information among companies in the health sector while protecting data confidentiality (Prior, 1996).

At the application layer, particularly in adding security to e-mail exchanges, PGP has been a popular choice. PGP is a well-developed collection of commercially supported encryption software that is now freely available for noncommercial use. This technology combines symmetric and asymmetric cryptography: symmetric cryptography is used to generate a session key for a multirecipient e-mail message, while asymmetric cryptography is used to encrypt the message for its transmission. Moreover, PGP is a generic set of encryption algorithms that can be conveniently extended to applications beyond e-mail.

Security measures can also be taken to protect data and knowledge elements embedded in e-mails rather than the entire e-mail message. Multipurpose Internet Mail Extension (MIME) is an extension of standard e-mail formats that supports different data forms, such as video and audio, that are not typically represented as ASCII text. A secured version of MIME (Secure/MIME, or S/MIME) supports the use of digital signatures to encrypt data in e-mail messages. S/MIME uses a hierarchical certificate authorization model and uses certificates based on the X509 (Version 3) standard. Extensions that incorporate MIME or S/MIME encryption technologies can also be added to existing videoconferencing standards such as H323.

H323 is a widely used set of recommendations for transporting multimedia information across a packet-based network such as the Internet. Following the publication of H323 (Version 1) in 1996, several versions have added improvements such as support for QoS and e-security. These improvements make H323 useful for e-health applications such as e-consultation and remote surgery. H323 (Version 2), for example, includes e-security features specified in the H235 standards to support authentication, nonrepudiation, data integrity, and confidentiality. H235 does not restrict the authentication and encryption technologies that may be used; it provides a generic mechanism to negotiate these and supports various combinations of symmetric and asymmetric cryptographic technologies. H235 requires call control channels to be secured—for example, using IPSec. To provide greater e-security, authentication is implemented through end user digital certificates rather than through end terminals. As multimedia e-networking advances, new versions are incorporating more complex e-security features to ensure the integrity and validity of the data exchanged and to deal with issues such as user privacy, security, and confidentiality on e-networks.

Given the many technological options available to support telecommunication and Internet-associated technologies, it is clear that a wide range of varying e-health services is possible. These services include those directed by surgeons and physicians such as remote surgical procedures and e-consultation as well as services such as on-line appointments and remote patient monitoring. Notable examples of current, potential, and sometimes very successful applications include remote assessment of patient problems; on-line diagnostic, therapeutic, and prognostic services; remote drug dispensing services; remote patient monitoring and sending of reminders; provider-to-patient and patient-to-provider consultation; physician-to-physician referrals; knowledge management capability in the form of automatic transmission of clinical data, texts, X-rays, CT scans, and other forms of imaging, as well as e-consumer informatics, interactive education, research, and distance training related to e-health care applications (Zhang and others, 2000).

Again, the e-networking requirements and standards we have reviewed so far can only function appropriately within the context of an open systems interconnect model and appropriate e-networking infrastructures. Accordingly, we now turn to these topics.

E-Networking Infrastructures

In this section, we focus on the concept of an open systems interconnect model and on two contrasting approaches to e-network infrastructures and configurations. Besides describing a case scenario using cellular infrastructure, we show how terrestrial networks can be extended in geographical scope through the use of satellite technologies for a low-bandwidth or a high-bandwidth satellite infrastructure. The latter configuration is also used to examine the bottlenecks of satellite communications and some suggested improvements.

Open Systems Interconnect Model

Health organizations are sometimes locked into the technologies of the past because of legacy systems that are poorly integrated, costly, difficult to maintain, and hard to change. One strategy for moving toward e-health care is to learn how to leverage these investments to take advantage of both existing and new technologies. Major problems often faced in connecting legacy systems with e-networks are hardware incompatibility, layering of complex protocols, and difficulty in understanding how data can be exchanged between two computer systems within a network. The *open systems interconnect* (OSI) model addresses these problems in large part by showing how many devices can exchange and communicate information via a hierarchy of seven layers. These layers—which roughly correspond to the three-tier connectivity concept of systems, applications, and physical connectivity that was discussed in Tan and Hanna (1994)—are the application, presentation, session, transport, network, data link, and physical layers. Understanding the way these layers work to execute the exchange of information between the network and the transmitting host system and user (source) on one end, and between the network and the receiving host system and user (destination) on the other end will assist us in designing better e-networks.

Essentially, when a source—that is, a transmitting host system—is preparing to send information out, the user will appear to work directly via e-mail, file transfers, or remote logins from the application layer of the source computer to the application layer of the destination computer, independent of the e-network architecture or configuration. While this may appear intuitively simple, the actual process is quite sophisticated; the data are physically and sequentially moved from the highest (application) layer to the lowest layer and are transformed into bits and bytes to be physically channeled through the nodes of a network. At the receiving end, these bits and bytes are moved in reverse from the lowest (physical) layer to the highest layer and transformed into appropriately coded and formatted data available to the user of the receiving system.

Below the application layer, the presentation layer insulates the destination user from the source user by presenting the data to be transferred to the destination user in an understandable format even when the different host systems use different data formats. The presentation layer also provides the necessary security measures.

Just below the presentation layer is the session layer. Here, applications on the two different host systems may engage in a logical connection through a synchronization of the session, specifying to the users at both ends when to send or to receive the message. The session layer also handles error recovery.

The transport layer is next; it deals mainly with the end-to-end communications by dividing the data into segments and then either sending or receiving the data.

The next three layers—the network layer, the data link layer, and the physical layer—have to do with the physical routing and the actual network navigational process. In the network layer, the optimal data routing is determined, including the switching elements that will be used to conduct the transmission. The data link layer then supervises the flow of information among and between nodes in the network, while the physical or electrical aspects of data communication and exchange are controlled in the physical layer.

While the OSI model has not been commercially adopted, the concept is nevertheless valuable for our understanding of how e-health data can be transferred from one end of an e-network, where the data are available, to the other end, where the data are needed. Moreover, the development of narrowband and broadband integrated services digital networks (ISDNs) was based on the OSI model. At this point, it is important to understand how e-health data can be transferred via e-networks, not only in the digital environment of ISDN network infrastructures but in the environment of wireless and mobile network infrastructures.

ISDN Infrastructures

Integrated services digital network (ISDN) technology enables the merging of separate networks into a single high-speed multimedia communications infrastructure through digital switching and digital transmission. ISDN networks can be divided into narrowband (an amalgam of circuit-switched and packet-switched signals) and broadband (high speed packet-switched network). The performance of these networks has received some attention in the literature, most prominently, those of the Clarke experiments discussed next.

Using the Advanced Informatics Distributed Medical Access Network (AIDMAN) to deliver e-health services to remote areas in Greece, Clarke, Fragos, Jones, and

Lioupis (2000) investigated the performance of three types of link protocols to determine how their characteristics affect the performance of e-health care applications when bandwidth is limited to 256 kilobytes per second. The three types of protocols that were tested are (1) a circuit-switched (or narrowband N-ISDN) network; (2) a packet-switched (or Transmission Control Protocol/Internet Protocol [TCP/IPv4]) network (analogous to broadband B-ISDN); and (3) a cell-switched (or Asynchronous Transfer Mode [ATM]) network (these differentiated terms are based on the bandwidth requirements and the type of technology used in the networks).

Figure 6.2 shows the different e-network configurations that were set up for the Clarke, Fragos, Jones, and Lioupis's investigation.

With the narrowband ISDN (circuit-switched) network shown in Figure 6.2a, videoconferencing and image transfers can be supported using the International Telecommunications Union H320 and T120 standards, respectively. These standards are useful for transferring images and sharing applications between videoconference participants. TCP/IP is not supported by H320, so applications based on the DICOM standard, such as X-ray transmission, cannot be used simultaneously with videoconferencing. The advantage of narrowband N-ISDN is that each application has exclusive rights to the full bandwidth, so performance is guaranteed.

ISDN allocates the entire bandwidth for an application, thereby enhancing performance. For the TCP/IP network shown in Figure 6.2b, videoconferencing is accommodated using the H323 standard, which also supports the T120 standard. In contrast to the narrowband ISDN network, TCP/IP applications can be used with

FIGURE 6.2. COMPARISON OF THREE E-NETWORK CONFIGURATIONS

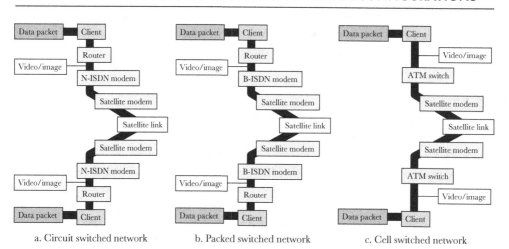

a. Circuit switched network   b. Packed switched network   c. Cell switched network

videoconferencing, but they must compete for bandwidth, which may affect the speed of the transfer. As shown, the key difference in the two network configurations is the use of N-ISDN in the former and the use of B-ISDN for greater bandwidth transmission in the latter.

The ATM network, shown in Figure 6.2c, differs from the TCP/IP network in its use of fixed-length cells (ATM uses 53-byte cells). Also, the ATM network implements QoS, which gives priority to specified streams of traffic such as voice and images over data.

A simulated typical e-consultation session was modeled and tested, using various combinations of traffic. The results showed that the narrowband ISDN network behaved almost perfectly during the simulation. The major drawback was that the narrowband ISDN link required separate transmission of X-rays over a TCP/IP connection, so the simulation could not transmit everything at the same time.

For the TCP/IPv4 network, with a satellite link bandwidth of 128 kilobytes per second which is no more than the 256 kbps limit set for the experiment, X-ray transmission and videoconferencing worked well separately, but the results were not encouraging when they were used together; the X-ray transfer time became unacceptably large, and the videoconference session suffered unacceptable delay and jitter. The slow start or latent time experienced in the transmission of the different types of data and global synchronization required of TCP in order to transmit both the X-ray and videoconference data resulted in X-ray transfers' using up most of the bandwidth. The transfer of maximum-length packets of TCP-based X-rays also caused intolerable delays in video transmission. An end delay as accumulated for video transmission was 244.5 milliseconds, significantly higher than the required 100 milliseconds.

The ATM network showed excellent performance at 128 kilobytes per second, which is again less than the 256 kbps limit set for the experiment. This is because the ATM network is based on small cells, which interleave much better than the large IP packets. Every stream is guaranteed bandwidth and given priority via ATM. The drawbacks of ATM, however, include its high cost and its lack of available tailored applications.

Clarke, Fragos, Jones, and Lioupis (2000) conclude that low-bandwidth satellite links can be used for e-health services that include videoconferencing and image transfer using TCP/IP. However, if the link is set at 128 kilobytes per second, they argue for the use of QoS to prioritize traffic. Even though the ATM network yielded excellent performance, it was not the recommended alternative, owing to its relatively high cost and lack of available applications. Because narrowband N-ISDN did not allow the simultaneous transmission of X-rays and videoconferencing, it was considered unacceptable.

To date, several solutions have been suggested to improve networking performance for e-health services. In addition to TCP spoofing, selective and forward acknowledgments have been proposed. TCP spoofing divides the TCP connection between a server and a client into two paths. One path connects the client to its gateway router, then to the satellite. The other path also emanates from the router, but traverses an Internet link. Both paths terminate at the destination client sites where information is to be sent or retrieved. Another solution is to pace TCP segments by appropriately spacing acknowledgments to control the rate at which data are put into the network so that the total capacity of the network is preserved at all times for optimizing data transmission.

Not surprisingly, various studies have also found that TCP/IP should be enhanced to give better performance for e-health care over satellite networks that allow a high rate of data transfer. Tyrer (2000), for example, claims that satellites should be used to provide the high-bandwidth infrastructure for e-health services because telephone companies and cable companies are not likely to be able to do so. He does not believe that TCP/IP performance in a satellite environment is adequate. Over a long propagation of transmission delay, the TCP features prove to be very inefficient. A minimum of 1 to 1.5 round-trip transmission times are required to establish network connections. Similarly, the long delay may hamper functionality, through such problems as congestion avoidance and slow start. Acknowledgments are delayed and loss recovery are also hindered.

Cellular Versus Satellite Infrastructures

A *cellular communication network* comprises many cells, or areas, each with limited signal coverage. Using a particular frequency channel repeatedly, the cells are just far enough from one another to be interference-tolerant. The repeated use of a particular frequency enables the network to support a large number of subscribers. Another important feature is the hands-off mechanism through which the frequency assigned for a call is seamlessly changed as the mobile terminal crosses cell boundaries.

Woodward, Istepanian, and Richards (2001) demonstrated one application of cellular communication technologies: transferring medical information and knowledge to remote areas. They used a 9.6-kilobytes-per-second global system for mobile communications (GSM) channel to send ten-minute electrocardiograms (ECGs) via cellular telephone. The ECG images were compressed, using wavelet techniques at ratios of up to 10:1, a ratio considered to yield acceptable quality as judged by a cardiologist. The data and knowledge elements were encrypted before the cellular phone signals were sent to a remote location via the GSM cellular network and the public switched telephone network (PSTN). A LAN server was then connected to the PSTN using a modem. Results of the experimental transmission via this cellular network infrastructure demonstrated that the main clinical features of the transferred images were retained.

The researchers hope that this cellular network system, when fully developed, will allow a doctor to monitor patients remotely while they are actively doing their jobs. A patient should be free to move around while being monitored, both at work and during sports and activities. Existing cellular technology can be used to create a very inexpensive setup that interferes minimally with the life of the patient or the doctor.

Communication satellite technology is another wireless or mobile network infrastructure that can be used to promote e-health services and products. A network consisting of satellites, a system control center, and gateways allows direct channels to users via links to air, marine, and land mobile terminals and connects feeder links to various land networks. Satellite infrastructure supports fixed wireless access, broadcast of e-health programs, and mobile health (m-health) services. Broadcast services are mostly offered through traditional geostationary earth orbit (GEO) systems, while global mobile satellite personal communications are mostly provided through low or mid-earth orbit (LEO/MEO) satellites. Satellite networks offer several advantages over cellular phones and the Internet, including wide bandwidth, guaranteed bit rate, broadcast and multicast capabilities, and secure connections (Wang, 1999).

Farserotu and Prasad (2000) note that the type of satellite used can make a difference. LEO satellites move at a lower altitude than GEO satellites and thus cost less to launch and have less round-trip delay. In contrast, GEO satellites have much greater coverage. The relatively limited coverage of LEO systems necessitates frequent handovers between ground terminals and satellites, as well as cross-links among neighboring satellites. This makes LEO systems more complex and more susceptible to delay jitter than GEO systems. E-health applications employ the latest in e-networking research and developments—specifically, integrated audio-video, telecommunication, and Internet-associated technologies; digital networks; and cellular technology and satellites—to provide e-clinical information and knowledge transfer services for geographically dispersed health care facilities operated by a network of multiprovider organizations catering to even more geographically dispersed populations. However, the medicolegal challenges to the future of e-networks must be overcome if e-health care is to flourish.

Conclusion

E-health encompasses a wide range of applications, from browsing for health information on the Web to remote surgical procedures. The e-networking requirements that these applications impose vary greatly. High-end applications such as e-consultation have stringent e-networking requirements. They require high bandwidth for the exchange of high-resolution medical imaging data. Real-time e-consultation and other interactive applications also demand low latency and possibly a symmetric transfer rate (upstream/downstream) that is not commonly supported in current access network infrastructures. Accessibility is a key requirement in some biomedical research projects, such as visualization of complex gene-based data as it provides a continuum of e-health care services for e-patients in remote and restricted areas.

In this chapter, we have demonstrated that e-health services can be provided using today's e-technologies, although many improvements in QoS guarantees and e-networking security need to be achieved in order to enable such services as remote surgery. As with traditional health care services, the success of e-health care depends on support from governments, e-vendors, e-providers, e-payers, and, most important, e-consumers.

Chapter Questions

1. Discuss the open system interconnect (OSI) model. What is its significance in e-networking, and how does understanding of this model help in designing e-networks for major classes of e-health applications?

2. How are ISDN and mobile e-network infrastructures different? What are some of the configurations of these e-network infrastructures that are used in e-health care applications?

3. What is the importance of understanding the e-networking requirements for major classes of e-health applications? What are some of the more complex e-health applications with advanced e-network requirements?

4. How do medicolegal considerations impede the diffusion of e-health services?

5. Imagine that you are a radiologist who has been hired to do a teleradiological reading in order to examine a child's state of health and susceptibility to a lung problem. From a medicolegal standpoint, what would your reaction to this request be if the request comes from potential adoptive parents of the child? Would you feel that you or the minor child had a right to keep your conclusions from the adoptive parents if the results were detrimental to the child's future? Who would be the best people to decide such an issue? Why?

References

Clarke, M., Fragos, A., Jones, R., & Lioupis, D. (2000). Optimum delivery of telemedicine over low bandwidth links. IEEE EMBS International Conference Proceedings. *Information Technology Applications in Biomedicine*, 32–37.

Daley, H. (2000). Telemedicine: The invisible legal barriers to the health care of the future. *Annual Health L., 9*, 73.

DICOM Standards Committee and Working Groups. (1998, December). *DICOM committee procedures*. Retrieved May 15, 2001, from Digital Imaging and Communications in Medicine Web site: http://medical.nema.org/dicom/wgs.html

Elsner, C., Kottkamp, H., & Hindricks, G. (2000). Introducing new telemedical services into clinical environments: A step-by-step approach at the Heart Center, Leipzig, Germany. *Computers in Cardiology*.

Farserotu, J., & Prasad, R. (2000, June). A survey of future broadband multimedia satellite systems, issues and trends. *IEEE Communications Magazine, 38*, 128–133.

Huang, H. K. (1999). *PACS: Basic Principles and Applications*. New York: Wiley.

Kleinke, J. (2000, November–December). Vaporware.com: The failed promise of the health care Internet; Why the Internet will be the next thing not to fix the U.S. health care system. *Health Affairs*.

Kontaxakis, G., Walter, S., & Sakas, G. (2000). EU-TeleInViVo: An integrated portable telemedicine workstation featuring acquisition, processing and transmission over low-bandwidth lines of 3D ultrasound volume images. *IEEE EMBS International Conference on Information Technology Applications in Biomedicine Proceedings*.

McDermott, W., Tri, J., Mitchell, M., Levens, S., Wondrow, M., Huie, L., Khandheria, B., & Gilbert, B. (1999, July–August). Mayo Foundation, optimization of wide-area ATM and local-area Ethernet/FDDI network configurations for high-speed telemedicine communications employing NASA's ACTS. *IEEE Network, 13*(4), 30–38.

McWherter, D., Sevy, J., & Regli, W. (2000, July–August). Building an IP network quality-of-service testbed. *IEEE Internet Computing, 4*(4), 65–73.

National Research Council Committee. (2000). *Networking health: Prescriptions for the Internet*. Washington DC: National Academy Press.

Pradhan, M. (2001). Retrieved from http://www-smi.stanford.edu/people/pradhan/articles/telemed.html

Prior, F. (1996). Communication technology for telemedicine. *Proceedings of the National Forum*.

Rickards, T. (1996). Retrieved from http://www.uni-mainz.de/Cardio/dicom/links/2106.htm

Sarek, M. (1997). The transfer of multimedia information in biomedicine. *Proceedings of the IEEE Engineering in Medicine and Biology Society Region 8 International Conference*.

Skolnick, A. (1998, March 11). Monitor passes first tests with flying colors. *Journal of the American Medical Association, 279*(10).

Tan J., & Hanna, J. (1994). Integrating health care with information technology: Knitting patient information through networking. *Health Care Management Review, 19*(2), 72–80.

Tarn, J., Wen, H. & Tan, J. (2001). Communications system architecture: Networking health provider organizations and building virtual communities. In J. Tan, *Health management information systems: Methods and practical applications* (2nd ed., pp. 179–203). Sudbury, MA: Jones & Bartlett.

Tyrer, H. (2000). Satellite wide-area-network for telemedicine. *IEEE Aerospace Conference Proceedings* (Vol. 1, pp. 141–148).

Wachter, G. (2000, March 26). *Two years of Medicare reimbursement of telemedicine: A post-mortem*. Retrieved May 15, 2001, from http://tie.telemed.org/legal/issues/reimburse_summary.asp

Wang, C. (1999). Security issues to tele-medicine system design. *IEEE Southeastcon '99 Proceedings*.

Woodward, B., Istepanian, R., & Richards, C. (2001, March). Design of a telemedicine system using a mobile telephone. *IEEE Transactions on Information Technology in Biomedicine, 5*, 13–15.

Zhang, J., Stahl, J., Huang, H., Zhou, X., Lou, S., & Song, K. (2000). Real-time teleconsultation with high-resolution and large-volume medical images for collaborative healthcare. *IEEE Transactions on Information Technology in Biomedicine, 4*(2), 178–185.

Mobile Health Networks Case: Unconfined Mobile Bluetooth Technology for E-Medical Services

Qiang Cheng, Huyu Qu, Yingge Wang, Joseph Tan

Most conventional telemedicine (or e-medicine) systems use fixed wired LAN, cable, DSL (Digital Subscriber Line), and other landline systems to transmit medical data or operations. As wireless LAN technology becomes increasingly pervasive, e-health professionals are considering wireless LANs for their mobile medicine systems.

However, both landline and wireless systems used today have limited real-world applications. Landline systems are restricted to indoor use—for example, in hospitals, clinical wards, or family rooms (in family nursing systems); when patients or physicians leave those small areas, they lose access to the system. Data transmitted through wireless channels are more vulnerable to eavesdropping or interception than data transmitted through wired channels. To enable secure, real-time, distant health care, we therefore propose a new wireless e-medicine system that combines wireless LANs with wireless WANs, mobile PSTN networks, or satellite communication networks. Using our system, patients, physicians, nurses, and health care workers would be able to get real-time medical service anywhere in the world. We also propose to build covert channels of wireless LANs into our system to transmit important medical data or operations, which would greatly enhance the security of e-medicine.

Background

E-medicine uses telecommunication technologies to provide conduits for information exchange between physicians, nurses, and patients. The recent development of remote patient monitoring systems using Bluetooth wireless LAN techniques has eliminated wire lines and given patients the freedom to move around inside a hospital, clinic, or patient ward (Woodward and Rasid, 2003; Hung and Zhang, 2002). We will use the term *mobile medicine* to describe such a system. In these systems, the patient's body is equipped with Bluetooth-enabled smart sensors. The signals from the sensors are transmitted via wireless to the nearest receiver, a Bluetooth access point to the central nursing system.

Although the major advantage of wireless medicine is its mobility, existing remote patient monitoring systems still restrict the patient to a ward unit or a hospital, so the patient has to pay expensive inpatient care fees. To address this problem, we propose a family nursing system. A Bluetooth access point could be installed inside the patient's home. Sensor signals collected from the patient's body would be conveyed from Bluetooth-enabled instruments to the central nursing system in the hospital via the access point and the Internet (Woodward and Rasid, 2003; Hung and Zhang, 2002). With this family nursing system, the patient could substantially reduce medical cost yet still receive quality health care service.

Some patients undergoing medical monitoring need to move around for work, travel, or other outdoor activities. Existing nursing systems, including family nursing, will not permit this freedom of movement (Woodward and Rasid, 2003; Hung and Zhang, 2002; Luo and Cheng, 2004). Keeping these patients (for example, those with chronic diseases who need long-term health services) in wards or at home all the time is undesirable; thus, mobile medicine or monitoring can play a useful role.

To this end, we propose a new mobile system to provide unconfined health care services, one that combines wireless LANs (WLANs) with wireless WANs, the public switched telephone network (PSTN), and the Internet or satellite communication networks. With the help of our proposed wireless system, patients, physicians, and nurses could be empowered to receive or provide real-time, distant health care services. Both patients and providers would have the freedom to be anywhere in the world while sending, receiving, checking, and examining medical data in a timely fashion. The proposed system provides, among other benefits, a technological solution to the long-term shortage of nurses in the United States (Luo and Cheng, 2004).

We first present the prototype of our unconfined mobile wireless medicine system and illustrate the application of such a system. Next, we discuss the security issues and propose a covert channel to enhance the security of the system. Finally, we discuss future research possibilities.

Prototype of a Bluetooth-Enabled Medicine System

With mobile medicine, reliability and security are key technical considerations. The two widely used WLAN standards are IEEE 802.11b and Bluetooth. In North America, WLAN systems operate in the unlicensed industrial, scientific, and medicine (ISM) band ranging from 2400 to 2483.5 MHz using Gaussian-filtered frequency shift keying (GFSK) modulation. To reduce the interference, spread spectrum (SS) techniques are used. For example, Bluetooth uses frequency-hopping SS with 1600 hops per second, and it hops among 79 channels spaced at 1 MHz; in contrast, IEEE 802.11b uses direct sequence SS for transmission. Bluetooth supports data transfer rates of less than 1 megabyte per second, while IEEE 802.11b supports up to 11 megabytes per second. Bluetooth forms networks on an ad hoc basis and covers short-range cells of less than 10 meters; IEEE 802.11b covers cells up to 20 meters in size (Molts, 2001; Haykin and Moher, 2003).

The IEEE 802.11b standard provides encryption and authentication mechanisms via the Wired Equivalent Privacy (WEP) protocol. WEP adopts the RC4 encryption algorithm to encrypt over-the-air transmissions (Molts, 2001; Haykin and Moher, 2003). RC4 concatenates a 128-bit secret key with a 24-bit random initialization vector (IV) and uses them to generate a pseudo-random sequence. This pseudorandom sequence is applied to the plain text to produce the cipher text. Upon receipt of the cipher text, the receiver uses the IV and the secret key to regenerate the pseudorandom sequence and reveal the original text. It is known that RC4 is vulnerable to various forms of attack based on statistical analysis (Knudsen et al., 1998; Xydis and Blake-Wilson, 2002).

There are also weaknesses in the key-scheduling algorithm of RC4, so related key attack can be mounted on RC4 cryptosystems (Fluhrer, Mantin, and Shamir, 2001).

Bluetooth is a low-cost, low-power, and short-range radio communication technology. The Bluetooth protocol has two types of link: a synchronous connection-oriented (SCO) link and an asynchronous connection-less (ACL) link. The SCO link supports time-bounded information and thus can be used in time-critical e-medicine applications, such as stethoscope examinations. The ACL link supports packet-switched connection so that the system can be used to transmit large volumes of non–time-sensitive information, such as electrocardiogram (ECG) and photoplethysmogram files.

Bluetooth is essentially a replacement for physical cables. Up to eight Bluetooth-enabled devices can automatically form a piconet on the fly. Each piconet consists of one master and up to seven active slaves. All devices in a piconet are synchronized, and the master determines the frequency-hopping pattern (Haykin and Moher, 2003; Rappaport, 2002). A piconet distinguishes itself from neighboring piconets by its hopping frequency. Transmission can happen only between a master and a slave; there is no direct communication between the slaves within a piconet. The transmission is full duplex, using a slotted time-division-duplex (TDD) access strategy. Master-to-slave transmissions always start in an even-numbered slot, while slave-to-master transmissions begin in an odd-numbered time slot. All security functions are performed at the link level, and the security is based on a 48-bit unique device address, a 128-bit pseudorandom private key for authentication, an 8- to 128-bit private key for encryption, and a 128-bit pseudorandom number generated by the device. The security of Bluetooth is superior to that of IEEE 802.11b based on current research evidence (Xydis and Blake-Wilson, 2002).

Bluetooth supports low-power transmission with a range of 10 meters or less, which is very limited for wireless medicine. The problem of the short-range radio link can be overcome by combining Bluetooth personal area networks (PANs) with mobile public switched telephone networks (PSTNs)—that is, via Bluetooth-enabled cellular phones. For better security and wide availability in portable consumer electronics, we employ Bluetooth techniques in our proposed mobile medicine system.

Exhibit 6.1 illustrates the proposed Bluetooth-enabled system to perform mobile medicine.

A Bluetooth piconet allows the creation of a set of wireless serial connections between a master and up to seven active slaves. In our proposed system, the access point—either the local area network (for example, a corporate intranet) or a Bluetooth-enabled mobile phone for remote area networks—is the master, and the Bluetooth-enabled medical instruments are slaves. A data collector, such as a personal data assistant (PDA), can collect data from the medical instruments and convey the data through the mobile phone.

With Bluetooth standards, the wireless network can be constructed in two ways: ad hoc or through infrastructure. In an ad hoc network, any node can communicate with other nodes in the Bluetooth piconet. In an infrastructure network, every Bluetooth node must link through a fixed access point to communicate with other nodes inside or outside the piconet. We adopt an infrastructure network and use the phone as the Bluetooth hub.

EXHIBIT 6.1. MOBILE BLUETOOTH TELEMEDICINE SYSTEM

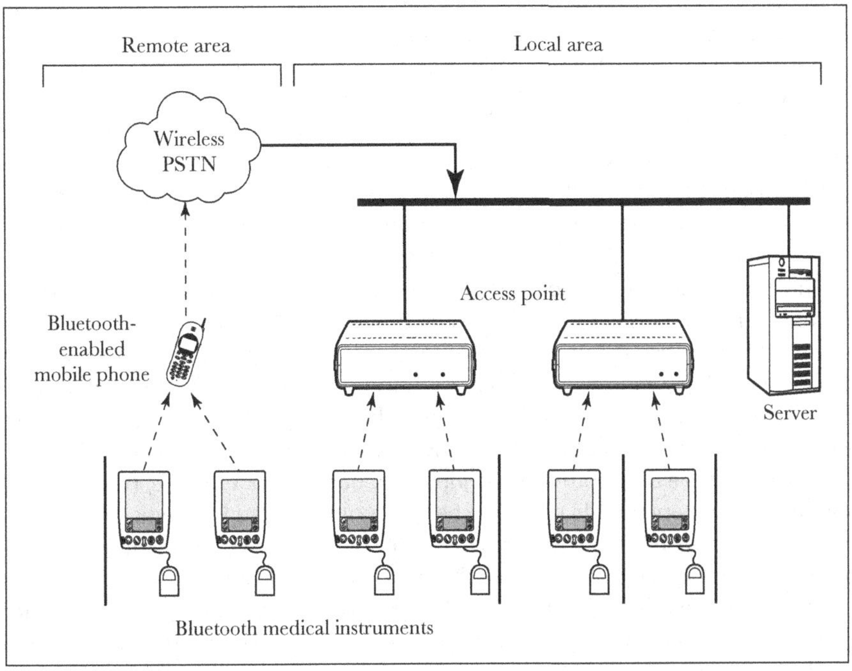

The medical instruments are based on an embedded computer running an operating system primarily designed to support real-time acquisition of data from biomedical sensors (Perez, 1998; Gomez et al., 1996; Banitsas, Tachakra, and Istepanian, 2002). Data can be stored in the instrument's memory or transmitted to a data collector for temporary storage, then sent to a central database server.

Two key parts of our unconfined mobile system are Bluetooth PANs or WLANs and wireless remote area networks. Many Bluetooth piconets cover a personal or local area environment—for example, a hospital or clinical ward unit or a home environment. The master of each piconet serves as the access point of a central medical database system, connecting wireless nodes in the sensor domain with the server or other nodes, either wired or wireless. A patient who is not bedbound can move around in the hospital or at home. The Bluetooth medical instruments worn by the patient send medical or patient data through a gateway (for example, a cellular phone) to the central database. Nurses or physicians can use their Bluetooth-enabled PDAs to access the central database to get data, including medical signals and images like ECGs and photoplethysmograms.

The patient can roam freely from one piconet to another. For unconfined wireless health services, we propose that the patient's cellular or mobile phone be exploited to collect data from the medical instruments, then the central database be accessed through a mobile PSTN or satellite network to store and retrieve data. The interaction of Bluetooth PANs and wireless remote area networks in a scalable and functional way is important, with the connectivity of the sensor domain and the remote area networks provided through packet translation, socket proxying, and so on.

In addition to connectivity, security is a key technical consideration as more than one server will be required to conduct secure wireless medicine. In this prototype, wireless service providers are given the responsibility of managing a central database for all of their cellular customers. The access control and authentication mechanisms currently used in cellular communication services are baseline security measures for a user (patient, physician, or nurse) to access the wireless database system. Additional security defenses will be needed, as we will discuss in the next section.

The rapid evolution of mobile and wireless telecommunication systems has given birth to faster data transfer rates and broader bandwidth. This evolution has facilitated our unconfined mobile medicine system, which requires high data transfer rates and on-line connection. Cellular telephones are commonplace today, and with improved services and increasing functionality, it would be practical for most patients to use cellular phones for the proposed unconfined mobile services. Several mobile phone models already have Bluetooth-enabled input and output—for example, Nokia's 7650. Adapting an ordinary mobile phone to be Bluetooth-enabled is technically straightforward, and the associated cost is moderate; thus, the cost of implementing our proposed system is expected to be within the reach of most people.

The volume of patient data could become large. If on-line monitoring is not necessary, home computers, PDAs, or dedicated electronic patient cards could be used to collect the medical data, which would then be periodically transmitted to the central database. If on-line monitoring is important, the cellular phone could send the medical data to the database in real time. Because it might be costly to store a lot of data in a wireless database maintained by the service provider, patients or physicians could regularly download the medical data from the central database. The diagnosis report and patient bills could also be uploaded from the hospital to the patient's account in the wireless database, and the patient could be informed via his or her cellular phone. A Bluetooth-enabled data container could be designed and dedicated to data storage; it would automatically download any relevant data from the wireless central database to the patient's data management system or collect data from the wireless sensors the patient wears.

Applications of Wireless Medicine

Our proposed mobile system has numerous prospective applications. It could be used for remote stethoscope diagnosis that is time-critical or for remote cooperative medical imaging diagnosis. (Woodward and Rasid, 2003; Hung and Zhang, 2002; Gomez et al., 1996).

Another simple yet important application is distant mobile nursing and daily data collection (Luo and Cheng, 2004). As previously mentioned, the serious shortage of nurses in the United States is unlikely to change in the near future. Wireless nursing systems provide more patients per nurse monitoring time (with physical attention given only to those who need help based on results of the remote monitoring) and can alleviate the shortage of nurses to a great degree; however, for any patient not physically in the hospital or at home, existing wireless nursing systems cannot work. In our proposed unconfined wireless medicine system, a patient's cellular phone collects medical or patient data from the Bluetooth-enabled sensors or instruments that the patient wears, then forwards them dynamically to the patient's account in the central database that is maintained by the wireless service provider.

Exhibit 6.2 shows the data flow of the unconfined mobile Bluetooth nursing system. The arrows denote communication. Medical data such as blood pressure, pulse, oxygen saturation, stethoscope signal, ECG, and other key measures can be sensed and conveyed to the cellular phone through Bluetooth links. The cellular phone then sends the data through the cellular or satellite networks to the central database, which is connected with the nurses or physicians. The patient is unconfined geographically. Neither are nurses or physicians limited to the wards. Nurses can monitor continually or check the medical data from the central medical database at regular times via their PDAs or wireless laptops. This way, one nurse can take care of more patients simultaneously.

EXHIBIT 6.2. DATA FLOW IN UNCONFINED MOBILE BLUETOOTH NURSING SYSTEM

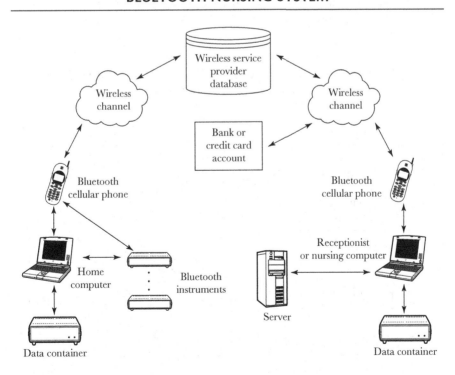

System Security Issues

For wireless medicine, security is critical (Banitsas, Tachakra, and Istepanian, 2002; Chakraborty, 1999). There are several ways to enhance the security of our proposed system: (1) designing access control mechanisms for the central database, including user authentication and authorization; (2) designing Bluetooth PAN or WLAN security based on secret keys and passwords or user biometrics such as retinal prints or other similar forms of identification useful for authentication so that the security will not be compromised even if the hardware is lost or stolen; (3) encapsulating PAN or WLAN security protocols with other security protocols like IPSec (Doraswamy and Harkins, 1999). Here, we will focus on the security of the Bluetooth protocol stack, because the stack is relatively vulnerable to both passive eavesdropping and active interfering, compared with the database or remote area networks.

The Bluetooth PAN or LAN offers both authentication and encryption at the baseband level (Gupta, Krishnamurthy, and Faloutsos, 2002). Exhibit 6.3 shows the security architecture for Bluetooth access.

In Bluetooth protocol, the commonly shared secret is called a *link key.* At initialization, the initialization key is the link key. Authentication is performed with a challenge-response scheme using the E1 algorithm, according to Bluetooth system specification. An encryption key is generated from the link key and a pseudorandom number, using the E3 algorithm. These mechanisms can be used to protect communications between two Bluetooth devices.

The security of Bluetooth is much better than that of IEEE 802.11b. The Bluetooth authentication never transmits the complete challenge-response pair. In addition, the

EXHIBIT 6.3. SECURITY ARCHITECTURE FOR BLUETOOTH LOCAL AREA NETWORK ACCESS

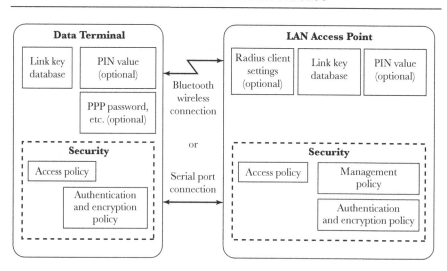

E1 algorithm is not easily invertible. Even if an attacker has recorded an authentication challenge-response session, this individual cannot directly use this information to compute the authentication key.

Typical Attacks on Bluetooth

Despite the security improvements of Bluetooth, there are still potential weaknesses. For instance, if an attacker can successfully get the personal identification number (PIN) code and especially the initialization key at initialization, then the protocol is vulnerable to attacks.

Several known Bluetooth holes include unique device address defined by IEEE, key management issues, PIN code but no support for user authentication. We will now consider three typical attacks exploiting these holes and suggest defenses. Then we will build a covert channel method to enhance the security.

Until a secure link is established, all exchanges between two devices are sent as plain text, including the variables for deriving the keys. The only defense is that a PIN and a device identity are used to generate an initialization key. All other link keys and authentication procedures depend on the initialization key. Thus, the initialization procedure is the most vulnerable. If an attacker can successfully guess or obtain the PIN, the initialization key and other link keys can subsequently be determined; furthermore, the attacker can decipher encrypted information from Bluetooth devices (Xydis and Blake-Wilson, 2002). The communications can then be subjected to eavesdropping and impersonation attacks. If an attacker has intercepted all information from the wireless channel at the initialization stage, then this individual may break the PIN code using brute force attacks. In many cases the PIN is a short number, so it is not that difficult to unlock. Thus, longer or random PINs should be used, and initialization should be performed only in a private place.

Because applications can choose to make a device connectable or discoverable (using Service Discovery Protocol), an attack on the Bluetooth system can be mounted by placing a rogue access point close to an existing WLAN. As wireless nodes usually associate with the access point that offers the best signal-to-noise ratio, they may connect to the rogue access point and lose contact with valid networks. Site survey can frequently be conducted to detect hidden access points.

Denial of service (DoS) is an active interfering attack that is very challenging to detect and prevent (Gupta, Krishnamurthy, and Faloutsos, 2002). An attacker can cause network congestion by generating an excessive amount of traffic either by itself or through other nodes. For the security of our proposed system, we need to consider both DoS attacks in wired networks, such as transmitting falsified route updates and reducing the time-to-live field in the IP headers causing data losses (Gupta, Krishnamurthy, and Faloutsos, 2002), and those in wireless networks. An attacker can send a message to keep the wireless channel busy, so that no other Bluetooth devices can use the channel. The attacker may use a particular node to continually relay spurious data so that the battery life of that node is drained. An end-to-end authentication may help prevent these attacks from being launched; however, DoS attacks will still be feasible if two legitimate nodes (one sender and one destination) collude.

Enhancing Security Using a Bluetooth Covert Channel

To defend against eavesdropping, interception, and impersonation, much attention has been given to encryption algorithms and sender/receiver authentications in the wireless networks.

For Bluetooth security in our proposed system, biometric authentication techniques are one promising approach. The patient's biometric traits such as blood type are entered into the cellular phone and verified on initialization of communication.

A complementary approach is to design three covert channels. These channels exploit the data frame headers of the Bluetooth protocol to transmit seemingly innocuous information between access points and sensor nodes. To guarantee the security of our covert channels, the sender can further encrypt or encode the covert messages. Many encoding algorithms—for example, the chaotic mixing algorithm—can be applied to our system (Qu and Cheng, 2004).

In the baseband layer, 13 bits can be transmitted as covert information; in the L2CAP layer, 8 or 9 bits (8 bits for signaling command packets, 9 bits for data packets); in the SDP layer, 16 bits. Thus, a 37-bit (or 38-bit) covert channel can be established in one Bluetooth packet. The covert channel can be exploited innocuously to transmit some information. Because only 37 or 38 bits can be sent per packet, this covert channel can send short yet critical information. We propose to send the activating share, a small number, via the designed covert channels, so that the pre-positioned secret-sharing mechanism (Simmons, 1989) can be enabled during Bluetooth key establishment. This is a particularly promising and powerful technique because it addresses holes in regard to PIN codes and user authentication. Moreover, the public-key method is less likely to be useful due to its high computational and associated architectural complexity. Our covert channel method combined with the pre-positioned secret sharing provides a solution. The covert channel method can also be applied to trace DoS attacks (Qu and Cheng, 2004).

Other security approaches relate specifically to medical image transmission. Some functional data are usually associated with the medical images, such as personal data of the patient and diagnosis results. Without the associated functional data, the medical image is of little use. One method to protect the security of these images is to selectively encrypt the image. The secret key can be established by using the secret-sharing scheme.

Exhibit 6.4 shows another method, in which the covert channel is used to transfer the patient's information, while the body field transfers the medical images. Encryption can be applied before the patient's data are sent through the covert channel.

Conclusion

Wireless medicine gives patients the freedom to go anywhere they like while receiving medical services and health care in a timely fashion. Our system minimizes interference in the patients' daily lives and empowers the medical providers as well. The system design and security issues can be managed, and a Bluetooth covert channel

EXHIBIT 6.4. USING A COVERT CHANNEL TO TRANSFER MEDICAL IMAGES

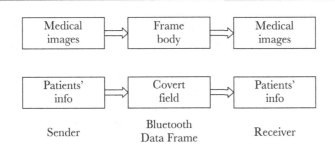

technique can enhance security. Miniaturized and portable medical instruments and sensors will further expand the application domains of our proposed system.

In mobile and wireless medicine, the power supply and battery life of the sensors or instruments are important and need to be studied. Hence, one fruitful research direction might be studying how to optimize the energy consumption of the proposed system. Another challenge is learning how best to incorporate advanced disease detection and prevention systems, which would be capable of analyzing automatically and reliably the medical data from Bluetooth-enabled sensors and providing warnings to both patients and physicians.

Case Questions

1. What other potential applications of the proposed mobile medicine system can you think of?
2. Besides the interoperability and security of PANs, WLANs, and remote area networks, what important technical issues do you feel should be considered in the proposed system?
3. Apart from technological issues, what are the social and economical implications of the proposed system? Imagine that you have been asked to evaluate the feasibility and acceptance of the proposed system among patients and providers. How would you go about doing this? What questions would you ask the providers and the patients?

References

Banitsas, K. A., Tachakra, S., & Istepanian, R.S.H. (2002, October). Operational parameters of a medical wireless LAN: Security, range and interference issues. In *Proceedings of the joint EMBS/BMES conference.* Houston, TX.

Bluetooth SIG Security Expert Group. (1999). *Specification of Bluetooth system.* (Vols. 1–2). Version 1.0, Part B.

Bluetooth SIG Security Expert Group. (2001, February). Baseband specification. *Specification of the Bluetooth system and core,* Version 1.1, Part B.

Bluetooth SIG Security Expert Group. (2002, April). *Bluetooth security white paper,* Version 1.0.

Chakraborty, S. (1999). Mobile multimedia: Concepts, services, and systems. In E. B. Furht (Ed.), *Handbooks of Internet and multimedia systems and applications.* CRC-IEEE Press.

Doraswamy, N., & Harkins, D. (1999). *IPsec: The new security standard for the Internet, intranet and virtual private networks.* Upper Saddle River, NJ: Prentice Hall.

Fluhrer, S., Mantin, I., & Shamir, A. (2001, August). Weakness in the key scheduling algorithm of RC4. In *Proceedings of the Annual Workshop on Selected Areas in Cryptography.*

Gomez, E.J., del Pozo, F., Quiles, J.A., Arredondo, M.T., Rahms, H., Sanz, M., & Cano, P. (1996). A telemedicine system for remote cooperative medical imaging diagnosis. *Computer Methods and Programs in Biomedicine, 49,* 37–48.

Gupta, V., Krishnamurthy, S., & Faloutsos, M. (2002). Denial of service attacks at the MAC layer in wireless ad hoc networks. In *Proceedings of MILCOM.*

Haykin, S., & Moher, M. (2003). *Modern wireless communications.* Upper Saddle River, NJ: Prentice Hall.

Hung, K., & Zhang, Y. T. (2002, October). Usage of Bluetooth in wireless sensors for tele-healthcare. In *Proceedings of the joint EMBS/BMES Conference.* Houston, TX.

Knudsen, L., Meier, W., Preneel, B., Rijmen, V., & Verdoolaege, S. (1998). Analysis method for (alleged) RC4. In *Proceedings of ASIACRYPT.*

Luo, X., & Cheng, Q. (2004, January). Unconfined mobile Bluetooth nursing and daily data collection. In *Proceedings of the IEEE Consumer Communications Networking Conference.* Las Vegas, NV.

Molts, D. (2001, December). Mobile and wireless technology. *Network Computing.*

Perez, R. (1998). *Wireless communications design handbook.* New York: Academic Press.

Qu, H., & Cheng, Q. (2004). *Enhancing Bluetooth security with covert channel signaling.* Unpublished manuscript.

Rappaport, T. S. (2002). *Wireless communications principles and practice* (2nd ed.). Upper Saddle River, NJ: Prentice Hall.

Simmons, G. J. (1989). Prepositioned shared secret and/or shared control schemes. In *Proceedings of Advances in Cryptology-EUROCRYPT.*

Woodward, B., & Rasid, M.F.A. (2003). Wireless telemedicine: The next step? In *Proceedings of the annual IEEE Conference on Information Technology Applications in Biomedicine.*

Xydis, T. G., & Blake-Wilson, S. (2002, February). Security comparison: Bluetooth communications vs. 802.11. *Bluetooth Security Expert Group.*

PART THREE

E-HEALTH DOMAINS
AND APPLICATIONS

The first two parts of this text provide a comprehensive overview and foundational knowledge of the early development (Part One) and continuing growth and development (Part Two) of the e-health field. Part Three begins by examining how various e-health domains and applications are interrelated. Chapter Seven highlights e-health domains as part of e-health landscapes and relates it to various e-health care services, providing an overview as well as a set of concepts that are explored in the other chapters of Part Three. Chapters Eight through Eleven focus on e-medicine, e-home care, e-diagnosis support systems (especially for back pain) and e-health intelligence through data mining and clustering.

CHAPTER SEVEN

E-HEALTH DOMAINS

Surveying the E-Health Landscape: Cases and Applications

Pam Forducey, Kawaljeet Kaur, Cynthia Scheideman-Miller, Joseph Tan

This chapter was made possible by grant number 5H2ATM00245–06 from the Advancement of Tele-health, Health Resources and Service Administration, U.S. Department of Health and Human Services.

Learning Objectives

1. Identify various models and modalities of the evolving e-health care system, including e-commerce, e-health, telemedicine, telehealth, e-home care (or telecare)
2. Illustrate the use of e-medicine, e-rehabilitation, e-home care, and e-disease management technologies and their significance for the future of e-health care development
3. Conceptualize e-learning and tele-educational models for intentionally affecting user (patient and provider) behavioral changes
4. Know the various facets of e-administrative and support services to which information technology and e-technologies are being applied
5. Understand e-rehabilitation as an application to illustrate a specific e-health domain

Introduction

Fifty-nine percent of Americans believe that our current health care system requires a major restructuring. This statistic is not surprising, given the stark reality that the annual health budget of the United States is now estimated at over a trillion dollars, while approximately 45 million Americans do not have health insurance.

Due to escalating costs of health care delivery, the Center for Medicare and Medicaid Services—a U.S. government agency—has imposed financial restrictions such as managed care and a prospective payment system (PPS). PPS essentially provides predetermined fixed-price payment rates for specific categories of illnesses or diagnostic related groups (DRGs). Because the PPS depended extensively on the use of averages to calculate reimbursements and payments to the health facility treating an insured patient, the system does not consider the severity of the patient's illness nor are the facilities being reimbursed if actual payments exceed those PPS-calculated payments. Moreover the lack of predictability of such payments, increased regulations due to the federal deficit reduction initiatives and other factors such as structural and educational payment changes make it difficult for hospitals and other health agencies to rely on traditional guarantees of payments for their services. PPS therefore mandates that health care facilities reexamine resource utilization and organizational effectiveness. Simply put, there is a serious and urgent need for a reevaluation of our health care system and exploration of alternative approaches to health care financing and delivery if we are to contain U.S. health care costs and prevent their further acceleration (Woods, 2001).

In Canada, the situation is perhaps equally serious; for example, hundreds of residents in the small town of Windsor do not have a family physician and rely on walk-in clinics. The Canadian shortage of doctors and nurses is causing delays and longer waiting times even for prescheduled surgical interventions, as well as an increasing number of bed closures, causing a continual shifting of services from primary care to secondary and tertiary care facilities. Health care costs for all parties including local government, providers and consumers alike have continued to rise in every Canadian province because of federal budgetary restraints, the aging population, and increasing dollars set aside for national security, public preparedness, and surveillance to defend against terrorist activities. Given the current unlimited wants and demands from all directions but only very limited health care resources to spare, it is critical for us to examine where-about (the domains) and how specifically (the applications) emerging e-technologies can maintain, even improve, the health status and future well-being of those living in countries such as the U.S. and Canada.

Emerging technologies and accompanying processes are being incorporated into mainstream health care on a daily basis. The expanding field of information and communication technology (ICT) is producing applications in e-commerce, e-health, telemedicine, telehealth, and e-home care (or telecare). *E-commerce* refers to the use of ICT to conduct business transactions, irrespective of physical or geographic boundaries. *E-health*, *telemedicine*, and *telehealth* all entail the application of the same principles to the health care field—that is, facilitating communications, collaborations, and e-commerce between health care providers and consumers without the limitations of time and location that are imposed by the traditional health care system. *E-home care (telecare)* is the application of the same technology for patient care, especially tele–home health care services. Despite fine semantic differences, many of these terms are sometimes used interchangeably.

There are two primary types of e-commerce transactions in health care: business-to-business (B2B) and business-to-consumer (B2C) transactions. *B2B transactions* are between the business entities, including the vendors, hospitals, insurance agencies, physicians' offices, and regulatory agencies. Consumers are not directly involved in these transactions. *B2C transactions* are between businesses or providers on the one hand and consumers on the other hand. In the context of e-health systems, these transactions may also be referred to as *patient-to-provider (P2P) transactions*. Another rapidly growing cluster of e-health care activities involves *consumer-to-consumer (C2C) applications* that have contributed to the creation of virtual communities, which have great potential to empower individuals and the public (Svensson, 2003).

A majority of e-health interactions use the World Wide Web as the infrastructure for business activities. The Web has the advantage of universal client software (Web browser) and a preexisting platform (the Internet). For e-commerce activities, eXtensible Markup Language (XML) provides a functional platform for transactional data exchange. The other major infrastructure used in e-health commerce systems is electronic data interchange (EDI), the exchange of data among organizations in a structured format (explained in Chapter One). However, due to high cost, the need for proprietary software, and trading volume requirements, EDI is rapidly declining in popularity, making way for Web-based, XML-functional e-health systems (Aggarwal and Travers, 2001). The theoretical perspectives for understanding and differentiating among the various e-commerce models discussed here have been explored to some extent in Chapter Three. Our focus in this chapter is on applications of e-health models and technologies.

Health care is a knowledge- and information-intensive industry, and e-health is changing health care. E-health has diverse applications, some of which have been studied and used extensively (for example, teleradiology, as discussed in the preceding chapter), while others are still in the experimental phase (for example, virtual reality which is discussed in Chapter Sixteen). Most e-health applications fit into three broad categories based on primary functions: (1) e-medical and direct patient care, (2) e-learning and tele-educational services, and (3) e-administrative and support services. This chapter is organized according to these three major service clusters. Once this background is in place, we examine the services performed at INTEGRIS Jim Thorpe Rehabilitation Center as a case study of e-health service domains.

E-Medical or Direct Patient Care Services

E-medical or direct patient care services involve the administration of direct patient care using ICT. These applications include the following:

- E-medicine, including e-diagnostic imaging
- E-home care and telemonitoring
- E-counseling
- E-disease management

E-medicine (or *telemedicine*) is the delivery of general and specialty e-clinical services to remote areas, using ICT and e-networking (see Chapter Six). In recent years, telemedicine has branched into various specialty disciplines that include the transmission of visual media in fields like teleradiology, teledermatology, telepathology, tele-ophthalmology, telesurgery, and robotics, as well as direct patient care and rehabilitation. Chapter Eight focuses on applications of e-medicine for both developed countries such as Canada and developing regions such as sub-Saharan Africa; Chapter Ten presents future developments in teleradiology; and Chapter Sixteen discusses virtual reality applications such as telesurgery and robotics.

Although it is increasing in popularity, e-medicine faces several challenges. First, e-medicine can require expensive infrastructure, making it difficult for underdeveloped or developing countries to adopt the technology. In addition, this same technology is not very useful for island states like Singapore because of its extent of urbanization, unless these city-states are used as centers for providing specialty e-medical care to less developed neighboring countries that have many rural settings. For example, Singapore could act as a hub, providing teleradiological services to other South-East Asian countries such as Malaysia, Vietnam, Cambodia, Thailand, Indonesia and the Philippines.

To be successful in teleradiology, however, as in any marketplace, a critical volume of services must be rendered in order to achieve cost-effectiveness and economies of scale. Difficulties also could arise due to different cultural and economic standards in neighboring countries; lack of equipment compatibility; uncertainty or lack of political will to participate in the program; socioeconomic complexities; cultural differences and regional relationships; legal procedures and policies regarding reimbursement for services; or currency valuation and monetary exchange policies, among other factors. Cooperation at national and international levels would be needed to realize such a vision. An official ceremony at which agreements of understanding are signed by the different heads of the countries is likely to be warranted, in order to promote sustained and meaningful collaborations among the countries.

E-medicine becomes truly cost-effective when it is planned and designed, just as with e-business, to become an integral part of the country's telecommunications and information technology infrastructure. Accordingly, e-medicine can then be available to serve a large geographical area in many health care specialty domains—for example, teleradiology and e-rehabilitation—where the costs of hiring specialists in these specific domain areas are prohibitive. Although e-medicine faces the problem of lack of physicality and direct human interaction, it is becoming increasingly popular as a means of providing care to the medically underserved and to areas experiencing health care shortages. Most e-medicine programs started as federally funded pilot projects to demonstrate the efficacy, viability, and feasibility of telemedicine networks. Concerted action is needed at both national and international levels to develop standards in order to reach network compatibility and build ethical frameworks (Stanberry, 2000; Terry, 2001; Mitchell, 2000).

E-medicine involves several components, all of which work together to create a strong consumer-oriented environment. *Teleconsulting* refers to the use of e-medical services by the patient to consult with a health care provider. *Teleconferencing* is the use of e-medicine by clinicians to confer with one another about a patient. *Telereporting* is the transmission of information about a patient to a remote site. *Telemonitoring* refers to monitoring a patient remotely by collecting patient information and analyzing it at a remote site.

Potential benefits of telemedicine include fewer office visits for patients; improved care for the elderly and people living in remote areas; convenience; and cost reduction. The disadvantages include missing the benefits of direct physical interaction; and costs associated with technology infrastructure setup. Challenges in implementing telemedicine include lack of consistency and quality in video links; patient confidentiality issues; need for support from management; and need for motivation on the part of patients and providers to try a new health care delivery model.

Tele-Ultrasound in Australia

Diagnostic ultrasound is an important component of health care services that is in great demand. In isolated and rural areas, however, a lack of local clinical expertise often limits its use. The Commonwealth Scientific and Industrial Research Organization's Telecommunications and Industrial Physics Center at Macquarie University in Sydney, Australia, has developed a high-performance, low-bandwidth, real-time tele-ultrasound device. This device transmits live ultrasound images to an expert consultant while the examination is in progress. The system operates under the control of the expert at the receiving end, which minimizes distractions from the ultrasound operator at the transmitting end and enables the expert to set transmission parameters.

Tele-ultrasound operates satisfactorily at a transmission rate of 128 kilobits per second because it uses compression technology with a "region of interest" within which the image is transmitted at high resolution and at relatively high frame rates. The remainder of the image is transmitted at a relatively low frame rate. The position and size of the region of interest is controlled by the consultant at the receiving end. The tele-ultrasound technique is compatible with all types of ultrasound equipment and is suitable for both color and gray-scale images (Tele-Health Applications, 2003).

E-Home Care Services at the University of Tennessee

E-medicine does not just include direct interaction through video modalities; it is increasingly being used for telemonitoring of patients in *e-home care* applications. For example, remote heart monitoring through halter devices is being used at several places in Europe; using devices such as mobile phones, data are transmitted in real time to the base station for analysis. Projects are also under way to develop sensing and storage technologies, which permit installation of simple devices in the home that link into a network for remote monitoring by health care professionals; medical interventions take place only when needed.

The telephone is the oldest tool for e-home care services. For example, University of Tennessee Home Care Services, along with the University of Tennessee Medical Center Telemedicine Network at Knoxville started providing e-home care in April 1998 as part of a federally funded demonstration project. The system uses a video camera, a video monitor, a speakerphone, and an electronic interface with the regular analog phone line at the patient's home. In addition, handheld digital monitoring devices such as glucometers, sphygmomanometers, pulse oximetry, spirometers, scales, and thermometers are used to check the patient's situation.

With these e-home technologies, nurses can now "see" their patients, evaluate medication compliance, read home monitors, and even check the dose in an insulin syringe. Skin tones and wounds can be assessed remotely. Based on the travel costs saved, the investment per home has been shown to be equivalent to the cost of about thirty home care visits. More intriguing is that the nurses were proficient with the system within just one week of training. It is conceivable that where there is a shortage of qualified nurses and doctors, paramedics and home caregivers can be trained to substitute for professional nurses, and residents and foreign doctors can substitute for licensed physicians. This will only work if the resulting home health care services are legal in the proposed jurisdiction.

In a study by Dimmick, Mustaleski, Burgiss, and Welsh (2000), nurses and some primary care physicians made about 444 tele–home care visits for conditions ranging from congestive heart failure to diabetes. The system had the benefit of low capital equipment cost and ease of use. Typically, the home care patient was called once or twice per week, depending on the patient's condition. Both the patient and the caregiver were trained in the use of the videophone and other equipment. Depending on the patient's hearing capabilities, the patient used either the speakerphone or the phone receiver. Telehealth has progressed considerably over the years (Durtschi, 2001), and as telephone technologies advance, new means of connecting with patients to enhance e-home care will naturally emerge. More recently, the concept of smart homes for the elderly and frail has brought together architects, building contractors, electrical and mechanical engineers, health care professionals and workers, owners of security management companies, and others to adapt existing houses to serve the needs of the e-home care industry. This topic is discussed further in Chapter Nine.

Other E-Home Care, E-Counseling, and E-Disease Management Applications

Studies similar to Dimmick, Mustaleski, Burgiss, and Welsh's have been conducted elsewhere. In the United Kingdom, researchers explored the management of chronic obstructive pulmonary disease through interactive video. The e-care providers were able to complete charts, assess oxygen saturation, evaluate peak expiratory flow rates, and measure temperature and pulse, all through interactive videos. The Harvard

Telepsychiatry Project investigated the use of videophones to provide telepsychiatric services in home health settings, with encouraging results. In North Carolina, the use of e-home care resulted in fewer long-term care placements and a reduction in the number of emergency room visits and in-patient hospitalizations (Dimmick, Mustaleski, Burgiss, and Welsh, 2000).

E-counseling (or on-line counseling) is another telemedicine modality that is gaining popularity as a means of reaching teenagers and other target populations who would not otherwise seek help. According to Xinhua News Agency, an on-line suicide intervention center was recently launched in China that connects patients with fifty psychiatrists from forty-four hospitals throughout the country. The Beijing Suicide Research and Prevention Center will provide services to a select population of 16 million Chinese who have various mental disorders. A recent survey in China revealed that about 90 percent of people with depression received no medical treatment, and only about 20 percent of those who sought treatment were treated appropriately. If anonymity and confidentiality can be ensured, the benefits of having a Web-based e-counseling service to serve these high-risk population groups far outweigh the costs of maintaining the Web site.

E-disease management is the last specialty domain of telemedicine that we will cover in this discussion. The concept of e-disease management is based on the fact that patients with chronic illnesses account for 70 percent or more of health care costs. In theory, therefore, an efficient e-disease management program could substantially reduce medical and administrative costs, resulting in trickle-down benefits for both patients and payers. E-patients who are interested in self-care can join a specific management program and report their vital readings via the Internet or phone on a daily basis. A nurse checks the readings regularly and alerts the patient if he or she notices any abnormality or change. Aggarwal and Travers (2001) argue that advertising, sponsorship, or subscription fees can generally be used to support or sustain these programs.

E-disease management systems range from sophisticated Web-based systems to text reminders on cell phones to networked hospital and community-based programs. Health Buddy, created by Health Hero Network in Mountain View, California, is a Web-based e-disease management tool that is being used for congestive heart failure (CHF) management. Health Buddy is a book-sized computer that asks the patient's weight and blood pressure. When directed by a nurse, it also has the capacity to ask the patient a set of questions (for example, what, when, and how various symptoms of the illnesses become aggravated or relieved). Such systems hold the promise of decreasing treatment costs, but they usually require costly, hard-wired computer systems that may be slow to change with changes in treatment protocols. Proponents of these e-disease management systems include vendors, application service providers (software vendors who also sometimes provide health computing consulting), and Web site developers. A conclusive business and clinical case for such e-disease management systems is still to be made (Joch, 2000).

LifeMasters is an example of a cost-saving e-disease management program for CHF patients. A controlled study revealed that the use of LifeMasters had resulted in savings of approximately $950 per month for CHF patients, with a 66-percent reduction in emergency room visits, compared with the control group. The referral process for patients wanting to be physically seen by their care providers involves about ten to fifteen steps, with the cost adding up to about $40 per referral. Many, if not all, of these steps can be bypassed if providers and patients are willing to go the electronic route (Goran and Standford, 2001).

E-LEARNING AND TELE-EDUCATION SERVICES

Electronic media and Web-based systems are increasingly being used for e-learning and tele-educational purposes, for patients as well as for health care professionals. Applications of e-health education include the following:

- Medical information Web sites
- Virtual communities
- Web-based databases
- E-learning

Medical and Health Information Web Sites

Access to medical information via the Internet has the potential to accelerate the transformation of the patient-physician relationship from that of physician authority ministering advice and treatment to that of shared decision making between the patient and the physician (Winker and others, 2000). According to analysis conducted by Mediametrix (mediametrix.com), the most frequently visited health sites on the Web include Intellihealth.com (Johns Hopkins), Mayohealth.org, and OnHealth.com. These sites provide health-related news and information in an interactive way (Cochrane, 1995). A survey by Harris Interactive (2003) indicates that the number of adults looking for health information on-line has been steadily increasing: 27 percent in 1998, 34 percent in 1999, 47 percent in 2001, and 53 percent in 2002. E-consumers with higher incomes and college or postgraduate degrees are more likely to use the Internet to find health information than their lower-paid or less educated counterparts. Hirsch (2000) argues that a better-informed patient will result in more time for the development of the doctor-patient relationship and thereby improve therapeutic compliance and outcome. E-physicians are also using Web-based information—for example, the "Harrison Online" Web site, where the information is provided mostly in the form of e-books, which are updated much more frequently than traditional paper publications (Selsky and others, 2001). Other sites such as "MDConsult" and "StatReference" also have full-text reference books with complete search capabilities. Most of these sites also contain practice guidelines and drug information or links to other sites that contain such information.

Virtual Communities

The creation of virtual on-line communities (e-communities) (see the case in Chapter Fifteen), so that people with similar interests could chat with one another, was one of the earliest uses of the Internet. This type of communication has become increasingly popular in health care, even among senior groups, minorities, and those living in rural and remote areas. Virtual communities serve as on-line support groups for both e-patients and e-caregivers. Numerous e-health companies are also promoting the concept of virtual communities as part of e-disease management programs. These communities provide consumers with general information, information about medical research on particular diseases, and information on available products and services specific to these diseases, as well as psychological support from affected patients facing the same condition. In addition, these communities provide a locus for patient advocacy.

Paradoxically, the patients who benefit the most from such communities are the ones with rare diseases, because virtual communities allow them to conveniently communicate with other people experiencing the same condition. For such patients, being a member of a virtual community can provide tremendous positive psychological effect (Patsos, 2001). A good example of such a support group is Alzheimer's Caregiver Support Online (2003). This community is the culmination of teamwork between the state of Florida's Department of Elders Affairs and the University of Florida's Center for Research on Telehealth and Healthcare Communications. The site presents scheduled expert presentations on topics relating to dementia care and provides a message board; a chat room for the users (this serves as a support group); and an e-library (electronic or digital library) that provides information on dementia, caregiving techniques, and research and developments in the field. The site also provides links to other state, federal, and community resources for dementia caregivers. The virtual class presentations are interactive and hosted by the staff, and they can be recorded so that viewers have the flexibility to view them at their convenience.

Web-Based Databases

As biological databases expand as a result of new research in genetics and other medical fields, a huge market is emerging in portal-based dissemination of biological content for the process of drug discovery testing, research and development. OVID, PubMed, and Medline are databases that store information in the form of journal articles, available on a subscription basis or otherwise (Jadad and Gagliardi, 1998; Razvi, 2000). Some of these databases include the Cumulative Index to Nursing and Allied Health Literature (CINAHL); Health and Psychosocial Instruments (HAPI); the Educational Resources Information Center (ERIC); Cancer Literature Online (CANCERLIT); AIDS Information Online (AIDSLINE); Online Mendelian Inheritance in Man (OMIM); and the Structure, Taxonomy, and Genome Databases.

In recent years, discussions have been ongoing to facilitate research and education; Internet2 is a consortium led by two hundred universities, in partnership with the government and industry, to develop advanced Internet technology and applications. It is a project of the University Corporation for Advanced Internet Development. Internet2 provides a leading-edge network capability for the national research community by linking research databases. Aside from increased speed and capacity compared to what are currently available in the Internet, Internet2 is designed to be reserved primarily for use in high-powered computing related research and development.

E-Learning

Although Web-based education is becoming commonplace in universities and colleges, its acceptance in the health care setting is still lagging, more in Canada than in the United States. Health care curriculum is different from that of most other fields, but e-learning has its place even in this specific context. Health care professionals can now attend classes, group meetings, workshops, conferences, and educational events online. With the expansion of voice and video capabilities, face-to-face interaction and learning are becoming easier (Hirsch, 2000; Herrin, 2001; Neuhauser, 2000).

In health care, e-learning has been primarily used for continuing medical education courses for professionals (e-CME) and administrative training in areas such as compliance. Many companies and physician portals provide such courses. The major ones are Healthstream, Physicians Online, Massachusetts General Hospital, Johns Hopkins, Mayo Clinic, and WebMD. These programs range from pure Web-based programs to hybrid Internet and compact disc (CD) modules that combine the record-keeping capabilities of the Internet with the bandwidth of CD media as data to be shared or integrated are either on the CD or on the Internet (Anderson and Stenzel, 2001).

E-learning also involves multimedia training systems and simulations. Computer simulation modeling has advanced considerably over the past twenty years and is now widely employed in various teaching settings. One example of a learning simulation is CathSim Intravenous Training System, which is used by nurses to learn how to perform intravenous annulations before they do the procedure on a real patient. CathSim is a computer-based system that has interactive multimedia instructions and a tactile feedback device. Feedback is provided on the final outcome as well as on the progression of the procedure. This simulation-based training improves nurses' experience and comfort level with doing the procedure, with resultant decrease in the rates of complications in the patients after intravenous annulations (Chang, Chung, and Wong, 2002). Surgeons at the University of Kentucky are developing computer-based simulators to train other surgeons to perform minimally invasive procedures. The simulators are based on the 3-D and other virtual reality technology previously used only in flight simulators.

Another example of an e-learning application would be the use of computer software in an easy-to-use educational module to help pregnant women who stopped smoking during pregnancy to avoid postpartum relapse. Such patients could be kept abreast of the latest research on the effect of smoking on childbirth and on their own health following childbirth. They could also be educated on strategies for overcoming the temptation to relapse.

The key to effective e-learning software is the design of the interface, because, to the user, the interface is simultaneously the computer, the counseling coach, and the motivating change agent. Understanding how best to present the information to users, how to design the interface so as to entice users to interact with the program regularly, and how to motivate the user in transforming their thoughts and behaviors as a result of their use of the software is a sure path to success. For example, the best marksmen among new military recruits were those who had previously played computer games, which provided them with virtual experience in shooting down enemies that dynamically move and disappear and reappear. This sort of training can be extended to health care providers for preparation of e-emergency services or e-hazard readiness.

E-ADMINISTRATIVE AND SUPPORT SERVICES

Health care providers use ICT and e-technologies for a variety of administrative and support services:

- E-prescription
- Electronic health records
- E-supply ordering, e-claims, and remittance
- E-decision support
- E-work

E-Prescription

Prescription drug business in the United States amounts to about $100 billion per year. Attempts have been and are still being made to "e-volutionize" this industry (Menduno, 1999a). Many new companies (some of which are offshoots of more established corporations) such as Allscripts, PocketScript, ePhysician, and iScribe are entering the market of *e-prescription* (electronic prescribing of drugs). Most of these companies use handheld devices for order entry. Automating order entry not only improves work flow but also saves a significant amount of physicians' and pharmacists' time. Medical errors are reduced significantly, resulting in better drug use information and improved patient satisfaction (Anderson and Stenzel, 2001).

Piloting online prescription drugs, Kinetra, based in Colorado, recently launched a pilot project with network service provider ProxyMed, linking nearly one thousand physicians to Walgreen's and Eckerd pharmacies. The project also included two managed care programs that collectively manage prescriptions for more than 100 million patients. The participating physicians logged into on-line formularies and entered their patient's drug histories whenever they wrote a prescription. Benefit managers could e-mail prescription renewal requests rather than calling the physician's office. The pilot has been a great success. Lower costs and reduced medical errors provide the biggest incentives for the project (Menduno, 1999a).

Most retail pharmacies also provide the option of ordering prescription refills online. The medicine can then be picked up from the pharmacy or mailed to the patient's home. Advantages of this practice include patient convenience and probable cost-effectiveness as no waiting time is involved and human transcription errors can be drastically reduced for patients on medications for chronic conditions. Virtual pharmacies also e-mail refill reminders and medication instructions that can lead to improved patient compliance. Unfortunately, patients may attempt to misuse the system by seeking to obtain drugs without an appropriate medical prescription, including unapproved or untested drugs or herbs. The process is expected to improve as specific guidelines and regulations are enacted and enforced. The American Medical Association plans to release ethics guidelines for e-physicians who intend to authorize on-line prescriptions.

Electronic Health Records

The use of electronic health records (EHRs) has grown and improved over the last thirty years, as Chapter Four discusses at length. Electronic records provide the advantages of storing patient information in a digital format, reducing medical errors, providing feedback and reminders, and aiding in outcomes analysis. Although most current programs are based on a mainframe or a client-server architecture, the focus is rapidly shifting to a Web-based application service provider model. Web-based applications have the advantages of open architecture, standard interfaces, and data transmission standards. EHRs are being increasingly subjected to security regulations, including the Health Insurance Portability and Accountability Act privacy rules, which regulate all health care electronic data interchange.

Some of the earlier EHR programs include Medscape's Logician for ambulatory care physician practices; Epic System's EpicCare for large, multisite practices; and Cerner's Millennium products, which combine clinical and administrative tasks for large health care systems. Kaiser Permanente, the nation's largest health care group, recently partnered with Epic Systems Corporation to initiate a paperless automated medical record system for its 8.4 million members nationwide. The system will be deployed during the next few years and will provide a clinical data repository for all patient data, which is being designed to be accessible twenty-four hours a day, seven days a week, from anywhere, with the hope of improving patient care through a reduction in administrative costs. These data will also be used for outcomes analysis, cost analysis, performance assessment, and trend analysis.

Wireless and handheld devices are increasingly being used in conjunction with EHRs to facilitate order entry, to increase efficiency, and to improve work flow by providing access to patient information from anywhere (Anderson and Stenzel, 2001). Tablet personal computers (PCs) are also gaining in popularity. They are smaller and lighter than a laptop computer, but have a bigger screen and provide easier data entry than personal digital assistants (PDAs). A growing number of vendors are developing programs specifically for tablet PCs and PDAs with enhanced features such as handwriting recognition and voice recognition. The development of wireless network infrastructure and the decreasing prices of these systems are stimulating the adaptation of these devices for regular patient care.

E-Supply Ordering, E-Claims, and E-Remittance

The supply industry is estimated to about $140 billion annually. Although on-line B2B health care supply procurement is in its infancy, it has already proved that it has several benefits. Real-time inventories and competitive pricing, which is not too different from traditional advertising, enable purchasing departments to compare prices on-line and plan their purchases electronically so that inventories can be filled just as they are needed to be filled (just-in-time inventory management). Orders can also be tracked digitally in order to support timely delivery. On-line ordering is a win-win situation for both purchasers and vendors; e-manufacturers can interact directly with e-purchasers, eliminating intermediaries. This direct interaction can ultimately reduce prices for the purchaser and increase profit margins for the manufacturer as the manufacturer will not over-manufacture certain parts and purchaser reduces holding costs in unwanted inventories.

Among other tangible benefits, a data warehouse can be used to track purchased items, and data mining can be applied to unravel usage patterns. Electronic auctions can be used for on-line trading of health care supplies and goods, as in supply chain management of any other business. Requests for proposals can be sent electronically, thereby saving time. Because hospitals often stock 100,000 units of popular items, e-procurement will work only if the searching for a match between supplier and purchaser is automated, which currently is not often the case (Arbietman, Lirov, Lirov, and Lirov, 2001; DeJesus, 1999; Menduno, 1999b).

The Alamo City Medical Group in San Antonio, Texas, comprises sixteen family physicians in eight different locations. According to their director of nursing, ordering supplies used to take about a day every month, filling out purchase orders for multiple vendors. The nurses at practice sites used to go through their supply closets to see what they needed. Since the group has switched to e-supply ordering, the process usually takes less than two hours every month. The on-line purchasing vendor has customized order forms for each practice site that are based on established ordering patterns. The nurses check off these forms, indicating what they need, and the order is entered via the vendor's Web site. Confirmation is instantaneous, and the order arrives within two days. The group reports a savings of about $8,000 every month due to savings in holding costs for inventories (35 to 40 percent of the medical supply budget) (Terry, 2002).

Increasing costs put pressure on health care providers and payers to improve decision-making processes and control expenses. The number of hospitals that submit their claims electronically has been rising over time generating an immediate effect on return on investment (ROI). According to John Glaser, vice president and chief information officer of Partners Health System, Boston, "The manual process of determining eligibility doesn't work well. We have a claim denial rate of 11 percent. Our goal is to reduce that to 5 percent. In large part that comes from online technologies for eligibility verification, pre-certificate referral authorization. The ROI is spectacular" (Solovy, 2000; Riley and Korpman, 2001).

E-Decision Support

E-decision support systems are data analysis and modeling tools that automatically track patterns and trends in a data repository or data warehouse (Tan with Sheps, 1998; Tan, 2001). The resulting analysis is then used to guide decision making. In essence, it is the process of converting raw data into useful information and then into rich and valuable knowledge. The primary types of e-decision support system (e-DSS) in health care include marketing, cost management, forecasting, and case-mix systems. Executive information systems are e-decision support systems that allow user-defined views of data. On-line analytical processing tools are becoming increasingly popular as a form of decision support. These provide the ability to slice and dice the data into various views and levels. The information obtained from these systems can be used to track outcomes, to develop clinical practice guidelines, or to develop e-disease management programs for target populations (Forgionne, Gangopadhyay, Klein, and Eckhardt, 1999).

Most health maintenance organizations structure their health plans by using an e-DSS to design benefits based on member characteristics, claims, and revenue information. Data patterns can also be used to detect possible fraud and system abuse (Callan, 2000). Clinical decision support systems have yet to gain much popularity. An example of such a system is Quick Medical Reference, which helps make clinical diagnoses based on signs and symptoms that have been entered into the system. Chapter Ten describes the application of an e-DSS to aid clinical diagnosis and management of lower back pain, while Chapter Eleven discusses the use of data mining and clustering methodology to detect hidden trends and data patterns.

E-Work

Now we will take a closer look at e-work in general, which has evolved from the use of information and communication technology and e-decision support systems for general e-health and other e-administrative and support applications. The users of these various e-technologies may be individuals, groups, organizations, or communities at large.

According to recent statistics, in 2000, nearly 80 percent of the world's largest companies used the Internet for recruiting, up from 60 percent in 1999 and 29 percent in 1998. On-line recruitment can translate into huge cost savings for an organization. According to a study by Creative Good, an e-commerce consulting firm in New York City, a facility can save up to $8,000 per person hired ($2,000 in advertising costs and $6,000 in time spent on interviewing on site because sending recruiters to various conferences and placement sites is costly) (Goldsborough, 2000). The health care industry has followed the general trend in this regard. Some popular recruiting sites include emedjobs.com, healthcareersonline.com, hospitalhub.com, medhunters.com, and nurserecruiter.com.

Advances in technology have removed the physical and geographic constraints that required workers to be at their workplace in order to accomplish productive work. E-work, or telework, is gaining popularity in administrative, research, and other support components of health care that do not require direct patient interaction. According to the International Telework Association and Council, on average, telecommuting increases productivity by 22 percent while decreasing employee turnover and absenteeism by 20 percent and 60 percent, respectively.

E-work or telecommuting options include working from home, working from a satellite office (a remote office location usually placed within an area of concentration of employee residences), a neighborhood work center that provides work space for employees of different companies in close proximity to the employees' residences, and a virtual mobile office that enable an e-worker to work from a car, an airport, a hotel, or any other location, as long as connectivity can be achieved. Employees may "e-work" part-time or full-time. E-work, however, entails specific challenges that need to be overcome, including management control issues, culture change for the organization, start-up costs, security issues, distractions, and lack of support services at home or in other locations where the e-work is to be performed (Dougherty and Scichilone, 2002). Examples of e-work include having online medical transcriptions performed and/or call centers manned by e-workers located in India and China.

TeleRehab™ at INTEGRIS Jim Thorpe Rehabilitation Center

Few e-medicine programs consist of only one application or discipline. Rather, most of them are a combination of the electronic clinical or administrative categories that we have just discussed. INTEGRIS Rural Health received a rural e-medicine grant (1997–2000 and 2000–2003) from the Health Resources and Services Administration in the Office of Advancement of Telehealth, a US government agency, to improve access to health care for rural individuals across the life span, to reduce isolation of rural medical practitioners, and to collect and disseminate resulting data. Under this grant, INTEGRIS Jim Thorpe Rehabilitation Center (IJTRC) provided e-rehabilitation services for physical therapy, occupational therapy, speech therapy, rehabilitation psychology, and vocational rehabilitation. Occasionally, other specialties such as psychiatry and pharmacology were included. E-health techniques were also used for administration, education, transfer of knowledge, and peer support services associated with the program.

IJTRC provides team-based, individualized restorative treatment for patients at all stages on the rehabilitation continuum of care. The IJTRC team has effectively used telerehabilitation to help individuals with disabilities reintegrate into their community in a variety of settings, including home, work, and school (Clark and Scheideman-Miller, 1999; Clark, Dawson, Scheideman-Miller, and Post, 2002; Dawson, Clark, and Scheideman-Miller, 1999). As is evidenced by the wide range of disciplines mentioned, e-rehabilitation lends itself to a multidisciplinary approach, probably more than traditional medical specialties limited to physical sites would allow. Table 7.1 depicts the range and scope of e-rehabilitation services offered at IJTRC.

E-rehabilitation sessions have been conducted using T-1 (high-speed leased network connection line) and the integrated services digital network (ISDN), as well as the "plain old telephone system" (POTS). T-1 and ISDN are used primarily to connect with rural school districts or hospitals because they provide better resolution and fewer transmission delays than low-technology systems. The POTS is the primary telecommunication technology used for therapy services to home-based patients.

Rehabilitation, much of which is usually conducted through touch, is often difficult to envision being delivered remotely. One of the reasons for the success of the

TABLE 7.1. E-REHABILITATION APPLICATIONS AT INTEGRIS JIM THORPE REHABILITATION CENTER

Type of Intervention	Purpose
Telementoring	Provision of training or expertise to distant or rural clinicians
Telemonitoring	Ongoing assessment of specified condition or situation
Teleconsultation	Provision of professional impressions or direction in regard to course of action or treatment planning
Tele-education	Continuing education, to develop content expertise
Telesupervision	Review of patient status or progress to satisfy regulation requirements
Teletherapy	
a. With physical intervention	Facilitation of patient's functional recovery through physical instruction
b. Without physical intervention	Facilitation of patient's functional recovery and improvement through suggestions

IJTRC program was a core group of clinicians and therapists who were able to focus on patient needs, putting aside uncertainties and barriers in order to address a growing underserved population. This driving purpose led them to devise safe and effective alternatives to traditional modes of delivery. A physical therapist, for example, might use a caregiver in a home situation as an assistant to lower the probability of patient falls, provide patient props, reinforce therapist instruction through cueing, and promote compliance with an in-home exercise regimen. A speech language pathologist might use toys such as an automated reader for joint play with the client in order to sequence language exercises to assist with reading skills. A psychotherapist could address adjustment to disability for the caregiver as well as the patient in the safety and anonymity of their home setting. This program has been developed over a period of three years. To date, a total of 3,711 consults have been provided through the use of e-rehabilitation technology, including 82 audio or verbal therapy consults, 39 occupational therapy consults, 126 physiatry consults, 539 physical therapy consults, 2,837 speech therapy consults, and three vocational rehab consults, in addition to other services (for example, adult mental health consults). Together, these sessions add up to 139,394 minutes of therapy as shown in Table 7.2.

The acceptance of e-rehabilitation is evidenced by improved outcomes such as better cognition, hearing and language skills. Over 67 percent of home care patients cite high satisfaction and say that they would use e-rehabilitation again.

TABLE 7.2. CLINICAL E-REHABILITATION ENCOUNTERS
AT INTEGRIS JIM THORPE REHABILITATION CENTER
(April 1999–August 2003)

Discipline	Number of Consults	Total Number of Minutes
Speech therapy	2,837	99,714
Physical therapy	539	28,255
Physiatry	126	1,920
Audio/verbal therapy	82	4,620
Occupational therapy	39	1,240
Adult mental health	85	3,495
Vocational rehabilitation	3	150
Total	3,711	139,394

Note: Clients were located in schools, hospitals, and residences during the encounters.

Conclusion

The health care marketplace is expanding and evolving at a rapid rate, and the focus is on automation, paperless offices, and increased efficiency and effectiveness of decision-making capabilities through the increasing use of information technology and e-technologies. According to Forrester Research, the health care purchasing market will reach $370 billion by the year 2004, and 35 percent of e-supply hospital procurement could be through the Web. Needs forecasting could be achieved by integrating e-supply acquisition and on-line inventory management with direct e-care (DeJesus, 2000). Combining the capabilities of the Internet with other interactive e-technologies such as voice recognition systems and telephone-based triage lines will continue to evolve and will greatly reduce unnecessary medical services and costs. E-medicine, e-commerce, e-clinical care, e-home care, e-learning, e-prescription, e-supply chain management, e-decision support, and e-work are all part of the larger e-health applications that can change the way health care products and services are to be delivered to e-consumers, the underserved, and the homebound.

The e-speech therapy case study at the end of this chapter supports the concept that telecommunications can be used to effectively deliver both articulation and language interventions to students in rural schools. The use of e-technology has resulted in the delivery of cost-effective, specialized health care to rural communities and is helping to bring rural schools into the new millennium on the cutting edge of specialized e-rehabilitation service delivery.

New technological standards such as XML are further simplifying e-health by permitting communications between and among parties independent of hardware platforms, operating systems, business applications, or database management systems. Instead, these standards use the local data definitions of the end user (Aggarwal and Travers, 2001). For patients, this will eventually translate into e-messages that will be used in medical triage, e-management of appointments and schedules, e-prescription refills, e-previsit preparation, and e-postvisit follow-up. The payoffs are in the form of more efficient use of time, documentation of all communications, fewer physical office visits, and improved visit quality (Joslyn, 2001). E-health is not the future but the present, and it will complement and not replace traditional health care services.

Chapter Questions

1. What general medical services lend themselves to electronic transmission of information?
2. What rehabilitation or ancillary services might be incorporated in e-medicine?
3. What adaptations could facilitate clinical and administrative acceptance of e-rehabilitation?
4. What are the external driving forces in your organization or community (for example, legislation, licensure, reimbursement, confidentiality) that contribute to either the potential success of or the existing barriers to the implementation of an e-health program?
5. What existing human resource capital could contribute to the operational implementation of an e-rehabilitation program in a health facility that you may have personally visited?

References

Aggarwal, A., & Travers, S. (2001). E-commerce in healthcare: Changing the traditional landscape. *Journal of Healthcare Information Management, 15,* 25–36.

Alzheimer's Caregiver Support Online. (2003). *Alzheimer's caregiver support online.* Retrieved November 18, 2003, from http://www.alzonline.net

Anderson, D.G.M., & Stenzel, C. (2001). Internet patient care applications in ambulatory care. *Journal of Ambulatory Care Management, 24,* 1–38.

Arbietman, D., Lirov, E., Lirov, R., & Lirov, Y. (2001). E-commerce for healthcare supply. *Journal of Healthcare Information Management, 15,* 61–72.

Callan, K. (2000). Preparing for a decision support system. *Topics in Health Information Management, 21,* 84–90.

Chang, K., Chung, J. W., & Wong, T. K. (2002). Learning intravenous cannulation: A comparison of the conventional method and the CathSim Intravenous Training System. *Journal of Clinical Nursing, 11,* 73–78.

Clark, P. G., Dawson, S. J., Scheideman-Miller, C., & Post, M. L. (2002). TeleRehab: Stroke teletherapy and management using two-way interactive video. *Neurology Report, 26,* 87–93.

Clark, P. G., & Scheideman-Miller, C. (1999). Telehealth "pre-pilot" successful in Oklahoma. *Advance for Speech-Language Pathologists and Audiologists, 9*, 18–19.

Cochrane, J. D. (1995). Healthcare at the speed of thought. *Integrated Healthcare Report, 1*(14), 16–17.

Dawson, S. J., Clark, P. G., & Scheideman-Miller, C. (1999). The new frontier: Telerehabilitation. *Physical Therapy Case Reports, 3*, 84–90.

DeJesus, E. X. (2000). Procurement e-bound. *Healthcare Informatics, 17*(11), 42–46, 48, 50–52.

Dimmick, S.L.P., Mustaleski, C. M., Burgiss, S.G.P., & Welsh, T. M. (2000). A case study of benefits and potential savings in rural home telemedicine. *Home Healthcare Nurse, 18*, 124–135.

Dougherty, M., & Scichilone, R. (2002). Establishing a tele-commuting or home-based employee program. *Journal of* American Health Information Management Association, *73*(7), 72A–72K.

Durtschi, A. (2001). Three patients' tele-home care experiences. *Home Healthcare Nurse, 19*, 9–11.

Forgionne, G. A., Gangopadhyay, A., Klein, J. A., & Eckhardt, R. (1999). A decision technology system for health care electronic commerce. *Topics in Health Information Management, 20*(1), 31–41.

Goldsborough, R. (2000). Job-hunting on the Internet. *RN, 63*, 21–22.

Goran, M., & Standford, J. (2001). E-health: Restructuring care delivery in the Internet age. *Journal of Healthcare Information Management, 15*, 3–12.

Harris Interactive. (2003). *No significant change in the number of cybercondriacs.* Retrieved October 22, 2003, from http://www.harrisinteractive.com

Herrin, D. (2001). E-learning: Directions for nurses in executive practice. *Journal of Nursing Administration, 31*, 5–6.

Hirsch, S. A. (2000). Academy introduces Web-based medical education for fellows and patients. *Journal of Bone and Joint Surgery, 82-A*, 1665–1667.

Jadad, A., & Gagliardi, A. (1998). Rating health information on the Internet: Navigating to knowledge or babble? *Journal of the American Medical Association, 279*, 611–614.

Joch, A. (2000, March). Can the Web save disease management? *Healthcare Informatics, 17*(3), 59–60, 62, 64–70.

Joslyn, J. S. (2001). Healthcare e-commerce: Connecting with patients. *Journal of Healthcare Information Management, 15*, 73–84.

Menduno, M. (1999a). Apothecary now. *Hospitals and Health Networks, 73*, 34–38.

Menduno, M. E. (1999b). E-commerce: Point, click, purchase. *Hospitals and Health Networks, 73*, 54–58.

Mitchell, J. (2000). Increasing the cost-effectiveness of telemedicine by embracing e-health. *Journal of Telemedicine and Telecare, 6*, 16–19.

Neuhauser, P. C. (2000). Culture.com: Leading the way to e-nursing. *Journal of Nursing Administration, 30*, 580–582.

Patsos, M. P. (2001). The Internet and medicine: Building a community for patients with rare diseases. *Journal of the American Medical Association, 285*, 805.

Razvi, E. (2000). E-commerce in biopharmaceutical industry. *Drug and Market Development, 11*, 241–245.

Riley, T., & Korpman, R. A. (2001). Beyond connectivity: What the success of one health plan's e-solution means for the future of the healthcare industry. *Journal of Healthcare Information Management, 15*, 37–49.

Selsky, D. B., Eisenberg, F. P., Spena, R. P., Hersh, W., Price, S. L., & Buitendijk, H. J. (2001). Knowledge integration: Insight through the e-portal. *Journal of Healthcare Information Management, 15*, 13–24.

Solovy, A. (2000). Is an e-commerce gap emerging among the nation's hospitals? *Hospitals and Health Networks, 74*, 30–41.

Stanberry, B. (2000). Telemedicine: Barriers and opportunities in the 21st century. *Journal of Internal Medicine, 247*, 615–628.

Svensson, P. (2003). *E-health applications in health care management.* eHealth Int. 2002; 1:5. Received June 23, 2002; Published online 2002 September 17 http://www.pubmedcentral. nih.gov/articlerender.fcgi?artid=135526

Tan, J. (2001). *Health management information systems: Methods and practical applications.* (2nd ed.). Sudbury, MA: Jones & Bartlett.

Tan, J., with Sheps, S. (1998). *Health decision support systems.* Sudbury, MA: Jones & Bartlett.

Tele-Health Applications. (2003). *CSIRO-Internet innovation center.* Retrieved November 5, 2003, from http://internet.csiro.au/Iapps/Telehealth1.htm

Terry, K. (2002). Should you order your supplies online? You bet! *RN, 65*, 2ON-4ON.

Terry, N. (2001). Access vs. quality assurance: The e-health conundrum. *Journal of the American Medical Association, 285*, 807.

Winker, M. A., Flanagin, A., Chi-Lum, B., White, J., Andrews, K., Kennett, R. L., DeAngelis, C. D., Musacchio, R. A. (2000). Guidelines for medical and health information sites on the Internet: Principles governing AMA Web sites. *Journal of the American Medical Association, 283*, 1600–1606.

Woods, D. (2001). Healthcare in the new millennium: Vision, values and leadership. *British Medical Journal, 322*, 243.

E-Speech Therapy for Children in a Rural Oklahoma School Case

Cynthia Scheideman-Miller, Pam Forducey, Sharon S. Smeltzer, Avery Clouds, Bob Hodge, David Prouty

Since the Individuals with Disabilities Education Act (IDEA) was implemented in 1990, schools have been required to supply specific specialty services such as speech therapy, occupational therapy, and physical therapy. Because of their geographic locations and sparse populations, many rural communities do not have the resources to provide these services to their students. Traveling to metropolitan areas where these services are more readily available is hard on the children and their families.

INTEGRIS Rural Telemedicine, INTEGRIS Jim Thorpe Rehabilitation Network, Choctaw Memorial Hospital, and the Hugo Public Schools collaborated on an initial e-speech therapy program in the spring of 1999 to see whether federally mandated speech therapy services could be delivered with two-way, interactive videoconferencing. This five-week pre-pilot program was conducted between the metropolitan and rural hospitals over a dedicated T-1 line. The effectiveness of this mode of delivery, including the success of the speech therapy and the satisfaction of the therapists, teachers, students, and parents, was measured.

Favorable results from the pre-pilot program led to an expanded program in which the services were delivered directly to the rural public school from the metropolitan hospital, using H323 and H320 videoconferencing equipment via OneNet, Oklahoma's telecommunications backbone.

Background

More than 51 million Americans live in areas classified by the U.S. Office of Management and Budget as nonmetropolitan. Rural populations, which constitute one-fifth of the U.S. population, frequently have difficulty in accessing adequate health care. Less than 11 percent of the nation's physicians are practicing in nonmetropolitan areas (Office of Rural Health Policy, 1997). Specialty services are even more limited than primary care and may be completely unavailable. Although the need for specialty services is high in rural areas, rural residents often go without these services. Geographic and financial barriers pose a threat to the provision of specialty care services for the rural population.

Populations in some rural communities fluctuate dramatically, contingent on recreational seasons and agriculture. When populations expand, demands for services, including special services for individuals with disabilities, also increase. At other times, a single individual may be the only one in the entire county with a specific medical condition and resultant physical or cognitive impairment.

IDEA guarantees all children with disabilities a free, appropriate public education, emphasizing special education and related services designed to meet their unique needs. All states are required to abide by this law; the states receive federal funding for special education, while the local education agency or school system is responsible for identifying, locating, and evaluating all children who require special education services. Under IDEA, schools must supply specific services such as speech therapy, occupational therapy, and physical therapy. It is often a struggle for school administrators to secure these services, and some rural schools may go for years without a speech language pathologist (SLP). Even when an SLP is hired, the newly hired professional often leaves for a metropolitan area where the caseload is lighter, pay is better, and peer support is available. One rural community offered wages that were 43 percent higher than the state average and still had difficulty obtaining a speech pathologist. Rural SLPs report many challenges: one SLP has to travel half of the day in order to work with children at geographically distant sites; another has trouble getting state universities to return calls or answer questions regarding students with complex medical conditions.

One alternative is for students to travel to a metropolitan area where these specialty services are more readily available. This incurs additional costs, since the schools have to pay for the trips. It also entails physical and financial stress on the children and their families, including lost work time and additional travel expenses. Children traveling such distances are more fatigued and less attentive to therapy, which lessens the sessions' effectiveness. Moving to a metro area where services are more readily available is a theoretical option, but most of the families make a living in agriculture-related fields. In addition, the family ties and social support of a rural area are usually strong, so that even if a family can move, the different culture of a metropolitan area and lack of family and community support create additional burdens. Financially viable alternatives that produce positive outcomes are clearly needed.

E-Speech Therapy Program Development for a Choctaw County School

Speech therapy primarily involves sessions of interactive speaking and visual cues in which a therapist assesses and guides a student. Two-way interactive videoconferencing has been used in Nebraska to deliver e-speech therapy to patients who had difficulty speaking subsequent to a stroke. This experiment brought specialty consultation and treatment to stroke patients who otherwise would not have had access to such care. Expanding on this idea, an e-speech therapy intervention for students in a rural Oklahoma school was developed and evaluated.

The first step was to determine whether e-speech therapy could be delivered in a cost-efficient and timely manner. It was also important that all the major stakeholders, including the therapists, administrators, parents, and students, be comfortable and supportive of the intervention. A pre-pilot program was planned to minimize technological and logistical problems. In order to eliminate as many extraneous variables as possible, the rural school needed an established relationship with the metropolitan hospital whose infrastructure would support the e-therapy sessions and carry the project to the next stage.

The selected site for the pre-pilot project was the town of Hugo, located in Choctaw County, Oklahoma. Choctaw County is located in the far southeast corner of Oklahoma, on the Texas border and near the Arkansas border. The population of Choctaw County is 15,302. The largest town, Hugo, has 5,978 residents. In Choctaw county, the poverty level is 49.3 percent; the child poverty level is 44.2 percent; and 80 percent of the children are on the school lunch program. Under federal guidelines, Choctaw County is both a medically underserved area (MUA) and a health professional shortage area (HPSA).

The Hugo Public School System has a school SLP, but at the time of the pre-pilot project, the number of students who needed speech therapy services was greater than the caseload allowed by the state. Supplemental services were required to meet federal mandates, but these services were difficult and expensive to secure. Choctaw Memorial Hospital in Hugo was part of the INTEGRIS Health System, a not-for-profit health care system based in Oklahoma. INTEGRIS Rural Telemedicine, INTEGRIS Jim Thorpe Rehabilitation Center (IJTRC), and Choctaw Memorial Hospital had a long-standing affiliation. Likewise, Choctaw Memorial Hospital and the Hugo Public Schools served the same community and had a strong alliance. The need for services, the availability of a rural SLP to help with monitoring, plus existing affiliations between facilities made Hugo an ideal site for the study. All four entities collaborated in the e-speech therapy study for four weeks in the spring of 1999.

E-Technology for an E-Speech Therapy Program

The initial program was conducted at the Choctaw Memorial Hospital. Southwest Medical Center, of which IJTRC is part, also participated via video bridge. The connection was bridged through INTEGRIS Baptist Medical Center (IBMC), which is the core of the

INTEGRIS Health System. Choctaw Memorial Hospital used an H320 videoconference unit connected via a dedicated T-1 line to the video bridge at IBMC.

Data and video services are distributed across the INTEGRIS Wide Area Network (WAN), which provides connections to over sixty locations throughout the state and access to specific extranets throughout the nation. The INTEGRIS WAN core is a Newbridge 3645 carrier-grade switch. This hardware allows INTEGRIS to port voice, video, and data over various bandwidths to remote locations. This site also houses a VTEL/EZENIA 320 standards-based video bridge capable of direct video connections to INTEGRIS facilities, as well as an EZENIA 320/323 gateway/gatekeeper. The gateway enables H320 or H323 connectivity throughout the network and beyond. An Ascend inverse multiplexer connected to an integrated services digital network (ISDN) primary rate interface gives the system the ability to connect both nationally and internationally.

Evaluation of E-Speech Therapy Sessions

INTEGRIS Rural Facilities was awarded a federal Rural Telemedicine grant from the Office for the Advancement of Telemedicine under the Human Resource and Services Administration. This grant supplied seed money and project oversight to help develop, oversee, and evaluate the pre-pilot e-speech therapy program. IJTRC, also part of the INTEGRIS System, employed board-certified SLPs to supply the needed services.

Education prior to each stage of program development was essential to ensure buy-in from key stakeholders and commitments from all partners. The Hugo Public School System was familiar with interactive technology, having used classroom video technology to share a language teacher for several years. This familiarity facilitated the implementation of the pre-pilot program. School administrators were brought in from the beginning and played an instrumental role in educating the school board and community members about the potential of this application. Presentations were made to the school board and to the Oklahoma Healthcare Authority (the state Medicaid agency that reimburses the schools for part of the services) prior to launching the project. An open house and technology demonstration was organized for potential participants in the program, their parents, teachers, school administrators, and hospital and school board members.

Once community orientation and informed consent procedures were completed, the five-week program commenced, using an intervention group of six students and a control group of three students. The intervention group consisted of three boys and three girls ranging in ages from three to nine. The control group consisted of one boy and two girls ranging in age from four to ten. The elementary-aged students' diagnoses ranged from mild to moderate articulation deficits. The prekindergarten group's diagnoses included cerebral palsy and cleft palate in addition to articulation disorders.

A hospital-based metro SLP from IJTRC conducted the interventions with the students. The students were transported to Choctaw Memorial Hospital in Hugo to use the videoconferencing equipment (VTEL FRED H320 unit) that was already in place. The metro SLP planned the sessions and conducted them over the INTEGRIS video network, using 384 kilobytes per second on a dedicated T-1 line from Oklahoma City. Hugo is approximately 178 miles, or a four-hour drive, from Oklahoma City. The Hugo school SLP was present in the Hugo conference room for all of the e-therapy sessions. This ensured that the student was receiving appropriate intervention, could understand what the metro SLP expected of them, and could respond appropriately. In addition, the metro SLP provided consultation services to the SLP in Hugo before and throughout the project. This added to the value of the relationship between a metro site and a rural site.

The therapy sessions were conducted in an area adjoining the cafeteria with an accordion room divider, which decreased visual but not auditory distractions. These distractions lessened the effectiveness of the therapy and raised the issue of confidentiality problems. This problematic setup would need to be improved for future implementations. Sessions must be held in a private area without extraneous disruptions.

Evaluation Outcomes

Due to the limited time frame and small number of students evaluated in the pre-pilot program, no major change in satisfaction levels was anticipated. Thus, organizers were pleasantly surprised to find that therapists and teachers saw significant improvement in the students' scores on a standardized pediatric rehabilitation assessment tool (WeeFIM) in the cognitive domains of social interaction, problem solving, and memory after they had participated in the e-speech therapy for only five weeks. Students less than seven years of age were found to be less attentive to the speech therapy sessions; as a result, it was decided to include only students seven years of age or older in the pilot study.

A nonstandardized customer survey tool was given to measure satisfaction. Satisfaction was high for all parties in regard to both the use of the technology and functional outcome measures, and it was highest for parents and students. Teachers found that e-therapy was beneficial because there were many observers, not just one therapist. Through the use of interactive video, multiple perspectives on the problems and treatment of each student emerged. The older children (second grade and above) responded better to the video interaction. One older child in particular thought that he was on a television program and made tremendous improvement, because he was doing his best while receiving individual care.

Feedback on the project from parents, students, therapists, and school administrators was favorable. The school board president informed his board that he was impressed when he saw an e-speech therapy session. He stated, "Through telemedicine, we are able to tap into the best of the best." Discussions were conducted among the stakeholders from both the rural and metropolitan areas. Meetings were held between the metro and rural SLPs on how to conduct sessions; strategies for incorporating a teacher's aide; the individual education plan (IEP) process; and selection of student candidates for the program. The school principal worked with the Rural Telemedicine Project and clinical directors on reimbursement, coding of medical data, and logistics. The project's technical director worked with the communications coordinator for the school's on-line hardware and software implementation and technology selection.

Expanded E-Speech Therapy Program

Favorable results from the pre-pilot program led to an expanded program, a collaboration between INTEGRIS Rural Telemedicine, IJTRC, and the Hugo Public School System, in the fall of 1999. Based on their IEP, eleven students were selected to participate in the expanded program. The project was initially approved for a duration of one school year (thirty weeks), but its success led to the approval of a second school year. The eleven students were in second grade or older, with either language or articulation deficits. During the two years of the pilot study, the students received individual one-hour speech therapy interventions as scheduled, resulting in almost a thousand virtual visits. Clinical outcomes, cost-effectiveness, and satisfaction of therapists and students with the telemedicine sessions were measured and reported elsewhere (Clark and Scheideman-Miller, 1999).

Implications for the Future

The e-speech therapy pilot project proved that telecommunications can be used to effectively deliver both articulation and language interventions to students in rural schools. This result was chronicled in a report to the American Speech-Language-Hearing Association's executive board. The Issues in Credentialing Team (1998) for that organization stated that it believed "that the remote delivery of audiology and speech-language pathology services through technology (telehealth) has the potential to become a more widely used mode of clinical service delivery and a rapidly expanding marketplace niche for our professions."

Future project directions include offering e-speech pathology services to additional schools—initially rural ones, then possibly metropolitan ones. Additional services—such as e-physical therapy, e-occupational therapy, and e-behavior modification therapy—are being explored. The use of e-technology has resulted in the delivery of cost-effective, specialized health care to rural communities in Oklahoma and is helping to bring Oklahoma into the new millennium on the cutting edge of specialized e-rehabilitation service delivery.

Case Questions

1. Why do you think students older than seven years of age in rural communities are more responsive than younger students to the e-speech therapy sessions?
2. Can you think of any way to improve this program so that it can provide other forms of therapies that rural children may also need in an e-health context?

3. What are some measurable clinical outcomes of e-speech therapy? How would you measure these outcomes?

4. If you were asked to evaluate an e-speech therapy program for an underserved population such as the one discussed here, how would you go about doing so? What criteria would you use? What do you think would be the impacts of your evaluation results?

References

Clark, P., & Scheideman-Miller, C. (1999). Telehealth "pre-pilot" successful in Oklahoma. *Advance for Speech-Language Pathologists and Audiologists, 9,* 18–19.

Issues in Credentialing Team, American Speech-Language-Hearing Association. (1998, August). *Telehealth issues brief: A report to the ASHA executive board from the Issues in Credentialing Team.*: American Speech-Language-Hearing Association.

Office of Rural Health Policy, Health Resources and Services Administration, U.S. Department of Health and Human Services. (1997, September). *Fact sheet—rural physician; facts about rural physicians.* Source 1. Rockville, MD: Author.

CHAPTER EIGHT

DIFFUSION OF E-MEDICINE

E-Medicine in Developed and Developing Countries

Joseph Tan, Mengistu Kifle, Victor Mbarika, Chitu Okoli

The authors would like to acknowledge the contributions of students, research assistants, and colleagues from their various universities, particularly graduate students at the University of British Columbia and Wayne State University, who have contributed to the literature searches and materials used in this chapter. Any omissions or errors remain the responsibility of the authors. This work was partially supported by grants provided to Joseph Tan by the Office of the President of Wayne State University.

231

Learning Objectives

1. Define e-medicine in the context of the different periods in the development and growth of e-medicine as a concept, a discipline, and a practice
2. Review challenges faced in the history of e-medicine
3. Understand the significance of diffusing e-medicine in Canada
4. Identify factors affecting the implementation and diffusion of e-medicine in developing countries, specifically Ethiopia
5. Recognize the relationships among the factors that affect the transfer of e-medicine as well as their potential impact on the success of e-medicine implementation

Introduction

E-medicine can be defined as the diffusion of medicine and health care services through the use of information and communications technologies. In mainstream medical, public health, and health services research literature, terms such as *telemedicine* (which literally means medicine at a distance) and *telehealth* are often used interchangeably to refer to e-medicine services, with the understanding that telehealth encompasses not only telemedicine services but also important e-health administrative and support services (see Chapter Seven). The application of telemedicine to deliver e-health care and e-health education is not new (Bashshur, 1997). Throughout this book, however, the term *e-medicine* is often used not only in a broad sense because it corresponds elegantly to the notion of e-health diffusion but also in a more restricted sense because it refers to a specific aspect of e-health diffusion: the diffusion of various specialties and subspecialties within the telemedicine domain. Specific examples of e-medicine include teleradiology, teledermatology, telepathology, tele-ophthalmology, tele-oncology, telepsychiatry, telecardiology, telenursing, and tele-accident and emergency support. E-medicine contributes to the sociopolitical, cultural, and economic infrastructure and development of a country. It can help provide multidisciplinary perspectives in health care delivery to individual citizens, selected groups and communities, and even entire populations.

In this chapter, we provide an overview of e-medicine, focusing on the history of and the driving factors in the diffusion of e-medicine technology. Next, we discuss e-medicine in Canada, focusing on the work of the Canadian federal government, provincial initiatives, and investigations by university researchers. We then highlight the diffusion of e-medicine in developing countries, pointing out the critical success factors and challenges. Finally, we move on to discuss the diffusion of e-medicine in less developed countries, using the specific case of Ethiopia and examining the factors influencing success in the implementation of e-medicine applications.

E-Medicine Overview

As we discussed in Chapter Seven, e-medicine technologies have been and are being used for e-clinical services, e-diagnostic and information services, e-learning, and e-administrative applications in the health care sector. *E-clinical applications* support the access and delivery of clinical care at a distance and capture, organize, store, and share clinical information among providers as well as between providers and patients. The information collected is typically needed for e-patient assessment, e-diagnosis, and e-treatment.

One application of e-medicine for e-clinical services is telesurgery. In *telesurgery*, surgeons control a robotic device to perform an operation at a remote location. This work is still in the very early stages, with feasibility studies being conducted on pigs. Another popular form of e-medicine, illustrated in the case discussion in Chapter Ten, is *teleradiology*, in which rural hospitals can obtain readings of teleradiological images from urban centers that are more likely to employ senior and highly qualified radiologists.

Within e-diagnostic and information services, the four subcategories are teleconsulting, teleconferencing, telereporting, and telemonitoring. In *teleconsulting*, a patient uses an e-medicine service to consult with a health care provider. A *teleconference* entails two or more health care workers communicating over a video link to share responsibility for the patient, who is usually not present. Both *telereporting* and *telemonitoring* involve the transmission of relevant health information by a clinician to a remote center for interpretation. The analysis is then fed back to the clinician. The only difference between these two subcategories is that in telemonitoring the patient data are collected continuously or at intervals, whereas in telereporting, the transmission is usually done once.

E-learning applications provide on-line, Internet-based, and remote delivery of training and education services such as continued medical education for physicians and other health care professionals. These applications can also provide consumer health information. For example, one of the authors generated teaching materials jointly with a team of experts from the University of British Columbia (UBC) and the University of Cape Town (UCT) for health planning modules for the maternal and child health program for residents and medical students being trained in South Africa. The materials developed were delivered on-line. Several issues were immediately apparent. For example, due to cultural, socioeconomic, and political differences between the countries, the materials did not address real-life scenarios encountered by the medical students in their workplace. In other words, the perspectives and experiences of the experts in British Columbia were not ideally meaningful to the medical students in Cape Town. Collaborative learning had to occur between developers of the materials from the two countries. Such difficulties and challenges were quickly resolved among the team members through videoconferencing over satellite channels rather than expensive overseas travel. Some medical students located at UCT were also able to access materials via the Internet, cutting across geographical barriers and providing opportunities for a dialogue between the students and the experts. Both experts and students learned from this process.

E-administrative support is the exchange of e-health information among payers, providers, employers, and consumers—for example, through electronic health records, administrative data warehouses, and clinical databases, as well as through public health networks. On-line business-to-business and business-to-consumer billing; on-line claims made by e-consumers on e-businesses and between business entities; e-inventory management by suppliers and retailers; and e-financial transactions between vendors and third-party payers are all examples of e-administrative processes. Detailed discussions and illustrations of these e-technologies are available in Chapter Seven and elsewhere in this text. We will focus our discussion at this point on the history of e-medicine.

The History of E-Medicine

The roots of e-medicine can be traced as far back as 1876, when the telephone was invented. Even as early as the 1920s and 1930s, the concept of linking patients and doctors without the physical presence of the parties in the same location had surfaced publicly. In 1924, a picture of a patient interacting with a doctor on television appeared on the cover of the magazine *Radio News*, with the title: "The Radio Doctor—Maybe!" (Field, 1996). Interestingly, the first television transmission did not occur until 1927.

Today, the telephone is still an important component of e-medicine. During the days when telephones were reserved mostly for those who could afford them, physicians and pharmacists used them to teleconsult with one another. Wealthy patients also used them to reach their physicians for emergency services. Eventually, telephones were used to transmit basic clinical information; for example, in 1948, X-ray images were sent between New York and Pennsylvania through telephone lines (Viegas, 1998). However, e-medicine today encompasses more than low-cost telephone technology.

A critical phase in the development of e-medicine was the emergence of radio at the end of the nineteenth century and television in the early twentieth century. Radio was first used to provide medical advice for seafarers who required medical attention while at sea; it is still being used on board aircraft to provide medical assistance to passengers. As for television, physicians used it to aid in neurological examinations, as well as to teleconsult with other experts (Field, 1996). Among the first demonstrations of the capability of interactive video for e-medicine was the use of a two-way closed-circuit television system to link the Nebraska Psychiatric Institute and Norfolk Hospital with the University of Nebraska.

Subsequent significant breakthroughs in the diffusion of e-medicine can be divided into three historical periods. The first period covers the 1950s to the early 1970s. The 1950s and 1960s were marked by an effort to improve e-clinical care in specialty areas, including teleradiology, telecardiology, teledermatology, and telepsychiatry. In the early 1970s, longer distances were being covered through the use of satellite signals instead of phone lines. The majority of projects undertaken during this era before mass computing, however, were mainly proof-of-concept research in the form of technological feasibility studies. Most of these projects were attempts to provide medical services to astronauts. Governments picked up the substantial expense of staffing and directing projects operated with standard analog televisions. However, when the funds were exhausted, the projects similarly dwindled.

Fortunately, the second e-medicine period, from the late 1970s to the early 1990s, was characterized by the development of digital technology. During this period, computers became commonplace and digital communication methods emerged. Soon it was discovered that interactive videos could be distributed over wide area surface networks at a much lower cost than with analog television systems. During this period, e-medicine projects made use of computer-based, digital teleconferencing systems. Among the most significant projects of this period were those examining the feasibility of e-medicine for rural areas. Here, it was argued that real cost savings would materialize because of reduced travel costs; in addition, better health outcomes for e-patients would result from more timely diagnoses of illnesses.

Some very challenging barriers to the diffusion of e-medicine also became obvious during the second e-medicine period. Barrett and Brecht (1998) list these barriers as technology and standards; liability, licensure, and confidentiality; and reimbursement. Even so, the large number of images and data to be transmitted in teleradiology and telepathology led to the development of the Digital Imaging and Communications in Medicine (DICOM) guidelines, the first set of standards, by the American College of Radiology and the National Electrical Manufacturers. At the same time, Internet use and communications via e-mail were proliferating among physicians and other health professionals, who were exchanging text, images, and video around the world (Viegas, 1998). Concerns over escalating health care costs in both the United States and Canada, coupled with the diffusion of e-technologies, gave rise to renewed interest in e-medicine.

Today, the key challenges we are facing involve the need for improved standards; the use of wireless technologies; security, confidentiality, and privacy issues; legal questions about jurisdictions and reimbursements for e-medicine services; and the need for large-scale formative and summative evaluation of e-medicine initiatives.

Challenges in Diffusing E-Medicine

At present, there are more Internet hosts and servers in Los Angeles than on the entire African continent and more hosts and servers in Singapore than in Vietnam or the numerous Indonesian islands. In most developing countries, many suburbs and villages still lack basic telephone service. Despite our heralding the news that the Internet will provide one of the cheapest and fastest solutions to improving the health and well-being of world populations, the grim reality is that we are not going to easily close the gap and erase the inequities caused by the current digital divide. In fact, because of differences in the level of education between the haves and have nots, it is generally expected that the poor will have less accessibility to computing power and Internet capabilities. For example, there are many more high-speed Internet connections within a city in developed and developing countries such as Singapore or New York than the entire state of an underdeveloped country or even the country itself such as Ethiopia. The evolution of the Internet itself may therefore have further widened the divide.

As we have noted, prior research in e-medicine has focused on a number of important themes discussed throughout this and other chapters of this text. Key research areas include the following:

- E-medicine services
- Technical aspects of e-medicine
- Cost-effectiveness of traditional medicine versus e-medicine
- Clinical effectiveness and satisfaction with mainstream medicine versus e-medicine
- Diffusion, implementation, and impact of e-medicine

Of these themes, the last is the least developed but will perhaps provide the most valuable insights into the future development of e-medicine. To develop a comprehensive design model for e-medicine services, further research needs to be completed on the implementation and installation of e-medicine services and their general effects. Very little research has been done on the implementation and installation of e-medicine services, especially in developing countries. The questions that need to be answered relate to the difficulties encountered with actual implementations and how these challenges can be overcome.

The main focus of this chapter will be e-medicine diffusion. Before we look at the diffusion of e-medicine in developed countries such as Canada and in developing countries such as those in sub-Saharan Africa, we will discuss the factors underlying the diffusion of e-medicine.

Factors Driving the Diffusion of E-Medicine

From our historical knowledge of e-medicine technologies and applications, we see that the diffusion of e-medicine is fueled by many factors, including growth in e-home care needs, new trends in consumer health informatics, changes in legislation, increased competition, market expansion, new technological breakthroughs, as well as other socioeconomic factors. Given an aging population, closures of hospital beds, and reduced inpatient stays for operative procedures, the market for e-health care is projected to grow rapidly. Advances in medical technologies and pharmaceutical products are making a wider range of diagnostic, therapeutic, and surgical procedures and services for e-home care possible (see Chapter Nine). New legislation and rising health care costs are forcing payers and administrators to seek new and innovative ways to provide adequate levels of services at lower costs (see Chapter Twelve). E-medicine appears to offer an intelligent solution for the redistribution of medical services especially among the unprivileged because they may be in more urgent needs of such services and promises to bring about new opportunities for increased competition and commercial partnerships in the expanding e-health marketplace (see Chapter Thirteen).

E-medicine represents a dramatic shift from traditional thinking about medicine, which focuses on transporting the patient to the site of the health practitioners. Instead, e-medicine transmits expert knowledge and know-how to patients and practitioners; simply put, it moves the information rather than the patient. E-medicine services have therefore been used partly to replace and augment face-to-face home care visits with teleconferencing and video visits for the chronically ill and elderly. E-home care telemonitoring of heart conditions and vital signs, including blood pressure; the use of laptop computers by e-home care workers to document, review, and check medication and progress on patient charts; the ability to e-communicate with home care teams; and emergency or alert systems linking homes with clinics or hospitals are all developments in e-medicine diffusion.

Increasingly, e-consumers are demanding high-quality and reliable health information of all sorts on the Internet. This demand has also strengthened the e-medicine model. Rapid access to the World Wide Web has enabled the diffusion of e-medicine expertise to individuals whose access to such services used to be restricted. Increasing sources of medical and health care information have also led to demand for better medical information and knowledge, faster and more efficient means of accessing evidence-based medicine electronically, and improved on-line medical bibliographic resources and health research networks.

E-home care needs and consumer health informatics are not the only factors contributing to the diffusion of e-medicine. Rapidly rising costs of health care and increased competition among health providers have also contributed. In this regard, the politics and economics of the managed care approach to health care delivery have become some of the most important factors driving the diffusion of the e-medicine perspective. In a managed care setting, a certain population within a geographic boundary is expected to be covered for medical services regardless of their geographic location. Insurance companies in many U.S. jurisdictions were at first unable to reimburse physicians for e-consultations and e-medicine services. In managed care, where the fee-for-service practice arrangement is no longer prevalent, e-medicine can play a much more significant role. In other words, in a competitive environment, e-medicine applications will be readily accepted by insurance companies if such use results in overall cost savings and increased market share for the e-health provider organizations.

Another important question about the diffusion of e-medicine is the way in which the market for e-medicine is developing. Perednia and Allen (1995) state that the market share of a product or service can be increased in two ways: (1) increasing the size of the total market—for example, by expanding the demand for bandwidth suitable for e-medicine applications; and (2) increasing market share through extensive marketing and product differentiation—for example, by offering e-services at a higher discounted rate for Internet services among seniors and the underserved. E-medicine applications create new demands not only by introducing new medical technologies but also by requiring faster and higher bandwidths. This is why many telecommunication carriers who control the distribution of bandwidth have also entered the e-medicine market; they have a vested interest in the widespread use of their products.

Finally, several other factors play a role in the promotion of e-medicine services, including direct and indirect costs related to obtaining health and medical care—for example, travel costs, time lost from work, and the mental stress of dealing with physical visits to obtain health care services. The e-medicine approach cuts down on duplication of services and paperwork; helps to reduce the number of harmful drug interactions and inappropriate prescriptions; improves public safety, security, health, and well-being; reduces patient and professional travels; speeds up availability and delivery of key patient information in emergency as well as non-emergency situations, and enables shorter hospital stays by integrating assisted home care and community services through e-networks (see also Chapters Four, Five, and Six). Advances in computer hardware and telecommunications, along with improved high-capacity storage technology, will soon permit the integration of different e-medicine applications within a single network. Ultimately, this will translate into new and expanded opportunities for e-medicine technology transfer and commercialization.

E-Medicine in Canada

In general, the technologies and systems used in e-medicine are designed to enable a two-way exchange of information between the general public on one hand and the health provider community on the other hand. The health care community essentially becomes an agent that gathers, processes, stores and disseminates data, information, and knowledge elements, using hardware and software components.

These components include a device or mechanism for receiving signals; a means to transfer the information captured via communication or e-network technologies; and a device or mechanism for representing, storing, and presenting the output information (Industry Canada, 1998). Input signals can be represented in data, audio, or real-time video format, and output devices can include video monitors, computer file servers, and data recorders. Data, information, and knowledge elements collected and processed become valuable aggregated information or organized knowledge to be shared with the general public or for a specific purpose—for example, customized therapeutic interventions for a patient or a group of patients. While the general public provides most of the base data, instructions and critical information provided by experts will eventually be needed to sustain the health and well-being of the public. Figure 8.1 depicts this simple conceptualization of e-medicine as an exchange of information.

Despite the proliferation of new technologies and applications, Canada's e-medicine industry is still relatively small and underdeveloped. Canada has a land area of approximately 3.8 million square miles. The majority of Canadians live in urban cities located within 155 miles of the country's border with the United States, and the rest of the country is sparsely populated. Owing to the size of the country and the difficulties of traveling in remote areas due to geography and bad weather,

FIGURE 8.1. E-MEDICINE AS AN INFORMATION CLEARINGHOUSE

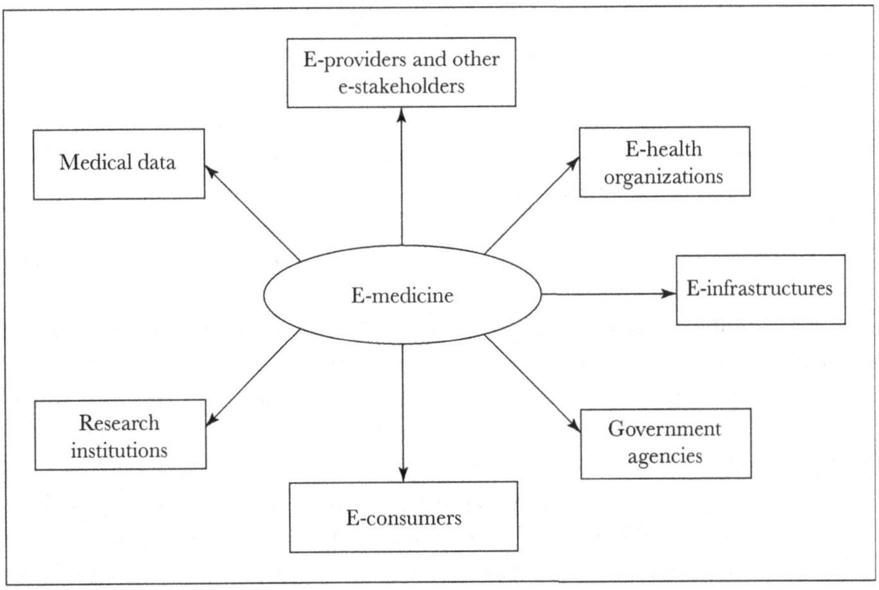

Canadians need to develop expertise in e-medicine technology if Canada is to play a key role in the global e-health marketplace. In fact, Canada was one of the first countries to use telecommunications technology to assist in the delivery of health care. In 1956, a neurosurgeon in Saskatoon used closed-circuit television to transmit live electrocorticography tracings, and a Montreal radiologist pioneered teleradiology in 1958 (Elford and House, 1996).

Canada also launched its first domestic telecommunication satellite, Anik A-1, in 1972. From 1976 to 1982, the Federal Department of Communications sponsored a number of projects that evaluated the use of satellite technology for e-medicine. In these projects, although e-medicine was found useful, satellite systems were not found to be cost-effective. In the following ten years, although they participated in a few international e-medicine projects, Canadian researchers basically lagged behind. Lately, however, there appears to be renewed interest in e-medicine across Canada (Watanabe, 1998), perhaps due to the development of provincial and national infrastructures for the health information highway, as well as pressure to deliver health care at a lower cost and with increased technological capacity and speed (Wright, 1998).

One reason that the Canadian e-medicine industry has grown very slowly over the years is that many potential users still have little knowledge about or experience in this field. Medicolegal, ethical, and administrative concerns also inhibit the growth of e-medicine. For example, telephone triage systems allow nurse practitioners to provide health care advice over the telephone, but there are potential liability issues such as medication errors due to human transcription errors. However, it is not clear what the legal implications would be if medication errors occur either because of nurse giving wrong advice or the patient having heard wrongly. As Blair and others (1998) point out, the issues of licensing and regulatory requirements for practicing across jurisdictional boundaries; responsibility for clinical care decisions and medical malpractice insurance coverage; and standards of care are all influencing the determination of physicians to practice e-medicine. In addition to these concerns, a number of ethical issues in regard to the health professional–patient relationship—such as privacy, confidentiality, informed consent, and security of transmitted data—are emerging. The Center for Bio-ethics at the Clinical Research Institute in Montreal is studying these issues (Industry Canada, 1997).

There is also a paucity of research showing the value of health care delivered via e-medicine. As a result, there is a need to assess the effectiveness of care delivery using various e-technologies, as well as the cost-effectiveness of these applications. A number of initiatives that focus on these topics are being undertaken by the University of Calgary in Alberta as well as the University of Victoria in British Columbia (see Tan with Sheps, 1998, Chapters Fifteen and Sixteen). In the United States, the National Academy of Sciences' Institute of Medicine (IOM) has also called on researchers everywhere to strengthen the evidence base for e-medicine. Field (1996) has suggested an evaluation framework for e-medicine applications in Canada and the United States that is based on the criteria of quality, accessibility, cost, and acceptability of health care services.

The Canadian Network for the Advancement of Research, Industry and Education is a government-funded initiative to help develop a national high-speed network and information-based technologies for many sectors, including health care. One ambitious project is the formation of a nationwide Asynchronous Transfer Mode (ATM) network (see Chapter Six). For this project, seven regional high-speed networks will be linked. The province of Nova Scotia has just implemented an e-medicine network, and other provinces—such as Quebec, Alberta, New Brunswick, and Ontario—are following in Nova Scotia's footsteps. Coalitions of private companies such as STENTOR are also working closely with provincial governments across Canada to research and develop advanced telecommunication and networking technologies, with an emphasis on e-medicine applications.

The Canadian Institute for Health Information (CIHI) has identified the need for standards in e-medicine, including standards for health information security and privacy, for information exchange and applications, and for linking provincial health care information systems (Industry Canada, 1997). British Columbia's Ministry of Health has instituted the British Columbia Health Information Standards Council (BCHISC). Comprising many stakeholder representatives from health care agencies, universities, governmental agencies, and user communities, the BCHISC identifies standards and sets guidelines to promote the effective and efficient sharing of health information in British Columbia. Joseph Tan, the editor of this text, was a member of this council for three years, participating in provincewide meetings on health information standards and related issues. In collaboration with the CIHI, the BCHISC works to improve the flow of e-health information to support new initiatives in different parts of the health care sector, including e-medicine. Although British Columbia has one of the most automated provincial health systems, including an on-line billing system for practitioners, PharmaNet/BC, and HealthNet/BC, the province still faces several challenges in developing and implementing e-clinical and e-medicine applications. Major barriers to the adoption of e-medicine practices are unresolved issues of professional acceptance, the ability and desire to change current practices, and reimbursement.

Watanabe (1998) argues that e-medicine will succeed in Canada only if "its development responds primarily to the needs of the health care sector and not simply to the availability of technology." The Health Association of British Columbia (HABC) has identified several key factors that are necessary for the successful implementation of e-medicine systems.

- Leadership from e-medicine champions in health care practice and government to build partnerships and a vision for the field

- A coordinating body with representation from all levels of the health care sector and from academia, industry, and government to provide harmonization of activities, a forum for communication, and act as a pool of information resources
- Government funding for the implementation, ongoing maintenance, and evaluation of innovative diffusion of technology in various regions

It is often exciting to cover e-medicine from the perspective of a developed country such as Canada because of the growing number of initiatives and activities that are developing as e-medicine moves to the forefront of health informatics. Yet the greatest needs for e-medicine technologies and applications are not in developed countries, where health care standards are usually established and citizens can expect a certain level of support for their health and wellness. Canada, for example, subscribes to the vision of universal health care, and all citizens, regardless of race, ethnicity, or religious beliefs, have equal rights to access the health care system. In developing countries, however, even basic infrastructures for health care may be lacking, so e-medicine strategies may be able to provide quality medicare conveniently available at reasonable costs. Therefore, we now turn our attention to a country where an understanding of the e-medicine diffusion process would be especially helpful in designing future e-medicine programs.

E-Medicine in Ethiopia

For the last decade, Ethiopia has been planning a long-term national health care strategy to increase the number of citizens receiving care and to decrease the subsequent health care costs. However, health problems such as HIV/AIDS and malaria, combined with high population growth rates (2.6 percent in 2002), have increased the demand for health care services and have resulted in more expensive treatments. Moreover, slow economic growth and funding of the health sectors have not kept up with these rising health care costs. This is true not only of Ethiopia but of most developing countries, especially in sub-Saharan Africa.

In addition to financial scarcity, the shortage of medical specialists in many developing countries has led to a high mortality of patients suffering from various diseases. In the specific case of Ethiopia, the country's inadequate transportation infrastructure and large geographical area makes it more difficult than usual to provide health care services in remote and rural areas, where 85 percent of the population lives. Where clinics and hospitals do exist, especially outside urban areas, they are often poorly equipped and below the standards set by the World Health Organization (WHO). In addition, extended drought and famine have resulted in food shortages, illiteracy, and poor socioeconomic conditions.

Nevertheless, buildings, medical equipment, medical staff, and drugs are essential to good health care and require a high level of investment. To meet this challenge, the Ethiopian government and its international donors must supplement the existing human, infrastructure, and financial resources with modern technology. E-medicine has been identified as a possible solution.

As we noted earlier in this chapter, e-medicine involves delivering health care using telecommunication equipment as simple as telephones and fax machines or as complex as Internet-connected personal computers with full-motion interactive multimedia (Huston and Huston, 2000). There is a critical need to better understand the factors affecting the diffusion of e-medicine in developing countries. Services such as teleradiology, teledermatology, telepathology, telecardiology, and tele-ophthalmology can be extended to underserved communities and individuals in both urban and rural areas. In addition, e-medicine can help attract and retain health professionals in rural areas by providing ongoing training and collaboration with other health professionals. Although e-medicine, like all information and communication technologies (ICTs), was developed and tested in developed countries, it has successfully addressed some medical problems in developing countries. However, many of these initiatives have been relatively small and isolated. Wright (1998) suggests that while developing countries' priorities in most cases may not be to finance e-medicine activities, despite their known potential, the governments of these countries could at least facilitate the provision and flow of medical information and health care, thereby reducing unnecessary health care expenditures (for example, providing online training of nurses and doctors on how to share information resources and use teleconsultations). Experience in the developed world demonstrates that most successful e-medicine applications require a change in the organization of health care delivery.

We address the lack of understanding of e-medicine diffusion in developing countries by focusing on a conceptual framework to measure e-medicine transfer outcomes relating to information technology, people, cultures, economics, and the social setting. The framework measures four areas: (1) ICT policies; (2) ICT infrastructure; (3) e-medicine implementation; and (4) culture-specific beliefs and values, and technological culturation. In explaining the framework, we present supporting arguments and insights on issues surrounding the diffusion of e-medicine in Ethiopia. We also highlight implications for research, practice, and other application domains.

Background on Ethiopia

Located in the horn of Africa, Ethiopia is the second most populous country in sub-Saharan Africa, with a population of 67.3 million. The country is made up of more than eighty ethnic groups who speak more than eighty languages. Ethiopia is not only populous, but it is a geographically large country (slightly less than twice the size of

Texas). The geography and lack of transportation infrastructure is challenging. Eighty-five percent of the population is rural, with agricultural production as their primary livelihood activity. Ethiopia is bounded on the north by Eritrea, on the east by Djibouti and Somalia, on the south by Kenya, and on the west by Sudan. The country is among the poorest in the world, with an annual income of less than $100 U.S. per capita, 51 percent health coverage, 19 percent and 40 percent literacy rate among women and men, respectively, and a life expectancy of 43.4 years. The country scores low in almost all social and economic indicators. For example, in 2001, it ranked 158th out of 162 countries on the global human development index.

Social poverty is on the rise; the majority of the population does not have access to education, health care, or safe water. The high prevalence of HIV/AIDS and malaria has also put a significant pressure on the economy and the social infra-structure. Nevertheless, the Ethiopian government's openness to improving the situation, focusing on long-term development through agricultural development–led industrialization, has resulted in some prospects for increased productivity, improve-ment of rural infrastructure, growing private investments, and mobilization of exter-nal resources such as financial aids from other developed countries. The focus on rural areas and small households has led to expansion of agricultural extension in the sense of improved technology and credit schemes, primary education, primary health care, rural water supply projects, and rural roads. For example, the gross enrollment in pri-mary education increased from 35 percent of eligible children in 1990 to 46 percent in 2000.

The health care infrastructure is spread thin and poorly equipped. Health care facilities, in the relatively few locations where they exist, are usually overcrowded and in need of physical repair. The human capacity problem is perhaps even more se-rious. There is one doctor for every 36,000 Ethiopians, and those doctors tend to be concentrated in Addis Ababa and the major towns. Ethiopia has three schools of med-icine, 87 hospitals with less than 12,000 total beds, 257 health centers, and 196 pri-vate clinics. Although Ethiopia's medical schools are turning out trained personnel, too many graduates (about 60 percent) leave after their required in-country service due to low pay, difficult working conditions, lack of opportunities for professional de-velopment, and insufficient autonomy. For example, the International Organization for Immigration ranked Ethiopia first among African countries in the number of em-igrant medical professionals.

Ethiopia is a typical developing country; its large proportion of children reflects high fertility rates and low life expectancy. The mortality rate for infants and those under the age of five started to decrease at the beginning of 1990s, but no further progress was recorded in later years. This may be due to the fact that HIV/AIDS is killing many children. Ethiopia has the lowest health progress in the region and around the globe, due to drought and famine, civil war, poor government, and political instability. Ethiopia has also the highest maternal mortality ratio in the world (800 per 100,000 live births), due to poor health infrastructure, scarcity of medical professionals and low rates of female education. Ethiopia is greatly affected by the HIV/AIDS epidemic, third in the world after only South Africa and India. Not only is this a serious health problem, but it is also becoming a developmental, social, psychological, and political problem. The problem is still increasing because of a lack of behavioral and lifestyle changes along with poor, voluntary counseling and testing. AIDS is sending Ethiopia's development backward and making a poor country even poorer.

Despite the obstacles, Ethiopia's health care spending has been increasing, particularly since the launch of the health sector development program in 1997. The total spending on health increased from 1 percent of gross domestic product (GDP) in 1992–93 to 1.4 percent in 1996–97. It then dropped back to 1 percent before it picked up to 1.8 percent and 2.1 percent of GDP in 2000–01 and 2001–02, respectively. A moderate increase in health accessibility has been recorded, from 49 percent in 1995–96 to 52 percent in 2000–01. Table 8.1 shows the major comparative socio-economic and health indicators of Ethiopia and sub-Saharan Africa.

Experts believe that the social and economic woes of Ethiopia are far from being resolved. Concerted efforts must be made to think out policies and strategies based on objective evaluation of the causes of rampant poverty, taking global dynamics into account. Agriculture, which contributes more than 50 percent of GDP, cannot save the country from poverty. Experts have argued that efforts should focus on untapped potentials such as tourism and ICTs. Introducing ICTs into health care services offers opportunities to improve the quality of care. Applications of ICTs not only will provide opportunities for Ethiopia to participate in the global economy but are also important in increasing people's ability to learn and change behavior.

The Ethiopian government has also shown its readiness to consider developing ICT policies and programs in order to address challenges in socioeconomic development. A broad-based national ICT policy development initiative began in early 1997. The first draft of an ICT policy was developed by a team of experts in June 2001 following a national workshop in November 1999. In early 2002, the Council of Ministers adopted the ICT policy, which emphasizes the need to harness ICTs in the health sector and build the necessary infrastructural capacity. The policy also discusses needs for human resource development and for building and strengthening institutions. A general description of ICT for health in Ethiopia is provided in Table 8.2.

E-medicine has been identified as a possible solution to some of Ethiopia's medical problems. Lessons from sub-Saharan African countries include some established standard practices for e-medicine diffusion (Mbarika and Okoli, 2003). E-medicine has already successfully addressed some clinical applications in Ethiopia, such as tele-ophthalmology, telecardiology, teleradiology, telepathology, and teledermatology. Following is a description of a teledermatology project.

TABLE 8.1. MAJOR SOCIOECONOMIC AND HEALTH INDICATORS OF ETHIOPIA AND SUB-SAHARAN AFRICA

	Ethiopia	Sub-Saharan Africa
Social and Economic Variables, 2002		
Population	67.3 million	680.0 million
Population growth (annual)	2.2%	2.2%
Life expectancy (years)	42.1	45.8
Illiteracy rate (age 15 and older)	58.5%	36.7%
Surface area (square kilometers)	1.1 million	24.3 million
Gross national income per capita (U.S. dollars)	$100	$450
Gross domestic product (U.S. dollars)	$6.0 billion	$318.6 billion
Contribution to Gross Domestic Product, 2002		
Agriculture	52.3%	15.7%
Industry	11.1%	27.7%
Service	36.5%	56.4%
Health Sector, 2002		
Population with access to health care	51.6%	59.0%
Access to an improved water source	13% rural	50% rural
	77% urban	86% urban
Access to improved sanitation facilities	6% rural	43% rural
	58% urban	73% urban
Doctor-to-population ratio	1:36,000	1:10,800
Health budget (percentage of national budget, 2001–02)	7.0%	N/A
Health expenditure per capita (U.S. dollars)	$1	$42
Corporations and third party expenditure on health (percentage of total expenditure)	60.6%	60.47%
Technology and Infrastructure (2001)		
Number of telephone lines and mobile telephones (per 1,000 people)	4.8	40.6
Paved roads (percentage of total roads)	14%	13.8%
Number of personal computers (per 1,000 people)	1.1	9.9
Number of Internet users	25,000	5.3 million

Note: N/A = not applicable.

Sources: World Development Indicators Database, August 2003; WHO/UNICEF Joint Monitoring Program, 2001; African Human Development Indicators—United Nations Development Program, 2001.

TABLE 8.2. INFORMATION AND COMMUNICATION TECHNOLOGY FOR HEALTH IN ETHIOPIA

Positive Factors
- The number of telephone subscribers has increased from 105,985 in 1987-88 to 283,683 in 2000-2001.
- Internet services, which were introduced in 1996-97 with 1,042 subscribers, have increased the number of subscribers to 6,487 in 2002.
- Internet services have been extended to twelve major towns, although about 96 percent of the total subscribers are from Addis Ababa.
- A mobile telephone system became operational in 1998-99 with 6,740 subscribers, rising to 27,532 subscribers in 2000-01.
- Mobile telephone services are expanding to other regions.
- There are no institutions that register the number of computers in the country; however, according to an estimate by the International Telecommunication Union, there were 75,000 computers in 2001.
- More than 75 percent of the health professionals have a telephone line at home.
- Mobile telephones are also commonly used among health workers.
- Availability of computers, direct telephone lines, and Internet connectivity has expanded, to about 33 percent, 96 percent, and 13 percent of hospitals, respectively.

Negative (Inhibiting) Factors
- The Internet bandwidth is very small: the bandwidth from Internet service provider (ISP) to the Internet backbone is only 4 megabytes for uploading and 10 megabytes for downloading.
- The maximum bandwidth from user to ISP is 56 kilobytes for dial-up access and 64 kilobytes for leased lines.
- The main Internet connection lines satisfy only 65 percent of the expressed demand of the country, and the proportion of the number of connections requested to the number of connections available was 55 percent in 2000-01.
- Information technology professionals constitute less than 0.3 percent of the total health staff.
- ICT investment and expenditures in the health sector are low.
- Sixty-one percent of computers are used as office tools—for example, for finance and administration.
- Seventy-one percent of Internet use is for e-mail.
- Tax rates in the country are high compared with some African countries.
- ICT skill and knowledge are weak among health care professionals.
- ICT related to health projects in Ethiopia is limited.

Source: SCAN-ICT Baseline Studies UNECA (Information and Communication Technologies, 2003).

In 1998, the Telecommunications Development Bureau (BDT) of the International Telecommunications Union (ITU) launched its first e-medicine project in sub-Saharan Africa. The connecting sites are the Tikur Ambessa hospitals, the Faculty of Medicine in Addis Ababa, and ten rural hospitals. The project was set up by a multidisciplinary group of partners that included the national e-medicine committee in close collaboration with domestic and international partners, including the WHO, European Community, United Nations Educational Scientific and Cultural Organization, E-Health Solution, WorldSpace, Tokai University of Japan, Addis Ababa University, Ethiopian Telecommunication Cooperation, and the Ethiopian Telecommunication Agency.

The project uses standard low-cost equipment, including e-networking via servers, digital cameras, and color scanners; e-medicine software; and telecommunication interfaces installed at the central studio and the remote hospitals. The Internet is used to connect hospitals, forming an e-medicine information network. The primary health care units will use e-mail to give the rural sites access to doctors' advice.

The teledermatology link between the teaching hospitals of Tikur Ambessa and ten regional secondary care hospitals throughout the country. The link allows the regional hospitals to exchange digital and video images of patients in rural areas who are suffering from skin disorders and then to send them, via the Internet, to doctors in the regional capital of Tikur Ambessa. The doctors consult among themselves and forward advice on treatment. These procedures considerably reduce patients' waiting time from six months to less than one week, and they also reduce unnecessary travel to a referral hospital. In addition, teledermatology has increased access to specialist health care.

Although these initial successes are promising, the projects are still relatively small and isolated. There is a critical need to better understand the factors affecting e-medicine transfer outcomes learned from the experience of other developed countries. In the next section, we present an ICT framework, identify and speculate on some of the positive and negative factors that have been found to influence e-medicine diffusion, and apply this thinking to Ethiopia.

Factors Affecting the Diffusion of E-Medicine in Ethiopia

For more than fifteen years, clinicians, health services researchers, and others have been investigating the use of ICTs to improve health care. E-medicine, representing an integration of the practice of medicine with the innovative applications of ICTs, is one area of such investigation. By drawing knowledge from various sources in technology diffusion research, we hope to develop an understanding of key factors that determine e-medicine transfer outcomes in a developing country.

Issues of technology transfer—that is, moving a given technology from creators to users—have been studied extensively, and the findings reveal major challenges, even in developed countries. Kwon and Zmud (1987), for example, argue that these challenges include difficulties in new technology implementation, which sometimes ends in failure. The problems become exacerbated when such transfers are attempted from developed to developing countries with significantly different socioeconomic and cultural environments.

We have identified four critical factors of e-medicine transfer to Ethiopia:

- National ICT policies
- ICT infrastructure
- E-medicine implementation factors
- Culture-specific beliefs and values and technological culturation—that is, cultural differences between the makers of the technologies, based in developed countries, and the users of the technologies, based in developing countries

Figure 8.2 depicts the impact of various constructs on e-medicine transfer outcomes. Some of these relationships are positive, while others are negative.

National ICT Policies. *National ICT policies* are both general policies and specific health and security policies tailored to e-medicine. Government policies have been found to be highly instrumental in the diffusion of computing within a society (Gurbaxani and others, 1990). In Ethiopia, the formulation and implementation of policies in the ICT sector is still very rudimentary. An integrated set of laws, regulations, and guidelines to shape the generation, acquisition, and utilization of ICTs does not yet exist. Nonetheless, the government controls most of the ICT infrastructures and upholds policies that influence the acquisition and use of these infrastructures by private

FIGURE 8.2. CONCEPTUAL FRAMEWORK OF ISSUES IN TELEMEDICINE TRANSFER IN ETHIOPIA

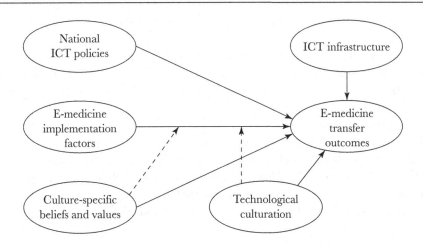

organizations. Policies such as these, which encourage computer ownership and investment, encourage the transfer of ICT to all segments of the population.

Another aspect of ICT policy issues in Ethiopia is privatization of ICT infrastructures. In Ethiopia, the government owns and manages the telecommunications operator that provides phone lines for Internet, fax, and e-mail access, which are important infrastructures for the transfer of e-medicine technologies. However, because Ethiopian government policies forbid or restrict privately owned telecommunication and Internet service provider services, lack of competition makes such services expensive and usually poor in quality. Hence, a policy that is not specific to e-medicine significantly affects e-medicine transfer through its effect on ICT infrastructures.

Like other health care systems, the health care system in Ethiopia deals with very sensitive and private data. Given that these data systems are increasingly interoperable yet the primary demands are that the data be correct, not corrupted, relevant, complete, and accessible only to authorized persons, the data systems must be secure. This gives rise to the need to address technological, legal, regulatory, ethical issues not only within a national context but also at the international level. A key strategic issue in any health care system is the technical, communications, and data standards, although in most instances these standards are not specifically directed at health care.

Figure 8.3 depicts the impacts that national ICT policies can have on e-medicine transfer outcomes.

Based on our understanding of national ICT policies in Ethiopia, we propose the following national policy directions in order to effect positive e-medicine transfer outcomes:

- Policies that favor the development of ICTs, to increase the level of ICT infrastructures and increase e-awareness in society, thereby encouraging foreign investment
- Policies that favor the development of e-health and technical standards and favor legal protection of providers
- Policies that favor the development of security, confidentiality, and privacy measures

ICT Infrastructures. *ICT infrastructures* are the telephone and telecommunication infrastructures, the information technology (IT) sector, electrical power, the Internet, and the extent of ICT penetration and ICT industry that facilitates data and image communications.

To enable the use of e-medicine, a country needs a solid ICT infrastructure. In the past, telecommunications infrastructure has usually been measured in terms of *teledensity*, the number of telephone landlines per capita (for a review, see Mbarika, Musa, McMullen, and Byrd, 2002). However, with the spread of wireless telecommunications, a broader perspective should be taken in identifying ICT infrastructure. Figure 8.4 depicts the impacts that ICT infrastructure can have on e-medicine transfer outcomes.

FIGURE 8.3. EFFECTS OF NATIONAL ICT POLICIES ON E-MEDICINE TRANSFER OUTCOMES

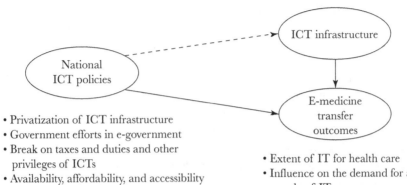

- Privatization of ICT infrastructure
- Government efforts in e-government
- Break on taxes and duties and other privileges of ICTs
- Availability, affordability, and accessibility of ICTs
- Sectoral development in health and education
- Awareness and efforts of ICTs
- Security, privacy, and confidentiality

- Extent of IT for health care
- Influence on the demand for and supply of IT
- Technological innovation
- Usability and timely delivery of services
- Success of e-medicine
- Standards and legal protection
- Mobilization of financial resources

FIGURE 8.4. EFFECTS OF ICT INFRASTRUCTURE ON E-MEDICINE TRANSFER OUTCOMES

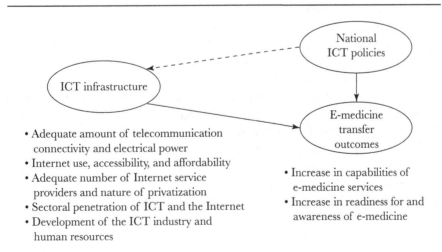

- Adequate amount of telecommunication connectivity and electrical power
- Internet use, accessibility, and affordability
- Adequate number of Internet service providers and nature of privatization
- Sectoral penetration of ICT and the Internet
- Development of the ICT industry and human resources

- Increase in capabilities of e-medicine services
- Increase in readiness for and awareness of e-medicine

Due to various socioeconomic and political problems, Ethiopia has been reported to have the lowest levels of most types of ICT-related infrastructures in the world (Goodman, 1991; Mbarika, 2001; Mbarika, Byrd, McMullen, and Musa, 2002; Mbarika, Byrd, and Raymond, 2002). Ethiopia's ICT infrastructure problems include a huge gap between supply and demand; a strong distribution imbalance that favors urban over rural areas; poor-quality service; long waiting times for new services; and peak traffic demands that exceed network capacity (Mbarika, 2001). One result is an extremely low level of basic telephone penetration: less than one phone line per 100 people (International Telecommunications Union, 2001).

Three aspects of how ICT infrastructures affect e-medicine diffusion should be addressed: (1) what ICTs are currently being employed in the practice of e-medicine; (2) what other ICTs could be employed in this effort; and (3) what enhancements to current infrastructures are necessary to enable other e-medicine practices. We propose that the following factors will have favorable impacts on e-medicine transfer outcomes in Ethiopia:

- More advanced and available telecommunication and electrical power infrastructure
- A more advanced and available IT sector
- More penetration of ICT in the health and IT sectors
- More advanced and available Internet infrastructure

Implementation Factors. E-medicine *implementation factors* include the involvement of technology champions or institutions, e-medicine policy, interoperability, e-standards, e-awareness, e-readiness, and e-acceptance.

Figure 8.5 depicts the potential impacts of key implementation factors on e-medicine transfer outcomes (Checchi, Sevcik, Loch, and Straub, 2002; Mbarika and Byrd, in press; Rogers, 1983).

Information systems researchers have identified a number of implementation factors for ICTs in general, including user training, project champions, and top management support (Checchi, Sevcik, Loch, and Straub, 2002; Culnan, 1986; Kwon and Zmud, 1987; Loch, Nelson, and Straub, 2000; Lucas, 1978; Robey and Zeller, 1978; Rogers, 1983). Traditionally, information system introduction failures are correlated with how the systems were implemented. For example, after researching user training in sub-Saharan Africa, Aynu, Okoli, and Mbarika (2003) argue that ICT training or human capacity development can play an important role in structuring sustainable ICT transfer. They further argue that although the development of ICT infrastructure is a fundamental need for effecting sustainable economic development in Ethiopia, the presence of substantial infrastructure is insufficient to yield economic development without the trained human capital to effect this conversion.

FIGURE 8.5. EFFECTS OF E-MEDICINE IMPLEMENTATION FACTORS ON E-MEDICINE TRANSFER OUTCOMES

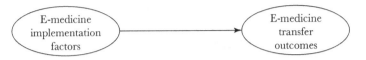

- Training, project champions, top management support
- Accessibility and reliability
- E-strategy for the health sector and readiness
- National e-medicine policy
- Recognition and adoption of standards
- Consideration of e-medicine within national health policies and strategies
- Involvement and determination of medical professionals
- Clear criteria for application of e-medicine
- Readiness of stakeholders for implementation of e-medicine

- Importance in terms of health gain
- Relevance in terms of access, equality, cost
- Seamless care across primary/secondary/ tertiary interface
- Exposure to telemedicine use

Factors that specifically affect e-medicine implementation include policies that maintain e-medicine initiatives, integration of e-medicine into mainstream health care services, and interoperability standards at all levels including technical, human, and operational. Many interfacing standards—for example, Health Level Seven (HL7), Digital Imaging and Communications in Medicine (DICOM), picture archiving and communication systems (PACS), ITU telecommunication standards (the H320 family), International Organization for Standardization standards (ISO 9000)—as well as safety regulations must be considered. In addition, relevant clinical application criteria such as health gain, volume, cost, access, and equity can all influence e-medicine implementation. Further, human factors—mainly awareness and acceptance of technology as well as willingness and e-readiness on the part of stakeholders—can also contribute to implementation success.

While efforts have been made to assess the level of a community's e-readiness, including issues of digital divide, based on available indicators (Dutta, Lanvin, Paua, and Cornelius, 2003), much information is still lacking on issues such as ICT use and health. However, it seems safe to assume that assisting a country's e-readiness will help maintain and develop the implementation of e-medicine.

We propose that the following implementation factors will have positive impacts on e-medicine transfer outcomes in Ethiopia:

- Factors that favor e-readiness and e-medicine implementation in general
- National health policies that favor the development of e-medicine
- Stakeholder awareness of, readiness for, and acceptance of the use of e-medicine services
- The presence of criteria for selecting clinical applications
- Clinical applications that have matured in technologically advanced nations
- Clinical applications that involve medical images

Culture–Specific Beliefs and Values and Technological Culturation. *Culture-specific beliefs and values* refers specifically to the effects of practitioner and patient attitudes toward e-medicine implementation, while *technological culturation* has to do with the influence of technologically advanced cultures on an individual's attitude toward technology. Culture is a complex notion that is usually assessed in terms of multiple variables. Its potential impact on e-medicine transfer outcomes in Ethiopia is shown in Figure 8.6.

Culture is a system of attitudes and traditions that are transmitted from one generation to another through learning. The health sector must take into account the issues of an individual's ethnic and cultural context. The poverty in Ethiopia means that many people simply cannot afford to expect, let alone demand a basic standard of health care. As a result, there is no standard of care, or the existing standard of care is inaccessible to the public at large. In summary, the health care situation in Ethiopia encompasses vulnerability marked by increasing poverty, and primitive sociocultural traditions with high illiteracy such as the dependency on village chiefs or priests rather than medical doctors to provide a cure; little health care treatment is therefore available. Participating in a clinical trial may be considered a privilege because trial patients are given the benefit of significantly better health care than the rest of the population.

Two levels of beliefs and values should be considered in e-medicine diffusion. On an individual basis, the issue is a person's beliefs and attitudes toward treatment providers and health care institutions. From an organizational standpoint, the focus is on a social system that involves different physician group behaviors as well as outcomes and performance of the wider health system. The nature of e-medicine is in networks—networking of both people and technology. Networking works well with developed power structures in which people have clear roles and responsibilities.

In Ethiopia, there are no clear job descriptions for physicians or other workers. Beliefs and values ingrained in people by their cultural context significantly affect their thinking and perspective, including their approach to using technology, for example,

FIGURE 8.6. EFFECTS OF CULTURE ON E-MEDICINE TRANSFER OUTCOMES

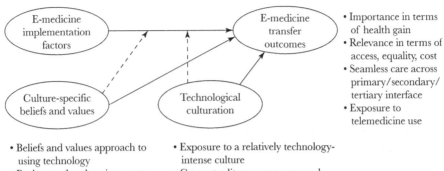

a stubborn preference for face-to-face interactions. In Ethiopia, as elsewhere, physicians working in an organization are often subject to cultural shock when networks replace hierarchies and when relationships become predominantly contractual rather than collegial. Hence, fear of change becomes a major factor in how physicians in Ethiopia may react to a specific project or need. It is easy to see that cross-cultural analyses are important in planning e-medicine systems, because what may work in one culture may not be appropriate in another.

Straub and others (2002) divided the construct of "culture" into two subconstructs:

- Culture-specific beliefs and values that a person might hold because of the influence of their cultural background
- Technological culturation, which describes a person's exposure to a relatively technology-intense culture

In the context of studying ICT diffusion in developing countries, technological culturation could indicate the degree to which a citizen of a developing country has been exposed to more technologically advanced cultures (Checchi, Sevcik, Loch, and Straub, 2002). Specifically looking at technology adoption at the individual level of analysis, McCoy (2002) tested a comprehensive model of the moderating effects of national and cultural dimensions on technology transfer. Researchers (for example, Checchi, Sevcik, Loch, and Straub, 2002; Straub and others, 2002; Straub, Loch, and Hill, 2001) have found that both of these cultural subconstructs have a mediating effect on ICT implementation. Put simply, beliefs, values, and technological culturation affect the effectiveness of ICT implementation, in addition to their direct effects on ICT outcomes.

Based on the above analysis, we identify the following cultural effects on e-medicine transfer outcomes in Ethiopia:

- Culture-specific beliefs and values consistent with e-medicine practice in technologically advanced nations will yield favorable outcomes.
- Social culture and behavior consistent with risk assessments, care-seeking experiences, and medical decisions within e-medicine practice will positively affect outcomes.
- Taking patient preferences and knowledge into account and building patient-provider relationships within the health service will yield favorable outcomes.
- Technological culturation of citizens will enhance the favorable effect of e-medicine implementation factors on transfer outcomes.

Research on the Diffusion of E-Medicine in Developing Countries

The study of e-medicine diffusion in developing countries should focus on national ICT policies, ICT infrastructures, e-medicine implementation factors, culture-specific beliefs and values, and technological culturation. National ICT policies reflect the aspirations of government policymakers in prioritizing ICT for national development. They reflect both general ICT policies and those specific to e-medicine. ICT infrastructures include computers, telephones, wireless networks, and telecommunication infrastructures that facilitate communications and data collection and storage. We expect both national ICT policies and ICT infrastructures to have a direct effect on e-medicine transfer outcomes, and we also expect national ICT policies to also have a direct effect on ICT infrastructure. *E-medicine implementation factors* refer to a set of antecedents, such as training; health policies; selection of e-medicine applications based on accessible technologies and needs; e-awareness; e-acceptance; e-readiness; and e-management support. This set of factors affects the effectiveness of e-medicine transfer. In regard to culture-specific beliefs and values and technological culturation, our analysis shows that cultural factors affect e-medicine transfer directly and also through their moderating effect on e-medicine implementation.

E-medicine outcome measures for projects in developing countries, like outcome measurements for any health technology or service, are essential for several reasons. Reviewing outcomes gives government policymakers the opportunity to form new insights into the effectiveness of various national ICT policies on e-medicine transfer to developing countries. Such insights could help policymakers fine-tune their policies in a bid to encourage further e-medicine investments by stimulating infrastructure development, increasing financial resources, mobilizing e-medicine programs, reducing policy barriers, as well as informing health managers about the feasibility, cost-effectiveness, and acceptability of clinical e-medicine and helping those who have invested in e-medicine identify problems and improve programs.

E-medicine infrastructure providers, such as equipment manufacturers and service providers, need an understanding of where the needs are and how best to base organizational practices strategically for both local and multinational organizations. For example, e-medicine equipment manufacturers (which are mostly based in Europe and North America) can develop systems that fit within the cultural and educational context of developing countries.

The requirements for e-medicine in developing countries are not the same as in developed countries, and the telecommunication infrastructure and resources also vary dramatically. The greatest need for e-medicine is in countries where a majority of rural community residents are deprived of efficient health services due to their location. For example, in Ethiopia there is a digital divide between the capital region and the rest of the country. Addis Ababa is comparatively well equipped with ICTs, but the rural areas are generally cut off from most information and communication facilities.

Moreover, four major trends are driving the need for and increasing the significance of ICTs in the health care sector for developing nations: (1) the need to curtail health care costs in general; (2) infectious diseases such as HIV/AIDS and malaria, with their more treatment dependent patients and higher care needs; (3) increasing focus on preventive care; and (4) political changes in the structure of health care systems. E-medicine may not solve all medical problems, and technical, clinical, organizational, behavioral, and cultural obstacles to e-medicine technologies will remain, as will policy impediments and uncertainties related to reimbursements, standards, security measures, licensure, medical liability, and other concerns. However, research on the transfer and diffusion of e-medicine is a starting point in efforts to reach Africans who live in areas with limited medical facilities and personnel. E-medicine research with a focus on developing countries could have far-reaching positive outcomes.

Conclusion

Rogers' studies revealed five major characteristics of an innovation that affect its diffusion: the innovation's relative advantage, its compatibility with mainstream technology, its complexity, the ability to apply the innovation, and the opportunity to effectively observe the innovation (Rogers, 1983). In the case of e-medicine, the diffusion process will affect not just individuals, groups, and communities but countries and continents. Hence, in addition to the significance of e-medicine's technological characteristics, we must also become aware of individual, group, community, and national characteristics, communications, and contextual factors (such as regulations and economics).

Chapter Questions

1. What is meant by diffusion of e-medicine? What is the significance of studying the diffusion process in the context of evolving e-health systems and environments?
2. How does e-medicine development in the United States and the United Kingdom compare with that in Canada?
3. What can developing countries learn from the diffusion process of e-medicine in developed countries? What differences between developed and developing countries should be considered when implementing e-medicine as a system of knowledge transfer?
4. In what ways is the diffusion of e-medicine similar in developed and developing countries? In what ways is it different? What are the reasons for these differences?
5. What do you think are the critical success factors for e-medicine diffusion in a country such as the one you live in? Have any of these factors changed over the years?
6. Imagine that you are the minister of health for a large geographical region. You have been allotted a large sum of investment money to develop e-medicine in your area. How would you go about planning, designing, and evaluating the success of an e-medicine program—for example, a tele-ophthalmology program?

References

Aynu, B., Okoli, C., & Mbarika, V.W.A. (2003, June 8–10). *IT training in Sub-Saharan Africa: A moderator of IT transfer for sustainable development.* Paper presented at the 4th Annual Global Information Technology Management World Conference, Calgary, Canada.

Barrett, J. E., & Brecht, R. M. (1998). Historical context of telemedicine. In S. F. Viegas & K. Dunn (Eds.), *Telemedicine: Practicing in the information age* (pp. 9–17). Philadelphia: Lippincott-Raven.

Bashshur, R. L. (1997). Telemedicine and the health care system. In R. L. Bashshur, J. H. Sanders, & G. W. Shannon (Eds.), *Telemedicine theory and practice* (pp. 5–36). Springfield, IL: Thomas.

Blair, P., Bambus, A., & Stone, T. H. (1998). Legal and ethical issues. In S. Viegas & K. Dunn (Eds.), *Telemedicine: Practicing in the information age* (pp. 49–60). New York: Lippincott-Raven.

Checchi, R. M., Sevcik, G. R., Loch, K. D., & Straub, D. W. (2002, December 1–3). *An instrumentation process for measuring ICT policies and culture.* Paper presented at the International Conference on Information Technology, Communications and Development, Kathmandu, Nepal.

Culnan, M. J. (1986). The intellectual development of management information systems, 1972–1982: A co-citation analysis. *Management Science, 32*(2), 156–172.

Dutta, S., Lanvin, B., Paua, F., & Cornelius, P. (2003). *The global information technology report 2002–2003: Readiness for the networked world.* Oxford, England: Oxford University Press.

Elford, R., & House, M. (1996). *Telemedicine experience in Canada (1956–1996).* Report of the Congress International Conference, Montreal, Canada. St. John's, Canada: Telemedicine Centre, Faculty of Medicine, Memorial University of Newfoundland.

Field, M. (1996). *Telemedicine: A guide to assessing telecommunications in health care.* Washington, DC: National Academy Press.

Goodman, S. E. (1991). Computing in less-developed countries. *Communications of the Association for Computing Machinery (CACM), 34*(12), 25–29.

Gurbaxani, V., Kraemer, K. L., King, J. L., Jarman, S., Dedrick, J., Raman, K. S., & Yap, C.S. (1990). Government as the driving force toward the information society: National computer policy in Singapore. *Information Society, 7*(2), 155–185.

Huston, T., & Huston, J. (2000). Is telemedicine a practical reality? *Communications of the ACM, 43*(6), 91–95.

Industry Canada. (1997). *Telehealth in Canada: Challenges on the road ahead.* Retrieved from http://strategis.ic.gc.ca

Industry Canada. (1998, September 18). *The definition, many applications.* Retrieved from http://strategis.ic.gc.ca

Information and Communication Technologies (ICT) Team of the Development Information Services Division (DISD), Third Meeting of the Committee on Development and Information (CODI 3), Addis Ababa, Ethiopia, from April 10-17, 2003.

International Telecommunications Union. (2001). *African telecommunication indicators.* Geneva, Switzerland: International Telecommunication Union.

Kwon, T. H., & Zmud, R. W. (1987). Unifying the fragmented models of information systems implementation. In R. J. Boland & R. A. Hirscheim (Eds.), *Critical issues in information systems research* (pp. 227–251). New York: Wiley.

Loch, K., Nelson, G., & Straub, D. W. (2000). *NSF project summary: IT transfer to Egypt: A process model for developing countries.* Unpublished manuscript.

Lucas, H. C. (1978). Empirical evidence for a descriptive model of implementation. *MIS Quarterly, 2*(2), 27–41.

Mbarika, V.W.A. (2001). *Africa's least developed countries' teledensity problems and strategies.* Yaoundé, Cameroon: ME and AGWECAMS.

Mbarika, V.W.A., & Byrd, T. A. (in press). Stakeholders' perceptions of strategies to improve the technological infrastructure for e-commerce in Africa's least developed countries. *European Journal of Information Systems.*

Mbarika, V.W.A., Musa, P., McMullen, P., & Byrd, T. A. (2002). Teledensity growth constraints and strategies for Africa's LDCs: "Viagra" prescriptions or sustainable development strategy? *Journal of Global Information Technology Management, 5*(1), 25–42.

Mbarika, V.W.A., Byrd, T. A., & Raymond, J. (2002). Growth of teledensity in least developed countries: Need for a mitigated euphoria. *Journal of Global Information Technology Management, 10*(2), 14–27.

Mbarika, V.W.A., Byrd, T. A., Raymond, J., & McMullen, P. (2001). Investments in telecommunications infrastructure are not the panacea for least developed countries' leapfrogging growth of teledensity. *International Journal on Media Management, 2*(1), 133–142.

Mbarika, V.W.A., & Okoli, C. (2003, January 6–9). *Telemedicine: A possible panacea for sub-Saharan Africa's medical nightmare.* Paper presented at the 36th Hawaii International Conference on System Sciences, Waikoloa Village, Hawaii.

McCoy, S. (2002). *The effect of national culture dimensions on the acceptance of information technology: A trait based approach.* Unpublished doctoral dissertation, University of Pittsburgh, Pittsburgh, PA.

Perednia, D. A., & Allen, A. (1995). Tele-medicine technology and clinical applications. *Journal of the American Medical Association*, *273*(6), 483–488.

Robey, D., & Zeller, R. L. (1978). Factors affecting the success and failure of an information system for product quality. *Interfaces*, *8*, 70–75.

Rogers, E. M. (1983). *Diffusion of innovations*. New York: Free Press.

Straub, D. W., Loch, K. D., Evaristo, R., Karahanna, E., & Srite, M. (2002). Toward a theory based definition of culture. *Journal of Global Information Management*, *10*(1), 13–23.

Straub, D. W., Loch, K. D., & Hill, C. E. (2001). Transfer of information technology to developing countries: A test of cultural influence modeling in the Arab world. *Journal of Global Information Management*, *9*(4), 6–28.

Tan, J., with Sheps, S. (1998). *Health decision support systems*. Sudbury, MA: Jones & Bartlett.

United Nations Development Program (UNDP). (2001). *The World Development Report—African Human Development Indicators*. New York: Author.

Viegas, S. F. (1998). Past as prologue. In S .F. Viegas and K. Dunn, (Eds.), *Telemedicine: Practicing in the information age* (pp. 1–8).Philadelphia: Lippincott-Raven.

Watanabe, M. (1998). Telehealth in Canada [Editorial]. *Telemedicine Journal*, *4*(3), 197–198.

World Development Indicators Database, World Bank, Washington, DC. August 2003; WHO/UNICEF Joint Monitoring Program, New York, 2001; *African Human Development Indicators*—United Nations Development Program, 2001.

Wright, D. (1998). Telemedicine and developing countries. *Journal of Telemedicine and Telecare*, *4*(2, Suppl.), 1–88.

E-Medicine Development in Taiwan Case

Paul Jen-Hwa Hu, Chih-Ping Wei, Tsang-Hsiang Cheng, Joseph Tan

E-medicine is an essential form of e-health, as is indicated by its inclusion as a core application in the Taiwan's National Infrastructure Initiative (NII), which was launched in 1995, and in similar national initiatives, including the National Broadband Experimental Network. Technology-enabled e-medicine allows service delivery and collaboration beyond geographic and temporal barriers. Government participation, particularly that of the Department of Health (DoH), Taiwan's supreme health authority and policymaker, is critical to the dissemination of e-medicine. According to DoH, the overarching goal of e-medicine in NII is to design, establish, and evaluate a wide array of services that jointly constitute a nationwide infrastructure for remote diagnosis and e-patient management.

The diffusion of e-medicine programs has been initiated and propelled chiefly by leading acute tertiary care centers and teaching hospitals, including the National Taiwan University Hospital, the Taipei Veterans' General Hospital, and the Taipei Military General Hospital. Initial motivation for e-medicine programs included enhancement of access to services and quality of care, particularly through vertical service integration that connects care providers in primary, secondary, and tertiary care sectors. Over time, additional services and support activities have been incorporated, including support for e-clinical training and continuing education.

At the time that this case study was completed, all existing programs were still largely in an experimental stage. In spite of adequate technology bases, the continued operation and services of most of these programs is greatly dependent on external resources and the voluntary participation of individual physicians and specialists, technologists, and academic or clinical researchers. While these programs have demonstrated clinical value and resulted in encouraging evaluations of the technical feasibility of e-medicine for patient care and service collaboration, efforts to make the transition from the current experimental stage to real-world clinical settings raise important challenges in program management. As Perednia and Allen (1995) commented, the ultimate success of an e-medicine program requires an adopting organization to address key challenges pertinent to both technology and management.

Major E-Medicine Programs in Taiwan

In 1995, the DoH released the first national blueprint for e-medicine in Taiwan, highlighting the use of adequate and available information and telecommunication technologies to enhance service accessibility, quality, timeliness, and cost-effectiveness. Both horizontal service extension to remote areas and vertical care integration to seamlessly connect care providers in the primary, secondary, and tertiary care sectors were identified as important e-medicine applications. Support for nonclinical services or activities was also emphasized. With partial funding by NII, the DoH provided pilot e-medicine programs with financial assistance for technology acquisition. Technologies supporting both synchronous and asynchronous services were targeted.

Videoconferencing systems with multimedia capability were commonly used with synchronous services, including real-time patient assessment, e-diagnostic services, and e-consultation. On the other hand, medical imaging transmission and display systems and electronic patient record systems were used with asynchronous services or consultations. A review of the services rendered found a mix of diagnostic, prognostic, and consultation services using medical images, particularly in such specialty areas as neurology, dermatology, and internal medicine.

Exhibit 8.1 highlights the major e-medicine programs in Taiwan. As shown in the exhibit, most Taiwanese e-medicine programs are based in Taipei, with the exception of the program housed at National Cheng-Kung University Hospital. All existing programs share an emphasis on enhanced patient care and management through vertical service integration. Typically, the e-medicine programs are housed at and managed by a tertiary or teaching hospital with a direct service link to a primary or secondary care facility; for example, an outpatient clinic or a regional general hospital. The point-to-point service arrangement is common, although it is not effective for creating a service network or community because of the increasing number of nodes needed to service a growing community. The existing programs focus primarily on the clinical aspects of e-medicine, although other services or activities are also supported.

EXHIBIT 8.1. MAJOR E-MEDICINE PROGRAMS IN TAIWAN

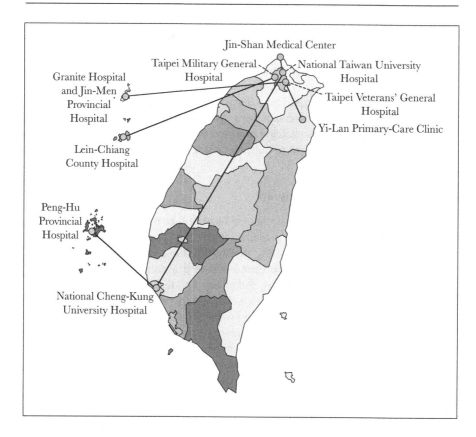

The National Health Insurance Scheme (NHIS) and the NII will both reimburse the cost of providing an e-medicine service. Specifically, the NHIS reimburses the services of on-site (local) attending care providers, while the NII partially reimburses services performed by the remote tertiary or teaching hospitals. Connection services are provided free of charge by the Bureau of Telecommunications, Taiwan's largest telecommunications service provider, which is primarily owned and controlled by the Ministry of Transportation. Depending on the requirements of the specific project, different connection services are available, including an integrated service digital network (ISDN) and a high-speed digital exchange network that supports frame relay and asynchronous transfer mode (ATM) transmissions.

Videoconferencing Project at National Taiwan University Hospital

Officially launched in 1995, this program connects the National Taiwan University Hospital (NTUH) and the Jin-Shan Medical Center, a primary care clinic located in rural

Taipei County. Using a state-of-the-art videoconferencing system in conjunction with a medical imaging transmission and display system and a multimedia patient record retrieval system, NTUH provides both synchronous and asynchronous services to patients located in the connected medical center. The services in high demand include remote patient assessment, diagnosis, and diagnostic or therapeutic consultation across a wide array of specialty areas.

In 1997, NTUH expanded its e-medicine program by connecting directly with National Cheng-Kung University Hospital, the most important e-medicine center in southern Taiwan. The connection between two major centers supports peer-to-peer consultation, collaborative patient management, and clinical case discussions among physicians and specialists located at different tertiary hospitals. In addition, this link will be the backbone of the nationwide e-health service network envisioned by the DoH.

Around-the-Clock Consultation Project at Taipei Veterans' General Hospital

Taipei Veterans' General Hospital (TVGH) is a modern tertiary hospital that serves both the military community and the general public. TVGH joined the NII e-medicine scheme in 1995, operating a direct service link to Granite Hospital, the largest military hospital on Jin-Men Island. Using the same designated ATM-T1 line, TVGH also offers services to patients at Jin-Men Provincial General Hospital. The e-medicine suite is located in Granite Hospital, so patients from the provincial hospital have to travel there. By design, the program uses integrated information and medical imaging technologies, including a videoconference system, a medical image transmission and display system, and the existing patient information systems and image archive database systems housed at TVGH. TVGH offers around-the-clock e-diagnostic and therapeutic consultation services to patients located at both of the connected hospitals on Jin-Men Island, especially to those in need of immediate medical attention or emergency care. In 1997, TVGH launched a second service link, providing similar services to a public primary care clinic in Yi-Lan County in eastern Taiwan.

Emergency Support at National Cheng-Kung University Hospital

National Cheng-Kung University Hospital (NCKUH) is the only tertiary teaching hospital that joined the NII e-medicine scheme at its commencement. Operating a direct service link to Peng-Hu Provincial Hospital, a general hospital located on the island of Peng-Hu, NCKUH provides mainly remote consultation and diagnosis support for emergency care. This program's technological requirements include a high-resolution image transmission and display system and a videoconferencing system. In addition to its primary concentration on emergency medicine, the program provides scheduled virtual outpatient clinic sessions to patients not in need of urgent care, as well as clinical case discussions and continuing education programs for health care professionals. Judged by the service volume and the range of activity supported, this program is arguably the most active e-medicine program in Taiwan, offering about six hundred remote clinical sessions and delivering continuing education to over five hundred individuals in a typical year.

Military Acute Care at Taipei Military General Hospital

Taipei Military General Hospital (TMGH) provides acute tertiary care to the military community. TMGH joined the NII e-medicine scheme in 1997, operating a direct ISDN line that connects to Lien-Chiang County Hospital on Ma-Tsu Island. The program is supported by a mid-range videoconferencing system and a medical image transmission and display system. Use of this program, which is mostly restricted to urgent patient care, has been limited.

Program Evaluation and Management Issues

A survey of the major e-medicine programs in Taiwan suggested several key issues and observations concerning program evaluation and management. Overall program planning has mostly been centralized, with the DoH playing a critical role in program (need) assessment and coordination. Each program is highly autonomous with respect to particular services and medical specialty areas offered. At the same time, the programs share a fairly sophisticated technology base that integrates the relevant information, telecommunication, and medical imaging technologies to different degrees. Typically, while each program acquires technologies from external vendors, technology transfer, testing, evaluation, enhancement, and integration are mostly undertaken and managed by in-house IT staff, especially in the tertiary (teaching) hospitals.

Most, if not all, of the existing programs concentrate on serving patients in rural or offshore areas and focus primarily on vertical service integration by connecting care providers in primary, secondary, and tertiary care sectors. The target service recipients and service focus are largely consistent with those commonly found in U.S. programs but distinctly different from those of urban-based programs in Hong Kong as these programs are centrally controlled and administered through the Hong Kong Health Authority (Sheng and others, 1997, 1998). Program and service financing is mostly supported by the NHIS or the NII.

Several issues pertinent to program management deserve highlighting. First, the provision of routine technology-enabled e-medicine services may require considerable learning or training on the part of physicians and specialists. That is, user training is essential. Kleinke (2000) surmised that physician resistance is a significant bottleneck in the adoption and diffusion of technology innovations in health care. Training should not be confined to technology use and operations but, when and where appropriate, should include training in verbal communication skills and in detecting or using important nonverbal expressions or cues in a virtual setting.

Technology management represents another key challenge, commencing with technology acquisition. Both system integration and interoperability are relevant and need proper attention. Integration includes interfacing with existing (legacy) systems and with multiple sources of information or data. The importance of system interoperability significantly increases when scaling services from a point-to-point configuration to a networked setting in which participating organizations use heterogeneous technologies. For instance, a medical image system whose storage format follows a Digital Imaging and Communications in Medicine (DICOM) standard is desirable. Similarly, transmission of medical images between or among service participants can be greatly supported when all connecting organizations have implemented a picture archiving communications system (PACS). Cross-platform system interoperability is also required in order to preserve the confidentiality of patient information at both the algorithm level (for example, encryption software) and in a particular communication layer (for example, Secure Socket Layer).

Service configuration is also important. In a nutshell, e-medicine should generally be network-based because the value of an e-medicine service may be perceived to be higher when it includes more participants, patients, or care providers. In this light, expanding e-medicine services from a point-to-point configuration to a network-based service community is desirable, especially when connecting a network of service providers (for example, physicians and specialists) with a network of service consumers (the general public). An expanded service configuration is also economically appealing because of the resulting economy of scale and probable economy of scope.

Finally, service diversity is also critical to the success of an e-medicine program. An organization that chooses to concentrate on the clinical aspect of e-medicine services nonetheless should not exclude alternative or expanded service applications. Basic clinical training and continuing education are fundamental nonclinical activities that may be better supported and enhanced in an e-medicine setting. Diversity in medical specialty areas is a useful goal. In short, e-medicine services may differ considerably in their respective requirements, but including more services in an e-medicine program contributes to the program's overall value and its likelihood of success.

Conclusion

In this case study, we have surveyed the development of e-medicine in Taiwan and highlighted some major and representative programs. Several implications for program evaluation and management are identified and discussed. Overall, we suggest that not only should program champions work to convince physicians and specialists in general about the clinical value and technical feasibility of e-medicine programs, but they should also demonstrate the common benefits of e-medicine services and their implications for professional authority or autonomy, together with adequate strategies for protecting stakeholders. In addition, concerns about service delivery, physician-patient relationships, system integration and interoperability, legal liability, and payment for services must be addressed in order for e-medicine programs to continue and grow.

Case Questions

1. Would you consider the dissemination of e-medicine in Taiwan similar to or different from that of other developed countries in Asia, Europe, or North America? Why or why not?

2. Based on this case, identify and discuss common barriers to the diffusion of e-medicine services within a health care system.
3. What are the core technologies that support e-medicine services in Taiwan?
4. Compare and contrast the different e-medicine programs highlighted in this case. Does one program appear to be more effective and successful than others? If so, which one, and why?
5. How are the surveyed e-medicine programs funded? What challenges do these programs face? What do you project for the future of these programs?

References

Kleinke, J. D. (2000, November–December). Vaporware.com: The failed promise of the health care Internet–Why the Internet will be the next thing not to fix the U.S. health care system. *Health Affairs,* Vol 19, Issue 3, 57-71.

Perednia, D. A., & Allen, A. (1995). E-medicine technology and clinical applications. *Journal of the American Medical Association, 273*(6), 483–488.

Sheng, O.R.L., Hu, P. J., Au, G., Higa, K., & Wei, C. (1997). Urban teleradiology in Hong Kong: Lessons learned and implications. *Journal of E-Medicine and Telecare, 3*(1), 81–86.

Sheng, O.R.L., Hu, P. J., Wei, C., Higa, K., & Au, G. (1998). Organizational adoption and diffusion of e-medicine technology: A comparative case study in Hong Kong. *Journal of Organizational Computing and Electronic Commerce, 8*(4), 247–275.

CHAPTER NINE

E-HOME CARE

REJUVENATING HOME HEALTH CARE AND TELE–HOME CARE

George Demiris, Joseph Tan

Learning Objectives

1. Identify the scope and boundaries of e-home care services in the context of the evolving e-health care system and environment
2. Define e-home care and discuss the significance of home health care in the context of the mainstream health care delivery system
3. Understand the trends and benefits of e-home care that arise from emerging technologies and applications
4. Identify the issues and challenges in e-home care applications
5. Understand the future possibilities for e-home care applications

Introduction

The *home health care* (HHC) industry has a century-long history. Beginning with wealthy families hiring live-in maids and nurses, as well as caregivers for family members who were either immobilized or homebound due to physical or mental disabilities, the cottage home health care industry soon grew to cater not just to the rich but to anyone who needed home-based services such as rehabilitation, massage, or physiotherapy; food preparation or meal delivery service; help with personal hygiene or moving around the house; arrangements for doctors' and nurses' visits; urgent and emergency responses; and even regular administration of medications. Over the years, the industry has diversified to provide a wide variety of services that are similar to those provided in long-term care facilities such as chronic care units, group homes, or residences for the elderly. Even hospitals are often involved in the delivery of some home care services.

E-home care services may include patient assessment; supervision of patient care; routine nursing care and health monitoring; medication administration and scheduled injections; or management of dietary needs, daily exercise, and lifestyle changes (for example, smoking cessation). Historically, family members performed most of these chores for homebound patients, but nowadays arrangements are often made to have caregivers, nurse's aides, or even professional nurses provide day care services several times a week.

In addition, with rapid advances in science and technology, many who need HHC services can now perform a number of these services independently, using assistive devices and equipment programmed with intelligent software and sensors. E-home care was built on this foundation, incorporating information and telecommunication technologies to support HHC services and community health care. Advancing technological applications that have contributed to the emergence of e-home care include the Internet and associated technologies such as intranets and extranets, videoconferencing

devices, personal data assistants (PDAs), and special remote patient monitoring equipment, including spirometers and electronic stethoscopes, that can send readings from
the patient's home to nurses, doctors or specialists.

E-medicine has been defined as the use of advanced information and communication technology (ICT) to bridge geographic gaps and improve care delivery and education (see Chapter Eight). Advances in ICT, such as portable monitoring devices
and wireless sensor applications like a "robotic dog" that can be easily installed and
operated at a patient's home, introduced a new era for home care. Such applications
reduce the cost of care and can enrich provider-patient communication and improve patients' quality of life. New applications of ICT and telehealth care have also
led to consumer-friendly, Web-based e-health services; applications that promote self-
care directly to consumers; e-clinical care via satellites or wireless technologies to support independent living; use of PDAs by home caregivers or by consumers directly for
teleconsultation (or e-consultation) with expert physicians; and use of automated intelligence, decision support technologies, and assistive devices for e-health monitoring
(Tan with Sheps, 1998). E-care technologies that support independent living include
telephone support, personal response systems, alarm monitoring systems, and assistive devices such as hand-held prescription reminders. Other e-technology systems that
can be incorporated into e-home care include e-nursing, e-learning, and remote patient monitoring systems. Several of these concepts have already been discussed and
illustrated in previous chapters. Here, we simply note that these e-technologies require
the use of e-networking applications to enable nurses and other caregivers to monitor
patients in their homes.

In this chapter, we will discuss the role and significance of e-home care in terms
of cost savings. In addition, we outline the trends driving e-home care in the context
of the evolving e-health care system and environment, review the range of e-home
care services, and highlight the benefits and challenges in e-home care. We close the
chapter with a look at the evaluation of e-home care technologies and their future
prospects.

E-Home Care Concepts

The goal of making e-health care systems sustainable in this era of health care reform
and fiscal constraints focuses on improving quality and health outcomes while delivering health care services using cost-effective methods. Providing responsive and dynamic health care requires the effective and coordinated use of new information
and communications technologies. E-home care is an innovative approach that has
the potential to improve our health care delivery system by meeting the growing need
of aging and homebound patients for improved access to health care while maintaining patient autonomy. Given the demographic trend toward an older population

in most developed countries, e-home care may become one of the fastest-growing domains in the e-health care marketplace.

Over the last few years, a growing number of health professionals and consumers have been using terms such as *tele–home care* and *telecare*, which were barely in use before the end of the twentieth century. *E-home care*, which encompasses those terms, is a relatively young concept, but with the increasing availability of e-technologies and the proliferation of assistive and remote home monitoring devices, it is being gradually incorporated into the mainstream. Home health care products and services are marketed via the Internet, e-health provider and community networks, and other wireless and handheld devices such as mobile telephones. More broadly, the underlying challenges for e-home care include the need to connect e-providers, home health caregivers, and e-patients; to educate and inform e-health care professionals, e-home health caregivers, and e-consumers who are homebound or simply prefer to have health care delivered to their home; and to stimulate innovations in e-home care delivery.

Patient empowerment, a concept that has emerged in the health care literature in the last few years, is based on the principle that patients are entitled to have access to health information and to make their own care choices (see also Chapter Three). Feste and Anderson (1995) argue that the empowerment model introduces "self-awareness, personal responsibility, informed choices and quality of life." Empowerment can be perceived as an enabling process through which individuals or groups take control over their lives and manage any diseases they may have. Thus, a key element for home care patients is taking responsibility for managing their own illnesses; this can be supported by e-health applications that allow them to stay at home while accessing specialized care and becoming active participants in their own health care management process.

E-home care uses clinical, administrative, and consumer health informatics to enable effective HHC delivery. E-home care is not, in itself, a product; rather, it is a means of accomplishing high quality, patient-centered community, and home-based care with the aid of emerging e-technologies. Its development is therefore a reflection of advances in e-marketing, e-health care, e-medicine, and increasing demand for affordable HHC services.

Significance of Home Health Care

Home health care is one of the fastest-growing areas in the health care industry. More than twenty thousand providers deliver home care services to approximately 8 million individuals diagnosed with acute illness, long-term health conditions, permanent disability, or terminal illness (National Association for Homecare, 2000). Annual expenditures for home health care in the United States alone were estimated to be $41.3 billion in 2001. According to a document produced by the Office of Health and the Information Highway of Health Canada, annual public home care expenses in

Canada reached just over $2 billion in 1997–98, representing a substantial increase of $1.1 billion (104 percent) from 1990–91 (Office of Health and the Information Highway, 1999). We can say with some confidence that unless more efficient and effective approaches are applied, the incremental costs of delivering HHC will continue to escalate because of an aging population, rising wages and antiquated technologies. Nevertheless, HHC is already saving the mainstream Canadian and the U.S. health care systems hundreds of millions of dollars annually if one considers what comparable care in a medical office or hospital would cost.

The first U.S. HHC agencies were established in the 1880s. Their number grew to 1,100 by 1963 and to more than 20,000 in 2001 (National Association for Homecare, 2000). Although HHC agencies have been providing services to Americans for more than a century, Medicare's decision in 1965 to make home care services widely available to the elderly fueled the industry's rapid growth (National Institute of Nursing Research, 1994). The goal of HHC is to optimize functional capability (National Center for Health Statistics, 1996), which requires the identification and management of not only medical but also environmental, behavioral, and psychosocial problems. Determining the proper diagnosis and developing a treatment plan often requires information about the patient's home environment and social resources (Ramsdell, Swart, Jackson, and Renvall, 1989). Home care nurses are likely to develop therapeutic relationships with their patients because they see them over extended periods of time and can provide a range of support services through continuity of care (Pesznecker, Patsdaughter, Moddy, and Albert, 1990). This continuity and the extended supervision enhance compliant behavior (McCord, 1986).

Studies suggest that home visits can lead to improved medical care through the discovery of unmet health care needs (Ramsdell, Swart, Jackson, and Renvall, 1989; Arcand and Williamson, 1981; Fabacher and others, 1994). One study found that home assessment of elderly patients with relatively good health status and function resulted in the detection of an average of four new medical problems and up to eight new intervention recommendations per patient (Ramsdell, Swart, Jackson, and Renvall, 1989). Kane and Kane (1987) reviewed several studies on the effects of HHC and found in many cases that home care patients had fewer hospital and nursing home admissions, shorter lengths of stay, fewer outpatient visits, and lower estimated total health care costs.

Home care enables providers to interact with their patients on an ongoing basis in the patients' homes and not a clinical setting. The importance of this interaction is documented in published literature: communicative features of medical consultations have been linked to various outcomes such as patients' satisfaction with care, understanding of medical information, adherence to prescribed regimens, and health improvement (Hall and Roter, 1988; Kaplan and Greenfield, 1989). Kane and Kane (1987) gathered studies that found positive attitudes in terms of satisfaction and perceived health in patient groups receiving home care services. Kaplan and Greenfield

(1989) found that "better health," whether measured physiologically (through blood pressure, blood sugar, and other measures), behaviorally (functional status), or more subjectively (evaluation of overall health status), was consistently related to specific aspects of provider-patient communication.

Nonetheless, especially in the United States, HHC faces several potential threats to its viability, given the combined effect of increased life expectancy, population growth, and funding limitations on the Social Security/Medicare situation. These new, challenging realities will lead to changes in the definition and focus of home care in this new millennium. People aged sixty-five years and older are projected to represent 20 percent of the population in the year 2030 (Economics and Statistics Administration, 1994). Social Security and Medicare programs could experience financial difficulties in the near future because the ratio of workers paying taxes to retirees drawing benefits has long been decreasing. The number of workers paying into Social Security per beneficiary is expected to decrease to 2.1 by 2020 (Social Security Administration, 2000).

Rationale and Trends for E-Home Care

E-home care can address the issues of cost of health care delivery and problematic access to traditional home care for both rural and urban underserved patients. The use of technology has the potential to decrease travel time and costs for nurses and increase the number of patients that an HHC nurse visits in a given day. E-home care, also known as *tele–home care*, uses telecommunication and videoconferencing technologies to enable a health care provider at a clinical site to make virtual visits to patients. In this context, the term *actual visit* is used to describe a traditional visit of a health care provider to a patient's home (face-to-face interaction).

A study conducted in 1997 by the Insight Research Corporation estimated that approximately 20 percent of home visits would use e-home care applications by 2001. The following observable trends in the U.S. and Canadian health care systems have contributed to the rapid development of e-home care:

- Integration of health care services, particularly e-health care services, to meet increasing community and primary care needs among underserved patient populations such as seniors, those living in rural areas, and those who have impaired mobility or who are homebound
- Increasing outpatient procedures, decreasing institutionalization, and shortened inpatient stays as a result of discharging patients from hospitals and clinics earlier, even when they require continuing care and regular clinical monitoring
- Demographic changes resulting from an increasingly elderly population, more advanced medical technology and procedures, health-promoting lifestyle and alternative medicine movements, and longer life spans

- Rising prevalence of chronic illnesses—such as diabetes, joint and lower back pain, heart problems, and mental health problems—that require regular therapy, long-term care, and regular monitoring of health status
- Increasing partnerships between the government, granting agencies, universities, health provider organizations, investors, venture capitalists, and private companies to develop e-technologies and innovative products that can be applied to HHC—for example, smart cards, smart cars, automated massage chairs, robot dogs, intelligent refrigerators, and smart homes
- Growth in home care across the continuum of care as a substitute for acute care and long-term care and as a preventive service
- Advances in decision support technologies, diffusion of Internet-related technologies, developments of smart interface technologies, and diffusion of e-health information on community and e-home care services, leading to better-informed patients and caregivers who want more flexible health care delivery

E-home care complements community health infrastructure and enables the system to address the issues raised by these trends.

E-home care can also lighten the burden of unnecessary expenditures and cut waste. First, it reduces unnecessary emergency room visits and decreases the burden on long-term care facilities and minimizes unscheduled visits to physicians. Many patients, especially in countries such as Canada where the government pays the bulk of health care costs, will simply go to an emergency room even though a non-emergency clinic would be more appropriate. Non-emergency patients going to an ER represents the use of inappropriate services that imposes an unnecessary, additional cost to the system. The same is true if a patient needing only non-specialist services insists on consulting with a specialist. Patients may miss prescheduled visits because of work responsibilities or transportation problems. A few simply forget their prescheduled visits.

Looking at statistics for the small Okanagan-Similkameen Health Region of British Columbia, we can see how e-home care services could result in significant cost savings. A spring 1999 report stated, "There is an immediate requirement in this small geographic area for over 900 long term care beds and escalating at a daily cost of between $90,000.00 and $110,000.00 [Canadian dollars] per bed depending on the level of care required." If we factor in the cost of day-to-day operations and extrapolate these numbers over a larger population, the figures for the province of British Columbia are overwhelming. The provincial government is not able or prepared to absorb all of the costs generated by the mainstream health care system. E-home care could substantially reduce use of traditional health care modalities; provide early intervention and prevention services, resulting in further savings; teach patients self-care and management of early symptoms, thus helping them to avoid health complications; provide round-the-clock information on vital sign fluctuations; and encourage the use of e-administrative and support services—for example, automatic recording of patient-submitted data, on-line payment and service reimbursements, and other critical administrative functions.

E-Home Care Applications

With the development of portable monitoring devices and the diffusion of the Internet, the number of e-home care applications started to increase in the 1990s. Sparks and others (1993) investigated the use of exercise monitoring via telephone as an alternative for cardiac rehabilitation patients who were unable to participate in a hospital-based program. The study was conducted as a randomized, controlled trial and provided indications that this kind of monitoring was an effective supplement to hospital-based monitoring. Turnin, Bolzonella-Pene, and Dumoulin (1995) developed and evaluated a telemedicine system for self-monitoring and dietary education of diabetic patients that had a positive impact on patients' nutritional knowledge and on some clinical outcomes (total cholesterol, cholesterol of low-density lipids). Evaluating the clinical usefulness of cardiac arrhythmia monitoring via telephone, Wu, Kessler, Chakko, and Kessler (1995) found it more effective than ambulatory electrocardiography in detecting arrhythmias. A randomized, controlled trial by Friedman, Kazis, and Jette (1996) demonstrated that automated patient monitoring and counseling via telephone had a positive effect on patient adherence to antihypertensive medications and on blood pressure control. Mehra, Uber, Chomsky, & Oren (2000) studied the efficacy of e-home monitoring for patients with chronic heart failure and identified a need to further investigate this approach. Comparing the use and costs of home care through remote video technology with those of traditional home care, Johnston, Wheeler, Deuser, and Sousa (2000) determined that the remote approach achieved cost savings and improved access to home care support while producing no differences in clinical outcomes.

It has been argued that the application of telehealth technology to home health care services will eventually prove both clinically and technologically sensible. However, the full impact and effectiveness of e-home care in the context of our traditional health care delivery system is far from being realized. The full potential of this technology will be accessible only when e-home care applications are integrated with the data analysis, business intelligence (the application of data mining methodologies to discover hidden trends or patterns for improving business performance), and decision support aspects of e-health, empowering home-based populations to live independently and receive quality care, as needed, in their own homes. One example of an effort to tap the potential of integrated e-home care is the work being done to integrate "smart home" technology with e-home care services, which will be discussed later in this chapter.

E-Disease Management

Disease management includes "a set of coordinated health care interventions and communications for populations with conditions in which patient self-care efforts are significant" (Disease Management Association of America, 2002). These interventions aim to enhance care plans and provider-patient relationships, emphasizing the prevention or delay of deterioration and complications through the use of evidence-based practice guidelines. Additional goals of disease management include improvement of outcomes, cost reduction, patient education, and patient monitoring.

The concept of *e-disease management* is defined by the utilization of ICT such as the Internet to allow patients with chronic conditions to stay at home and be involved in the care delivery process. Such e-technologies can help co-ordinate e-home care with hospital and ambulatory care and facilitate information exchange and communications between and among patients, family members, and care providers. If an e-patient has to be attended by specialists, for example, in the case of a cardiac arrest, linking e-home care with hospital and ambulatory care would prove more efficient and beneficial in the treatment of the e-patient. E-patient education is an essential component of e-disease management and can be easily supported by the transmission of tailored health information or automated reminders to patients or their caregivers. The integration of commercially available household items such as television sets, mobile phones, videophones, medication dispensing machines, and handheld computers introduces new communication modes and new tools for patient empowerment into e-disease management programs.

The Internet is being used for e-disease management applications in different clinical areas. In e-disease management for asthma patients, for example, the home asthma telemonitoring (HAT) system assists in early detection of allergies and timely intervention to prevent asthma attacks (Finkelstein, O'Connor, G., and Friedmann, 2001). HAT assists patients with the daily routine of asthma care through personalized interventions and alerts health care providers when patients require immediate attention. Web-based management of diabetes can also enhance care delivery because of the disease's requirements for long-term prevention and intervention of other associated illnesses. The Center for Health Services Research of the Henry Ford Health System in Detroit, Michigan, developed a Web-based system to support care delivery to diabetic patients (Baker and others, 2001). The system was evaluated within a nonrandomized, longitudinal study, and findings suggested that Web-based systems integrating clinical practice guidelines, patient registries, and performance feedback can improve the rate of routine insulin testing. A distributed computer-based system for the management of insulin-dependent diabetes was developed and evaluated within the Telematic Management of Insulin-Dependent Diabetes Mellitus project, which was funded by the European Union. The objective was to use Internet technology and monitoring devices to support the normal activities of physicians and diabetic patients by providing a set of automated services enabling data collection, transmission, analysis, and decision support (Riva, Bellazzi, and Stefanelli, 1997).

E-disease management applications can also be developed for post-transplant care. Regular spirometric monitoring of lung transplant recipients, for example, is essential in early detection of acute infection or rejection of an allograft. A Web-based e-monitoring system that provided direct transmission of home spirometry to a hospital was developed and evaluated, demonstrating that home monitoring of pulmonary function in lung transplant recipients via the Internet is feasible and accurate (Morlion, Knoop, Paiva, and Estenne, 2002).

Another application using low-cost, commercially available monitoring devices and the Internet was developed for the TeleHomeCare Project at the University of Minnesota, aiming to enable patients with congestive heart failure, with chronic obstructive pulmonary disease, or requiring wound care to interact from their homes with health care providers at the agency. Personalized Web pages encouraged patients to fill out daily questionnaires, answering questions about vital signs (such as weight, blood pressure, or temperature), symptoms, and overall well-being and nutrition. Alerts were triggered and care providers were instantly notified when a patient's entry required immediate medical attention, which was determined by predefined, personalized rules (Demiris, Finkelstein, and Speedie, 2001).

E-Medicine in Hospice Care

Hospice care is a concept based on the provision of comfort and support to patients and their families when a life-limiting illness no longer responds to cure-oriented treatments. Thus, hospice care neither prolongs life nor hastens death but rather aims to improve the quality of dying patients' last days by offering comfort and dignity, focusing on palliation, individual control, and relief of suffering. Hospice care deals with the emotional, social, and spiritual impact of the disease on the patient and the patient's family and friends through interdisciplinary teams composed of physicians, nurses, social workers, chaplains, aides, and volunteers.

While the number of hospice agencies has increased greatly in the last ten years, less than 25 percent of dying patients in the United States currently use hospice services. Many elderly patients approach the end of life in isolation. Several barriers to the provision of hospice services, especially in rural communities, have been identified—for example, inadequate reimbursement, restrictive regulatory definitions of service areas based on mileage and driving time rather than care outcomes, and shortages of nurses, aides, and social workers interested or willing to work in this area. The same issues are found in other developed countries such as Canada and the United Kingdom.

In the United States, the Institute of Medicine has identified systemic deficiencies in end-of-life care (Field and Christine, 1997) including legal, organizational, and economic obstacles to palliative care and the systemic lack of appropriate education of and effective communication between health care providers. Telemedicine can eliminate some barriers to quality end-of-life care. Hospice services via telemedicine (e-hospice) can be delivered directly into a patient's home through videoconferencing. This is of particular significance for underserved patients in rural and urban sites and for patients with limited caregiver support.

The director of the Hospice Association of America has urged the House Committee on Small Business of the U.S. House of Representatives to further develop initiatives in e-hospice care and services. Interestingly, the incorporation of telemedicine into palliative care has been successfully implemented in many different countries, including Spain (Riano, Prado, Pascual, and Martin, 2002), the United Kingdom (Regnard, 2000), Australia (Elsey and McIntyre, 1996), and Japan (Oyama, Wakao, and Okamura, 1997), as well as in the American states of New York (Oyama, Wakao, and Okamura, 1997), Kansas, and Michigan, (Coyle, Khojainova, Francavilla, and Gonzales, 2002). An e-hospice application can support an agency's commitment to be accessible to patients and caregivers twenty-four hours a day, providing outpatients with one of the advantages of inpatient care.

Other E-Home Care Technologies

Other e-technologies that can be used within an e-home care context include the following:

- Portable monitoring devices
- Videophones
- Wearable sensors
- PDAs
- Smart shirts
- Smart home technologies

Several commercially available *portable monitoring devices,* such as pulse oximeters, blood pressure monitors, spirometers, weight scales, and glucose monitors can be used for e-home care applications. These devices are tested for accuracy and are approved by the Federal Drug Agency before they become available on the market. In some cases, data are stored in the device and retrieved later; in other cases, they are displayed on a monitor at the completion of the test session. Devices that allow the automatic transmission of data over regular phone lines or in accordance with the system's transmission architecture are preferred over devices in which the patient has to read the results and announce them to a nurse during a virtual visit, which can impose a burden on elderly or visually impaired patients and affect accuracy.

Videoconferencing at patients' homes without any cost for upgrading the existing infrastructure has been enabled by International Telecommunication Union—Telecommunication Sector (ITU-T) standard H324 for multimedia conferencing on plain old telephone service. H324 defines standards for transmitting video, audio, and other data over one analog telephone line. Because local and wide area networks use the same interoperable substandards as H324, significant interoperability among videophones with different features and by different manufacturers can be achieved. Videophones can be installed in patients' homes and operated over regular phone lines. Training required for patients is often minimal because videophones operate like regular phones with the addition of a screen. Some of these devices can also be connected with television sets or other monitors (for example, on a personal computer) to achieve a higher-resolution display. Depending on the application, the camera embedded in the videophone can be sufficient. In cases where providers wish to assess the home environment, a portable camera can be easily integrated into the system. The H324 standards allow low-cost e-home care solutions. However, if low cost is not a priority, there is always the option of using an advanced infrastructure, if one exists, or upgrading the existing one to achieve maximum video and audio quality (for example, by installing ISDN, DSL, or T-1 lines) (see Chapters Six and Seven). As ICT and e-technologies advance, e-networks can be expanded, and the level of achievable audio and video quality of videoconferencing sessions will increase, leading to more creative and appealing interfaces.

Physical, chemical, and biological *sensors* can also be used to enhance e-home care applications. A physical sensor will measure physical parameters such as temperature or pressure, whereas a biological or chemical sensor involves a receptor (for example, an enzyme or antibody), which binds with an analyte (that is, a target molecule). The signal produced by the sensor is transferred to a circuit and digitized. The resulting digital data can be stored or displayed. Sensors can be incorporated into watches, items of clothing, and eyeglasses. One could argue that wearable sensors function as non-invasive in vitro diagnostic tools, because they are capable of analyzing human sweat, tears, stress, strain, pH increases, and more.

An example of a *wearable sensor* is the "intelligent knee sleeve" that monitors knee strain or injury (University of Wollongong, 2001). Originally designed for football players, this device is strapped to the knee and provides feedback to the user by emitting an audio tone. It can be a useful application for e-home care patients with mobility impairments or during rehabilitation. Another wearable sensor is a small portable detector in the form of a wristwatch, which provides cystic fibrosis test results in minutes rather than the twenty-four hours that is the typical response time for a laboratory test (Lynch, 2000). The wristwatch device uses an electric field to push pilocarpine nitrate into the skin, thereby dilating the pores. Sweat is then absorbed and stored in a duct in the watch. A sensor analyzes the sample and records the levels of sodium, chloride, and potassium ions. Other wristwatch devices include meters that measure glucose in the interstitial fluid as a low electric current pulls glucose through the skin (Tamada, Lesho, and Tierney, 2002) and a blood oxygen monitor (Wahr and Tremper, 1995).

PDAs are now being used in dietetics and nutritional screening. Two studies at California State University, Los Angeles, have found PDA use in nutritional screenings to be readily adaptable to ongoing efforts by dietitians. The PDAs were found to be useful in identifying potential indicators of poor nutritional status in institutionalized elderly patients as people can check the nutrient content of their food by accessing their PDAs. Food service supervisors can learn to use them in a relatively short time, allowing an increase in the number of nutritionally relevant variables to be assessed and improving the quality of documentation in the medical record.

As new technological innovations continue to arise, the possibilities for sensor use in e-home care become seemingly endless. In the last few years, the *smart shirt* has been introduced. The smart shirt incorporates technology into the design of clothing to monitor the wearer's heart rate, electrocardiogram (ECG), respiration, temperature, or vital functions, alerting the wearer or physician if there is a problem (Georgia Institute of Technology, 2004). Smart shirts also can be used to monitor the vital signs of military personnel, chronically ill patients, firemen, or frail elderly persons living alone. The U.S. Navy initially funded the smart shirt project in October 1996; in 2000, the Georgia Tech Research Corporation licensed the technology to a private company in order to manufacture and market the product (Georgia Institute of Technology, 2004).

A *smart home* is a residence equipped with a set of advanced electronics and automated devices that are specifically designed for care delivery, remote monitoring, early detection of problems or emergencies, and maximization of patient safety. A smart home is usually linked with a local processor that analyzes sensor data and detects critical situations; the smart home is also connected to a remote control center that notifies the appropriate emergency service such as the health agencies, police, and the fire station in the case of a fire. Smart home features usually include motion-sensing devices for automatic lighting control; motorized locks; door and window openers; and motorized blinds and curtains; smoke and gas detectors; and temperature control devices (Elger and Furugren, 1998). Such an infrastructure aims to address problems associated with neurological and cognitive disorders in the elderly and to enhance patients' ability to function independently within their own residence.

The Swedish Handicap Institute operates a demonstration apartment as part of the so-called SmartBo project (Elger and Furugren, 1998). This project focuses on solutions for visually impaired, hearing-impaired, and mobility-impaired residents and residents with cognitive disabilities. It is based on the integration of visual and tactile signaling devices, a text-enlargement program, a speech synthesizer, and a Braille display for visually impaired residents. Another smart home project is PROSAFE, which uses a set of infrared motion sensors connected to either a wireless or wired network to support automatic recognition of resident activity and possible falls and, when appropriate, triggers alarms, aiming to accommodate patients with Alzheimer's disease (Chan and others, 1999; Chan, Bocquet, and Steenkeste, 1999). Finally, the Aware Home Research Initiative is an interdisciplinary research initiative at Georgia Tech that addresses the fundamental technical, design, and social challenges associated with smart home technologies (Kidd, Orr, Abowd, and Atkeson, 1999).

E-Home Care Issues and Challenges

The success and diffusion of e-disease management systems in particular and e-home care applications in general depends on the following critical factors:

- Privacy and confidentiality
- Accessible design
- Reimbursement

Privacy and Confidentiality

As a result of recent technological advances, the health care sector faces many challenges in guarding the privacy and confidentiality of individuals' health information. Information privacy refers to patients' right to control the use and dissemination of their personal information. Confidentiality is a tool for protecting privacy. In 1998, the "Notice of the Proposed Rule from the Department of Health and Human Services Concerning Security and Electronic Signature Standards" was introduced in the United States as part of the Health Insurance Portability and Accountability Act (HIPAA) that was passed in 1996 (U.S. Department of Health and Human Services, 1999). This proposed rule became law in the United States in 2000 and proposes standards for the security of individuals' health information and electronic signature use for health care providers, systems, and agencies. These standards refer to the security of all e-health information and have a great impact on the design and operation of e-home care applications such as ensuring that home-based electronic prescription services are not misused.

Privacy issues related to video and audio recording, maintenance of tapes, storage and transmission of still images, and other types of patient records have yet to be codified, and efforts must be undertaken to address these challenges fully. The transmission of information over communication lines such as phone lines and satellite or other channels raises concerns about possible privacy violations. An additional concern in some cases is the presence of technical staff assisting with transmission procedures at the clinical site (or at both ends of the transmission), which could create a perceived or actual loss of patient privacy. In addition, patients' unfamiliarity with the technical infrastructure and operation of the equipment can lead to misperceptions of the possibilities of privacy violation during a videoconferencing session.

In the context of Web-based e-disease management, issues of access to and ownership of the data have to be addressed. In many e-home care applications, patients record monitoring data and transmit these daily to a Web server, which is owned and maintained by a private third party, that allows providers to log in and access their patients' data. Such an application calls for discussion and definition of the issue of data ownership and patients' rights to access parts or all of their records. Implications include not only possible threats to data privacy but also ethical debates about the restructuring of the care delivery process and introduction of new key players.

Accessible Design

Many patients requiring e-home care services or e-disease management interventions are elderly and in some cases have functional limitations due to aging, illness, or injury. A functional limitation is a "reduced sensory, cognitive or motor capability associated with human aging, temporary injury, or permanent disability that prevents a person from communicating, working, playing or simply functioning in an environment where other people in the population can function" (Telecommunications Industry Association, 2004).

While many argue that the Internet and advanced e-technologies have the potential to empower patients and even revolutionize the process of health care delivery, the fastest-growing segment of the U.S. population (people over the age of fifty) are at a disadvantage because software and hardware designers often fail to consider them as potential users, although usability and accessibility are important quality criteria for Web-based interventions (Bellazzi, Montani, Riva, and Stefanelli, 2001). Designing an intelligent Web-based interface that targets users who are inexperienced with the technology and who may have functional limitations can be a real challenge. Systems targeting e-home care patients should provide a high level of functional accessibility (Demiris, Finkelstein, and Speedie, 2001) and should have undergone rigorous usability tests. Several design considerations should be taken into account when developing systems for patients with functional limitations (Demiris, Finkelstein, and Speedie, 2001). For example, an interface that could be activated via a person's eye movements would be suited to assist someone who may be deaf and mute.

Reimbursement

The Health Care Financing Administration has initially denied Medicare reimbursement of e-home care, emphasizing that it has not been proven cost-effective. Some evidence demonstrates the cost-effectiveness of traditional disease management (for example, a retrospective analysis of 7,000 patients found a savings of $50 per member per month in diabetes treatment costs over twelve months and an 18 percent decrease in hospital admissions) (Georgia Institute of Technology, 2004). As yet, there is little evidence on cost-effectiveness or even possible reduction of long-term costs through the use of the Internet or other advanced ICT and e-technologies in e-disease management and e-home care applications.

The U.S. Balanced Budget Act (BBA) of 1997 allows reimbursement for telemedicine services in specific cases, especially for rural locations, which the BBA has defined to mean health professional shortage areas (HPSAs). In these cases, reimbursement is provided for Medicare patients who stay at home and receive HHC services via telemedicine. In 2000, a new means of paying for home care, the Prospective Payment System (PPS), went into effect. This system apportions payment per episode of care (using sixty-day periods) instead of per "physical" visit, allowing e-home care agencies to integrate "virtual" visits to be counted as part of the total treatment episode within the care plan.

Cost analyses and cost-effectiveness studies will contribute to discussions of reimbursement issues in regard to Web-based monitoring services and will further address the question of which party or parties should bear the costs of implementing and maintaining the requisite systems.

E-Home Care Evaluation

In evaluating the merit of e-home care applications, a number of criteria should be examined, including clinical outcomes, clinical processes, costs of care, and access to care, as well as acceptance by providers, patients, and family members.

Clinical Outcomes and Processes

The measured outcomes of e-home care should be the same or better than those of traditional care. This question has been investigated to some extent, but there is a need for large randomized clinical trials. Johnston, Wheeler, Deuser, and Sousa (2000), for example, studied the effect of e-home care on medication compliance and ability to provide self-care in a quasi-experimental study with a control group that received traditional home care and an intervention group that received access to a remote video system in addition to traditional care; they found no statistically significant difference between the two groups. Jerant, Azari, and Nesbitt (2001) conducted a one-year randomized trial to assess the effectiveness of e-home care delivered via a two-way videoconferencing device with an integrated e-stethoscope and found that this technology could reduce hospital readmissions and emergency visits for patients with congestive heart failure.

The premise of most e-home care applications is that the enabling e-technologies can yield more intensive and frequent physiological monitoring, which can lead to early detection of health problems and appropriate intervention. In addition, these technologies can be used as tools to monitor medication compliance and promote patient education. As mentioned earlier, the time has come to move from small-scale feasibility studies to large clinical trials.

It could be argued that video-mediated communication alters the relationship between nurse and patient and decreases the quality of care due to the lack of personal contact. Face-to-face interactions are considered "more spontaneous" and "free-flowing" than videoconference interactions (O'Conaill, 1997). Therefore, it might be expected that the range of issues addressed during a virtual visit and the communication between the participants in general differ from those of an actual visit. One could also argue that the use of e-home care technology might intimidate patients and result in limited participation during the virtual visit. The lack of patient participation is potentially significant because patients tend to value the opportunity to express their concerns, questions, and opinions when seeking care (Street, 1992; Ende, Kazis, Ash, and Moskowitz, 1989). Furthermore, patient participation in medical care often contributes to improved postconsultation outcomes such as greater satisfaction with care (Lerman and others, 1990), greater adherence to treatment recommendations (Rost, Carter, and Inui, 1989), a stronger sense of control (Street and Voigt, 1997), and more successful disease management overall (Kaplan and Greenfield, 1989).

Moreover, addressing technical issues, such as focusing the camera or adjusting the audio, constitutes an additional theme of communication that does not take place in an actual visit and that could dominate the virtual visit. Thus, the study of the e-home care delivery process versus traditional care delivery is important. The nature of communications in virtual home care visits has been examined to some extent. In a study conducted by Demiris, Finkelstein, and Speedie (2001), 122 virtual visits were reviewed, and a content analysis was performed. Time was apportioned among the following categories of communication: assessing the patient's clinical status, promoting compliance, addressing psychosocial issues, general informal talk, education, administrative issues, technical issues, assessing patient satisfaction, and ensuring accessibility. While some activities clearly cannot be conducted during a virtual visit, these findings indicate that e-home care has the potential to enrich the care process. Further studies and direct comparisons between actual and virtual visits will provide clearer insight into the process of virtual visits. It has yet to be determined whether telemedicine enhances or inhibits patients' communication about their discomfort, symptoms, and emotional state or whether it encourages or inhibits doctors' communication of instructions or expressions of empathy (Bashshur, 1995).

Costs of Care and Access to Care

Virtual visits should provide a cost-effective alternative to traditional home care. The economic analysis of an e-home care system is a comparison of specified sets of inputs and outputs in the provision of health care. Inputs involve the level of medical expertise, facilities, technology, service personnel, and client characteristics. The focus is on assessing the effects of known quantities of health care, such as episodes of care and hospital stays or the length and quality of the care process. If e-home care increases costs but produces only the same clinical outcomes as traditional home care, it will fail to address the challenges of home care services.

Cost savings from the use of e-home care systems can be realized if the following outcomes can be demonstrated:

- Reduction of unnecessary visits to the emergency room
- Reduction of unnecessary or unscheduled visits to the physician's office
- Early detection of health problems, allowing early intervention
- Prevention of repeat hospitalizations or overall reduction of rehospitalization rates
- Patient education that leads to improvement of lifestyle choices and medication compliance

Many argue that substituting virtual visits for actual visits, which would reduce travel time and its associated costs, could in some cases reduce the number of actual visits. Using portable devices and ICT applications, vital signs data can be collected and interpreted several times a day rather than only during scheduled weekly visits. This may result in earlier detection of health problems and earlier intervention in some cases, while signs of deterioration or problems may be missed or identified later if patients are monitored less frequently.

HHC agencies and patient advocate groups need to determine whether e-home care increases access to care for rural and urban underserved home care patients. The question of whether e-home care provides the means for more frequent monitoring of patients or whether it could be claimed as a cost-saving method and used as an excuse to deprive patients of actual home care visits also needs to be addressed. Specifically, such an investigation should aim to study how e-home care services address issues associated with the decreased use of traditional services, particularly at the entry to care, and the associated structural, financial, or personal barriers.

Acceptance by Providers, Patients, and Family Members

The success of e-home care depends largely on the acceptance of care providers, because they are often the ones who determine how the care process is to be conducted. An e-home care intervention alters the practice patterns of providers and has an impact on their work flow. Nurses, for example, who will be conducting virtual visits, have to accept this mode of care delivery and be comfortable using the required equipment and interacting with their patients by using videoconferencing technology. As with all technological innovations, stakeholders' commitment is essential to the optimum system use.

One unique aspect of e-home care is the fact that the required technology is installed and used in homes and will be operated by the patients or their surrogates. In this sense, the success of e-home care depends not only on its acceptance by the care providers but also on acceptance and technological competence on the part of patients and their family members. The way in which patients understand e-home care will influence its level of acceptability and, consequently, its rate of diffusion. Therefore, patients' perceptions should be investigated before and after they have participated in an e-home care system, and the features they perceive differently after experiencing it should be identified. The acceptance of the technology by patients and their family members will also be contingent on the satisfaction with the e-home care system.

There is a lack of consistent effort among researchers to develop valid and reliable instruments to measure patient perceptions of or satisfaction with e-home care. One such instrument is the Telemedicine Perception Questionnaire (TMPQ) (Demiris, Speedie, and Finkelstein, 2000). This instrument has been extensively tested and shows a high level of internal consistency and very high test-retest reliability. The TMPQ covers domains such as perceived effect on quality of and access to health care; time and money, including time expenditure for the patient and nurse and costs for the patient and the health care agencies; factors related to the conduct of a virtual visit, including ease of equipment use, equal acceptability of virtual and real visits, protection of privacy and confidentiality, lack of physical contact, reduced sense of intimacy, and the patient's ability to explain medical problems during a virtual visit; and general impression of the concept of e-home care and its role in the future (Demiris, Speedie, and Finkelstein, 2000).

Conclusion

The Center for Medicare and Medicaid Services estimates that total U.S. spending for health care will rise to $2.1 trillion by 2007, which represents almost 17 percent of the gross domestic product (Centers for Medicare and Medicaid Services, 2003). As the health care sector aims to curtail expenditures, emphasis is being placed on outpatient services; as a result, especially given the increase in life expectancy and in the aging population, the number of patients being cared for at home is increasing. As HHC services become more costly and the shortage of home health providers continues, e-home care technology has the potential to provide a cost-effective alternative modality, thereby increasing the likelihood of quality care for rural and urban underserved populations as well as the general population.

Modern ICT and e-networking technologies are believed to have the potential to contribute to the "ability of patients to actively understand, participate in and influence their health status" (Bruegel, 1998). Patients are viewed as consumers of health care who can participate in their own disease prevention and treatment. The success of e-medicine, e-health, e-disease management, e-clinical care, e-learning, and other e-technological applications in the area of e-home care will be determined by the extent to which the necessary technologies are integrated into the process of care delivery, meet the needs of the users, and achieve acceptance among the general public.

Several factors must be considered in determining whether the use of technology is ethical and appropriate for a particular patient. These include the following:

- Stability of the patient's disease processes
- Level of the patient's functional limitations
- Infrastructure at the patient's home (depending on the type of application, a phone line, a phone, or a television might be required)
- Patient's mental state
- Patient's attitude toward the system and willingness to provide informed consent

The American Telemedicine Association (ATA) (2004) has produced a set of clinical guidelines for the development and deployment of e-home care applications. These guidelines include patient, provider, and technological criteria. The patient criteria involve the need for informed written consent, selection of patients able to handle the equipment, and training. The health provider criteria cover the need for plans of action, training issues, and after-hours technical support. The technological criteria encompass the operation and maintenance of equipment, establishment of clear procedures and safety codes, and protection of patient privacy and record security. The ATA initiative indicates one important factor to take into consideration when implementing e-home care applications: determining the appropriateness of the innovation.

Based on the patient's primary diagnosis, stability, and ability to use the system, the health care provider should determine the type of virtual visit and the visit pattern. Patients challenged by medication compliance or at risk of adverse drug reactions, for example, might benefit from an application that provides frequent monitoring and different types of medication reminders, as well as assistance in the retrieval of relevant education materials on the patient's diagnosis and nutritional needs.

Chapter Questions

1. How will the familiarity of the younger generation with technological innovations affect the diffusion of e-home care as they grow older?
2. What are some possible ethical concerns associated with the installation and maintenance of medical sensors and assistive devices in a patient's home and the "medicalization" of their residence?

3. Consider an e-home care network in which e-health care providers from the acute care institution from which the patient was discharged, the home care agency, out-of-state family members, and social workers are linked and able to interact with the patient via videoconferencing and transmit data from one site to another. What considerations need to be addressed, given that each institution has its own computerized patient record? What implications does this application have for security and confidentiality of patient data? Suggest guidelines for protection of the patient's privacy rights and auditing methods that will ensure confidentiality of patient data.

References

American Telemedicine Association. (2004). *ATA adopts telehomecare clinical guidelines.* Adopted by the ATA Board of Directors: October 17, 2002. Retrieved March 4, 2004 from http://www.americantelemed.org/icot/hometelehealthguidelines.htm.

Arcand, M., & Williamson, J. (1981). An evaluation of home visiting of patients by physicians in geriatric medicine. *British Medical Journal, 283,* 718–720.

Baker, A. M., Lafata, J. E., Ward, R. E., Whitehouse, F., & Divine, G. (2001). A Web-based diabetes care management support system. *Joint Commission Journal on Quality and Safety, 27*(4), 179–190.

Bashshur, R. (1995). On the definition and evaluation of telemedicine. *Telemedicine Journal, 1,* 19–30.

Bellazzi, R., Montani, S., Riva, A., & Stefanelli, M. (2001). Web-based telemedicine systems for home-care: Technical issues and experiences. *Computer Methods and Programs in Biomedicine, 64*(3), 175–187.

Bruegel, R. (1998). Patient empowerment—a trend that matters. *Journal of the American Health Informatics Association, 69*(3), 30–33.

Centers for Medicare and Medicaid Services. (2003). *National health accounts.* Retrieved March 4, 2003, from http://cms.hhs.gov/statistics/nhe/

Chan, M., Bocquet, H., Campo, E., Val, T., & Pous, J. (1999). Alarm communication network to help carers of the elderly for safety purposes: A survey of a project. *International Journal of Rehabilitation Research* (London), *22,* 131–136.

Chan, M., Bocquet H., & Steenkeste, F. (1999). *Remote monitoring system for the assessment of nocturnal behavioral disorders in the demented.* Paper presented at the European Medical and Biological Engineering Conference, Vienna, Austria.

Coyle, N., Khojainova, N., Francavilla, J. M., & Gonzales, G. R. (2002). Audio-visual communication and its use in palliative care. *Journal of Pain Symptom Management, 23*(2), 171–175.

Demiris, G., Finkelstein, S. M., & Speedie, S. M. (2001). Considerations for the design of a Web-based clinical monitoring and educational system for elderly patients. *Journal of the American Medical Informatics Association, 8*(5), 468–472.

Demiris, G., Speedie, S. M., & Finkelstein, S. M. (2000). An instrument for the assessment of patients' impressions of the risks and benefits of home telecare. *Journal of Telemedicine and Telecare, 6,* 278–284.

Demiris, G., Speedie, S., & Finkelstein, S. M. (2001). The nature of communication in virtual homecare visits. In *Proceedings of the AMIA Symposium* (pp. 135–138).

Disease Management Association of America. (2002). *Definition of disease management.* Retrieved September 25, 2002, from http://www.dmaa.org/definition.html.

Economics and Statistics Administration, U.S. Department of Commerce. (1994). *How we are changing: The demographic state of the nation.* Report P23–188. Washington, DC: U.S. Census Bureau.

Elger, G., & Furugren, B. (1998). SmartBo—an ICT and computer based demonstration home for disabled people. In *Proceedings of the 3rd TIDE Congress: Technology for Inclusive Design and Equality Improving the Quality of Life for the European Citizen, Helsinki, Finland.*

Elsey, B., & McIntyre, J. (1996). Assessing a support and learning network for palliative care workers in a country area of South Australia. *Australian Journal of Rural Health, 4*(3), 159–164.

Ende, J., Kazis, L., Ash, A., & Moskowitz, M. A. (1989). Measuring patients' desire for autonomy: Decision-making and information-seeking preferences among medical patients. *Journal of General Internal Medicine, 4,* 23–30.

Fabacher, D., Josephson, K., Pietruszka, F., Linderborn, K., Morley, J., & Rubenstein, L. (1994). An in-home preventive assessment program for independent older adults: A randomized controlled trial. *Journal of the American Geriatric Society, 42,* 630–638.

Feste, C., & Anderson, R. M. (1995). Empowerment: From philosophy to practice. *Patient Education and Counseling, 26,* 139–144.

Field, M. J., & Christine, K. (Eds.). (1997). *Approaching death: Improving care at the end of life.* Washington, DC: National Academy Press.

Finkelstein, J., O'Connor, G., & Friedmann, R. (2001). Development and implementation of the home asthma telemonitoring (HAT) system to facilitate asthma self-care. *MedInfo, 10*(Part 1), 810–814.

Friedman, R., Kazis, L., & Jette, A. (1996). A telecommunications system for monitoring and counseling patients with hypertension: Impact on medication adherence and blood pressure control. *American Journal of Hypertension 9,* 285–292.

Georgia Institute of Technology. (2004). *From research to market: Smart shirt moves.* Retrieved March 5, 2004, from http://www.gatech.edu/news-room/archive/news_releases/sensatex.html

Hall, J., & Roter, D. (1988). Meta-analysis of correlates of provider behavior in medical encounters. *Medical Care, 26,* 657–675.

Jerant, A. F., Azari, R., & Nesbitt, T. S. (2001). Reducing the cost of frequent hospital admissions for congestive heart failure: A randomized trial of a home telecare intervention. *Medical Care, 39*(11), 1234–1245.

Johnston, B., Wheeler, L., Deuser, J., & Sousa, K. H. (2000). Outcomes of the Kaiser Permanente Tele-Home Health Research Project. *Archives of Family Medicine, 9*(1), 40–45.

Kane, R. A., & Kane, R. L. (1987). *Long-term care: Principles, programs and policies.* New York: Springer-Verlag.

Kaplan, S., & Greenfield, S. (1989). Assessing the effects of physician-patient interactions on the outcomes of chronic disease. *Medical Care, 27,* S110–S127.

Kidd, C., Orr, R., Abowd, G., & Atkeson, C. (1999). The aware home: A living laboratory for ubiquitous computing research. In *Proceedings of the Second International Workshop on Cooperative Buildings, CoBuild.*

Lerman, C., Brody, D. S., Caputo, G. C., Smith, D. G., Lazaro, C. G., & Wolfson, H. G. (1990). Perceived involvement in care scale: Relationship to attitudes about illness and medical care. *Journal of General Internal Medicine, 5*, 29–33.

Lynch, A., (2000). Point-of-need diagnosis of cystic fibrosis using a potentiometric ion-selective electrode array. *Analyst, 125*(12), 2264–2267.

McCord, M. (1986). Compliance: Self-care or compromise? *Topics in Clinical Nursing, 7*, 1–8.

Mehra, M. R., Uber, P. A., Chomsky, D. B., & Oren, R. (2000). Emergence of electronic home monitoring in chronic heart failure: Rationale, feasibility and early results with the HomMed Sentry Observer System. *Congestive Heart Failure, 6*, 137–139.

Morlion, B., Knoop, C., Paiva, M., & Estenne, M. (2002). Internet-based home monitoring of pulmonary function after lung transplantation. *American Journal of Respiratory Critical Care Medicine, 165*(5), 694–697.

National Association for Homecare. (2000). *Basic statistics about homecare.* Retrieved February 5, 2004, from http://www.nahc.org/Consumer/hcstats.html

National Center for Health Statistics. (1996). Advance data: Vital and health statistics of the centers for disease control and prevention.

National Institute of Nursing Research. (1994). *Long term care for older adults.* National Nursing Research Agenda. U.S. Department of Health and Human Services.

O'Conaill, B. O. (1997). Characterizing, predicting, and measuring video-mediated communication: A conversational approach. In K. E. Finn, A. J. Sellen, and others (Eds.), *Video-mediated communication* (pp. 107–131). Mahwah, NJ: Erlbaum.

Office of Health and the Information Highway. (1999). *Canadian health infoway: Paths to better health.*: Health Canada.

Oyama, H., Wakao, F., & Okamura, H. (1997). Virtual reality support system in palliative medicine. *Stud Health Technol Inform, 39*, 60–63.

Pesznecker, B., Patsdaughter, C., Moddy, K., & Albert, M. (1990). Medication regimens and the homecare client: A challenge for health care providers. *Home Health Care Services Quarterly, 11*, 9–68.

Ramsdell, S., Swart, J., Jackson, J., & Renvall, M. (1989). The yield of a home visit in the assessment of geriatric patients. *Journal of the American Geriatric Society, 37*, 17–24.

Regnard, C. (2000). Using videoconferencing in palliative care. *Palliative Medicine, 14*(6), 519–528.

Riano, D., Prado, S., Pascual, A., & Martin, S. (2002). A multi-agent system model to support palliative care units. In *Proceedings of the 15th IEEE Symposium on Computer-Based Medical Systems* (pp. 35–40).

Riva, A., Bellazzi, R., & Stefanelli, M. (1997). A Web-based system for the intelligent management of diabetic patients. *MD Comput, 14*(5), 360–364.

Rost, K., Carter, W., & Inui, T. (1989). Introduction of information during the initial medical visit: Consequences for patient follow-through with physician recommendations for medication. *Soc Sci Med, 28*, 315–321.

Rubin, R. J., Dietrich, K. A., & Hawk, A. D. (1998). Clinical and economic impact of implementing a comprehensive diabetes management program in managed care. *J Clin Endocrinol Metab, 83*(8), 2635–2642.

Social Security Administration. (2000). *The future of Social Security.* Publication No. 05–10055. Baltimore, MD: Author.

Sparks, K., Shaw, D., Eddy, D., Hanigosky, P., & Vantrese, J. (1993). Alternatives for cardiac rehabilitation patients unable to return to a hospital based program. *Heart and Lung, 22,* 298–303.

Street, R. L., Jr. (1992). Communicative styles and adaptations in physician-parent consultations. *Soc Sci Med, 34,* 1155–1163.

Street, R., Jr., & Voigt, B. (1997). Patient participation in deciding breast cancer treatment and subsequent quality of life. *Medical Decision Making, 17,* 298–306.

Tamada, J. A., Lesho, M., & Tierney, M. J. (2002, April). Keeping watch on glucose: New monitors help fight the long-term complications of diabetes. *IEEE Spectrum,* pp. 52–57.

Tan, J., with Sheps, S. (1998). *Health decision support systems.* Sudbury, MA: Jones & Bartlett.

Telecommunications Industry Association. (2004). *Resource guide for accessible design of consumer electronics: Linking product design to the needs of people with functional limitations—A joint venture of the electronic industries alliance and the electronic industries foundations.* Retrieved March 5, 2004, from http://www.tiaonline.org/access/guide.html

Turnin, M., Bolzonella-Pene, C., & Dumoulin, S. (1995). Multicenter evaluation of the Nutri-Expert Telematic System in diabetic patients. *Diabetes and Metabolism, 21,* 26–33.

University of Wollongong. (2001). *Intelligent knee to save costly sporting injuries.* Retrieved on March, 5, 2004, from University of Wollongong (Wollongong, Australia) Web site at http://www.uow.edu.au/science/research/ipri/kneesleeve.html

U.S. Department of Health and Human Services. (1999, November 3). Standards for privacy of individually identifiable health information: Proposed rule. *Federal Register, 64*(212), 59917–60016.

Wahr, J., & Tremper, K. (1995). Non-invasive oxygen monitoring techniques. *Critical Care Clinics, 11*(1), 199–217.

Wu, J., Kessler, D., Chakko, S., & Kessler, K. (1995). A cost-effectiveness strategy for transtelephonic arrhythmia monitoring. *American Journal of Cardiology, 75,* 184–185.

The OliverHome Case

Joseph Tan, George Demiris, Joshia Tan

Steven, a seventy-two-year-old home care patient, was discharged from the hospital only a few months ago. Since his home care agency suggested that Steven be enrolled in an experimental project to adapt his home into a smart house named "OliverHome," he has dramatically transformed his daily routines. The main concept of OliverHome is to provide Steven, who is heavily disabled and also becoming hard of hearing, with access to special functions installed as additions to the existing basic infrastructure of his house. Indeed, Steven had already spent much of his hard-earned savings to convert his house to facilitate his movement around the bedrooms and kitchen. Such costly but necessary renovations included special handles and locks for easy accessibility to closets and toilets, resizing of the bathtub and shower stand so that all of the switches and vital controls can be reached effortlessly, and installing easy-to-use remote-controlled doors, lighting, and other accessories. Now the OliverHome Project promises to help Steven take the next step in independent living.

The OliverHome Project

The OliverHome Project evaluates e-home care equipment and provides a model for consultancy in the area of smart housing. Steven's home (OliverHome) is now equipped with an electronic central bus system for control of particular functions. Because Steven must use a wheelchair, some of the controls of these functions have been integrated and placed conveniently on Steven's wheelchair. In essence, there is a separate bus for mobile environment control. Because Steven is a successful fiction writer who writes about future worlds, abduction of human earthlings, and visits from extraterrestrials, it is hoped that further development of OliverHome will apply laboratory-tested e-work technologies to support Steven in working at home; for example, integrating his television and his computer would allow Steven to complete his novels and transfer his final drafts directly to his publishers for further editing, production, and printing. The monitor for the computer would not have to be a television; instead, it could be a common display that would integrate work and entertainment interfaces. Other types of display units can address visual limitations of impaired individuals that common computer monitors or television sets cannot.

The OliverHome Project supports individuals such as Steven who are disabled or chronically ill who want to continue to e-work meaningfully in their own homes. The idea is to equip the house with a number of stand-alone e-home care applications, such as an e-paging system and optical signaling (good for Steven and others who are hard of hearing). It is important to note that a person like Steven, who suffers from cognitive impairments, may be physically capable of bathing, showering, doing housework, and even preparing meals, but impaired memory will limit his ability to perform these activities. Other home management functions enabled by the OliverHome Project include a security system and a temperature maintenance system that also includes humidity controls, which not only improve comfort levels but also protect Steven's grand piano. Ongoing plans for OliverHome include continued development of ways to integrate home management functions with external services such the police, the fire station and ambulance services.

Nowadays, as soon as he wakes up, Steven transfers into the wheelchair at his desk and near the television. He measures his blood pressure, his lung capacity, and his weight using networked devices. He controls these devices from an OliverHome centralized remote control system that he can take with him around the house; many of the more critical functions are also available from the operating system installed directly on Steven's wheelchair so he can complete these without having to access the centralized remote in order to do them. More important, Steven knows that Oliver-Home will automatically transmit all these measurements to his agency for monitoring and analysis, and thus his medical record is always updated. Steven uses a medication-dispensing machine attached to the OliverHome network system to take his morning pills. He knows that he will be notified if he forgets to do so. Then he fills out an on-line questionnaire, reporting symptoms, problems, and nutrition. Twice a week, he has a virtual visit with his home care nurse; during these visits, he can see her on his television screen while talking to her on the phone. Although Steven e-mails questions and general observations that he wants to share with his nurse on a regular basis, much more information is shared during these visits.

Development of Steven's OliverHome

Steven's home was completely rewired to convert it into OliverHome so that he can live in his own home despite his diagnosis, his daily needs, and his changing health status. When he first became homebound, Steven was concerned about his location in a rural area, miles away from the town. Since he has no family members and he was in a frail state, he was concerned about isolation. Thanks to smart home technology and the OliverHome Project, his home care agency does not seem so distant anymore, which helps Steven manage his concerns about isolation.

With the help of a central data highway (network) acting as the control bus, the old house that Steven lives in is now wired to allow intelligent remote transmission of health monitoring data. Within the area of Steven's control, each device or system to be controlled in OliverHome, such as Steven's television, his computer, and other health-monitoring gadgets, is interfaced or networked to the central bus. Although the controls are not difficult to use, Steven did get on-line training from his home care agency. The agency will be automatically notified of any malfunction of the control systems and will then check out what is going on in OliverHome. Because of the system's complex interface, Steven also needs access to the controls in other environments, such as when he is moving around, in public places, or during an emergency by accessing his PDA linked to his wheelchair, his pager and other sensors installed in his vehicle.

Theoretically, Steven can manage three different levels of OliverHome control systems: his direct mobile environment; the fixed environment (that is, OliverHome); and the distant environment. When Steven is in his wheelchair away from the OliverHome centralized control system, a local bus permits him to interact with local, directly coupled input devices such as the keyboard on his laptop, the joystick attached to the game system linked to his wheelchair, and various switches and output devices such as a telephone handset, personal communication systems such as a pager, a PDA, and other mobility controllers. When Steven is at home, OliverHome's centralized bus systems permit varying levels of control of the home environment. The features that would allow interaction with the distant environment are still in development, because this set of controls involves local authorities, mobile and telecommunication equipment providers, and large corporations such as banks.

OliverHome Applications

The OliverHome Project aims to cover three major areas of e-home care applications. The first is *safety*—for example, reducing the risk of Steven falling when he tries to get out of bed at night. *Cueing* is the second application, which provides Steven with assistance for daily living tasks such as moving around the house, personal hygiene, basic housekeeping, meal preparation, and remembering to eat his meals. Finally, *supervision,* which enables remote monitoring by e-caregivers and e-health care professionals, is the application that is most significant to e-home care. The remote monitoring activities of Steven and his agency have already been discussed, so we will now focus on how OliverHome handles safety and cueing.

When Steven gets out of his bed during the night, lights in his bedroom and the adjoining hall come on at a low level of illumination, increasing to a full level after a few minutes. Steven's bathroom light is automatically switched on when his footsteps or the movements of his wheelchair trigger the sensors.

After Steven leaves the bathroom, the bathroom light automatically switches off. After he gets back into bed, his bedroom light gradually dims from a full to a half level after one minute or so and then switches off automatically. If Steven does not leave his bathroom after 20 minutes or so, OliverHome alerts the HHC agency, which then beeps the bracelet sensor that he always wears on his left wrist. If Steven does not respond by pressing a sequence of buttons on this wired bracelet, an alarm is activated and a home care nurse is dispatched to OliverHome. If Steven responds correctly, the HHC will expect a report from Steven via e-mail in the next twenty-four hours, explaining why his bathroom trip took so long. Steven can choose to delay the alerting system while in the bathroom by temporarily bypassing the "set alert system" timing. The system, however, will default to the original timing two hours after each temporary bypass is initiated. Of course, all data sent back to the agency are kept for further analysis.

If Steven forgets to do his stretching as scheduled, he may be prompted with a familiar voice, or music may play in the family room. Following the music, a tape used for his regular stretching routine will be played, and illumination will be automatically increased to get Steven started with his routine. The exercise equipment machines, once selected, will automatically move to Steven's timing. Sensors in the machine record how long it took Steven to complete his movements. This information is eventually transmitted to his HHC agency. Because OliverHome's control system learns from Steven's previous actions and commands and behaves intelligently according to past patterns of Steven's actions and stored commands, if Steven were out of the house, this action sequence would not be initiated. At the end of the routine, Steven may move on to the computer in his office to get on with his work. The illumination in the family room will be dimmed, and the tape will stop playing.

Conclusion

E-home care systems have the potential to revolutionize the field of home health care. In fact, e-home care providers can provide better-quality care through frequent monitoring, increase patients' access to care services, increase visit frequency, and ensure quick response to early detection of any health problems. The success of any e-home care system depends to a large extent on providers' ability to communicate with patients and to effectively monitor them in spite of geographic distance. E-home care applications can empower patients and provide them with increased knowledge, autonomy, control, involvement in their care, and satisfaction with delivered care services. The challenge for researchers, designers, and users of such systems will be to acknowledge the system's limitations and to address the need for extensive formative and summative evaluation of its operation.

Case Questions

1. What benefits does this e-home care program provide to Steven, as opposed to staying in a long-term care facility?
2. Why is OliverHome considered a smart home?
3. Do you see any ways to improve the services provided by OliverHome?
4. Imagine that Steven's home health care agency wants you to assist in evaluating OliverHome. How would you go about this, and what questions would you ask Steven? Discuss the impact of OliverHome on traditional long-term care facilities.

CHAPTER TEN

E-DIAGNOSIS SUPPORT SYSTEMS

An E-DSS for Lower Back Pain

Lin Lin, Paul Jen-Hwa Hu, Olivia R. Liu Sheng, Joseph Tan

Learning Objectives

1. Learn the SOAP process for lower back pain diagnosis
2. Recognize the challenges in designing an e-DSS for lower back pain
3. Understand the systems architecture, knowledge representation, and knowledge inference mechanisms for e-DSS design for lower back pain
4. Identify the components and functions of an e-DSS evaluation framework in an e-health system and environment
5. Identify some future directions of e-DSS research

Introduction

Over the years, the use of decision support systems (DSS) in clinical health care has received varying levels of attention from information systems researchers and practitioners (Berner and Ball, 1998; Buchanan and Shortliffe, 1975; Heckerman, Horvitz, and Nathwani, 1992; Leaper, Horrocks, Staniland, and deDombal, 1972; Vaughn and others, 1998, 1999; Waddell, 1987). Of particular interest is diagnosis decision making, a fundamental aspect of clinical health services. From a clinical information management perspective, *diagnosis* refers to a classification process in which a service provider assigns a clinical case to one or more prespecified illness or disease categories (using, for example, ICD-10 or mix-group classification), based on the patient's symptoms and information collected for the case (Suojanen, Andreassen, and Olesen, 2001). Obviously, an incorrect or inadequate diagnosis can adversely affect subsequent patient treatment or management plans. In many cases, a clinical diagnosis decision requires complex and highly specialized knowledge that may not be readily available or accessible. In this context, the value of an electronic diagnosis support system (e-DSS) that is designed to encompass pertinent diagnostic knowledge and to make that knowledge available to care providers and patients is significant.

This chapter discusses the development, implementation, and evaluation of an e-DSS for clinicians to help them address or resolve problems with lower back pain (LBP). LBP prevents many adults from being able to work or live a normal lifestyle (Waddell, 1987). Diagnosis of LBP problems requires understanding a complex anatomical and physiological structure, factoring in several diverse considerations, and juggling with nonstandardized terminology (Danek, n.d.). Jackson, Llewelyn-Phillips, and Klaber-Moffett (1996) report that only about 15 percent of LBP patients receive accurate diagnoses with some degree of certainty. Because clinicians' acquisition of complex diagnostic knowledge is mostly experiential and entails an intensive and time-consuming process, the use of an e-DSS to support a clinician's diagnosis is both beneficial and justifiable. The primary focus of this discussion is e-DSS design challenges, architecture, implementation, and evaluation. Aside from highlighting the challenging characteristics of LBP diagnosis, we describe how multiple methods are employed to acquire the targeted knowledge from two highly experienced experts who practice in different clinics and geographic regions. Following this, evaluation of the e-DSS— including its verification, validation, clinical evaluation designs, and important results— is documented. Finally, the chapter raises a series of questions that still need to be asked or answered in establishing future directions for this domain.

The e-DSS presented here is Web-based. Architecturally, the system consists of a knowledge base, an inference engine, a case repository, and two interfaces for convenient system access and knowledge update. The case repository uses a star schema–based data warehouse designed to support clinicians' ability to reference and analyze previous clinical cases. To ensure the system's validity and utility, evaluations of the e-DSS include knowledge base verification, system validation, and clinical efficacy assessment.

Overview of Lower Back Pain

Anatomically, the term *lower back* refers to a complex structure of vertebrae, disks, spinal cord, and nerves. LBP is a physiological and medical condition often accompanied by or resulting from common colds and other illnesses. According to Waddell (1987), four out of five adults will experience significant LBP in their lifetime. Diagnosis of LBP problems is challenging. The underlying pathology of a persistent and oppressive LBP problem is not always easily identified (Nachemson, 1985). Often, clinicians have to evaluate physical, social, behavioral, and environmental issues. In addition, LBP patients often exhibit other symptoms commonly noted in individuals who are free of LBP (Bounds, Lloyd, Mathew, and Waddell, 1988).

LBP patients are treated by different groups of clinicians, including physical therapists, orthopedists, general practitioners, chiropractors, and pain specialists (for example, physiatrists). These care providers differ subtly, if not noticeably in their training and in their approaches to pain epidemiology, diagnosis decision making, therapeutic protocol and selection, and overall patient management plans. Of these specialists, physical therapists probably are the most sought-after care providers for LBP problems; therefore, the e-DSS was developed with physical therapy as the main treatment modality.

The SOAP Process

SOAP (subjective testing, objective testing, assessment, planning) is a common service process used by physical therapists to manage LBP patients; it consists of four phases (see Figure 10.1).

FIGURE 10.1. SOAP: A COMMON SERVICE PROCESS FOR MANAGING PATIENTS WITH LOWER BACK PAIN

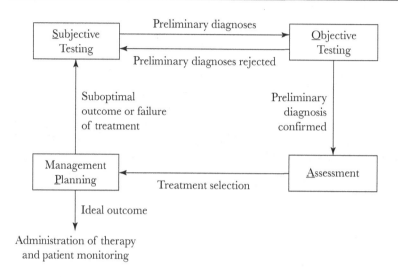

Phase 1, **S**ubjective testing, entails qualitative tests to obtain relevant patient history and clinical information. This phase includes a question-and-answer session using mostly programmed question items to identify the nature of the pain and its probable causes. Based on the patient's responses, the therapist collects information such as pain description, location, activation, severity and frequency, together with important patient or case symptoms. The therapist also acquires information on the patient's assessment of and concerns about the pain in relation to his or her clinical history. By documenting and analyzing such information, the therapist then generates one or multiple preliminary diagnoses.(For convenience, we will use the plural term *diagnoses* throughout this chapter, with the understanding that some LBP patients may have a simple single diagnosis.)

Phase 2, **O**bjective testing, involves physical examinations to confirm or refine the preliminary diagnoses. This testing usually proceeds in an iterative fashion and thus may require additional subjective question-and-answer sessions, especially when the objective results do not support the preliminary diagnoses. Phases 1 and 2 are knowledge-intensive, and their effectiveness demands considerable experience on the part of the therapist.

In Phase 3, **A**ssessment, the therapist confirms his or her diagnoses and proceeds with an evaluation of pain epidemiology and severity and plausible therapeutic protocols.

Phase 4, the final phase, is **P**lanning for patient management, in which the therapist designs, selects, and administers therapeutic treatments. The attending therapist continually monitors and evaluates the patient's response and revises the diagnosis and treatment plan accordingly. This process terminates when the therapist observes satisfactory patient response and recovery.

Essential in the SOAP process are the care provider's preliminary diagnoses, which are generated during subjective testing and which have significant effects on subsequent patient assessment, therapeutic protocol selection, and overall treatment plan. Obviously, inadequate preliminary diagnoses are likely to result in unnecessary testing and an ineffective treatment plan, thus diminishing service quality and adversely affecting the patient's well-being.

Designing an E-Diagnosis Support System for Lower Back Pain: Key Challenging Characteristics

From a clinical decision-making perspective, diagnosis of LBP has a number of challenging characteristics that have a significant impact on designing an effective e-DSS product:

- Effective LBP diagnosis requires both highly specialized knowledge and wide-ranging considerations on the part of the therapist.
- A therapist may develop multiple preliminary diagnoses partially because of incomplete patient or case information.
- Experienced therapists often find it difficult to articulate their underlying diagnostic knowledge for the benefit of newer therapists.
- Accessible diagnostic knowledge tends to be limited to sources in close geographic proximity or personal networks; timely sharing or reuse of large-scale knowledge is rare.
- Coupled with the stringent time constraints common to clinicians, all of the impediments on this list are likely to result in a reduced or suboptimal level of service.

The clinical significance of LBP and limited support for diagnostic knowledge sharing and reuse beyond geographical constraints make a knowledge-based e-DSS approach desirable and justifiable, though not easy. Yet an adequately designed and implemented e-DSS for LBP could facilitate and enhance clinicians' acquiring, sharing, and using the specialized knowledge that is indispensable in the effective care and management of LBP patients.

In this context, an e-DSS that incorporates pertinent LBP diagnostic knowledge and demonstrates sufficient validity and efficacy through rigorous evaluation would be of great value. Supported by an adequately designed e-DSS, clinicians would become increasingly effective and efficient in collecting and interpreting patient and case information and making appropriate diagnosis decisions, ultimately leading to improved service quality and patient outcomes. Three major challenges of e-DSS design are diagnosis involving uncertainty, clinical decision making involving multiple diagnoses, and completeness of an e-DSS.

Diagnosis Involving Uncertainty

Uncertainty, which is common to many clinical diagnostic tasks, represents a fundamental challenge to e-DSS design. Several methods have been proposed to represent or reason about uncertainty. For example, researchers have used a certainty factor scheme to represent or model the confidence level of a system-recommended solution or diagnosis (Buchanan and Shortliffe, 1975). The exact certainty value associated with a particular rule is usually determined by the presence of specific evidence suggested by experts or the extant literature. The overall *degree of belief* for a particular diagnosis is then calculated, using a probabilistic summation that combines all relevant evidence (Buchanan and Shortliffe, 1975). *Bayesian theory,* based on Bayes' Theorem and probabilistic chain rules, has also been applied to represent and reason about uncertainty. Typically, the underlying causal relationships among the evidence and diagnostic variables are modeled using a directed acyclic graph in which each node incorporates the respective prior and posterior probabilistic distributions (Przytula and Thompson, 2000). A set theory concept known as *belief function* has also been employed (Dempster, 1967; Shafer, 1976). A belief function models the interaction of independent criteria. Despite the differences in their representation or modeling specifics, all of these methods would typically require substantial numerical probability estimates by LBP experts.

Numerical probability estimates from LBP experts can be difficult to obtain and prone to bias, especially when there is a lack of adequate anchors or calibration (Kahneman, Slovic, and Tversky, 1982). The likelihood of unsystematic or inconsistent assessments tends to increase with the sheer volume and complexity of knowledge. Previous work has examined different methods for eliciting such probability estimates, ranging from probability scales for predicting assessments to risk-laden gambling (van DerGaag and others, 2002). However, none of these methods can be directly applied to LBP diagnosis, for the following reasons: First, therapists are not experienced in numerical probability assessment, making the use of a probability scale to articulate, visualize, and interpret conditional probabilities difficult and unlikely to be effective. Second, from a human reasoning perspective, the probabilistic combination of individual rules in LBP diagnosis differs from that common in diagnostic tasks examined by previous e-DSS projects. For instance, with LBP, the presence or absence of a particular piece of evidence can completely rule out one or more diagnoses, whereas in other situations, this is more likely to merely affect respective degrees of belief. To address this "exclusive negation or elimination" characteristic the proposed LBP project uses a certainty factor scheme that is based on an intuitive and easy-to-use uncertainty representation and reasoning framework, which could reduce the cost of soliciting probability assessments from LBP experts. Hence, the suggested approach is based on accumulated experiential knowledge or predetermined verbal probability estimation (van DerGaag and others, 2002) that is intuitive and capable of facilitating domain experts' estimates significantly, compared with methods based on Bayesian theory or belief function. The performance of the resulting system is still robust and does not require (and is not highly sensitive to) precise estimates for each individual rule. Hence, the suggested approach is computationally unique and differs from previous use of a certainty factor or its modifications (Cabrero-Canosa and others, 2003).

Clinical Decision Making Involving Multiple Diagnoses

The support of simultaneous *multiple decision outcomes* has been identified as a challenge to DSS development (Suojanen, Andreassen, and Olesen, 2001). Earlier work—for example, Pathfinder (Heckerman, Horvitz, and Nathwani, 1992)—bypassed this challenge by assuming that a patient at any given point in time can suffer from only one disease from a prespecified, mutually exclusive set. Accordingly, each disease can be modeled as a single state of a discrete stochastic variable. Other case studies—such as MUNIN (Suojanen, Andreassen, and Olesen, 2001)—modeled each disease as a stochastic variable and therefore were able to accommodate simultaneous multiple diagnoses.

Owing to the rule-based approach employed in the LBP project, using a single stochastic variable to represent diagnosis is inadequate as in all of the approaches described so far. We addressed the multiple-diagnosis requirement by examining the confidence level of each individual diagnosis independently—that is, allowing these to compete on the basis of certainty. Theoretically, rule-based systems using a certainty factor scheme support such competitions among individual rules. However, a review of previous research cases in the literature suggested no explicit efforts toward addressing the reasoning of multiple decision outcomes. In fact, evaluation of previous cases focused predominantly on accuracy-based metrics (metrics that focus on "accuracy" as the main scoring criteria), which are insufficient for assessing the performance of a system designed to support multiple diagnoses simultaneously. This, clearly, is another limitation of previous cases.

Completeness of a Clinical Decision Support System

Judged by scope and clinical readiness, most systems reported in previous research cases are of limited *completeness*, particularly with regard to system evaluation (Shortliffe and Davis, 1975; Smith, Nugent, and McClean, 2003). A review of these cases revealed a focus on modeling, algorithm development, or computational performance enhancement. While interesting, the resulting systems were a long way from clinical deployment and use. In addition, previous system evaluations were mostly ad hoc and focused predominantly on output performance assessment, that is, evaluation of primarily the accuracy of the predicted diagnoses, and thus incomplete with respect to fundamental dimensions of system evaluation. Engelrecht, Rector, and Moser (1995) suggest that evaluation of a DSS include verification, validation, and impact assessments at individual and organizational levels. Shortliffe and Davis (1975) advocate evaluating a system's clinical efficacy using real-world cases and settings. Chau and Hu (2002) reported that health care professionals tend to exhibit a tool-oriented view of technologies and are likely to accept a system only when it offers considerable utility in patient care and management. Thus, evaluation of an e-DSS must include assessment on fundamental dimensions, using clinical cases; in this particular case, evaluation should include knowledge base verification, system validation, and clinical efficacy.

A Web-Based e-Diagnosis Support System for Lower Back Pain

An intelligent, Web-based e-DSS was designed, implemented, and evaluated to support clinicians' diagnosis of LBP problems. Key objectives of this design included verifiable knowledge, validated system utility and clinical efficacy, and user-friendly interfaces for knowledge access and update. The Web is a prevailing platform that allows round-the-clock access to the e-DSS, without geographic constraints (Bharati and Chaudhury, in press); in addition to assisting clinicians' diagnoses, this system will also support self-service by patients to access information from the database.

Compared with most previous developmental projects, our e-DSS is more complete and clinic-ready, due to careful attention given to key issues in problem analysis, uncertainty modeling and reasoning, system design, implementation, and evaluation. Drawing on Engelrecht, Rector, and Moser's (1995) and Shortliffe and Davis's (1975) analysis, the e-DSS evaluation presented here includes knowledge base verification, system validation (using a modified Turing test), and a clinical efficacy assessment using 180 cases collected from real-world clinical settings.

E-DSS System Architecture

As shown in Figure 10.2, the e-DSS system architecture consists of a knowledge base, an inference engine, two Web-based interfaces for knowledge access and update, and a case repository.

The *knowledge base* consists of a total of 140 rules and uses a modified certainty factor scheme specifically designed to relieve burdensome probability estimation requirements previously placed on domain experts. The rules were extracted from two

FIGURE 10.2. ARCHITECTURE OF A WEB-BASED DIAGNOSIS SUPPORT SYSTEM

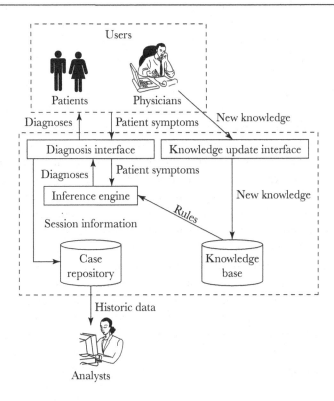

highly experienced therapists and stored in a relational database that was developed using MySQL. Simultaneous multiple diagnoses are supported by an *inference engine* enabled by an algorithm built on a consensus model for combining individual rules, which will be explained in more detail later in the chapter. The inference algorithm also captures the exclusive negation or elimination property of LBP diagnosis. The inference engine was implemented using ANSI standard Java 2. Based on the factual data and clinical evidence provided by a clinician or patient and the subsequent activation of the relevant rules in the knowledge base, the e-DSS generates one or multiple diagnoses of varying certainty values. The diagnoses of the highest certainty value or the ones with certainty values exceeding a prespecified threshold are then recommended to the user.

The e-DSS includes two user interfaces. The graphic design of the *diagnosis* interface allows a clinician or patient to describe and visualize relevant symptoms using nonmedical terminology. Guided by the sequenced question items, the user provides information on symptoms or pain assessments. Upon completion, the user submits his or her responses to the inference engine, which, in turn, generates preliminary diagnoses. A clinician can override the system recommendation by submitting his or her own diagnoses. In addition, a clinician can activate the explanatory panel to review the system's decision-making process. The entire diagnostic session, including the final diagnoses reached, is stored in the case repository for future training or data mining purposes.

The e-DSS also has a second interface, *the knowledge update interface*, which allows clinicians to update the knowledge base. Using a graphics tool, a clinician can add, remove, or modify an existing rule, in terms of its left-hand or right-hand side or both. Allowing clinicians to update the knowledge base is important because the diagnostic knowledge or heuristics may evolve dynamically over time. This e-DSS therefore allows individual clinicians to update the knowledge base without needing to become familiar with the knowledge representation schema of the system in any detail. Both interfaces were implemented using JavaServer Pages and Java servlets technology.

The *case repository* was implemented as a data warehouse. A star schema was employed, with the fact table providing the session information and dimensions representing key factors that included patient demographics and symptoms. By slicing and dicing the data, clinicians can gain insights into existing diagnostic knowledge or discover new information—for example, significant indicators suggesting a particular diagnosis, diagnostic patterns specific to a clinician or a group of clinicians, or relationships between particular demographic variables and diseases. Implemented in Oracle, this repository also serves as a data cleansing and preparation mechanism for data mining.

Knowledge Acquisition and Representation

Domain knowledge was solicited from two highly experienced therapists. One is a European therapist and the other practices in the United States. Each one has more than fifteen years of clinical experiences in diagnosing and treating LBP problems. Using multiple methods that included unstructured and structured interviews, field observations, and scenario-based case reasoning and analysis, three knowledge engineers worked closely with both experts for six months. Fourteen common diagnoses, or decision outcomes, were identified, as shown in Table 10.1.

Also identified were fifteen questions that are critical to therapists' diagnosis of LBP problems. Table 10.2 summarizes these question items, which can be broadly characterized as involving patient demographics, current symptoms, clinical history, and follow-up items specific to gender or pain description. Jointly, the experts singled out 152 legitimate responses to these question items. On average, a question has approximately ten conceivable responses.

TABLE 10.1 DECISION OUTCOMES INCLUDED IN
DIAGNOSIS SUPPORT SYSTEM

Diagnosis Category	Description
1	Acute disk-related pain
2	Acute disk-related pain with radiculopathy or myelopathy
3	Chronic disk-related pain (degenerative disk disease or instability)
4	Chronic disk-related pain with radiculopathy or myelopathy
5	Stenosis, osteoporosis, or compression fracture
6	Acute facet joint–related pain
7	Chronic facet joint–related pain (degenerative joint disease)
8	Neuropathy of a peripheral nerve, such as the sciatic or cluneal
9	Sacroiliac joint-related pain and other pelvic ring–related conditions
10	Hip joint–related pain
11	Miscellaneous musculoskeletal pathologies, including muscle, tendon, or ligament strains or sprains, bursitis, compartment syndromes, fractures, and kissing spine
12	Nonmusculoskeletal internal pathologies, including neoplasms
13	Gynecological
14	Inappropriate illness behavior

Analysis of therapists' diagnosis of LBP problems suggested several challenging characteristics. First, therapists usually make diagnostic decisions by combining evidence or information acquired in the question-and-answer session in some additive fashion. Hence, a diagnosis supported by more evidence (for example, positive responses to multiple questions) is seen as more likely than one supported by less evidence. This suggests independent contributions of the respective pieces of evidence toward recommending a particular diagnosis, without considerable interactions among them. Hence, an additive method for combining relevant evidence can represent and address the uncertainty associated with individual rules.

Moreover, therapists often find it difficult to estimate uncertainty in diagnosis. Unlike the case of MYCIN, in which those assisting in its development were able to estimate certainty with impressive precision (a certainty factor of 0.525) (Buchanan and Shortliffe, 1985), the domain experts for LBP found it difficult to assess or estimate the numerical probability of individual rules, in spite of the different methods that the knowledge engineers had attempted to apply. Previous human probability judgment

TABLE 10.2. QUESTION ITEMS INCLUDED
IN DIAGNOSIS SUPPORT SYSTEM

Category	Item	Description
Demographic	Gender	Patient's gender
	Age	Patient's age
Current symptoms	Pain location	Body parts that have the pain
	Pain pattern	How the pain changes throughout a day
	Pain feeling	How the pain feels
	Pain duration	How long the patient has had the pain
	Alleviating position	Positions that make the pain feel better
	Worsening position	Positions that make the pain feel worse
Clinical history	Pain start	How the pain started: suddenly or gradually
	Cause of pain	Whether a trauma caused the pain, and type of trauma
	Pain history	Number of pain episodes the patient has had before
	Fracture history	Types of fractures the patient had before
	Surgery history	Types of surgery the patient had before
Follow-up questions	Female-related pain (if gender is female)	Pain patterns that might appear with pregnancy
	Numbness or tingling (if pain feeling is numbness or tingling)	Regions where the patient has numbness or tingling

research suggests that individuals might feel more comfortable rendering verbal probability expressions (for example, "maybe" or "possibly") than numerical probability estimates (van DerGaag and others, 2002). To physical therapists, certainty values may be more natural, meaningful, and comprehensible when expressed by using a verbal probability scale than when expressed numerically. Based on results of the knowledge elicitation process, certainty was thus defined at three verbal levels: "impossible," "neutral," and "likely." Here is a sample rule:

If observation shows patient age is between 30 and 40

Then recommend diagnosis "Chronic Disc Degenerative" with certainty level of "likely"

As well, a therapist often excludes a particular diagnosis on observing evidence that suggests its impossibility, regardless of other evidence supporting that diagnosis. In regard to decision modeling, this characteristic is unique and has not been examined previously. An intuitive schema for addressing this uncertainty characteristic was therefore advanced, based on the verbal probability estimation method just described. Structurally, knowledge in the format of an "if-then" production rule was implemented—that is, "*if* response, *then* diagnosis," with a certainty level based on the underlying verbal probability estimation.

Knowledge Inference

The *knowledge inference* in the e-DSS was based on a voting scheme in which a rule with a probability of "likely" generates one vote toward the diagnosis or diagnoses it recommends. A rule with a probability of "neutral" has no effect on the voting, whereas a rule with an "impossible" verbal probability invalidates all votes that its recommended diagnoses receives from other rules. In other words, an exclusive negation or elimination effect completely removes diagnoses from consideration. According to this scheme, the votes received by each diagnosis are summed; those receiving the most votes or exceeding a prespecified threshold are then recommended to the user.

Theoretically, this scheme is based on consensus-based modeling and differs from the probabilistic summation approach used in previous research cases (Buchanan and Shortliffe, 1985). The central principle of a consensus-based model is the theoretical adequacy of a consensus position established by the voting of multiple experts or participants. We represent the LBP diagnosis using a consensus model primarily because each response independently affects the likelihood of a diagnosis instead of being simply an additive factor, as in the probabilistic summation approach. For details about the consensus model and a formal mathematical proof of our inference algorithm, please refer to Appendix A.

As an illustration, consider a patient with three symptoms, A, B, and C. Let's assume that there are three possible diagnoses, x, y, and z. (The actual number of possible diagnoses is often much larger.) We have the following set of rules:

If A, then x	likely	If B, then x	neutral	If C, then x	likely
If A, then y	likely	If B, then y	likely	If C, then y	impossible
If A, then z	impossible	If B, then z	neutral	If C, then z	likely

When combining all evidences, diagnosis x receives two votes. Although diagnosis y also receives two votes, symptom C makes it an impossible choice. Similarly, symptom A makes diagnosis z an unlikely outcome. Therefore, in this case, diagnosis x wins out.

Two important prerequisites have to be met for the above algorithm to work. First, each of the rules must have high level of credibility (the rule should have higher than a 50 percent chance of being true). Second, the prior probabilities of the diagnoses should be similar, if not the same as this is an important assumption for the algorithm to work accurately in the computation software. This indicates that all diagnoses should have similar incidence rates in the general population. Although this is unlikely in the real world, the algorithm can easily be modified to adapt to more complicated scenarios in which each diagnosis has a different incidence rate and the rates are known. This further permits complex simulation of the system to be performed, allowing us to study the behavior of complex system variations and generate theoretical principles for related scenarios.

A FRAMEWORK FOR EVALUATION OF AN E-DIAGNOSIS SUPPORT SYSTEM

As previously noted, the e-DSS evaluations were designed to include knowledge base verification, system validation, and clinical efficacy and to use real-world test cases. Five therapists, all clinically active and with at least ten years of experience in LBP diagnosis and treatment, participated. Three of them practice in a nationwide pain clinic in the United States; the other two practice in Europe. The inclusion of therapists who practice in different regions extends the generality of the evaluation results.

Table 10.3 summarizes the evaluation framework, showing the method of evaluation and metrics for each area of evaluation. The design and key analysis results of each evaluation are discussed in the sections that follow.

TABLE 10.3. EVALUATION FRAMEWORK FOR AN E-DIAGNOSIS SUPPORT SYSTEM

Evaluation Focus	Evaluation Methods	Evaluation Metrics
Knowledge base verification	• Preliminary completeness verification • Face value verification • Completeness verification • Check for developer-induced errors	• Usefulness • Completeness
System validation	Modified Turing test	System performance benchmarked by experts' performance
Clinical efficacy	Test using 180 real-world clinical cases	• Recall rate • Precision rate • Accuracy

Knowledge Base Verification

Verification refers to ensuring a system's compliance with its defined requirements and specifications (Kak et al., 1990). For knowledge base verification, the focus was on validating each stored rule, including its left- and right-hand sides and their pairing or mapping using the relevant medical foundation. The criteria included consistency and completeness. More simply, the aim was to detect and correct any syntactic or semantic errors that would adversely affect the knowledge base's consistency or completeness.

Using a questionnaire, each therapist verified the usefulness and completeness of the rules by examining each rule's left-hand side (that is, patient responses) and right-hand side (that is, diagnoses). Based on the collective assessment results, the knowledge base was verified as satisfactorily complete, containing the decision variables and diagnoses essential to the physical therapists' clinical services. The evaluators made few suggestions to include an additional diagnosis, remove an existing diagnosis, or allow additional responses to a decision variable. As a group, the therapists discussed the few suggestions face to face and recommended against any changes.

The therapists were then asked individually to verify each rule at face value, with particular emphasis on the mapping or pairing of its left- and right-hand sides. When examining a rule, a therapist reported his or her assessment of its left- and right-hand side pairing scores, together with a confidence level of the assessment. Once individual assessments were completed, the therapists reviewed the assessments collaboratively in panel meetings. A revised certainty level was suggested for 8 of the 140 rules stored in the knowledge base, using the confidence value suggested by the group. Overall, the face-value verification was satisfactory, suggesting that the system embraces verified or verifiable knowledge for LBP diagnosis.

The completeness of the e-DSS knowledge base was also assessed by examining whether the system was able to reach some diagnosis for all clinical cases tested. All of the 180 real-world clinical cases received at least one diagnosis recommendation from the e-DSS. While not exhaustive, our test cases were sizable in number and exhibited considerable diversity.

In addition, potential developer-induced errors in the rules implemented in the back-end database were examined. Judged by our knowledge representation scheme and the integrity constraints enforced by the relational data model, the knowledge base appeared to have no serious syntactic or semantic problems stemming from system development errors.

System Validation

Validation verifies that the system performs at a level that is acceptable to domain experts or users (Biswas, Abramczyk, and Oliff, 1987; Kak et al., 1990). The e-DSS was validated through a modified Turing test that involved all five therapists and twenty clinical cases. Commonly used to validate knowledge-based systems, a Turing test (Walczak, Pofahl, and Scorpio, 2003) can generate artifacts of a system, whereby the system's intelligence or performance is assessed. In spite of the concerns raised by some researchers, a Turing test is generally considered to be a valid method and particularly effective for evaluating a system's performance with respect to domain experts' expectations (Gordon and Shortliffe, 1985). Accordingly, a modified Turing test was designed and used to validate the e-DSS, with a particular focus on system efficacy.

The validation approach used twenty previously diagnosed clinical cases. Several considerations were crucial to case selection:

- A minimum of one case for each diagnosis supported by the e-DSS was included for validation.
- The selection aimed at preserving the case distribution in clinical settings; in particular, the diagnoses of test cases had to exhibit a distribution comparable to that in the underlying case population. Accordingly, based on a sample population of 180 clinical cases, the diagnosis distribution was analyzed and 20 test cases were selected. This fairly large sample population was randomly collected from a national clinic so that it would resemble, to some degree, the underlying diagnosis space.
- The choice of how many test cases to include was based on a trade-off between data requirements for the intended analysis and the risk of overwhelming the five participating therapists.

First, using the modified Turing test procedures described next, each expert's competence was estimated. It should be noted that all experts would not be equally competent for a particular case; similarly, an expert would probably not be equally competent across all clinical cases. Hence, the unit of analysis was an expert's diagnosis of a test case.

The modified Turing test used consisted of four phases. In the case-solving phase, each expert (along with the e-DSS) diagnosed each case assigned. In the second phase, the identity of the expert who rendered each diagnosis was removed. This allowed the other experts to conduct a blind evaluation of each diagnosis recorded for each case. In the third phase, each expert rated each diagnosis. Using a rating r and a certainty factor c, each expert gave an explicit assessment of each presented diagnosis, together with his or her self-reported confidence in the assessment made. Each r and its certainty factor $c(r)$ were measured by using a seven-point Likert scale, with 1 being "not certain or confident at all" and 7 being "very confident or certain." Thus, the experts assessed one another as well as the e-DSS. In the final phase, the e-DSS was evaluated by producing a validity measure for each test case. This validity measure was calculated as the average rating of the system's diagnoses by the human experts, taking into account each expert's competence and subjective certainty assessment. The global validity of the system was then rated by averaging its validity score over the test cases under examination. In short, if the system "fools" the experts into thinking that it is a real expert (indicated by comparing the validity score it receives with those received by real experts), we can conclude that the system *behaves* like an expert, hence validating its performance. For mathematical details about the Turing test, please refer to Appendix B.

Evaluation of Clinical Efficacy

The e-DSS's *clinical efficacy* (that is, its utility in relation to domain experts' expectations) was further evaluated, using 180 real-world cases randomly collected from a nation-wide pain clinic in the United States. Two highly experienced therapists examined each case before its inclusion in the clinical efficacy evaluation. Only one of the two therapists had actively participated in the development of the e-DSS.

Three measurements were used for this evaluation:

- *Recall rate:* the portion of an expert's diagnoses that are correctly recommended by the e-DSS. As defined here, with a focus on false negatives, recall rate measures the e-DSS's power.
- *Precision rate:* a system's efficiency, mainly anchored in false positives. In this case study, *precision rate* is defined as the portion of the diagnoses recommended by the e-DSS that are actually made by an expert.
- *Accuracy:* a measurement based on primary diagnosis. Results from previous field observations and interviews with numerous therapists suggested that a therapist often first pursued the primary diagnosis—that is, the one in which he or she was most confident. Hence, primary diagnosis is relatively more important clinically than other diagnoses. A 100 percent accuracy is therefore assigned when the primary diagnosis of an expert is included in the system's recommendation, and 0 percent otherwise.

Each therapist individually reviewed the diagnoses documented for each test case and rendered his or her diagnoses if it differed from the ones documented. Together, the experts reviewed, discussed, and consolidated their individual assessments and diagnoses to produce a "gold standard" diagnosis for each test case. The resulting diagnoses were then used as the "correct diagnoses," which in turn were used to evaluate the e-DSS's clinical efficacy. The overall performance of the e-DSS, as shown in Table 10.4, is similar to that of the five experts.

TABLE 10.4. COMPARATIVE ANALYSIS OF PERFORMANCE: E-DIAGNOSIS SUPPORT SYSTEM VERSUS HUMAN EXPERTS

Test Case	System	Expert 1	Expert 2	Expert 3	Expert 4	Expert 5
1	0.77	0.72	0.93	0.97	0.93	0.97
2	0.87	0.74	0.63	0.72	0.32	0.22
3	0.81	0.74	0.79	0.74	0.56	0.43
4	0.63	0.64	0.83	0.88	0.82	0.79
5	0.62	0.72	0.70	0.71	0.74	0.71
6	0.39	0.76	0.71	0.79	0.69	0.55
7	0.72	0.55	0.44	0.44	0.62	0.61
8	0.40	0.68	0.53	0.73	0.53	0.69
9	0.84	0.93	0.93	0.93	0.89	0.90
10	0.82	0.81	0.81	0.86	0.53	0.76
11	0.83	0.81	0.85	0.28	0.74	0.41
12	0.48	0.63	0.67	0.77	0.78	0.39
13	0.50	0.62	0.48	0.67	0.61	0.62
14	0.86	0.80	0.83	0.83	0.79	0.86
15	0.70	0.90	0.90	0.72	0.86	0.84
16	0.49	0.41	0.66	0.52	0.63	0.62
17	0.92	0.80	0.80	0.94	0.90	0.90
18	0.86	0.62	0.64	0.49	0.86	0.86
19	0.75	0.60	0.70	0.49	0.50	0.55
20	0.63	0.63	0.43	0.56	0.65	0.58
All cases	0.69	0.71	0.71	0.70	0.70	0.66

Table 10.5 shows that the e-DSS averaged 75.82 percent in recall, 64.56 percent in precision, and 73.08 percent in accuracy. Overall, the measures suggested that the e-DSS exhibited reasonably satisfactory efficacy, particularly when compared with the disappointingly low likelihood of LBP patients' receiving adequate diagnoses (Jackson, Llewelyn-Phillips, and Klaber-Moffett, 1996).

The analysis also revealed a number of interesting observations. For example, the test set included one case for acute facet joint–related pain (diagnosis category 6) and one case for gynecological pain (diagnosis category 13), reflecting the infrequent occurrence of such cases in clinical settings. That both cases were diagnostically challenging was suggested by the system's poor performance (0.00) in each category. This may indicate a need to further evaluate and enhance our diagnostic knowledge of these LBP problems.

The system's performance in the acute disease categories (for example, categories 1 and 2) also suggested a need for further evaluation of the assumption that all LBP diagnosis categories have comparable or identical clinical occurrence rates. Without

TABLE 10.5. SUMMARY OF CLINICAL EFFICACY EVALUATION RESULTS FOR E-DIAGNOSIS SUPPORT SYSTEM

Diagnosis Category	Number of Test Cases	Distribution of Test Cases (Percentage)	Recall Rate (Percentage)	Precision Rate (Percentage)	Accuracy (Percentage)
1	16	8.79	46.88	46.88	56.25
2	16	8.79	40.62	37.50	50.00
3	46	25.27	86.17	74.47	89.36
4	45	24.73	81.11	64.44	62.22
5	10	5.49	80.00	60.00	60.00
6	1	0.55	0.00	0.00	0.00
7	3	1.65	100.00	66.67	100.00
8	3	1.65	66.67	33.33	33.33
9	11	6.04	90.91	72.72	90.91
10	13	7.14	73.08	76.92	92.31
11	14	7.69	92.86	82.14	92.86
12	3	1.65	50.00	50.00	33.33
13	1	0.55	0.00	0.00	0.00
14	0	0.00	0	0	0
Overall	182	100.00	75.82	64.56	73.08
Total with categories 6 and 13 excluded	180	98.90	76.67	65.28	73.89

categories 1 and 2, our system averaged 82.67 percent in recall, 69.33 percent in precision, and 77.33 percent in accuracy. Based on equation (2) in Appendix A, our algorithm has a tendency to favor diagnoses with high prior probabilities. That is, a diagnosis with high prior probability has a higher posterior probability for being true, even if it receives the same number of votes as other diagnoses.

A comparative analysis of the system's performance on chronic (for example, categories 3, 4, and 7) and acute (for example, categories 1 and 2) LBP problems suggests that chronic problems might have had a higher prior probability than acute ones, thus biasing our system. Findings from an interview with a senior therapist supported this speculation. The differential performance might also be partially attributed to potential biases in expert selection; for example, our selected therapists were more experienced in diagnosing chronic LBP problems than acute LBP problems. This suggests that the prior probability (p) might not be constant across different diagnosis categories. A refined knowledge representation and reasoning approach is needed to examine these concerns further.

Conclusion

Lower back pain is a common physiological and medical condition among adults, often depriving them of the ability to pursue routine activities and normal lifestyles. Recognizing the scarcity of key diagnostic knowledge and the frequency with which patients do not receive adequate care for LBP problems, we report on the development of an e-diagnosis support system to support clinicians in effective LBP diagnosis and its clinical evaluation.

Previous work on diagnostic support systems has uncovered important challenges. For example, different methods have been proposed for modeling, representing, or processing clinical reasoning under uncertainty, including applied machine learning algorithms (Bounds, Lloyd, Mathew, and Waddell, 1988; Graham and Espinosa, 1989; Vaughn and others, 1999), certainty factors (Buchanan and Shortliffe, 1975, 1985), Bayesian theory (Andersen, Olesen, Jensen, and Jensen, 1989; Przytula and Thompson, 2000), belief functions (Dempster, 1967; Shafer, 1976) and fuzzy logic (Zadeh, 1983). By and large, these methods require significant probability estimations by domain experts and thus are likely to create bottlenecks in an already time-consuming and tedious knowledge acquisition process. Another major challenge to designing and implementing diagnosis support systems in clinical health care (Suojanen, Andreassen, and Olesen, 2001) is the fact that clinical diagnosis may simultaneously involve multiple decision outcomes. While most prior cases addressed tasks involving single decision outcomes (Bounds, Lloyd, Mathew, and Waddell, 1988; Graham and Espinosa, 1989; Vaughn and others, 1999), the LBP problems presented here involve simultaneous multiple preliminary diagnoses. Findings from interviews with therapists and observations of their practice suggested that a therapist is likely to generate one to three preliminary diagnoses when examining a LBP patient. As noted, these preliminary diagnoses vary in certainty in ways that that require proper representation and reasoning. A final challenge is that a clinically viable system needs thorough evaluation in order to be widely accepted and used by targeted clinicians.

Motivated by the need for a system-based approach to support clinicians' diagnoses of LBP problems, we report on a Web-based e-DSS that addresses the challenging characteristics of LBP diagnosis. The e-DSS uses an intuitive and easy-to-understand framework for representing and reasoning about the uncertainty embedded in simultaneous multiple decision outcomes. Evaluations of the e-DSS addressed knowledge base verification, system validation, and clinical efficacy. As noted, analysis of these evaluations using multiple performance metrics revealed that the e-DSS does embrace important and verifiable diagnostic knowledge, provides a performance level similar to that of domain experts, and exhibits adequate clinical efficacy.

Despite the initial success reported by this system, several questions have emerged that require continued attention and serious investigation. First, how can the work presented here be more or less extended to enhance our understanding of other similarly rich and potentially difficult e-health related cases—for instance, the electronic diagnosis, prevention, and treatment management of many other ailments of a physical, cognitive, mental, psychological, or chronic nature, such as carpal tunnel syndrome, arthritis, multiple sclerosis, migraines, and depression?

Second, how might the intelligence of the e-DSS be enhanced? For example, can the system be designed to provide reasoning capability, such as the ability to identify the reasons behind the observed differential e-DSS effectiveness across LBP diagnosis categories? By understanding the source of inconsistent performance, we can further explore the assumption adopted (that is, identical prior probability of all diagnosis categories) and at the same time shed light on plausible boundaries of the proposed framework for representing and reasoning about uncertainty. A refined framework may then be analyzed and developed.

Finally, knowledge replenishment may be another area worth exploring. Although it allows the knowledge base to be updated by individual clinicians, the current e-DSS offers limited support for systematic knowledge replenishment. Such support is essential because clinicians' diagnostic knowledge is likely to evolve dynamically over time. In light of this, an automated machine learning or data mining approach may be able to adapt to important changes in knowledge instead of experts' having to repeat the tedious, expensive, and time-consuming knowledge engineering process. Such automated approaches would allow desirable integration or fusion of knowledge extracted or discovered through different methods, improving the quality of the knowledge base. For instance, the knowledge revealed by such data mining techniques could be used as anchors (data which are used as starting point for human experts to generate required estimation and projection) to complement the knowledge of human experts. Hence, the use of a Bayesian network to support knowledge integration is an appealing possibility. An investigation of the use of a Bayesian network to combine the diagnostic knowledge from different sources has been initiated, using the existing rule base, inference engine, case repository, and knowledge update module to support a hybrid DSS (Lin, Sheng, Hu, and Pirtle, 2002).

Chapter Questions

1. Would you argue that the SOAP scheme recommended for lower back pain diagnosis could be used for other types of chronic ailments? If so, give instances and discuss how this scheme would assist in guiding the therapists. How can e-technology be applied in automating such a scheme?

2. What are key features in the design of the e-DSS for LBP as discussed by the authors? Can you think of any other factors that may be important to consider? If you were asked to participate in the e-DSS design, what other concerns would you feel should be addressed?

3. What is the significance of evaluation of the e-DSS? What type of feedback is important, and how do you think the feedback assists in the evaluation? Please discuss.

4. In this chapter, we learned that knowledge acquisition and representation play vital roles in the design of a Web-based e-DSS for LBP. How do these considerations differ in the design of traditional health care systems?

5. Imagine that this e-DSS for lower back pain is available to an occupational therapist in your workplace. How might people who may have LBP problems benefit from such a system? Please discuss its socioeconomic value.

Appendix A: Formal Proof of a Consensus Model–Based Inference Algorithm

Using Bayes' theory, we formally prove the consensus model–based inference algorithm presented in this chapter:

Assuming n independent observations $o_1, \ldots, o_n$ and for each observation o_i, there exists a rule r_i in the format of "if o_i, then x" with a verbal probability $p(r_i), p(r_i) \in \{impossible, neutral, likely\}$.

Let p_i be the probability that rule r_i is correct $(1 \leq i \leq n)$ and P_x be the prior probability that diagnosis x is true.

Also, consider the following additional assumptions:

1. If $p(r_i) = $ impossible, $P(x \text{ is true} \mid R) = 0$, where R is any set of observations that contains o_i. That is, the presence or absence of certain evidence can rule out a diagnosis completely.

2. $p_i = p_j = p, \forall\, 1 \leq i,\ j \leq n$—that is, the prior probability for each rule being correct is identical. This assumption is reasonable, in part because of the comprehensive and nondiscriminant nature of therapists' practices in diagnosing and treating patients with various LBP problems. In this context, the decision rules extracted from their diagnostic knowledge should have a comparable baseline of correctness.

Assumption 1 implies that x cannot be true when there exists any observation on the left-hand side of a rule with a certainty level of "impossible." Hence, we consider only cases associated with rules with certainty levels of "neutral" or "likely." Assume there are m rules with a certainty level of "likely" $(m <= n)$ and all other rules are "neutral." According to Bayes' Theorem, we then can derive the following proposition:

Proposition 1

When $p > 0.5$, $P(x \text{ is true} \mid m \text{ likely rules})$, 5 is monotonically increasing in m—that is, the more "likely" rules there are, the higher the likelihood that x is true.

Proof:

$P(x \text{ is true} \mid m \text{ likely rules})$

$$= \frac{P\left(m \text{ likely rules} \mid x \text{ is true}\right) \cdot Px}{P\left(m \text{ likely rules} \mid x \text{ is true}\right) \cdot Px + P\left(m \text{ likely rules} \mid x \text{ is false}\right) \cdot (1 - Px)}$$

$$= \frac{p^m (1-p)^{n-m} P_X}{p^m (1-p)^{n-m} P_X + p^{n-m} (1-p)^m (1 - P_X)}$$

$$= \frac{1}{1 + \left[\left(\dfrac{p}{1-p}\right)^{n-2m} \cdot \left(\dfrac{1-P_X}{P_X}\right)\right]} \tag{1}$$

As shown, the Bayesian probability under discussion monotonically increases in m when $p > 0.5$.

Given the domain experts' extensive clinical experience, the assumption that $p > 0.5$ is reasonable. For single-diagnosis problems, our voting scheme suggests an increasing likelihood of accepting a diagnosis when it receives more "likely" votes.

To extend this illustrative example to multidiagnosis scenarios, assume that there are l diagnoses $d_1, \ldots, d_l$. For each observation o_i, there are l rules $r_{ij} \left(1 \leq i \leq n, 1 \leq j \leq l\right)$ in the format of "if o_i, then d_j" with a verbal probability $p\left(r_{ij}\right)$, $p\left(r_{ij}\right) \in \{$impossible, neutral, likely$\}$.

Let p_{ij} be the probability that r_{ij} is correct, and Pd_j be the prior probability that diagnosis d_j is correct. Including the two assumptions from the previous illustration and focusing likewise on scenarios involving no rules with a certainty level of "impossible," we arrive at the following proposition:

Proposition 2

$\forall j, k, 1 \leq j, k \leq l$, for an observation set R, if the following are true:

1. $p > 0.5$
2. $Pd_j = Pd_k$
3. Based on R, d_j receives n_j votes and d_k receives n_k votes, where $n_j > n_k$,

then $P\left(d_j \text{ is true} \mid R\right) > P\left(d_k \text{ is true} \mid R\right)$—that is, based on the same set of observations, the diagnoses that receive more votes are more likely to be true.

Proof:

Based on (1),

$$P\left(d_j \text{ is true} \mid R\right) = \frac{1}{1 + \left[\left(\dfrac{p}{1-p}\right)^{n-2n_j} \cdot \left(\dfrac{1-P_{d_j}}{P_{d_j}}\right)\right]}, P\left(d_k \text{ is true} \mid R\right) = \frac{1}{1 + \left[\left(\dfrac{p}{1-p}\right)^{n-2n_k} \cdot \left(\dfrac{1-P_{d_k}}{P_{d_k}}\right)\right]} \tag{2}$$

Since $\forall j, k, 1 \leq j, k \leq 1$, $Pd_j = Pd_k$, in light of the monotonic characteristic of the function, proposition 2 is proved.

Appendix B: Formal Description of the Modified Turing Test

For n experts e_i ($1 <= i <= n$) and m test cases t_j ($1 <= j <= m$) on the panel, let Sol_{ij} represent the solution by expert i for case j. The e-DSS was denoted as expert$_{n+1}$. The modified Turing test that was used consisted of four phases. In the case-solving phase, each expert (including the e-DSS) diagnosed each of the m cases assigned, resulting in a total of $m \cdot (n + 1)$ diagnoses. In the second phase, the identity of the experts who rendered the diagnoses were removed. This allowed the other experts to conduct a blind evaluation of each diagnosis recorded for each case. In the third phase, each expert rated each diagnosis presented. Using a rating r and a certainty factor c for each rating, each expert gave an explicit assessment of each presented diagnosis, together with his or her self-reported confidence in the assessment made. As a result, an $m \cdot (n + 1)$ rank matrix r_{ijk} was produced for expert e_i for evaluating the diagnosis by expert e_k for case t_j (Sol_{kj}), or $r_i(Sol_{kj})$. Each r and its certainty factor $c(r)$ were measured by using a seven-point Likert scale, with 1 being "not certain or confident at all" and 7 being "very confident or certain." The e-DSS was evaluated in the final phase of the modified Turing test and produced a validity measure $V_{sys}(t_j)$ for each test case. This validity measure was calculated as the average rating of the system's diagnoses by the human experts, taking into account each expert's competence and subjective certainty assessment. The global validity of the system V_{sys} was then rated by averaging its validity score over the test cases under examination.

Essentially, sources of individual competence estimation and the specific measurements used in the e-DSS evaluation were as follows:

a. *Certainty:* an expert's certainty while rating other experts' diagnoses. In particular, the certainty of an expert i on case j is denoted *Certainty* (e_i, t_j), which is calculated as his average certainty ratings ($c(r)$) on all other experts' diagnoses of case j (including the e-DSS's diagnosis):

$$Certainty\left(e_i, t_j\right) = \frac{\sum\limits_{k=1, k \neq i}^{n+1} c_{ijk}}{n} \tag{3}$$

b. *Consistency:* an expert's confidence in making a diagnosis, signified by the rating an expert specifies for his or her own diagnosis:

$$Consistency\ (e_i, t_j) = r_{iji} \tag{4}$$

c. *Stability:* the certainty of an expert's rating of his or her own solution:

$$Stability\ (e_i, t_j) = c_{iji} \tag{5}$$

The performance of each expert (including the e-DSS) on a given case is thus measured by the average rating received from other experts (including the e-DSS) weighted by their respective certainty.

$$Performance\left(e_i, t_j\right) = \frac{\sum\limits_{k=1, k \neq i}^{n+1} c_{kji} \cdot r_{kji}}{\sum\limits_{k=1, k \neq i}^{n+1} c_{kji}} \tag{6}$$

Fundamental to our competence estimation is (a) intentional self-reflection based on certainty, (b) unintentional self-reflection based on consistency and stability, and (c) external competence based on performance. If equal weights are assigned for these different sources for competence estimation, then we have the following equation:

$$Competence\left(e_i, t_j\right) = \frac{1}{3}\left[Certainty\left(e_i, t_j\right) + \frac{Consistency\left(e_i, t_j\right) + Stability\left(e_i, t_j\right)}{2} + Performance\left(e_i, t_j\right)\right] \tag{7}$$

Using the metrics presented, the human experts' average rating of the e-DSS's diagnoses on a specific case can then be calculated, weighted by their respective estimated competence and certainty level specified, as:

$$V_{sys}\left(t_j\right) = \frac{\sum\limits_{i=1}^{n} Competence\left(e_i, t_j\right) \cdot c_{ij}\left(n+1\right) \cdot r_{ij}\left(n+1\right)}{\sum\limits_{i=1}^{n} Competence\left(e_i, t_j\right) \cdot c_{ij}\left(n+1\right)} \tag{8}$$

Thus, the overall e-DSS validity can be estimated by averaging across the validity score for each case.

$$V_{sys} = \frac{\sum\limits_{j=1}^{m} v_{sys}\left(t_j\right)}{m} \tag{9}$$

In fact, comparative scores rather than actual values were used for rating and confidence, to ease interpretation of these measurements. Also, all of these rating or confidence measurements were normalized—that is, divided by 7 because of the seven-point Likert scale used. As a result, V_{sys} is inclusively bounded between 0 and 1.

Consistent with Knauf, Gonzalez, and Abel (2002), it is further argued that a single V_{sys} cannot accurately reflect the system's performance. Use of a single measurement is inadequate for comparing a system's performance with that of human experts. Indeed, deliberation of a system's capability requires careful interpretation and comparison of the system's performance by human experts.

To take human experts' performance into consideration, we modified Knauf, Gonzalez, and Abel's approach by introducing V_{exp}, which is defined as follows:

$$V_{exp}\left(t_j\right)_i = \frac{\sum\limits_{k=1, k \neq i}^{n} Competence\left(e_k, t_j\right) \cdot c_{kji} \cdot r_{kji}}{\sum\limits_{k=1, k \neq i}^{n} Competence\left(e_k, t_j\right) \cdot c_{kji}} \tag{10}$$

$V_{exp}(t_j)_i$ reflects expert i's performance on case j as evaluated by his or her peers. Expert i's overall performance can be then calculated as follows:

$$V_{expi} = \frac{\sum\limits_{j=1}^{m} V_{exp}\left(t_j\right)_i}{m} \tag{11}$$

References

Andersen, S. K., Olesen, K. G., Jensen, F. V., & Jensen, F. (1990). HUGIN: A shell for building Bayesian belief universes for expert systems. Morgan Kaufmann Publishers Inc., San Francisco, CA, USA. In *Proceedings of the Eleventh International Joint Conference on Artificial Intelligence* (pp. 332–337).

Berner, E. S., & Ball, M. J. (1998). *Clinical decision support systems: Theory and practice*. New York: Springer-Verlag, 1999.

Bharati, P., & Chaudhury, A. (in press). An empirical investigation of decision-making satisfaction in Web-based decision support systems. *Decision Support Systems*.

Biswas, G., Abramczyk, R., & Oliff, M. (1987). OASES: An expert system for operations analysis—The system for cause analysis. *IEEE Transactions on Systems, Man, and Cybernetics, 17*(2), 133–145.

Bounds, D. G., Lloyd, P. J., Mathew, B., & Waddell, G. (1988). A multilayer perceptron network for the diagnosis of low back pain. In *Proceedings of IEEE International Conference on Neural Networks* (Vol. 2, 481–489). San Diego, CA.

Buchanan, B. G., & Shortliffe, E. H. (1975). A model of inexact reasoning in medicine. *Mathematical Biosciences, 23*, 351–379.

Buchanan, B. G., & Shortliffe, E. H. (1985). *Rule-based expert systems: The MYCIN experiments of the Stanford Heuristic Programming Project*. Reading, MA: Addison-Wesley.

Cabrero-Canosa, M., Castro-Pereiro, M., Graña-Ramos, M., Hernandez-Pereira, E., Moret-Bonillo, V., Martin-Egaña, M., & Verea-Hernando, H. (2003). An intelligent system for the detection and interpretation of sleep apneas. *Expert Systems with Applications, 24*(4), 335–477.

Chau, P., & Hu, P. J. (2002). Examining a model for information technology acceptance by individual professionals: An exploratory study. *Journal of Management Information Systems, 18*(4), 191–229.

Danek, M. S. (n.d.). *Causes of low back pain*. Retrieved from http://www.back.com/causes.html

Dempster, A. P. (1967). Upper and lower probabilities induced by a multi-valued mapping. *Annals of Mathematical Statistics, 38*, 325–339.

Engelrecht, R., Rector, A., & Moser, W. (1995). *Assessment and evaluation of information technologies*. Amsterdam, Netherlands: IOS Press.

Gordon, J., & Shortliffe, E. (1985). A method for managing evidential reasoning in a hierarchical hypothesis space. *Artificial Intelligence, 26*, 323–357.

Graham, J. H., & Espinosa, A. (1989). Computer assisted analysis of electromyographic data in diagnosis of low back pain. *IEEE International Conference on Systems, Man and Cybernetics, 3*, 1118–1123.

Heckerman, D. E., Horvitz, E. J., & Nathwani, B. N. (1992). Toward normative expert systems: Part I: The Pathfinder Project. *Methods of Information in Medicine, 31*, 90–105.

Jackson, D., Llewelyn-Phillips, H., & Klaber-Moffett, J. (1996). Categorization of low back pain patients using an evidence-based approach. *Musculoskeletal Management, 2*, 39–46.

Kahneman, D., Slovic, P., & Tversky, A. (1982). *Judgment under uncertainty: Heuristics and biases*. Cambridge, England: Cambridge University Press.

Kak, A. C., Andress, K. M., and others. (1990). Hierarchical evidence accumulation in the PSEIKI system and experiments in model-driven mobile robot navigation, North-Holland, pp. 353–370. In *Uncertainty in Artificial Intelligence*. New York: Elsevier.

Knauf, R., Gonzalez, A. J., & Abel, T. (2002). A framework for validation of rule-based systems. *IEEE Transactions on Systems, Man and Cybernetics, 32*(3, Part B), 281–295.

Leaper, D. J., Horrocks, J. C., Staniland, J. R., & deDombal, F. T. (1972). Computer assisted diagnosis of abdominal pain using estimates provided by clinicians. *British Medical Journal, 4,* 350–354.

Lin, L., Sheng, O.R.L., Hu, P., & Pirtle, M. (2002). Adaptive medical knowledge management: An integrated rule-based and Bayesian network approach. In *Proceedings of the Tenth Annual Workshop on Information Technologies and Systems.*

Nachemson, A. L. (1985). Advances in low-back pain. *Clinical Orthopedics and Related Research, 200,* 266–278.

Przytula, K. W., & Thompson, D. (2000). Construction of Bayesian networks for diagnostics. *IEEE Aerospace Conference Proceedings, 5,* 193–200.

Shafer, G. (1976). *A mathematical theory of evidence.* Princeton, NJ: Princeton University Press.

Shortliffe, E. H., & Davis, R. (1975). Some considerations for the implementation of knowledge-based expert systems. *SIGART Newsletter, 55,* 9–12.

Smith, A. E., Nugent, C. D., & McClean, S. I. (2003). Evaluation of inherent performance of intelligent medical decision support systems: Utilizing neural networks as an example. *AI in Medicine, 27*(1), 1–27.

Suojanen, M., Andreassen, S., & Olesen, K. G. (2001). A method for diagnosing multiple diseases in MUNIN. *IEEE Transactions on Biomedical Engineering, 48*(5), 522–532.

van DerGaag, L. C., Renooij, S., Witteman, C.L.M., Aleman, B.M.P., & Taal, B. G. (2002). Probabilities for a probabilistic network: A case study in oesophageal cancer. *AI in Medicine, 25*(2), 123–148.

Vaughn, M. L., Cavill, S. J., Taylor, S. J., Foy, M. A., & Fogg, A.J.B. (1998). Interpretation and knowledge discovery from a MLP network that performs low back pain classification. *IEEE Colloquium on Knowledge Discovery and Data Mining,* pp. 2/1-2/4.

Vaughn, M. L., Cavill, S. J., Taylor, S. J., Foy, M. A., & Fogg, A.J.B. (1999). Using direct explanations to validate a multi-layer perceptron network that classifies low back pain patients. In *Proceedings of the 6th International Conference on Neural Information Processing* (Vol. 2, pp. 692–699).

Waddell, G. (1987). A new clinical model for the treatment of low back pain. *Spine, 12*(7), 632–644.

Walczak, S., Pofahl, W. E., & Scorpio, R. J. (2003). A decision support tool for allocating hospital bed resources and determining required acuity of care. *Decision Support Systems, 34*(4), 445–456.

Zadeh, L. A. (1983). The role of fuzzy logic in the management of uncertainty in expert systems. *Fuzzy Sets and Systems, 11,* 199–227.

Teleradiology Case: Present and Future

Yao Y. Shieh, Mason Shieh

We have introduced a case on "Teleradiology" here as this technology often incorporates the use of e-DSS and e-diagnosis on the part of teleradiologists. However, the case is an expansion of e-medicine and telemedicine discussion, a central theme of the e-health domains explored throughout Part Three of this text.

Telemedicine can be defined in a broad sense as any medicine-related interaction between a user and a provider that is not done face-to-face. The provider can be either a human being or an intelligent entity such as a search engine, an interactive video demonstration program, or a rule-based inference engine. The communication channels do not have to be identical in both directions. For instance, the user can send image data to a provider via satellite, and the provider can respond with a diagnostic report by telephone. Among others, telemedicine covers the following important scenarios:

- *E-consultation:* A patient (or a generalist) taps into the expertise of a physician (or a specialist) located at a geographically distant site.
- *On-line scheduling:* An informed e-patient consults Web sites such as CSS Credentialing (www.tese.com) and Certified Doctor (www.certifieddoctor.com) for relevant information, leading to an on-line appointment with a prospective physician.
- *Decision support:* A patient uses software as an aid in choosing among treatment options. Examples of such software include an interactive video program provided by Duke University Medical Center or the Comprehensive Health Enhancement Support System produced by University of Wisconsin.
- *Remote patient monitoring:* Health status signals of patients with chronic illnesses are sent to a monitoring center for regular monitoring.
- *E-learning:* A physician takes on-line continuing medical education courses, or an e-consumer surfs the Internet for on-line health information.

Of the five scenarios, e-consultation receives the most attention and is therefore the focus of this case discussion.

Teleradiology: A Booming Niche in Telemedicine

Despite its great potential, telemedicine, by and large, has had minimal usage. In addition to the cost of technology and the lack of third-party reimbursement, limited usage of telemedicine has been attributed to cultural factors such as a lack of education in the use of telemedicine equipment and a lack of communication between physicians and videoconferencing engineers. However, one telemedicine niche, teleradiology, is an exception; it has enjoyed rapid proliferation in the past decade. Following two decades of research on the display and management of digital medical images, teleradiology is moving ahead of most other e-subspecialties.

Four elements separate teleradiology from other telemedicine services:

- Endorsement of the Digital Imaging and Communications in Medicine (DICOM) standard by the American College of Radiology ensures interoperability among products from different vendors. Open competition made possible by standardization has driven rapid advancement of technologies and provided large cost reductions.

- Teleradiology comes as a free by-product of picture archiving and communications systems (PACS). Many radiology departments have gradually abandoned film-based operation to embrace soft-copy reading because of PACS. As a result, a radiologist can read images anywhere, anytime, as long as he or she has access to a reading station that is connected to a PACS server. Consequently, there is no additional cost in supporting a teleradiology operation. In contrast, nonradiologic telemedicine is very different from routine, daily medical practice and therefore requires an additional investment for videoconferencing equipment as well as additional personnel support.

- Teleradiology is non-interactive by nature. Most telemedicine services require that the physician interact with the patient in real time. Thus, telemedicine demands extra effort to coordinate participants, which can be very frustrating and resource-consuming. In contrast, requests for teleradiology consults can be answered when it is convenient for radiologists.

- Teleradiology enjoys exceptional acceptance as far as reimbursement is concerned. Private insurance companies and government agencies such as Medicare and Medicaid have been reluctant to reimburse for general telemedicine services. In contrast, teleradiology has been fairly uniformly recognized by third parties (Thrall and Boland, 2002).

Teleradiology has come a long way from its initial status as a low-end system to supplement evening and weekend coverage. In the past few years, teleradiology has evolved into a core technology of virtual radiology departments in which radiologists can read images anytime, anywhere within an institution. With the rapid growth of the Internet, teleradiology faces the new challenge of being a potential core technology in a global e-health care infrastructure, readily accessible at an affordable cost to patients and health care providers.

Challenges that teleradiology faces as it progresses toward fulfilling its potential include the following:

- Digitization across the spectrum of modalities
- Evolution into a multisite, multispecialty teleradiology network
- Evolution into cross-disciplinary telemedicine
- Equitable teleradiology service for the underserved
- Telecommunication networks
- Sophisticated data compression
- Reimbursements to promote remote teleradiology
- Patient confidentiality and security

Each of these challenges is discussed in the following sections.

Digitization Across the Spectrum of Modalities

Mammography is the last remaining modality that needs to be converted into digital format to achieve total digitization of radiology. Although a small number of digital mammography products have received clearance from the Food and Drug Administration, digital mammography remains immature. Standard mammography provides higher resolution, which is important in detecting early breast cancer. In addition, digital mammography costs about four to five times more than standard mammography. It will take time for the technology to mature and the cost to drop so that digital mammography can be widely accepted.

Evolution into a Multisite, Multispecialty Teleradiology Network

Teleradiology was first developed in the 1980s in order to supplement evening and weekend coverage. It was meant for casual use that involved relatively small amounts of image and text data, with no long-term image archiving or automatic pre-fetch of previous studies for comparison. Since the advent of PACS, teleradiology operation has become routine within many hospitals, even to the extent of crossing organizational, regional, and national boundaries.

The radiology departments of Texas Tech University Health Sciences Center (TTUHSC) at Lubbock and El Paso are networked by permanent T-1 links to form a multispecialty radiology entity. The two campuses, which are 300 miles apart, benefit from complementing each other's subspecialties (X-Rays, MRI, CT Scanning, Digital Imaging) as well as workload sharing. Routine teleradiological interpretation service is also provided by TTUHSC to Lubbock Cancer Center. The ultimate goal is to achieve a global teleradiology network from which patients, radiologists, health care staff, and researchers in any part of the world can benefit.

Evolution into Cross-Disciplinary Telemedicine

Over the past decade, the technology of teleradiology has matured; it can now provide advanced functions such as work lists related to the patient's images to be analyzed, long-term archiving, and pre-fetching of earlier studies within the jurisdiction of the radiology department. In the modern information era, however, a radiologist also needs relevant clinical information generated outside the radiology department, such as laboratory test results, electrocardiography reports, pharmacy reports, and medical histories, in order to deliver optimal health care. Unfortunately, during the past few decades, clinical data have been fragmented and isolated in the health care departments where they are collected. Consequently, these data often are incompatible and cannot be exchanged efficiently.

Electronic health records (EHRs) enable effective data sharing between different departments by creating a centralized repository of electronic health records. A patient's data, collected from multiple sources, are filtered and translated by an interface engine into a common format before they are deposited into EHRs. With this technology, the patient's data can be accessed and viewed from any application program.

An even more ambitious concept called a *virtual medical record* (VMR) has also been proposed. A VMR would assemble a patient's medical record from various sources without drawing from a centralized repository, thus enabling collection of patient medical information that spans institutional, regional, and even national boundaries. However, VMRs require that all participating systems adopt a common methodology for linking various databases. This is the next step that TTUHSC is considering.

Recently, the Integrating the Healthcare Enterprise (IHE) initiative, sponsored by the Radiological Society of North America and the Healthcare Information and Management Systems Society, has been promoting the use of established standards such as DICOM and Health Level Seven (HL7) in order to support optimal patient care. Encouraged by their initial success with Health Information System, Radiological Information System, and PACS integration in support of optimal radiology operations, IHE sponsors are now trying to extend this initiative to other medical fields.

Equitable Teleradiology Service for the Underserved

Since the late 1970s, the World Health Organization has promoted the concept of equitable primary health care: provision of essential health care, using practical and scientifically and socially sound methods and technologies, to those who need it, at an affordable price. Although teleradiology has flourished in the past few years, most of its growth has been confined to metropolitan areas. Little progress has been accomplished in rural areas, where teleradiology service arguably is needed the most.

Radiology service in remote or rural areas often suffers from the problems of out-of-date radiology equipment, inadequately trained technologists, and lack of access to modern telecommunication infrastructures. Due to the low volume of radiographic examinations at any one site, it is difficult for a typical remote clinic to bear the financial burden of maintaining modern radiographic equipment. A more practical approach is sharing of costs by multiple clinics in the same general region.

Cost sharing can be done either with mobile modality equipment or with a hub-spokes topology. A *mobile modality* truck can travel from one town to another on a round-robin basis. The TTUHSC's mobile mammography service in the West Texas region provides a working example. Other popular mobile modalities include computed tomography, magnetic resonance, and positron emission tomography. Each clinic would contribute in proportion to the image volume it generates. A recent study showed that hospitals must have an annual volume of 1,500 to 2,000 magnetic resonance procedures to hold their cost per procedure to that of a mobile company (Fratt, 2002).

A *hub-spokes topology* stations modality equipment in a specific clinic, preferably one located in the geographic center of the region. This clinic is the hub, and the other clinics are the spokes. Instead of traveling a long distance to a metropolitan clinic, patients in the region travel a shorter distance to this hub to have radiological procedures done. Presumably, the hub clinic would contribute more financially than other clinics because of the special convenience it enjoys.

Between 1996 and 1998, the TTUHSC Radiology Department maintained an innovative teleradiology service in a triangular rural area in West Texas surrounding three rural hospitals, none of which had a resident radiologist. A radiologist recruited from that region hopped from one hospital to the next. While he was working at one hospital, images generated at the other two hospitals could be sent to him to read. This arrangement gave the radiologist the opportunity to perform special procedures, as well as to build good personal relationships with local referring physicians.

Traditionally, remote clinics have trouble retaining skillful radiologists because the low revenues generated by these clinics often cannot support technologists' high salaries. Combining the volume of procedures from several clinics, however, can generate sufficient revenues to recruit and retain registered technologists. Continuing education to keep technologists current on procedures and technology can be accomplished by allowing technologists to take on-line courses instead of having to travel long distances for training.

Telecommunication Networks

Extensive high-bandwidth telecommunication networks have been built worldwide, but populations in remote areas still have limited or no access to this type of infrastructure. Broadband telecommunication services such as direct subscriber lines (DSL) and integrated services digital networks (ISDN) are only available in select urban areas. Generally speaking, remote areas are limited to network service with bandwidth limited by regular telephone lines. The same factors, such as the high costs of installing fiber-optic cables, that limit bandwidth make populations in these areas the ones who need teleradiology service the most. Thus, in teleradiology, the notion of remoteness has more to do with affordable access to advanced network infrastructure than with geographic distance. For instance, a patient in Los Angeles can tap into the expertise of the M. D. Anderson Cancer Center in Houston through teleradiology much more easily than a patient in rural West Texas can, even though the patient in Los Angeles is several times farther away. The adoption of teleradiology in remote and rural primary health care settings requires equitable access to high-bandwidth network infrastructure, which thus is a limiting factor in the growth of the field.

Satellite communication presents a viable alternative in remote areas where no wired infrastructure exists. According to experts' forecasts, the satellite communication business will expand very rapidly to provide faster and cheaper communication service in the near future (Lamminen, 1999). Wireless technology is becoming popular in delivering e-health care. Some teleradiology functions can be performed using wireless personal digital assistants (PDAs). Wireless telephones with interactive video capability are already available in Japan. Given the rapidly advancing technology, it is expected that patient medical data will be exchanged routinely through wireless handheld devices in the near future.

Sophisticated Data Compression

The transmission of a typical radiographic study incurs significant latency if there is no high-bandwidth communication channel between the originating site and the consulting site. Data compression techniques aimed at reducing transmission time can be classified into two categories: lossless and lossy. Lossless compression results in a very moderate compression ratio and therefore is of limited help. Lossy compression can be done at a very high compression ratio, at the expense of losing diagnostically significant detail. Essentially, lossy compression is a low-pass filter technique that preserves the gross features and eliminates high-contrast details.

An ideal compression scheme would allow areas containing diagnostically significant details to be compressed losslessly while areas containing no diagnostically significant details are compressed lossily. Since decision making occurs mainly at the consulting site, this scheme can be implemented in an asymptotic manner by a process of iterative refinement. First, a small image, created with a very high and lossy compression ratio, along with a detailed description of symptoms, is transmitted to the radiologist. The radiologist examines the image and requests more detail on certain areas of interest. On receiving the one-level-enhanced version of these areas, the radiologist may then zero in by requesting further detail on an even smaller area. The process can be repeated until the radiologist is comfortable with the level of detail and can make a diagnosis. The success of such an approach hinges on the existence of a user-friendly interface—for instance, a system that allows freehand drawing with a mouse, which allows the radiologist to easily highlight the areas for which more details are being requested, along with an intelligent program at the originating site that can correctly interpret the radiologist's commands and respond interactively.

Reimbursements to Promote Remote Teleradiology

Medicare reimbursement rates are set by the Center for Medicare and Medicaid Services, and their regulations are complex. Levin, chairman of the Radiology Department at Thomas Jefferson University Hospital, describes the reimbursement situation: "The big problem is that reimbursements have not been keeping pace with the cost of running a radiology practice" (Fratt, 2001). The situation is more severe in remote areas because of higher utility costs—for example, for electricity, phone service, and other telecommunication equipment maintenance and service. Many experimental projects have terminated as soon as external funding was withdrawn. This pattern suggests that teleradiology service in rural areas generally has not been self-sustainable. The government's reimbursement policy should provide special incentives to encourage teleradiology operations in rural areas to promote the vision of equitable primary health care.

Patient Confidentiality and Security

The Health Insurance Portability and Accountability Act of 1996 (HIPAA) provides nationwide protection of the confidentiality and security of patient medical information. But HIPAA only covers health care providers, health plans, and health care clearinghouses that transmit patient information in electronic form. Other entities, such as secondary users (for example, researchers) who have access to such data, are not restricted by HIPAA. In a manual record-keeping environment, the enormous effort required to retrieve information recorded on paper creates a natural barrier against misuse of records. But in an electronic medical record environment, unauthorized retrieval of a patient's information can be accomplished almost instantly if no proper access controls are in place.

Protection of patient confidentiality and security of patient medical records requires a solid security infrastructure as well as a proven security policy. A *security infrastructure* covers the issues of login authentication, cryptography, access control, antivirus precautions, risk assessment, auditing, alert for medication errors, and disaster recovery. A *security policy* should clearly define the guidelines for creating, accessing, and maintaining the integrity of patient e-health data and the scope of accountability for each responsible party. The objective of instilling security awareness in employees involved in teleradiology operations—including explicit discussion of disciplinary measures for security violations—should inform the policy.

With the growing trend toward collaborative teleradiology consultation across institutional boundaries, the principles of data and information ownership tend to become entangled, because medical records of episodes may be compiled from a number of distinct data sources. Even when the originator practices good stewardship of its own database, the data being electronically transmitted elsewhere may subsequently be inappropriately exposed to unauthorized entities. Consequently, it is important that specification of security responsibilities for each party be part of any collaborative contract.

Radiology has pioneered the bridging of information technology and medical applications, primarily because of its demanding and enormous needs for computing power, storage capacity, networking bandwidth, and display speed and resolution, compared with other clinical applications. The IHE initiative demonstrates the leadership of radiology in enlisting the support of other clinical disciplines to promote an interoperable health care enterprise. Teleradiology has become the model for establishing a global, equitable, high-quality, affordable, and clinically effective e-health care system and environment.

Case Questions

1. Why do you think teleradiology is among one of the most successful, diffused, and accepted forms of telemedical services?
2. What kinds of e-networking infrastructure or configurations are suitable for supporting teleradiological services for underserved urban, rural, and remote areas?

3. Why are standards so critical to the diffusion of an e-technology like teleradiology? Who determines these standards? Why?
4. What is collaborative teleradiology? What are its benefits as an e-health service? What trends will affect collaborative teleradiology in the future?

References

Fratt, L. (2001). Trends in reimbursement: The downs and ups. *Medical Imaging, 16*(8), 68–74.

Fratt, L. (2002). Mobile equipment on the road again. *Medical Imaging, 17*(3), 62–70.

Lamminen, H. (1999). Mobile satellite systems. *Journal of Telemedicine and Telecare, 5*(2), 71–83.

Thrall, J. H., & Boland, G. (2002). Teleradiology. In K. J. Dreyer, A. Mehta, & J. H. Thrall (Eds.), *PACS: A guide to the digital revolution* (pp. 315–348).

CHAPTER ELEVEN

E-HEALTH INTELLIGENCE

A Multiple-Level Clustering Approach for E-Health Data Mining

Chih-Ping Wei, Paul Jen-Hwa Hu, Liang-Ming Kung, Joseph Tan

Learning Objectives

1. Identify the meaning of data mining and its relevance and value in e-health care
2. Know the clustering analysis approach and identify the elements and boundaries of clustering analysis in emerging e-health care data systems and applications
3. Understand what a concept space is and realize the significance of distinguishing it from a description space in the context of constructive clustering analysis techniques
4. Articulate a constructive clustering analysis algorithm that automatically selects the optimal concept space and the optimal number of clusters
5. Comprehend the issues and challenges in e-health data mining research
6. Appreciate the value of data mining in e-health systems and environments

Introduction

Health care is one of the fastest-growing and largest sectors in many developed countries, including the United States, Canada, the United Kingdom, and Taiwan. The role of information technology (IT) in health service provision and delivery has increased significantly, particularly in e-health. IT investments in health care in the United States alone are estimated to be between \$13 to \$15 billion dollars each year, with a projected annual growth of over a billion dollars (Raghupathi and Tan, 2002). Further exponential growth is expected as the health care industry implements integrated databases, e-health networks, enterprise resource planning systems, and enterprise data warehouses; provides remote diagnostics and e-clinical care via e-medicine and e-home care services; sets up intranets and extranets for sharing e-health information; and uses the information superhighway, including the Internet, to disseminate e-health-related information. Central to leveraging the rapidly expanding corpus of information and fast-growing e-health databases and data warehouses is the discovery of the knowledge, data regularities, or high-level information essential to supporting e-health intelligence, selecting desired service alternatives, making complex judgments, and predicting uncertain future events or individual behaviors (Chen, Han, and Yu, 1996; Cabena and others, 1997; Frawley, Piatetsky-Shapiro, and Matheus, 1992).

Based on the intended function or purpose, data mining can be broadly classified into several categories, including classification, clustering, association rule, sequential pattern, data visualization, and link analysis (Berry and Linoff, 1997; Chen, Han, and Yu, 1996; Wei, Piramuthu, and Shaw, 2003). Among these categories, *clustering* is a data mining technique that is appropriate and effective for undirected knowledge discovery or unsupervised learning. Due to its undirected nature, clustering is often an adequate first technique for analyzing a large, complex data set characterized by many variables and diverse internal structures. In a nutshell, in *clustering analysis,* a set of objects is partitioned or grouped into several clusters in which all instances in one cluster are similar to one another and different from the instances of other clusters, based on some Euclidean distance metric (Kaufman and Rousseeuw, 1990; Luger and Stubblefield, 1993; Ng and Han, 1994; Spath, 1980; Zait and Messatfa, 1997). Clustering analysis has been applied to a wide array of applications, including customer profiling, target marketing, cross-selling, hospital case mix analysis, and customer retention (Cabena and others, 1997).

Existing clustering analysis techniques generate clusters based on *description spaces,* which initially define the attributes of the objects. Results of clustering analysis may become inadequate or even misleading if the description spaces of attributes included in the analysis are of poor quality. However, even when the original description spaces are inadequate, it may be possible to transform them by incorporating them into a concept space at a higher level of abstraction, in which the clustering analysis can yield data regularities of increasing quality or actionability. Toward this goal, one logical and intuitive approach is to introduce new descriptions by combining or aggregating existing descriptions. The new descriptions represent concepts at a higher abstraction level than those described by the original descriptions. This process is commonly referred to as a *constructive approach* (Bloedorn and Michalski, 1991; Kramer, 1994; Wnek and Michalski, 1994).

The constructive approach has been applied to several data mining techniques, including classification, association rule, and sequential pattern analysis. DBLearn (Cai, Cercone, and Han, 1990; Han, 1995), AQ17-DCI (Bloedorn and Michalski, 1991), AQ17-HCI (Wnek and Michalski, 1994), and CN2-MCI (Kramer, 1994) are examples of constructive classification analysis techniques. Han and Fu (1995) extended the association rule analysis technique by using the constructive feature and proposed a multiple-level association analysis technique. Based on a user-defined taxonomy for items, Srikant and Agrawal (1996) generalized the sequential pattern analysis algorithm by allowing sequential patterns to include items across different abstraction levels. Results from these and other studies suggest that constructive data mining techniques broaden the scope of knowledge discovery and are capable of generating comprehensible knowledge not attainable by nonconstructive techniques.

Although it is applied in several data mining techniques, the constructive approach has not yet been incorporated into clustering analysis. The objective of this research is to propose a constructive clustering analysis algorithm to complement rather than substitute for existing clustering techniques. In this chapter, we first review the related literature, including clustering analysis fundamentals and the representations commonly adopted by existing constructive data mining techniques. Next, we describe the details of the proposed constructive clustering analysis algorithm, providing illustrations. Following this, we report an empirical evaluation based on a real-world application and highlight important analysis results. We then conclude the chapter with a discussion of current research contributions to data mining and single out some future research directions.

Fundamentals of Clustering Analysis Techniques

Clustering analysis is the process for partitioning a set of objects (described by a set of attributes) into clusters. The objects in a resulting cluster are more similar to one another than to those in other clusters.

Attribute Types and Distance Measures

A *clustering analysis algorithm* relies on some measure of distance that describes and assesses the similarity or dissimilarity between objects. Typically, attributes describing objects are of one of the following types:

- *Interval:* An interval attribute is defined by a continuous linear scale divided into equal intervals.
- *Ordinal (or rank):* An ordinal attribute has more than two states, which can be ordered in a meaningful sequence. The distance between two states increases when they are further apart in the sequence, although the intervals between these consecutive states may not be equal.
- *Nominal (or categorical):* A nominal attribute takes on multiple states, but these states are not ordered in any way.
- *Binary:* A binary attribute is a nominal attribute that has only two possible states.

Based on the attribute type, different distance measures have been developed. For example, Manhattan, Euclidean, or Minkowski distance can be used to measure the distance between objects that are described by interval attributes. Kaufman and Rousseeuw (1990) proposed a distance measure for attributes of different types, which can be described as follows:

Suppose the objects to be clustered are described by p attributes. The distance $d(o_i, o_j)$ between object o_i and o_j is calculated as follows:

$$d\left(o_i, o_j\right) = \frac{\sum_{f=1}^{p} \delta\left(f\right)_{ij} d\left(f\right)_{ij}}{\sum_{f=1}^{p} \delta\left(f\right)_{ij}}$$

$\delta\left(f\right)ij$ is equal to 1 if both measurements x_{if} (that is, the value of the fth attribute of object o_i) and x_{if} are not null—that is, not missing. Otherwise, it is equal to 0; that is, the measurement x_{if} or x_{if} is missing. $d(f)_{ij}$ characterizes the contribution of the fth attribute to the distance between objects o_i and o_j. If the fth attribute is of the binary or nominal type, then

$$d(f)_{ij} = 1 \quad \text{if } x_{ij} \neq x_{if}$$
$$\quad\quad = 0 \quad \text{if } x_{if} = x_{if}$$

If the fth attribute is interval-scaled, then

$$d(f)_{ij} = \frac{|x_{if} - x_{jf}|}{R_f}, \text{ where } R_f \text{ is the value range of the } f\text{th attribute.}$$

If the fth attribute is of the ordinal type, the measurements x_{if} and x_{if} in the previous equation are replaced by their respective numeric ranks, and $d(f)_{ij}$ is calculated as it is for interval-scaled attributes. Since each $d(f)_{ij}$ is between 0 and 1, regardless of attribute type, the resulting distance $d(o_i, o_j)$ is also bounded between 0 and 1.

Common Clustering Analysis Approaches

Common clustering analysis approaches include partition-based, hierarchical, and Kohonen neural network, each of which uses a specific distance measure. *The partition-based approach*, including k-means (Anderberg, 1973) and partitioning around medoids (PAM) (Kaufman and Rousseeuw, 1990; Ng and Han, 1994), segments a set of objects into multiple non-overlapping clusters. Given a specified number of clusters, a partition-based technique creates an initial partition and then attempts to improve the partition iteratively by moving objects between or among clusters. For example, the PAM algorithm partitions n objects into k clusters by first finding a representative object for each cluster. A representative is the most centrally located object in a cluster and is often called a *medoid*. Once k medoids have been selected, each nonselected object is classified into the cluster of the closest medoid, based on the distance measure of choice. The algorithm then repeatedly tries to make a better choice by substituting a nonselected object o_h for medoid o_i whenever such substitutions would improve the clustering quality. For each nonselected object o_j, the effect on o_j of substituting o_h for o_i is C_{jih}, which is defined as follows:

$$C_{jih} = d(o_j, o_p) - d(o_j, o_q)$$

where $d(o_j, o_p)$ denotes the distance between o_j and o_p, o_p is the medoid closest to o_j after o_h is substituted for o_i, and o_q is the medoid closest to o_j before o_h is substituted for o_i.

The total cost of substituting o_h for o_i is then given by the following equation:

$$TC_{ih} = \sum_j C_{jih}$$

$TC_{ih} > 0$ means that replacing the medoid o_i with o_h would result in a greater distance between an object and the medoid of its cluster. Therefore, o_h will not be selected to replace the medoid o_i if $TC_{ih} > 0$.

The *hierarchical clustering approach* builds a binary clustering hierarchy, or tree, in which leaf nodes represent objects to be clustered. Hierarchical clustering methods can be further classified into *agglomerative* or *divisive* clustering, depending on whether the clustering hierarchy is formed in a bottom-up or top-down fashion. The hierarchical agglomerative clustering (HAC) algorithm (Kaufman and Rousseeuw, 1990) exemplifies a bottom-up strategy, starting with as many clusters as there are objects. Based on an intercluster similarity measure of choice (for example, single link, complete link, group-average link, Ward's method), the two most similar clusters are then merged to form a new cluster. This merging process continues until either a hierarchy emerges (in which a single cluster remains at the top of the hierarchy containing all the target objects) or the process reaches a specified termination condition (for instance, intercluster similarity less than a specified threshold). In contrast, the hierarchical divisive clustering algorithm (Kaufman and Rousseeuw, 1990) employs a top-down strategy, starting with all the objects in one cluster. The cluster is then subdivided into its two most distinct clusters. The division process is repeated until either each object is part of a distinct cluster or the process reaches a specified termination condition (for example, intracluster similarity of each cluster greater than a specified threshold).

A *Kohonen neural network,* also known as a self-organizing map, is an unsupervised two-layer neural network (Kohonen, 1989, 1995) in which each input node corresponds to a coordinate axis in the input attribute vector space. Each output node corresponds to a node in a two-dimensional grid. The network is fully connected; that is, each output node is connected to each input node with a connection weight. During the training phase, all objects to be clustered are fed into the network repeatedly in order to adjust the connection weights in such a way that the distribution of the output nodes represents that of the input objects. The input vector space distribution serves as the criterion.

Determining Number of Clusters

Many clustering analysis algorithms (for example, k-means, PAM) assume the number of clusters to be known. But what is the optimal number of clusters for a given set of objects? The *silhouette measure,* proposed by Kaufman and Rousseeuw (1990), measures the degree of cluster separation and therefore can be used to determine the optimal number of clusters. Let the cluster to which object o_i is assigned be A. Let $a(i)$ be the average distance of o_i to all other objects in the cluster A. For any cluster C different from A, let $d(o_i, C)$ be the average distance of o_i to all objects in C. The smallest $d(o_i, C)$ among all clusters is selected and denoted as $b(i) = \min_{C \neq A} d(o_i, C)$. The cluster B for which this minimum is attained—that is, for which $d(o_i, B) = b(i)$—is called the *neighbor* of object o_i. Cluster B can be viewed as the second-best choice for o_i. The silhouette of o_i, $s(i)$, is then obtained as follows:

$$s(i) = 1 - \frac{a(i)}{b(i)} \qquad \text{if } a(i) < b(i)$$

$$= 0 \qquad \text{if } a(i) = b(i) \text{ or the object } o_i \text{ is the only object in the cluster } A$$

$$= \frac{b(i)}{a(i)} - 1 \qquad \text{if } a(i) > b(i)$$

$s(i)$ measures how well the object o_i matches the cluster to which o_i is currently assigned. Evidently, $s(i)$ is bounded between -1 and 1. When $s(i)$ is close to 1, this implies that the "within" distance $a(i)$ is much smaller than the smallest "between" distance $b(i)$. In this case, o_i can be regarded as well classified. When $s(i)$ is close to -1—that is, when $a(i)$ is much larger than $b(i)$—it suggests that o_i lies on the average much closer to cluster B than to cluster A. Hence, it would seem more natural or appropriate to assign o_i to cluster B. The average of $s(i)$ for all objects in the data set is called the *average silhouette width* of the data set under a predefined k, denoted by $\bar{s}(k)$. This calculation can be used to find the optimal number of clusters. If n is the number of objects, for $k = 2, 3, \ldots n-1$, the optimal number of clusters is the k that results in the maximum $\bar{s}(k)$. The maximum $\bar{s}(k)$ is called the *silhouette coefficient* of the data set.

Representation of Constructive Data Mining Techniques

Two approaches for constructing new description spaces have been proposed:

- Applying mathematical operators on original descriptions
- Applying logical operators that aggregate existing descriptions (original or constructed) into higher-level abstractions

Adopted from Bloedorn and Michalski (1991), the following example illustrates the concept of the first approach. Suppose there exist two sets of boxes, each of which is described by three attributes: height, length, and width. Sample data are as follows:

Class 1				Class 2		
Height	Length	Width		Height	Length	Width
2	12	2		12	4	2
6	4	2		4	12	2
3	8	2		8	6	2
4	4	3		4	8	3

The rules describing the characteristics of each class of boxes are fairly complex:

If [height = 2 or 3] or ([height = 4 or 6] and [length = 4]), then Class 1

If ([height = 4 or 8] and [length = 6 or 8 or 12]) or [height = 12], then Class 2

To generate more comprehensible rules, a new attribute can be constructed as a mathematical function of a set of original or constructed attributes. In our example, a volume attribute height × length × width of the box is constructed and found useful. Based on this constructed attribute, the original rules can be transformed or simplified as follows:

If [volume = 48], then Class 1

If [volume = 96], then Class 2

The second approach applies logical operators in order to aggregate existing descriptions into a higher level of abstraction. The most commonly adopted representation is a concept hierarchy, which represents a generalization process. *A concept hierarchy*, defined on one or more attribute domains, organizes concepts in a hierarchical form or a certain partial order, with higher-level nodes being more general concepts created by grouping several lower-level concepts under a unique name (Carter and Hamilton, 1995; Han, Cai, and Cercone, 1992; Han and Fu, 1994). The most general concept in a concept hierarchy is the *null description* (described by "any"). Figure 11.1 shows some examples of concept hierarchies.

The second approach provides a more semantic-oriented and structured representation than the first approach. We therefore adopt this approach and its underlying representation (that is, concept hierarchy) because it is more intuitively meaningful. In our future research, we plan to develop a more generalized representation capable of expressing both mathematical and logical operators.

FIGURE 11.1. EXAMPLES OF CONCEPT HIERARCHIES AT A UNIVERSITY

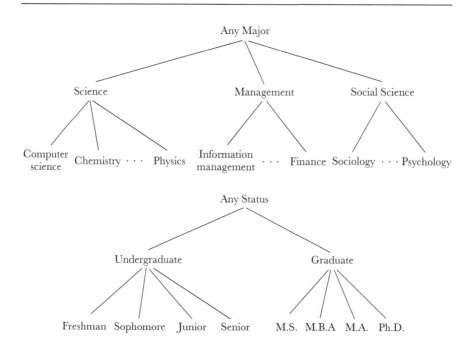

Development of Constructive Clustering Analysis Technique

The traditional clustering problem that uses the silhouette measure for determining the optimal number of clusters can be formulated as follows:

Given	a set of objects described by a set of attributes
Determine	the optimal number of clusters and the characteristics of each cluster

Additional input is required for constructive clustering, including the user-defined concept hierarchies. Therefore, the formulation of a constructive clustering problem is extended as follows:

Given	(1) a set of data, each of which is described by a collection of attributes
	(2) user-defined concept hierarchies

Determine

      (1) the optimal concept space

      (2) the optimal number of clusters within the optimal concept space

      (3) the characteristics of each cluster

In our study, a concept space is different from the description space that is defined for each attribute and that refers to the value domain of the attribute. If a concept hierarchy is provided for an attribute, this attribute essentially consumes multiple description spaces, each of which corresponds to a level in the concept hierarchy. Hence, *a concept space* is a relation of a specific description space for each attribute used to describe objects:

$CS: DS_1 \times \ldots \times DS_n$

where CS denotes the concept space of objects,

      DS_i denotes a specific description space of the attribute i,

      n denotes the total number of attributes used to describe the objects.

Measure for Determining Optimal Concept Space

Based on the described formulation of constructive clustering problems, an important research challenge is how to automatically determine the optimal concept space instead of needing to have that space specified by domain experts. Given a specific concept space that encompasses specific attributes of objects in a data set, the silhouette coefficient can be used to determine the optimal number of clusters, as described earlier. When a higher level of the concept hierarchy is superimposed on an attribute—that is, the attribute ascends one level in its concept hierarchy—the description space of that attribute is transformed into a more generalized description space. If the generalization of the concept space does not always result in increasing or decreasing the average silhouette width of the data set, that measure would be appropriate for selecting the *optimal concept space*—that is, the optimal configuration of concept hierarchies. The optimal concept space results in the maximum silhouette coefficient among all possible concept spaces.

In general, the attributes included in a clustering analysis consist of the following types: binary, nominal, ordinal, and interval. When an attribute moves up one level in its concept hierarchy, what will its attribute type become? This is important because the distance measures for different attribute types are different. For example, the higher concept governing a binary attribute must be "any," because a binary attribute can have only two possible values. When an attribute has the same value for all objects, this attribute makes no contributions to the distance between any two objects. Therefore, the attribute type for the ascent of a binary attribute need not be defined. This can also be applied to any attribute type when the governing concept immediately above it is "any." On the other hand, because a nominal attribute does not imply any order of its values, the ascent of this attribute should not place any demand for order on the generalized values. As a result, the ascent of a nominal attribute also results in a nominal attribute. In addition, the ascent of an ordinal or interval attribute results in an ordinal attribute in which the property of value ordering is preserved, although an equal distance between any two consecutive values may not be required. Table 11.1 summarizes types of original attributes and their ascents.

To show that the generalization of the concept space does not always result in increasing or decreasing the silhouette measure, one has to know whether the ascent of an attribute will bring two objects closer. Properties 1 and 2 address this question. Properties 3 and 4 show the relationship between the generalization of a concept space and the resulting average silhouette width.

Property 1. The ascent of a nominal attribute in its concept hierarchy results in identical or decreased distance between any two objects.

Proof:

Assume the kth attribute to be the target attribute that will ascend one level in its concept hierarchy. The distance measure between objects o_i and o_j can be rewritten as follows:

$$d\left(o_i,o_j\right) = \frac{\sum_{f=1,f\neq k}^{r}\delta\left(f\right)_{ij} d\left(f\right)_{ij}}{\sum_{f=1}^{p}\delta\left(f\right)_{ij}} + \frac{\delta\left(k\right)_{ij} d\left(k\right)_{ij}}{\sum_{f=1}^{p}\delta\left(f\right)_{ij}}$$

If the kth attribute of o_i or o_j contains a missing value, then $\delta\left(k\right)_{ij} = 0$ (that is, the kth attribute does not make any contribution to the distance between o_i or o_j). Thus, the ascent of this attribute (whether it is nominal or not) in its concept hierarchy will result in an identical distance between o_i or o_j. If the kth attribute of either o_i or o_j is a

TABLE 11.1. TYPES OF ATTRIBUTES AFTER THEIR ASCENT IN THE CONCEPT HIERARCHY

Original Attribute Type	Attribute Type After Ascent
Binary	—
Nominal	Nominal
Ordinal	Ordinal
Interval	Ordinal

nonmissing value, the distance between them after the kth attribute ascends one level in its concept hierarchy can be represented as follows:

$$d'\left(o_i, o_j\right) = \frac{\sum\limits_{f=1, f \neq k}^{p} \delta\left(f\right)_{ij}\, d\left(f\right)_{ij}}{\sum\limits_{f=1}^{p} \delta\left(f\right)_{ij}} + \frac{\delta\left(k\right)_{ij}\, d'\left(k\right)_{ij}}{\sum\limits_{f=1}^{p} \delta\left(f\right)_{ij}}$$

Since $\delta(k)_{ij} = 1$, the difference between $d(o_i, o_j)$ and $d'\left(o_i, o_j\right)$ is the difference between $d(k)_{ij}$ and $d'(k)_{ij}$.

Because the kth attribute is nominal, the following characteristics hold:

- $d(k)_{ij}$ is either 1 or 0.
- If the objects o_i and o_j have identical values on the original kth attribute, o_i and o_j will have identical values on the kth attribute after it ascends one level.
- If o_i and o_j have different values on the original kth attribute, o_i and o_j can have either different or identical values on the kth attribute after it ascends one level.

Accordingly, the following can be derived:

- If $d(k)_{ij} = 0$, then $d'(k)_{ij} = 0$.
- If $d(k)_{ij} = 1$, then $d'(k)_{ij}$ or $d'(k)_{ij} = 1$.

Thus, $d(k)_{ij} \geq d'(k)_{ij}$, which means that $d\left(o_i, o_j\right) \geq d'\left(o_i, o_j\right)$ in the case of nonmissing values on the kth attribute. Consequently, it can be concluded that the ascent of a nominal attribute in its concept hierarchy results in identical or decreased distance between any two objects.

Property 2. The ascent of an interval or ordinal attribute in its concept hierarchy results in identical, decreased, or increased distance between any two objects.

Proof:

Assume the kth attribute to be the target attribute that will ascend one level in its concept hierarchy. As proven in property 1, if the kth attribute of either of the objects o_i and o_j contains a missing value, the ascent of this attribute (interval or ordinal) in its concept hierarchy will result in an identical distance between o_i and o_j. Moreover, as described in property 1, if the kth attributes of both objects contain nonmissing values, the difference between $d(o_i, o_j)$ and $d'(o_i, o_j)$ is the difference between $d(k)_{ij}$ and $d'(k)_{ij}$. For example, consider a set of objects whose values of the kth attribute and of the ascent of the kth attribute are represented as follows:

Object	*k*th attribute	Ascent of *k*th attribute
a	1	I
b	2	I
c	3	II
d	4	II
e	5	III

Assume the range of the *k*th attribute in its original description space to be 4 and the range of the *k*th attribute after ascent to be 2. Thus,

$$d(k)_{ac} = \frac{2}{4} = \frac{1}{2} = d'(k)_{ac}$$

$$d(k)_{bc} = \frac{1}{4} < \frac{1}{2} = d'(k)_{bc}$$

$$d(k)_{ad} = \frac{3}{4} > \frac{1}{2} = d'(k)_{ad}$$

From the examples above, it is evident that the ascent of an interval or ordinal attribute in its concept hierarchy results in identical, decreased, or increased distance between any two objects.

Property 3. The ascent of a nominal attribute in its concept hierarchy results in a decreased, increased, or identical average silhouette width for the data set.

Proof:

Recall from our earlier formulation that the silhouette of an object o_i is given by:

$$s(i) = 1 - \frac{a(i)}{b(i)} \qquad \text{if } a(i) < b(i)$$
$$= 0 \qquad \text{if } a(i) = b(i) \text{ or the object } o_i \text{ is the only object in the cluster } A$$
$$= \frac{b(i)}{a(i)} - 1 \qquad \text{if } a(i) > b(i)$$

Assume a set of objects to be classified into two clusters *A* and *B*. According to property 1, the ascent of a nominal attribute in its concept hierarchy will result in identical or decreased distance between any two objects. As illustrated in Figure 11.2, it is possible that, after the ascent of a nominal attribute, the distance of any two objects within cluster *A* or cluster *B* will remain the same while the distance between any object in cluster A and any object in cluster B will decrease. We further assume that the resulting clusters remain the same after the ascent of the nominal attribute. Put simply, one cluster moves toward the other cluster. In this case, for any object o_i in *A* or *B*, $a(i)$ will be the same while $b(i)$ decreases. Thus, $s(i)$ decreases for any object o_i, and the average silhouette width decreases as well in this case.

Another extreme case is where the distance between any two objects in the cluster A decreases while the distance between any object in A and any object in B remains the same after the ascent of a nominal attribute. As shown in Figure 11.3, the area of cluster A shrinks. In this case, most silhouette widths will increase; clusters A and B appear further apart.

It is also possible that the distance between any two objects in the entire data set would remain the same after the ascent of a nominal attribute; that is, $a(i)$ and $b(i)$ would not change. Thus, the silhouette widths would be identical after the ascent of a nominal attribute.

Thus we conclude that the ascent of a nominal attribute in its concept hierarchy would result in a decreased, increased, or identical average silhouette width for the data set.

FIGURE 11.2. ONE POSSIBLE SCENARIO AFTER THE ASCENT OF A NOMINAL ATTRIBUTE (CLUSTER *B* MOVES TOWARD CLUSTER *A*)

Clustering before
the ascent of a
nominal attribute

Cluster A   Cluster B

Clustering after
the ascent of a
nominal attribute

 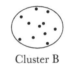

Cluster A   Cluster B

FIGURE 11.3. ANOTHER POSSIBLE SCENARIO AFTER THE ASCENT OF A NOMINAL ATTRIBUTE (CLUSTER *A* SHRINKS)

Clustering before
the ascent of a
nominal attribute

Cluster A   Cluster B

Clustering after
the ascent of a
nominal attribute

Cluster A   Cluster B

Property 4. The ascent of an interval or ordinal attribute in its concept hierarchy results in a decreased, increased, or identical average silhouette width for the data set.

Proof:

According to property 2, the ascent of an interval or ordinal attribute in its concept hierarchy results in identical, decreased, or increased distance between any two objects. Three possible scenarios after the ascent of an interval or ordinal attribute are shown in Figure 11.4. These scenarios correspond respectively to decreased, increased, and identical average silhouette width for the data set after the ascent of an interval or ordinal attribute. The proof is similar to that of property 3.

FIGURE 11.4. THREE POSSIBLE SCENARIOS AFTER THE ASCENT OF AN INTERVAL OR ORDINAL ATTRIBUTE

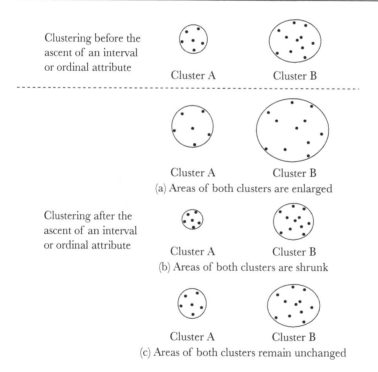

◆ ◆ ◆

In sum, properties 3 and 4 indicate that the ascent of an attribute may result in decreased, increased, or identical average silhouette width of a data set. Hence, the measure of average silhouette width appears appropriate for determining the optimal concept space. The optimal concept space results in the maximum silhouette coefficient among all possible concept spaces.

Constructive Clustering Analysis Algorithm

A constructive clustering analysis algorithm based on the silhouette coefficient measure for selecting the optimal concept space and the optimal number of clusters is presented in Figure 11.5. As shown in the figure, any existing nonconstructive clustering analysis algorithm such as PAM or k-means can be adopted as the core clustering technique of the proposed constructive clustering analysis algorithm. Moreover, the proposed algorithm employs the exhaustive strategy in searching for the optimal concept space and the optimal number of clusters for a specific concept space. The exhaustive search guarantees an optimal solution at the cost of long search time. In fact, a heuristic search strategy can be adopted to find a near optimal solution without incurring an expensive search cost.

FIGURE 11.5. CONSTRUCTIVE CLUSTERING ANALYSIS ALGORITHM

```
Set Optimal-Concept-Space = nil;
Set Best-SC be the lowest possible value;
Set max-clusters = number of objects in the data;
Set Best-cluster-no = 1;
/* Using the exhaustive search to find optimal concept space and optimal cluster number */
For each possible concept space CS_i (including the original concept space)
        Transform data based on CS_i;
        Set Cluster-no = 1;
        Repeat /*find the optimal number of clusters */
                Increment Cluster-no by 1;
                Apply a non-constructive clustering algorithm (e.g., PAM) on the transformed data to cluster
                data into Cluster-no clusters;
                Calculate the average silhouette width on the transformed data;
                If the average silhouette width > Best-SC
                Then    Best-cluster-no = Cluster-no;
                        Best-SC = the average silhouette width;
                        Set Optimal-Concept-Space be CS_i;
                End-if;
        Until Cluster-no > max-clusters;
End-for;
```

Empirical Evaluation

A real-world application has been selected to illustrate the proposed constructive clustering analysis technique, together with encouraging empirical results yielded by the proposed technique. The purpose of the evaluation is not to prove that constructive clustering will always generate better results than nonconstructive clustering techniques. Rather, our intent is to show that the constructive clustering analysis may generate increasingly comprehensible results. Toward this end, we adopted an external criterion approach by measuring the degree of correspondence between the clusters obtained from clustering algorithms and those produced by domain experts.

Application Overview

The Bureau of National Health Insurance (BNHI) in Taiwan is a public health care insurance organization operating six branch offices in different regions of Taiwan. To reduce fraud, reimbursement of claims submitted by health care service providers requires investigative analysis that can be costly. A common strategy for reducing analysis costs is to thoroughly scrutinize claims submitted by less credible service providers and analyze samples of those submitted by other, more credible service providers. To use this strategy effectively, it is essential to discover the inherent structures of the health care providers, based on attributes that are potentially relevant to the credibility assessment.

The data set collected for this study contains 138 health care providers. Each health care provider is represented by eight attributes. The meanings of these attributes are described in the following list and their types as well as their ranges are summarized in Table 11.2.

- *Number of claims:* total number of claims in the past six months
- *Growth rate of claims:* percentage change in the number of claims over the past six months
- *Total claim amount:* total cost of claims (in National Taiwan (NT) dollars) in the past six months
- *Growth rate of claim amount:* percentage change in claim amounts over the past six months
- *Average charge per patient visit:* average charge to a patient per visit (in Taiwan dollars) in the past six months
- *Average prescription charge per patient visit:* average charge for prescription drugs (in Taiwan dollars) per patient visit in the past six months
- *Average diagnosis charge per patient visit:* average charge for diagnosis (in NT dollars) per patient visit in the past six months
- *Disapproval rate:* ratio of total cost of disapproved claims to total cost of claims in the past six months

TABLE 11.2. ATTRIBUTES OF HEALTH CARE PROVIDERS

Attribute	Attribute Type	Range
Number of claims	Interval	613–33,457
Growth rate of claims	Interval	–23.21%–48.84%
Total claim amount	Interval	$208,122–$26,097,418
Growth rate of claim amount	Interval	–74.67%–102.03%
Average charge per patient visit	Interval	$276.47–$1,190.85
Average prescription charge per patient visit	Interval	$7.68–$132.82
Average diagnosis charge per patient visit	Interval	$11.42–$5,005.48
Disapproval rate	Interval	0–0.1

The relevant concept hierarchies provided by the domain experts for the "growth rate of claims" attribute and the "growth rate of claim amount" attribute are shown in Figure 11.6.

Evaluation of Clustering Results

Table 11.3 summarizes the clustering results for health care providers in different concept spaces. Accordingly, when both the growth rate of claims and the growth rate of claim amount ascend one level in the content hierarchy, the silhouette coefficient will be maximal (0.352517). In this case, 138 health care providers are segmented into two clusters. As shown in Table 11.4, in the optimal concept space, health care providers are better separated than in the original concept space because the standardized means of the number of claims, the growth rate of claims, the total claim amount, the growth rate of claim amount, and the average charge per patient visit attributes in the two clusters of the optimal concept space are further apart than those in the two clusters of the original concept space.

To perform the evaluation based on an external criterion approach, BNHI staff, provided with the same set of attributes, were asked to assign a credibility score between 0 and 100 for each health care provider. The resulting credibility scores range from 32.5 to 100. If the average score of one cluster is well separated from that of another cluster, then the concept space used to derive those two clusters better matches experts' decisions than does another concept space in which the clusters are not as well separated. As can be seen in Table 11.5, the clusters of the constructive concept space have more separated means (a difference of 23.9278) and smaller standard deviations (approximately 12 and 17) than those of the original concept space (difference in means of 3.0728; standard deviations of approximately 19 and 17). Thus, evaluated against this external criterion, the constructive clustering analysis technique provides a more conceptually intuitive and interpretive clustering result than the nonconstructive clustering analysis technique in this set of sampled data.

FIGURE 11.6. CONCEPT HIERARCHIES FOR CLUSTERING HEALTH CARE PROVIDERS

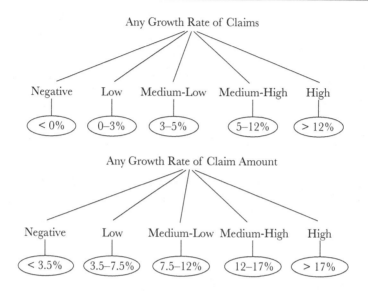

TABLE 11.3. RESULTS OF CLUSTERING HEALTH CARE PROVIDERS

Concept Space	Optimal Number of Clusters	Silhouette Coefficient
Original	2	0.347938
Growth rate of claims[a]	4	0.336275
Growth rate of claim amount[a]	4	0.302334
Growth rate of claims[a] and growth rate of claim amount[a]	2	0.352517[b]

[a]Attribute ascends one level in its concept hierarchy

[b]Maximum silhouette width across different concept spaces

Conclusion

Clustering analysis is one of the few data mining activities that can properly be described as undirected knowledge discovery or unsupervised learning. Due to its undirected nature, clustering is often the best first technique to turn to when dealing with a complex data set with many variables and many internal structures. Once the clustering analysis has discovered regions of the data space that contain similar records, other data mining techniques have a better chance of discovering rules or patterns within them (Berry and Linoff, 1997). Therefore, the quality of clustering analysis is essential because it may affect the results of subsequent analyses based on

TABLE 11.4. COMPARISON OF THE CLUSTERING RESULTS OF ORIGINAL AND OPTIMAL CONCEPT SPACES

Characteristics of Clusters

		Cluster 1		Cluster 2	
Concept Space	Attribute	Mean Value of Attribute	Standardized Mean Value	Mean Value of Attribute	Standardized Mean Value
Original	Number of claims	6887.92	0.19	5225.89	0.14
	Growth rate of claims	3.56%	0.33	−0.81%	0.26
	Total claim amount	5188117	0.19	2991045	0.11
	Growth rate of claim amount	7.34%	0.46	5.27%	0.45
	Average charge per patient visit	521.39	0.27	527.11	0.27
	Average prescription charge per patient visit	35.94	0.23	44.77	0.30
	Average diagnosis charge per patient visit	419.18	0.08	196.23	0.04
	Disapproval rate	−0.40	0.96	−7.81	0.22
Growth rate of claims[a] and growth rate of claim amount[a]	Number of claims	4831.63	0.13	8063.73	0.23
	Growth rate of claims	1.33	0.08	4	0.75
	Total claim amount	2956620	0.11	6090697	0.23
	Growth rate of claim amount	1.29	0.07	3.90	0.73
	Average charge per patient visit	504.51	0.25	549.34	0.30
	Average prescription charge per patient visit	40.63	0.26	38.03	0.24
	Average diagnosis charge per patient visit	290.82	0.06	379.43	0.07
	Disapproval rate	−4.37	0.56	−2.12	0.79

[a]Attribute ascends one level in its concept hierarchy

TABLE 11.5. AVERAGE AND STANDARD DEVIATION OF CREDIBILITY SCORES

Concept Space	Cluster	Average Score	Standard Deviation
Original	Cluster 1	74.0549	19.4470
	Cluster 2	70.9821	17.4165
Growth rate of claims[a] and growth rate of claim amount[a]	Cluster 1	83.0380	12.1599
	Cluster 2	59.1102	16.9988

[a]Attribute ascends one level in its concept hierarchy

other data mining techniques. If the description spaces of attributes used to characterize objects to be clustered are inadequate to reveal the complex inter-attribute structure in the data set, the clustering result as well as subsequent data mining results may also be inadequate. Although the original description spaces may be inadequate, it is possible to transform the original description spaces into concept spaces with higher-level abstractions in which the clustering result exhibits stronger regularity. This approach is referred to as the *constructive clustering analysis.*

The goal of our research is to develop a constructive clustering analysis technique to complement existing clustering techniques. An attribute may be associated with a concept hierarchy. Each level in a concept hierarchy represents a description space with a higher level of abstraction than the one below. An empirical evaluation study, based on a real-world application, shows the usefulness of the proposed constructive clustering analysis technique for generating more interpretative knowledge in order to make credible judgments or predictions about the large number of claims submitted. In the future, an e-health paradigm for processing and analyzing an even larger quantity of such claims data from e-health care providers can also be supported. It is conceivable, for example, that when these claims data are captured on-line directly from various sources, the data can be streamlined, cleaned, and stored in a large-scale data warehouse, in which the data could then be ambitiously mined, sliced, and diced in multiple ways on an automated basis to yield further insights into the nature and credibility of the claims.

Future research work may include an attempt to evaluate the performance of the proposed technique under different core clustering analysis algorithms and search strategies. Also, experts in this research were assumed to know the concept hierarchies, but it would be desirable to generate such hierarchies or adjust predefined concept hierarchies automatically and dynamically based on the characteristics of data encountered. As always, there are many possibilities for combining and integrating different e-health data mining techniques to provide meaningful tools to aid policymakers and e-health decision makers, as shown in the case scenario presented next.

Chapter Questions

1. What is data mining? Why is data mining important in health care and in e-health?
2. What are the critical factors in designing and executing successful data mining projects in e-health care?
3. Analyze key benefits and costs associated with a data mining project, from the perspective of a Web-based health-oriented organization.
4. What are the additional challenges of conducting data mining in e-health care, compared with those commonly observed in business settings?
5. Imagine that you are asked to examine the data of a health care organization in order to differentiate among the case-mix groupings found in the data so as to identify which services are bringing in the most revenues, and why. How would you go about applying the clustering analysis approach to help you perform this task? Discuss the potential limitations of data mining techniques.

References

Anderberg, M. (1973). *Cluster analysis for applications.* New York: Academic Press.

Berry, M., & Linoff, G. (1997). *Data mining techniques: For marketing, sales, and customer support.* New York: Wiley.

Bloedorn, E., & Michalski, R. (1991). Data-driven constructive induction in AQ17-Pre: A method and experiments. In *Proceedings of the Third International Conference on Tools for Artificial Intelligence* (pp. 30–37).

Cabena, P., Hadjinian, P., Stadler, R., Verhees, J., & Zanasi, A. (1997). *Discovering data mining: From concept to implementation.* Englewood Cliffs, NJ: Prentice Hall.

Cai, Y., Cercone, N., & Han, J. (1990). An attribute-oriented approach for learning classification rules from relational databases. In *Proceedings of the Sixth International Conference on Data Engineering* (pp. 281–288), Los Angeles, February.

Carter, C., & Hamilton, H. (1995). A fast, on-line generalization algorithm for knowledge discovery. *Applied Mathematics Letters, 8*(2), 5–11.

Chen, M., Han, J., & Yu, P. (1996). Data mining: An overview from a database perspective. *IEEE Transactions on Knowledge and Data Engineering, 8*(6), 866–883.

Frawley, W., Piatetsky-Shapiro, G., & Matheus, C. (1992, Fall). Knowledge discovery in databases: An overview. *AI Magazine,* pp. 213–228.

Han, J. (1995). Mining knowledge at multiple concept levels. In *Proceedings of 4th International Conference on Information and Knowledge Management* (pp. 19–24), Baltimore, Maryland, November 29 through December 2, 1995.

Han, J., Cai, Y., & Cercone, N. (1992). Knowledge discovery in databases: An attribute-oriented approach. In *Proceedings of the 18th International Conference on Very Large Data Bases* (pp. 547–559), Vancouver, British Columbia, Canada.

Han, J., & Fu, Y. (1994). Dynamic generation and refinement of concept hierarchies for knowledge discovery in databases. In *Proceedings of American Association for Artificial Intelligence '94 Workshop on Knowledge Discovery in Databases* (pp. 157–168), Burnaby, British Columbia, Canada.

Han, J., & Fu, Y. (1995). Discovery of multiple-level association rules from large databases. In *Proceedings of the 21st VLDB Conference* (pp. 420–431), British Columbia, Canada.

Kaufman, L., & Rousseeuw, P. (1990). *Finding groups in data: An introduction to cluster analysis.* New York: Wiley.

Kohonen, T. (1989). *Self-organization and associative memory.* New York: Springer.

Kohonen, T. (1995). *Self-organizing maps.* New York: Springer.

Kramer, S. (1994). CN2-MCI: A two-step method for constructive induction. In *Proceedings of Workshop on Constructive Induction and Change of Representation* (pp. 33–39). New Brunswick, New Jersey, 1994.

Luger, G., & Stubblefield, W. (1993). *Artificial intelligence: Structures and strategies for complex problem solving.* Menlo Park, CA: Benjamin-Cummings.

Ng, R., & Han, J. (1994). Efficient and effective clustering methods for spatial data mining. In *Proceedings of International Conference on Very Large Data Bases* (pp. 144–155), Santiago, Chile, September 1994.

Raghupathi, W., & Tan, J. (2002). Strategic IT applications in health care. *Communications of the ACM, 45*(12), 56–61.

Spath, H. (1980). *Cluster analysis algorithms: For data reduction and classification of objects.* New York: Wiley.

Srikant, R., & Agrawal, R. (1996). Mining sequential patterns: Generalizations and performance improvements. In *Proceedings of the Fifth International Conference on Extending Database Technology*, pp. 487–499, Santiago, Chile, September 1994.

Wei, C., Piramuthu, S., & Shaw, M. (2003). Knowledge discovery and data mining. In C. W. Holsapple (Ed.), *Handbook of Knowledge Management* (Vol. 2, pp.157–189). New York: Springer-Verlag.

Wnek, J., & Michalski, R. (1994). Hypothesis-driven constructive induction in AQ17-HCI: A method and experiments. *Machine Learning, 14*(2), 139–168.

Zait, M., & Messatfa, H. (1997). A comparative study of clustering methods. *Future Generation Computer Systems, 13*, 149–159.

E-Patient Image Retrieval Case: Incremental Neural Net Learning

Lin Lin, Olivia R. Liu Sheng, Chih-Ping Wei, Paul Jen-Hwa Hu, Joseph Tan

E-health intelligence is about the dynamic evolution of knowledge in health care practice. An e-health care decision support system (DSS) that cannot adapt to knowledge change will fail to provide accurate decision support, resulting in possible misdiagnoses and financial loss. Incremental learning in an e-health DSS involves the ability to adaptively acquire new knowledge from changes in data by reusing the knowledge structure that resulted from previous knowledge discovery activities. By saving the time needed to design a new round of knowledge discovery activity, incremental learning allows the construction of more adaptive knowledge discovery systems.

Neural network technology has been applied to a variety of classification problems. However, past research has not fully explored the area of *incremental neural net learning* (Craven and Shavlik, 1997), which is especially useful when one considers the time-consuming process of neural network training. A *multilayer neural network* is composed of an input layer that represents the properties of the real-world objects, an output layer that represents the outcome such as a classification, prediction or diagnosis, one or more hidden layers, and the weight matrices between these layers that capture the mapping from input space to output space (Hammad, 1998).

Neural net incremental learning can be categorized into two types: nonstructural and structural. *Nonstructural learning* focuses on setting new weight matrices based on previous ones, without changing the input or output layer structures of the previously built neural net. Nonstructural learning is applicable to problems that have unchanged input attributes and output classes but experience frequent knowledge pattern changes—for example, handwriting recognition. Several algorithms have been proposed for nonstructural learning (Fritzke, 1994; Hebert and others, 1999; Fu, Hsu, and Principe, 1991; Platt, 1991). *Structural learning* reuses a previously built neural net to construct changed input or output layer structures. It deals with real-world problems that have changing input attributes or output classes. Access to previously unavailable data may lead to the addition of new input attributes. New decision classes or new categorization standards can lead to the addition of new output classes.

Little attention has been given to structural learning. In this case study, we propose a structural incremental neural net learning procedure based on a hidden layer activation model (Ramani, 1992). We demonstrate that this procedure can perform incremental learning when new output classes are added in an intelligent patient image retrieval problem. Incremental structural learning is essential to this problem because of changes in retrieval behavior over time in a neural network. In addition, we present the analysis of results from experiments employing the proposed incremental neural network learning procedure with 200 clinical reading cases.

Intelligent Patient Image Retrieval: Motivation for Incremental Learning

The ability to refer to prior images of a patient is critical to a radiologist's ability to interpret the images generated as part of a radiological examination. Given a set of input attributes such as patient information (age, disease, and so on), reasons for exam, and image information (for example, modality), radiologists must decide which prior images to retrieve. A prior image can be characterized by its relationship with the current examination in terms of anatomical part, modality, and time or sequence. Jointly, these dimensions can construct radiologists' decision outcome classes for underlying image retrieval knowledge. Mapping from input attributes to outcome classes could then be accomplished by classification techniques such as neural networks and decision trees (Sheng, Wei, and Hu, 1998).

Challenges in the use of these classification techniques are posed by several special characteristics associated with image retrieval, such as incomplete input information and multiple decision outcomes (that is, retrieving multiple images in each image-reading instance) (Sheng, Wei, and Hu, 1994). In addition, patient image retrieval is a dynamic and evolving process. The structure of the whole learning task may change. New outcome decision classes may result from the addition of new diagnostic standards and use of new equipment.

We built a back-propagation neural network that achieved effective image retrievals comparable to those based on the knowledge-based approach where case reasoning may be used as the basis of retrieval behavior (Sheng, Wei, and Hu, 1994, 1998). This network also had high noise (that is, uncertainties) tolerance and could deal with multiple outcome problems. However, it did not address the incremental learning issue and could not adapt to dynamic changes in knowledge retrieval. Consequently, when new outcome decision classes were identified in radiologists' evolving image retrieval behavior, the trained neural net had to be discarded and a new network had to be retrained from scratch. The long training time required for a neural network makes this approach extremely expensive.

Among several proposed incremental neural net models, most have dealt with the *catastrophic interference problem.* Briefly, this refers to the situation in which a network "forgets" the solution to task A when it is trained to solve task B based on its previous training in solving task A (McCloskey and Cohen, 1989). A conceivable solution is to restrict each node in the hidden layers within localized regions of the input space so that training may be restricted to specific tasks. Radial basis functions (RBF) networks (Poggio and Girosi, 1990) were derived from this idea, and several constructive extensions to RBF nets have been proposed (Fritzke, 1994; Platt, 1991). Hebert and others (1999) proposed combining a feed-forward network and a self-organized map as an alternative solution based on a similar theoretical foundation. Yet by assuming a fixed neural net architecture (that is, nonstructural incremental learning), almost all the research cited demonstrated seriously limited learning ability of the networks when a new input or output class appeared. For the patient image retrieval process, this limitation is severe.

Ramani (1992) proposed an incremental learning method based on a *hidden layer activation mechanism* that enabled a trained neural net to be reused in building a new net with more output nodes. Neural nets built using this incremental approach performed similarly to the standard trained nets, but the training effort was reduced by a factor of about five. However, the problem addressed (fish classification) was a single-outcome problem (that is, each instance is classified into one outcome class only). Therefore, when samples belonging to the new outcome class were added, the number of samples belonging to old outcome classes was not affected. We wanted to examine how this algorithm performs in a multiple-outcome problem, where adding samples belonging to new outcome classes may also affect the number of samples belonging to old outcome classes. In addition, in Ramani's original experiment, only one set of data belonging to the new class was added to the original data set. As a result, it is not possible to determine whether the size of a sample (that is, the number of instances corresponding to the new class) had an effect on the performance of the incremental learning. Intuitively, it seems that the size of a newly added outcome class should affect the learning performance.

Here, we describe a neural network based on the hidden layer activation mechanism in order to address two research questions:

- Will this algorithm work for a multiple-outcome learning problem in which the addition of samples belonging to new outcome classes may affect the distribution of data in other output classes?
- Will the size of a new class affect incremental learning performance?

Hidden Layer Activation for Incremental Learning

Our incremental learning algorithm is based on the fact that the hidden layer in a three-layer neural net acts as a feature detector by means of pattern recognition and classification. We keep all the weights from input layer to hidden layer intact, even if a new output class is added. However, one additional output node will be in the output layer, and we still need to modify the weight matrix between the hidden layer and the output layer.

The proposed procedure is as follows: (1) Use the original data set to train a neural network. (2) Add the examples that contain the new output class into the data set, then use the whole set (the original set plus the new class) to compute the activations of the hidden layer. (3) Using these values as training data, train a two-layer network. (If the original neural network contains h hidden layer nodes and o output layer nodes, this two-layer net should contain h input layer nodes and $o+1$ output layer nodes.) (4) Replace the second half (hidden and output layers) of the original network with the newly trained two-layer net to get the desired new three-layer neural net.

Theoretically, a network created this way should perform as well as a new network created from scratch, but because the number of weights to be updated is much smaller, training time should be considerably shorter.

Evaluation of the Incremental Learning Procedure in E-Patient Image Retrieval Problem

In the following section, we turn to the evaluation of the incremental learning procedure in our e-patient image retrieval experiments.

Data. The data set in our experiments included two hundred cases for which clinical readings had been performed by radiologists or residents at University Medical Center, University of Arizona (Sheng, Wei, and Hu, 1998). Each case contained sufficient information to code the fourteen input attributes and twenty-six outcome classes derived from previous studies. The input attributes describe the characteristics of the patient, his or her disease, and the current examination. The output attributes include information such as recency, anatomical part, and modality of the retrieved images. Detailed descriptions for all twenty-six outcome classes are provided by Sheng, Wei, and Hu (1998).

Neural Network Models. In this study, we used three-layer neural networks to capture image retrieval knowledge. Two-layer neural networks were also used in the
process of incremental learning in previous research. Input attributes and output classes
were represented with a local scheme—that is, a one-to-one matching between an
input attribute value (or output class) and an input node (or output node). As a result,
there were sixty-four input nodes and twenty-six output nodes in the network that
was trained with the 200-case data set. Input nodes could take values of either 0 or 1,
and output nodes had activations between 0 and 1, inclusive. We set a *threshold value*
to decide whether the image represented by a certain output node would be retrieved
(1) or not (0). There were forty-five hidden layer nodes. In order to simulate the learning capacity of the net, all weights were initialized to random values between –0.05
and +0.05. We used a search-then-converge strategy in which the initial learning
rate r_0 remained constant for *T* epochs (search time) and then became $\frac{r_0}{1 + \frac{t}{T}}$, where
t was the current number of epochs. We chose an initial learning rate of 0.5, a search
time of 32 epochs, and a momentum of 0. The threshold was set to 0.5. We adopted
all these parameters on the basis of a series of Turing experiments, which are reported
in Sheng, Wei, and Hu (1998).

Procedure. To simulate the incremental learning problem, we eliminated all instances
in the 200-case data set that contained a certain outcome class. We then had a data
set with only twenty-five outcome classes. A neural net was trained with this data set.
The examples that had been removed were then added back to the data set as the
twenty-sixth class. This whole data set was then used to train two neural networks,
one built from scratch, the other built using the incremental procedure. The perfor-
mances of these two nets were then analyzed.

Because a single train-and-test process may generate misleading performance estimates when the sample size is relatively small, the data set was divided into four equal
parts, three to be used for training and one for testing. This is to ensure that the neural
net is properly and adequately trained. Thus, the experimental process was repeated
four times, once for each quarter of the data set. The learning performance was estimated by the average of the performance results from four individual processes.

For each of the six output classes we chose to perform the incremental learning,
we followed the training and testing procedures just described. The reason for choosing these six classes is given in the results section below.

Performance Evaluations. The effectiveness of our network was measured by two
variables, precision rate and recall rate. The *precision rate* is the percentage of images
that the network suggests that were actually referenced by a radiologist. Thus, the precision rate demonstrates the efficiency of the learning system and is closely related to
its level of false positives. The *recall rate* is the percentage of the images referenced by
a radiologist that the network correctly suggests. It demonstrates the power of the learning system by revealing its level of false negatives. To measure the training effort of the
neural network, we defined a *time reduction factor,* the training time of a net built from

scratch divided by the training time of the incremental net. Given the fact that all experiments were done on the same machine with no other process running in the background, this ratio could roughly reflect the difference in training effort.

In our data set, the number of samples in each outcome class varies. To detect whether the size of samples in a new outcome class has an effect on the incremental learning performance, we also included a variable named *incremental ratio,* the number of samples in the new output class divided by the total number of samples in all old output classes. For example, if there are 150 examples in the original data set, and 50 examples belonging to a new class are added, then the incremental ratio for this new class is 50/150 = 33.33 percent.

Experiment Results. The incremental rates of the twenty-six output classes in the 200-case data set mostly were less than 5 percent. We postulated that the addition of these classes would not typically be a problem. Six outcome classes had more significant incremental ratios, between 5 percent and 60 percent. We further divided the six classes into three categories: classes with an incremental ratio of more than 50 percent are *strong incremental* classes; classes with a ratio between 15 percent and 50 percent are *moderate incremental* classes; and classes with a ratio between 5 percent and 15 percent are *weak incremental* classes. Each category contains two outcome classes. We then performed six groups of experiments—one for each of the six outcome classes—following the procedure as discussed previously.

Exhibit 11.1 summarizes our experimental results. Comparing the performance of the neural nets that were trained by using our incremental strategy with the performance of nets built from scratch, we find a slight decrease in precision rate and a slight increase in recall rate. The decrease in precision rate corresponds to an increased average number of images retrieved and might be a direct result of the increased total number of output classes.

In examining the time reduction ratio for each of the six incremental learning procedures, we observed a fourfold reduction in training time in all six experiments, as shown in Exhibit 11.2. The theoretical foundation for the reduction in training effort is based on the smaller number of weight updates required. To train a neural net of x inputs, y hidden nodes, and z outputs, a total of $y \cdot (x + z)$ weights need to be updated in a single training run. The weight updates needed for a single training run in the incremental process is only $y \cdot (z + 1)$. Using the same training procedures, the time reduction factor should be about $\frac{(x + z)}{(z + 1)}$. Although this is a simplified estimation(the number of training epochs may be different), it should predict the time reduction ratio to some extent.

Using this estimation, the expected time reduction factor in Ramani's problem domain is about 27, but the result reported in his work showed a reduction factor of only 5. In our study, the expected time reduction factor was about 3.46; the incremental procedure results exceeded our expectation. The different results might be due to different calculation power. In the Ramani study, the calculation power may be the speed-limiting step.

EXHIBIT 11.1. PERFORMANCE OF INCREMENTAL NEURAL NETWORKS IN SIX EXPERIMENTAL GROUPS

Experiment	Output Class Added	Precision Rate of the Incrementally Trained Nets (percentage)	Precision Rate of the Net Built from Scratch (percentage)	Recall Rate of the Incrementally Trained Nets (percentage)	Recall Rate of the Net Built from Scratch (percentage)
1	2	76.73		76.58	
2	3	75.43		75.35	
3	6	70.79	78.22	66.64	71.84
4	7	79.32		75.12	
5	11	76.80		72.18	
6	16	77.58		73.32	
Average		76.11	78.22	73.20	71.84

EXHIBIT 11.2. INCREMENTAL RATIO AND TIME REDUCTION RATIO OF THE TESTED CLASSES

Category	Class	Incremental Ratio	Training Time for the Old Neural Network	Time Reduction Ratio
Strong Incremental	2	58.73		4.9101
	6	53.85		4.2256
Moderate Incremental	7	21.21		4.6789
	11	15.03	1,057,000.17 ms	4.4442
Weak Incremental	3	11.11		4.2459
	16	9.29		4.0343
Average				4.4232

Conclusion

In our case study, an incremental neural net learning procedure was applied to build an adaptive intelligent e-patient image retrieval system. The results led to the following conclusions. First, the incremental learning procedure we applied decreased the training effort by a factor of approximately four without hurting the performance of the network. Second, the multiple-outcome nature of the image retrieval problem has no significant effect on the performance of the incremental learning. This strongly supports our hypothesis that the hidden layer activation acts as a feature detector. Third, the performance of the incremental learning process was not affected by the sample size of the new output class, as reflected by the incremental ratio. Finally, we witnessed similar time reduction, precision rates, and recall rates in the three incremental training groups.

We observed a slight increase in recall and decrease in precision in the nets trained by the incremental learning procedure. Sheng, Wei, and Hu (1998) indicate that recall rate is a more important index than precision rate in patient image retrieval. Whether this increase in recall is a random phenomenon is still to be investigated. An interesting finding is that the incremental ratio, which to some extent reflects the impact of new samples on training effort, does not significantly affect the performance of the incremental learning procedure, perhaps because of the small amount of data. Larger samples are being used in an investigation currently under way. Indeed, several alternative incremental learning approaches do not employ neural networks (for example, Bayesian approaches, incremental decision trees). Hence, one future research direction would be to compare the performance of the incremental neural net with one of these other methods.

Case Questions

1. In this case, we demonstrate how machine learning algorithms (specifically, those in neural networks) can help radiologists in their decision-making processes. Identify two other decision-making processes that are common in health care practice.
2. For each of the decision-making process you named in question 1, identify potential inputs (for example, patient information) and decision outcomes (for example, a particular diagnostic decision).
3. Discuss the potential of using a classification algorithm such as a neural network to aid the decision-making processes you discussed in questions 1 and 2.
4. In the decision-making processes that you identified, does practitioners' knowledge evolve over time?
5. What is structural learning? What is nonstructural learning? What types of knowledge evolution problems do they deal with?
6. In the decision-making processes that you identified, is the application of structural learning or nonstructural learning necessary? Why?

References

Craven, M. W., & Shavlik, J. W. (1997). Using neural networks for data mining. *Future Generation Computer Systems, 13,* 211–229.

Fritzke, B. (1994). Growing cell structures: A self-organizing network for unsupervised and supervised learning. *Neural Networks, 7*(9), 1441–1460.

Fu, L., Hsu, H., & Principe, J. C. (1991). Incremental backpropagation learning networks. *IEEE Transactions on Neural Networks, 2*(3), 334–345.

Hammad, T. (1998). Computational intelligence: Neural networks methodology for health decision support. In J. Tan with S. Sheps, *Health decision support systems.* Sudbury, MA: Jones & Bartlett.

Hebert, J. F., Parizeau, M., Ghazzali, N. (1999). Cursive character detection using incremental learning. In *Proceedings of the Fifth International Conference on Document Analysis and Recognition* (pp. 808–811).

McCloskey, M., & Cohen, N. J. (1989). Catastrophic interference in connectionist networks: The sequential learning problems. *Psychology of Learning and Motivation, 24,* 109–165.

Platt, J. C. (1991). A resource–allocation network for function interpolation. *Neural Computation,* NC-3, 213–225.

Poggio, T., & Girosi, F. (1990). Networks for approximation and learning. *Proceedings of IEEE, 78*(9), 1481–1497.

Ramani, N. (1992). Incremental learning using hidden layer activations: Tests on fish identification data. In *Proceedings of International Joint Conference on Neural Networks* (Vol. 1, pp. 640–645), INSPEC Accession Number: 4417423, Baltimore, MD, USA.

Sheng, O. L., Wei, C. P., & Hu, P. J. (1994). Engineering patient image retrieval knowledge. *Journal of Knowledge Engineering and Technology, 7*(2), 44–60.

Sheng, O. L., Wei, C. P. & Hu, P. J. (1998). Neural network learning for intelligent patient image retrieval. *IEEE Intelligent Systems, 13*(1), 49–57.

PART FOUR

E-HEALTH STRATEGIES AND IMPACTS

Part Three highlighted how various e-health domains and applications are interrelated, with a focus on e-medicine and associated processes (for example, e-diagnosis). Part Four shows how the management of e-health affects the health care and health services industry. Chapter Twelve provides a comprehensive review of e-health strategies and applies e-business models and e-marketing concepts to e-health services. Chapter Thirteen focuses on e-health care technology management, covering the benefits and challenges of e-surveying health administrators and executive team members in order to generate a management perspective and measure success factors in e-health care technology management. Chapter Fourteen reflects the concern that all e-health stakeholders share in regard to the privacy and security issues involved in e-health data integration and aggregation. Chapter Fifteen articulates the positive impacts of e-technologies in many areas of the health care and health services sector. Chapter Fifteen also discusses the stages of e-health evolution and the future of e-technologies in the health care industry.

CHAPTER TWELVE

E-HEALTH STRATEGIES

Reshaping the Traditional Health Care System

H. Joseph Wen, Joseph Tan

Learning Objectives

1. Identify the e-stakeholders in the emerging e-health care system and environment
2. Conceptualize a general framework for mapping e-health strategies based on e-health business structures and their value propositions
3. Identify opportunities and challenges in e-health business strategies
4. Apply e-business models and e-marketing services concepts to e-health services, and understand the complexity of applying these concepts to e-commercialize health care products and services
5. Recognize the range and scope of e-health services

Introduction

E-consumers today have unprecedented access to volumes of information on almost every health topic that one can imagine. Use of the Internet has become pervasive and routine in no more than eight years. By comparison, television took almost twenty-six years to achieve similar penetration among U.S. consumers (Chin, 2000). One of the most remarkable health revolutions in this era is the availability and accessibility of e-health information on the Internet and the World Wide Web. Health care organizations that maintain Web sites run the gamut from networks of alternative, complementary, and integrative medicine practitioners and users (www.pandamedicine. com, www.healthpyramid.com) to pharmaceutical giants (www.merck.com) and health e-commerce aggregators (www.webMD.com). This wide-ranging array of e-health data resources offers the layperson access to more information, and possibly education, than ever before. The AltaVista search engine, for example, returns over 45,000 hits on the comparatively obscure subject of endocarditis. Any popular search engine will yield a comparatively large number of hits on almost any health topic. Even rare ailments and diseases will return at least a few hits.

This new phenomenon of widely available consumer health information has given rise to increase expectation for greater access to better-quality e-health information, education, and services. Where patients previously had the two alternatives of following a doctor's advice blindly or spending countless hours in a library trying to make sense of scholarly medical journals, now most health care consumer–focused sites feature detailed and readily comprehensible content tailored to a largely layperson audience. Nonetheless, e-consumers want and continue to expect to have much more control over their health than they do today. This chapter discusses means of bridging the gaps between what e-consumers want and what they are getting.

As indicated in Part One of this text, a successful e-health strategy must take into consideration the following components of an e-health system: (1) the *community* of e-stakeholders, (2) the *characteristics* of the e-health service model, (3) the *value propositions* of the e-health business, (4) the potential for a *critical mass* of transactions to be processed to ensure revenue generation and sustainability, and (5) the *potential to accommodate future developments* of the e-health business service. E-providers will need to continually rethink their e-health strategies in order to capitalize on the changing dynamics of e-health perspectives and infrastructures (Part Two), e-technologies and applications (Part Three), and the e-health marketplace (Part Four). In this chapter, our focus will be on e-health strategies, the opportunities and challenges facing e-stakeholders, and the steps needed to move from traditional brick-and-mortar health care business models to viable e-health care business models and services.

E-Health Strategic Framework

With escalating costs in health care, increasing turbulence in the Internet commerce environment, and growing uncertainties, traditional health care providers are under enormous pressure to provide new ideas and innovative ways of delivering health care products and services. As we have seen throughout this text, many would-be e-care providers are still struggling with a very basic yet difficult question: What is an appropriate e-health strategy to satisfy an identified e-health service need? Health care planners, administrators, and managers today are challenged to rethink, redesign, and reshape the current health care system. The e-health market system facilitates rapid access to information for all stakeholders involved in e-health care processes—for example, e-patients, e-physicians, e-care providers, e-vendors, and e-insurers or e-payers. Figure 12.1 depicts the relationships among e-stakeholders in a consumer-centered e-health marketplace.

Use of e-technologies enables e-caregivers not only to retrieve but also to process information on the Web. Like other e-commerce ventures, e-health services must provide e-consumers with what they want, when they want it in order to proliferate and become successful. For instance, a consumer-oriented e-prescription solution must offer patients who need prescription refills the opportunity to register, order, pay, and request additional services on-line. Comparatively few applications (beyond content) have actually been used by physicians or patients even though many companies and traditional health care organizations have great ideas about potential e-health strategies. In other words, while a lot of health-related content exists on-line, there is not a lot of e-health commerce in place (Fotsch, 2002; Allsop and Taket, 2003; Trevor Rohm, 2002). For the most part, health-related sites are not generating revenue; they are merely providing information.

As patients and e-consumers become informed and thus more able to make informed choices about their health and alternative modes of health care services, a new marketplace for e-health-related services will emerge. Indeed, a large portion of

FIGURE 12.1. STAKEHOLDERS IN THE E-HEALTH MARKETPLACE

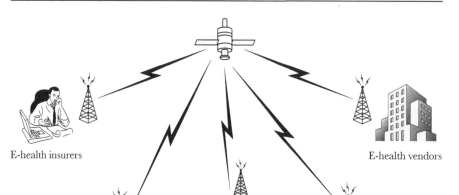

revenues for many health Web sites has come from advertising and spending on on-line health-related services will soon exceed several hundred million dollars (Haugh, 2001). Through the evolution of e-health, health care industry leaders who understand and respond to the needs and wants of e-consumers will prosper and expand services (www.WebMD.com) while others teeter on the brink of failure and bleed millions of dollars (www.drkoop.com). Continued success will go to those whose sites embrace, serve, and focus on the needs of the growing population of sophisticated e-consumers.

This section proposes a basic e-health care framework to enhance our discussion on e-health strategies, including designing, planning, and implementing nontraditional e-health care delivery modalities. Basically, a strategic e-health care framework may be thought of as a unique coupling of an organization's e-health business structure (supported by a proven business model) to satisfy the identified business needs or to leverage on strategic opportunities with a set of value propositions. Popular e-business structures include business-to-consumer (B2C) or business-to-business (B2B) service models whereas the value propositions can be some or a combination of specific performance benefits and/or goals such as achieving greater efficiency, convenience, effectiveness, affordability, accessibility, and intelligence. For instance, business-to-business (B2B) channels have been used widely by e-vendors in different ways to satisfy the need for connectivity between suppliers and purchasers. In this regard, health care procurement is an area ripe to benefit from e-technologies. For years, hospital procurement processes have been tedious, notoriously inefficient, and paperwork-intensive. Efficient B2B relationships with adequate technology can better fulfill health care system supply needs. The typical hospital purchases supplies from several hundred suppliers. E-vendors who bring together numerous suppliers can offer convenient one-stop shopping solutions for health care organizations. Auctions and reverse auctions of medical supplies and diagnostic equipment are becoming another popular alternative to traditional procurement methods. Hospitals can bid on a wide variety of items and potentially save large sums. Reverse auctions allow health care organizations to post lists of the supply items that they require and watch as vendors bid down the price to supply their needs. For example, an urban teaching hospital that has purchased a magnetic resonance imaging device to replace aging X-ray machines may want to sell those machines cheaply, while a small rural hospital may be looking for just those machines.

We now turn to a very general discussion of the similarities and differences between a typical virtual doctor visit and its traditional counterpart to further illustrate our strategic e-health framework concept. As we have noted, virtual visits represent a particularly attractive service strategy in today's e-health marketplace.

Most physician e-consultations begin with a patient having a health problem—for example, arthritis, hair loss, back pain, or some other symptom. A request for an e-consultation is initiated when the patient logs into the servicing Web site. For first-time visitors, the Web site can prompt for answers to some background questions; this is not much different from a physical doctor's office visit. Even when consulting in person, physicians depend on the honesty and accuracy of patient self-reports in order to dispense the proper treatment. Of course, visible physical ailments can be detected in person but are difficult and often impossible to perceive in e-consultations. In the future, e-technologies such as inexpensive, interactive Web-based videoconferencing may diminish this difference between physical and virtual consultations.

Another key step is for the e-patient to provide acceptable information on means of payment. Again, this is no different than checking in at the doctor's office and providing a health insurance card. After the payment information is received, the fees are displayed. Once the e-patient has been accepted for e-consultation and has agreed to the fee structure, he or she will be asked to describe current medical problems, including precise information about symptoms—that is, how often, where, and when the problems occur, what solutions have already been tried (if any), what makes the problems worse, what medications have previously alleviated the problems, and what treatments have been arranged to resolve the problems. This information completes the initial e-patient record.

After the patient profile is submitted, the site matches the e-patient with a local, experienced, board-certified physician from nationwide e-physician networks. Within twenty-four hours, the e-patient receives an e-mail notification from the Web site that connects the patient to an on-line physician for e-consultation. When the patient is back on the site, he or she will receive a message from the e-physician outlining the treatment plan or a request for more information. The interactions between the e-patient and the e-physician will continue asynchronously until the e-consultation process is completed. As a further enhancement, virtual doctor sites can be programmed to provide e-patients with the opportunity to choose a language other than English for their health communications. Additional features can include a quick link to on-line pharmacy chains coordinated with the patient's country of residence, a toll-free telephone number in countries where that service is available, as well as on-line customer service representatives to help e-patients get through the e-prescription process.

Placing this in our e-health strategic framework, we may argue that here, the e-business structure has been conceived as a business-to-consumer (B2C) service model. Moreover, its value propositions are many, especially when compared with traditional doctor visits—for example, greater convenience, faster accessibility, more efficient patient data collection and processing, more intelligent knowledge management capability, improved payment and cost billing processes, and time savings for e-physicians in interacting with e-patients. Like traditional office visits, e-consultation sessions will provide valuable information flow from e-patients to e-physicians and vice versa. E-consultation is also an affordable and economical solution for non-emergency problems from the standpoint of third-party payers, regardless of the geographic locations of the patients.

We will now look at how different e-health strategies support various e-health business structures. The discussion will then be extended to include e-business value propositions.

E-Health Business Structures

A simplified categorization of e-health business structures (Bernard, 2000; Goldstein, 2000) divides them into "click-and-mortar" e-health models and virtual business models and services as shown in Table 12.1.

Click-and-mortar corporations are mostly traditional health care product and service providers. These organizations use the Internet ("click") to support but not replace their company's main business activities (which take place in brick-and-mortar facilities); hence, the term *click-and-mortar* is used to describe them. They do not limit themselves to just marketing on the Web. In fact, they often primarily use traditional advertising and marketing strategies in order to meet their business goals and marketing objectives. The "E-Health Models and Services" section later in this chapter offers some examples of click-and-mortar e-health models.

The *virtual e-health business models and services,* in contrast, use the Internet to build a virtual organization—an independent, profitable venture that exists mainly on the

TABLE 12.1. E-HEALTH BUSINESS STRUCTURES

	Click-and-Mortar E-Health Models	Virtual E-Health Models and Services
Definition and Characteristics	Use the Internet as a supplement to traditional marketing, delivering additional benefits to customers and building relationships with them	Use the Internet to construct an independent, profitable venture that exists mainly on the Internet.
Competitive Strategies	• Build brand awareness and improve image • Use the Web as a cost-effective way to augment core products with related information and service functions • Obtain cost savings from automating routine customer services	• Provide convenience to customers that competitors cannot match • Provide extra information in a form that competitors cannot imitate • Use the Internet to produce superior economic benefits for customers that competitors cannot imitate
Merits	• Provide large quantities of information to customers • Give a company an instant global presence and attracts people who are not the company's current customers but potentially will be • Open a new communication channel, allowing a company to develop further relationships with customers All at a reasonable cost	• Provide a larger or more specialized selection of products than competitors can offer • Offer higher-quality information, more economic benefits, and more convenience than competitors can offer • Provide a sense of community for customers

Internet. Visitors can browse through the catalogue and order products on-line. Although there are still some obstacles (for example, data standards, information privacy and confidentiality, and transactional security), it seems that most organizations are likely to benefit directly from transacting business on the Internet, especially small and medium-sized health care organizations. Some successful cases of virtual e-health organizations are mentioned later, in the "E-Health Models and Services" section.

E-Health Business Value Propositions

E-health business *value propositions* define the relationship between e-provider offerings and e-consumer purchases by identifying how the e-provider fulfills the customer's needs across a range of tasks, functions, and activities (Band, 2000; Clarke, 2001; Porter, 1998). In e-health care, consumers can include not only individual purchasers (for example, a patient, a home caregiver, or a physician) but also large group purchasers such as business organizations (for example, a health care retailer, a hospital, or a health maintenance organization such as the Henry Ford Health Systems); communities or e-communities (for example, a senior group, a virtual community, or a sociopolitical advocacy group such as Greenpeace); and even multinational corporations (for example, General Motors).

E-providers and e-suppliers perceive value arising out of reduced consumer search costs, product and service promotion costs, and business transaction costs. Similarly, e-consumers perceive value arising out of reduced product and service search costs and transaction costs. In addition, customer-focused e-health services also provide improved shopping experiences and user convenience.

Health care institutions have been slow to migrate to automation and invest in e-technologies because of their lack of understanding of e-health strategic frameworks, among other reasons, not to mention the tremendous cost of major system planning and implementation in a period when the rapid migration to managed care has left many health care organizations struggling just to keep the lights and heat on. To invest in multimillion-dollar computing hardware and infrastructure development, knowing that the system will begin moving toward obsolescence before it is even implemented, is a terrifying proposition. Moreover, after seeing many of their competitors take the initiative in making significant investments in technology infrastructures and not realize any significant returns over several years, health managers and administrators have been very hesitant to plunge into e-health strategic development. In light of this, we look next at e-health strategic opportunities and challenges.

E-Health Strategic Opportunities and Challenges

While some data demonstrate that e-health investments have reduced the cost of doing business, demonstrable returns on e-health have not been widespread, perhaps because hospitals are just beginning to experiment with the Internet and because few truly effective and integration-friendly systems are available to e-providers. Most traditional hospitals and health maintenance organizations (HMOs) are burdened with old and inflexible legacy systems that were created before many of today's Web programmers were born. Major health care information system vendors and companies such as Eclipsys, McKesson Corporation, and Siemens Health Services are still scrambling to adapt their proprietary mainframe information systems for the Web.

To make the most of the Internet, however, both traditional and e-health providers need to look beyond the short-term challenges of cost cutting and staff reductions to embrace long-term vision and commitment to the opportunities offered by e-health initiatives. A successful e-health strategy needs to emphasize the primary benefits that e-health offers to the business goals of the organization. Customer acquisition and re-tention, customer satisfaction, relationship building, and provision of better-quality health care are but a few of the many benefits that await e-providers with the proper vision.

Physician-Patient Relationship Management

The cornerstone of the health care industry is the physician-patient relationship. Doctors make up the front line of health care and are the key gatekeepers to health services delivery systems for patients. Since the days of Hippocrates, the relationship between patient and physician provider has been close and very personal. The Internet is poised to change this relationship forever; it is hoped that this change will be for the better.

An increasing number of e-consumers are planning to change health plans and physicians in order to fulfill their desire to receive health care services on-line. Recently, the consulting firm Deloitte & Touche conducted three studies of e-health and health consumer desires. About 25 percent of respondents stated that they would be willing to switch to a health plan that offers on-line health benefits management, and a sim-ilar number indicated a willingness to switch physicians in order to establish on-line communication links regarding health concerns. Moreover, almost 35 percent of the re-spondents stated their willingness to pay up to $5 per month for the convenience of managing benefits on-line, while almost 25 percent expressed willingness to pay an ad-ditional amount for on-line physician interaction (Baldwin, 2001).

Today, although the house call is no longer practical, the Internet is enabling home health care monitoring and telecare delivery (see Chapter Nine). Health Hero Network of Mountain View, California, now markets a device called the Health Buddy, which is essentially a terminal connected to a central server via the Internet. This device monitors homebound patients by asking them questions throughout the day—for example, "How do you feel?" and "Have you taken your medication?" Assistance for the e-patient may then be followed-up or dispatched based on certain answers or a lack of response. Other advanced e-technologies that are coming to market will allow e-patients to digitally transmit blood sugar readings or peak flow data to health care providers.

Another application that offers great value to e-patients and e-providers is e-medicine services, which support two-way video and audio links that bring the ex-pertise of medical specialists to rural and underserved areas. One of the most suc-cessful subspecialties in this area is teleradiology (see the case in Chapter Ten). When e-medicine is implemented, health care quality is greatly improved for the populations served at a very reasonable cost. Virtual doctor visits, or e-consultations, are probably the most promising proposed e-health service application (Parente, 2000). Here, e-patients with non-emergency problems visit a virtual doctor. A compendium of health problems and solutions will be discussed in on-line forums for e-physicians to help with their diagnoses. The site will customize its information based on needs of the e-patient, classifying patients according to DRGs. E-consultations will also offer a great opportunity to up-sell (introduce higher-priced products or services) or cross-sell (introduce products or services related to the customer's original purchase) to patients. For instance, owners of e-consultation Web sites might strike a deal with drug and medical supply superstores and other sites to encourage customers to shop on the same visit when they connect with the virtual doctor. In return, owners of their sites might get free samples of medical supplies that they could ship to new online customers in order to build customer loyalty. Finally, given that employees can choose a virtual doctor visit instead of taking half a day off to see a doctor, employers are likely to be big supporters of the new technology. Many employers, in the service of increasing productivity and reducing absenteeism, will probably push their employees to buy in to e-consultation systems.

Opportunities to Meet Physician Needs

The Internet has also revolutionized medical education via e-learning, opening up a global learning community that allows quick and easy communication and collaboration among e-health providers. Broadband Internet connections support the transmission of large amounts of data, allowing e-physicians to participate in multimedia learning experiences with colleagues around the country and the world. Busy physicians can also use prepackaged computer-based education sessions at their convenience to increase skills and gain medical continuing education units. As well, personal data assistants (PDAs) are increasingly used to access computer-assisted instruction programs and as repositories for medical reference materials.

Physicians are increasingly embracing on-line technologies. One reason is that technology companies are recognizing the uniqueness of a physician's work flow and developing systems customized to that pattern. In fact, a few major players have joined forces specifically to cater to this market; Pfizer, IBM, and Microsoft have formed a joint venture to provide customized information technology services to physician practices as an application service provider. The new company will provide practice management solutions, registration, scheduling, billing, and a suite of integrated clinical applications served via Microsoft's new .NET Enterprise Server platform, Windows 2000, and wireless devices (Fonseca, 2001; Hill, 2001; Perkins, 2001). This alliance has the potential to revolutionize physician practices and bring the physician community squarely into the e-health arena. The company faces an uphill battle against the reluctance that the profession has exhibited toward information technology ventures in the past. Success in this market will require strong leadership and dedication to educating skeptical physicians.

E-Health Opportunities for E-Stakeholders

We will now discuss e-health opportunities and challenges from the perspectives of e-providers, e-vendors, e-payers, and other e-stakeholders.

At the e-health provider level, great potential exists for positive gains if e-technology is leveraged appropriately. These gains will accrue not only to the health care system through reduced costs and increased efficiencies but also more generally to the e-consumers.

Despite the use of computers, most hospitals and health provider organizations remain paperwork-intensive organizations. While many clinical information and order management systems exist to deal with the countless orders and requests for pharmacy, radiology, dietary, and other services, nurses, doctors, and other practitioners still complete much of their key documentation on paper forms. In the average physician's office or hospital, you will be asked to fill out paper after paper, repeating your health insurance or social security number and personal information for almost every provider or referral service that you encounter.

E-providers must build a virtual presence in the e-health marketplace that appeals to e-consumers. This virtual environment would eliminate the repetitive paperwork because information would be linked automatically in the new environment. As this is a new marketplace where dynamic changes can be expected, among the first learning steps will be to building a virtual presence. This may include learning from other successful e-businesses such as Amazon.com; offering more customization and personalization on existing Web sites; building valuable and sustainable long-term customer relationships through virtual connectivity; and becoming more acceptable to the public by pre-marketing survey of proposed business model. For many e-providers, a change in culture and attitude may be necessary. E-providers will be able to realize true value from e-health only when and if they can leverage their massive stores of patient and health information to give e-consumers the services that they want through a convenient and easy-to-use interface. One good example is the e-commercialization of drug prescription orders among physicians, patients, and retailing pharmacies.

In part because little regulation is in place, prescribing drugs over the Internet is controversial. Nonetheless, on-line prescriptions for pharmaceuticals such as Viagra are already available through Web sites such as viagrapurchase.com, which promises forty-eight-hour delivery. Other e-prescription sites include at-cost-drugs.com, e-scripts-md.com, drugsexpress.net, birthcontrol.com, getthepill.com, mammaknows.com, and kwikmed.com. Pharmaceutical refills have been identified as a high-volume, high-dollar niche market that may be just right for the Internet. Mail-order pharmacies may rapidly become obsolete in the face of Internet competitors. CVS (www.CVS.com), a drugstore chain, offers on-line prescription pharmaceutical purchases. Firms such as drugstore.com are just getting started. Selling pharmaceuticals requires state licenses, which has slowed but not halted the arrival of on-line access to drug refills. On-line prices are competitive with the deepest discounts available elsewhere and offer the convenience of next-day home delivery. The nation's most active health Web site, drkoop.com, offers pharmaceutical refills and free "drug checker" software to screen for drug compatibility. Other prescription sites include WebRx.com, HomeCareAmerica.com, and MedQue.com.

Hospitals are also exploiting network-based materials management systems from companies such as Pyxis and McKesson HBOC, removing human interaction from much of the supply cycle. These network-based systems hold supplies and drugs and dispense them to e-providers on a patient-by-patient basis, maintaining par levels and providing continual updates to the central supply department. Servers replace technicians' counting supplies with clipboard in hand. Increasingly, these systems are linked to on-line suppliers via the Internet. Orders for items are transmitted to suppliers to allow just-in-time inventory fulfillment. In this way, hospitals can maintain smaller, more focused, and more cost-efficient inventories.

Pharmaceutical companies have made tremendous inroads and corresponding investments in e-technologies and have realized significant gains from their investments. A KPMG survey showed that the pharmaceutical industry is aggressively moving into e-health and e-commerce. Although as of 2004, only about 21 percent of pharmaceutical companies have e-commerce offerings, over 82 percent expect to offer at least limited e-commerce transactions within the next eighteen months. Pharmaceutical industry executives expect their overall on-line sales to increase to 14 percent of their total sales, up from the current 3 percent (Adams, 2000).

The pharmaceutical industry is not just benefiting from new marketing channels and B2C Web sites such as the Merck-Medco managed care pharmacy site; the Internet has also provided an ideal medium for conducting and monitoring clinical trials and drug studies. In the past, clinical trials required numerous researchers deployed at hospitals around the county to recruit study participants, monitor trials, and compile data. Today, pharmaceutical companies are increasingly using the Internet to recruit study participants and monitor their participation. This streamlined approach to clinical trials speeds the testing and approval process and brings new drugs and therapies to the marketplace much more quickly.

Another benefit accruing to the pharmaceutical industry is increased access to physicians and reduced marketing costs. Sales representatives still call on the top physician prescribers, but the Web gives companies the opportunity to reach physicians who prescribe at lower volumes in a very cost-effective way. One key method for accessing this large market of physicians is to provide on-line information to satisfy physician wants. For example, the on-line Merck Manual provides constantly updated versions of this traditionally essential hard-copy resource. Once a physician is on the site, Merck offers the opportunity to sign up for personalized clinician information and starts building a relationship. The cost of building and maintaining this relationship is much lower than that of having a drug company representative make office or hospital visits. It also tends to be more enduring because a physician who finds the site useful may visit several times each day. Each visit is an opportunity to build and nurture the relationship and market Merck products.

The pharmaceutical industry is also enticing physicians to technology with free PDAs that are used as prescribing devices. These devices provide a handy, up-to-date drug information tool. Prescriptions entered into the device can be checked immediately for drug interactions and side effects. The drug companies benefit from the two-way communication link to the physician. They also have the opportunity to gather vast amounts of information about individual physicians' prescribing habits. These data are invaluable in developing more focused and effective marketing and development efforts.

At the e-payer level, health care insurers also have the potential to achieve huge cost savings and significant benefits from e-technologies. The Web offers e-payers a direct line to thousands of subscribers. Currently, most insurer Web sites offer health information and information on health claims and physicians. This is only the tip of the iceberg of potential value additions to these sites. As technologies advance, insurers will be able to provide patients with links to their electronic health records and thus become a key player in the health maintenance of their subscribers. Insurers will also be able to gather information on their subscribers and provide focused education based on the subscriber's age, sex, medical history, and medical record. This will help to increase subscriber satisfaction and reduce costs by keeping participants healthier. Participating subscribers can make more informed decisions about the level of health care they need and can find assistance in managing their chronic conditions.

Many insurance and B2B Web sites are developing e-commerce applications in order to process health insurance claims on the Internet. Increasingly, companies are developing easily accessible sites that allow individual plan subscribers to complete claim forms electronically. Completed claims are securely transmitted to the carrier for eligibility verification, processing, and adjudication. Subscribers can also receive explanation-of-benefit documents and confirm payments on-line. California consumers are currently empowered to use the Internet to check eligibility and apply for public health insurance. The system, Health-e-App, is being tested in San Diego County and is designed to make it easy for low-income children and expectant mothers to be enrolled in Medi-Cal and the Healthy Families Children's Health program. If it is successful, this California Health Care Foundation program will be rolled out to the entire state in order to facilitate access to public health insurance for these populations. As insurance companies embrace e-technologies and move away from their current paper-intensive processes, they will realize significant time and cost savings as well as human resource economies. Quicker response times for approval and payment of claims will also make for a more satisfied subscriber population.

Employers are also demanding or, in some cases, deploying their own interactive e-health management sites for their employees. The cost of providing and administering health benefits is significant for companies of all types and sizes. In particular, annual open enrollment periods, during which employees can elect to modify their health care and other benefits choices have been costly and labor-intensive for employers and insurers alike. The trend is to move open enrollment to interactive Web sites, which present participants with their current elections, allow them to get automated information about their benefit choices, and change their benefit elections. As an extension of these sites, many companies have also allowed employees to log on at their convenience to make benefit changes for life events such as marriage and childbirth. Most of these corporate health Web sites also include popular health promotion offerings such as health search engines and access to personalized information. Companies that have invested in such sites have not only saved money by reducing the cost of transactions but also increased employee satisfaction by providing greater interactivity and responsiveness to individual employees. When you add the employee relationship benefits to the huge cost savings realized, companies have a win-win solution. In addition, more companies are using health Web sites to host employee health questionnaires, gathering aggregate data on employee health habits that allow companies to identify areas of health risk and tailor their health promotion efforts to respond more effectively to those risks.

As summarized in Table 12.2, e-health opens up a world of opportunities for health care stakeholders. However, any new e-health application needs to do a prudent job of protecting patient information privacy and security while improving health care service quality. The next section takes up these challenges in detail.

E-Health Challenges for E-Stakeholders

One of the main challenges to the viability of e-health is the slow rate of adoption of new technologies among e-providers and e-consumers. Many physicians and other health care providers are entrenched in their paperwork worlds and are slow to adopt new techniques and technology. As well, some consumers are reluctant and sometimes afraid to lose the face-to-face care they have traditionally received from care providers.

Moreover, the U.S. Health Insurance Portability and Accountability Act (HIPAA) of 1996 offers some unique challenges to e-providers and e-payers (insurance companies) who want to migrate to Web-enabled subscriber management. The HIPAA rules establish federal policies and guidelines for managing and ensuring the security of confidential patient information. Because many sections of HIPAA are still being finalized, stakeholders have been hesitant to move quickly with Internet-based transactional sites for mediation of health care and medical claims. Once these regulations

TABLE 12.2. OPPORTUNITIES FOR E-STAKEHOLDERS

Stakeholder	E-Health Opportunities
Health care consumers	• Health care consumers have access to volumes of information on almost every health topic. • Consumer-focused e-health sites feature easy-to-read and readily comprehensible content that is tailored to a largely nonmedical audience. • E-health empowers consumers and bridges the gaps between what e-health consumers want and what they are getting. • Consumers are becoming better informed and thus more able to make informed choices.
Physicians	• The Internet enables home health care monitoring and telecare delivery. • Broadband connections allow physicians to participate in multimedia learning experiences with distant colleagues. • Telemedicine brings the expertise of physicians to rural and underserved areas.
Health care providers	• E-health can reduce costs and increase efficiencies. • The Internet offers significant value as a strategic tool for health care providers in terms of online marketing and business execution. • E-health provides an opportunity for on-line surgical procedures auctions via e-patient and e-physician willingness to bid on specific surgeries to be performed. • Reverse auctions allow hospitals to post the supply items that they require and watch as vendors bid down the price to supply their needs.
Health care vendors	• The Internet enables business-to-consumer sales and business-to-business procurement. • Vendors are able to provide hospitals with inexpensive just-in-time inventory service. • Pharmaceutical vendors offer on-line pharmacies and fully searchable product catalogues. • The pharmaceutical industry is able to increase its access to physicians with fewer marketing costs.
Health care insurers	• Health care insurers have the potential to achieve huge cost savings by offering their Web site to thousands of subscribers. • E-health enables insurers to gather information on their subscribers and provide focused health education based on the subscriber's age, sex, medical history, and medical record. • Web-based subscriber management can help insurers implement some part of the Health Insurance Portability and Accountability Act as providing the necessary forms online to be signed off by e-patients.

are better defined over the coming years, acceleration in the movement to on-line transactions is expected to occur (Lazarus, 2001; Sedkowski, 2001; Wilcox, 2001).

Among e-vendors, the pharmaceutical industry is especially noted for its slow adoption of e-medicine. This industry is conservative in general, and it also has specific concerns, including security. Data pertaining to trials and product strategy are sensitive, and companies are afraid that their competitors will be able to gain access to this information if it is transmitted and captured via the Internet. In addition, in the pharmaceutical industry, as elsewhere, leakage or sharing of patient information is not only inadvisable but illegal (Fisher, 2001; Terry, 2001).

Yet another issue hindering the adoption and diffusion of new and emerging technologies is the fact that the Internet's audience crosses national and governmental boundaries. For instance, if the U.S. Food and Drug Administration has not approved a drug for a particular indication but European authorities might accept this application of the drug, consumer confusion is likely and illegal prescription is possible. Thus, when visiting a site containing product information, visitors often must be directed differently on the basis of their stated nationality.

E-consumers also face significant limitations to the widespread adoption and use of e-health resources. While some 52 million Americans and a large share of Canadians (that is, over 50 percent of Internet users) have accessed health information on the Internet, significant barriers still exist for a large majority of people. Steven O'Dell cites six major factors that limit e-health adoption: (1) access and bandwidth, (2) awareness, (3) ease of use, (4) knowledge of usage patterns, (5) security and privacy, and (6) perception of value. In regard to access and bandwidth, a significant portion of the North American population, let alone the world's population, is still not on-line or lacks high-speed access. With so many options available on-line, many e-consumers have little awareness of the full breadth of on-line or e-health choices available. In addition, many e-health sites lack the integration and ease of use that has become commonplace in other e-commerce pursuits. No doubt this is because many hospitals and other providers are still struggling to figure out how individual users exploit the Internet and what they want from e-health applications. Major security violations in regard to personal information have occurred through the Internet in recent years, giving rise to growing concerns about whether e-health providers can be trusted with consumers' personal information. Finally, most health care organizations have yet to convince e-consumers that their e-health offerings have value. Table 12.3 summarizes the challenges faced by various e-health stakeholders.

The power of e-health depends on the extent to which e-consumers are ready to receive their health care services on-line. While concerns such as those about privacy and security may prevent many people from investing in e-health initiatives, forward-looking stakeholders who are already planning and strategizing about the best mix of e-technologies and applications to service the growing population of information-hungry e-consumers will have a competitive advantage.

TABLE 12.3. CHALLENGES FOR E-STAKEHOLDERS

Stakeholders	E-Health Challenges
Health care consumers	• Consumers are reluctant or afraid to lose face-to-face care, which is difficult to duplicate on the Internet. • Consumers are not on-line or lack high-speed access. • Many consumers have little awareness of the full breadth of choices available from providers and insurers. • Security and privacy of personal information on the Internet is a growing concern.
Physicians	• Physicians are well entrenched in their procedures and are slow to adopt new techniques. • E-health could depersonalize physician-patient relationships and remove much of the physicality and compassion from the healing arts.
Health care providers	• The rapid migration to managed care has left many providers with little way to pay basic operating costs, let alone the tremendous cost of major e-health implementations and upgrades. • The huge and growing number of health care provider Web sites makes regulation and monitoring difficult. • Demonstrable returns on e-health have not been widespread because hospitals are just beginning to experiment with the Internet and because there are few truly effective and integration-friendly systems available to health care providers.
Health care vendors	• Sensitive data pertaining to trials and product strategy are strictly confidential, and Internet security poses a challenge. For competitive reasons, companies are afraid to transmit and capture information via the Internet. • Another challenge is patient privacy. Leakage and sharing of patient information is illegal.
Health care insurers	• E-health has the potential to remove much of the "care" from health care. • An e-health vision requires a significant commitment of capital and effort. For many insurers, a change in organizational culture and attitude would also be necessary.

At this point, we return to our discussion of the different e-health models and services used by various e-stakeholders to plan, develop, and maintain a virtual presence.

E-Health Models and Services

Several strategic e-health service models and solutions that are gaining attention in the e-health marketplace were highlighted earlier in the chapter. Table 12.4 lists specific examples of these models and relates the e-health business structures to their e-health value propositions to yield e-health service solutions.

Business-to-Consumer Models and Services

B2C models and services are among the most widely accepted and practiced service models currently proliferating in the e-health marketplace. Examples include the following:

- Virtual doctor visits
- E-prescriptions
- On-line medical suppliers
- E-disease management
- Health insurance services

One of the most promising e-health value streams is the virtual doctor visit strategy. A new computer service from San Francisco-based Medem, "Online Consultation," offers a case example. This site allows patients to e-consult with their doctors. The system directs e-patients to use encrypted e-mails to interact with their doctors about symptoms and medications, or to set up appointments or refill prescription orders. Depending on the question or the issue, doctors may charge $15 to $30 per on-line consultation.

Virtual Medical Group (virtualmedicalgroup.com) provides virtual non-emergency doctor visits. This strategy shows great potential to reduce costs through remote diagnosis, use of electronic patient information, e-case management and monitoring, and e-consultation. VirtualMedicalGroup consists of Board Certified physicians who are licensed in any particular home state, treat minor, non-emergent medical conditions in the privacy of your home or office. The intent of the certification of physicians is to provide assurance to the public that a physician certified by a Member Board of the American Board of Medical Specialties has successfully completed an approved educational program and evaluation process which includes an examination designed to assess the knowledge, skills, and experience required to provide quality patient care in that specialty.

TABLE 12.4. E-HEALTH VALUE PROPOSITIONS

E-Health Value Proposition	E-Health Business Structure	
	Click-and-Mortar Models	Virtual Business Models and Services
Virtual doctor visits and on-line prescriptions	CVS.com riteaid.com Walgreens.com	virtualmedicalgroup.com at-cost-drugs.com e-scripts-md.com drugsexpress.net birthcontrol.com kwikmed.com
On-line medical suppliers	Merck-Medco.com advanceparadigm.com	PlanetRx.com ExpressScripts.com Neoforma.com drugstore.com drkoop.com
Disease management	accordant.com OnHealth.com	MSWatch.com Arthritissupport.com Alzheimersupport.com
Electronic medical records	WellMed.com ImpactHealth.com	WebMD.com Medscape.com PersonalMD.com
Hospital and physician procurement	Pyxis.com MedicalBuyer.com Promedix.com	Medpool.com Medsite.com MDLinx.com
Provider and physician directories		iEnhance.com healthstream.com physicians-background.com
Connecting e-health stakeholders		Healinx.com VirtualMedicalGroup.com usmddirect.com ehealth careconnections.com
Consumer health portals	KPOnline.org MayoHealth.org FDA.gov AmericanHeart.org	Achoo.com doctor.com doctorslink.com helioshealth.com healthanswers.com americasdoctor.com cbs.healthwatch.com doctorpage.com
Health insurance services	IntelliHealth.com oxhp.com AetnausHealthcare.com	Vivius.com HealtheCare.com HealthMarket.com
Mobile solutions		ePhysician.com e-MedSoft.com
Automated services	HealthHero.com athenahealth.com eHealthEngines.com	UnitedHealth care.com softwatch.com healthit.com

One limitation of virtual doctor visits is the doctors' inability to see (in most cases, although a small number of virtual visits occur through video monitors) or touch the patient. This leads to fears on all sides of misdiagnosis due to lack of information from a physical examination. In addition, patients resist paying the full price of an office visit for a cross between a telephone call and a face-to-face visit.

Among the more successful e-health business services gaining the attention of e-consumers, we find on-line medical consultation (e-consultation) and e-prescriptions (Siau, Southard, and Hong, 2002; Bogen, 1999). All types of medication, including Viagra (for problems with male sexual function), Propecia (hair loss), Zyban (smoking cessation), Retin-A (skin care), and the "morning after pill" (pregnancy prevention after sexual intercourse), are offered to e-consumers on e-prescription sites. The competitive advantage of these sites over traditional brick-and-mortar health care retail outlets is the ease and convenience of purchasing prescription drugs on-line at prices comparable to those of retail stores. E-prescription sites have grown in popularity partly because many people are embarrassed or even ashamed to ask their physicians face to face about some medications.

Another appealing area of e-health products and services is medical supply and specialty superstores. These sites feature items such as vitamins, medical devices, test kits, ointments, baby products, and over-the-counter remedies (Coile, 2000). These sites usually offer volume discounts and easy access to newly released products. What seems to be of most value is the information that these sites make available to e-consumers. With timely and relevant information, many e-patients are empowered to make the best decision or choice at the point of purchase.

As described earlier, on-line medical supply sites offer medical supplies and other related items at discounted or introductory prices. This strategy offers convenience, speed, the opportunity to compare items, access to hard-to-find items, and low prices. The suppliers provide an electronic catalogue with an almost limitless range of products. The value stream combines comparative product information with discount outlet prices. E-health consumers receive detailed product descriptions from search engines and can purchase name brands on-line, often at substantial savings. Neoforma.com provides on-line solutions that simultaneously enable buyers to lower product procurement costs and suppliers to access a highly efficient direct marketing channel.

E-disease management offers searchable, detailed medical information on a given disease. Patients can also find related articles and information on treatment, complications, exercise, diet, and medications. Disease management sites allow patients to track their medications, test results, and other information with the involvement of their physicians. OnHealth (OnHealth.com) provides consumer-oriented health information through standard medical references as well as original content from the site's writers and editors. The site features a personal tracker designed to identify specialized content in a subscriber's area of interest. OnHealth derives its revenue primarily from advertising. The firm is clearly focused on building brand-name recognition and developing a loyal customer base.

Accordant (www.Accordant.com) is a care management company that provides comprehensive patient care services by leveraging the Internet. The company offers on-line and off-line disease-specific training, clinical tools, and assistance from health care professionals.

Other examples of disease management sites include DiabetesWell.com, MSWatch.com, Arthritissupport.com, Alzheimersupport.com, and breathefree.com. One key ingredient of many such services is the community spirit that is encouraged through secure e-mails, chat areas, or on-line message boards.

Another e-health strategy is to allow insured patients to look up the status of a claim, find or change doctors within a network of doctors (through a provider directory), read up on special features of their health plan, and order refills of mail-order prescriptions. E-health help desks assist consumers in navigating through the health system, finding a suitable physician or specialist, and checking on health plan benefits. United Health Care offers Optum Health Forum (UnitedHealthcare.com), a sophisticated Web site where United enrollees can search for key policy information, ask about benefits, or check their doctor's status as a participating provider. Some sites also offer plan enrollment on-line. Aetna (www.IntelliHealth.com) has invested heavily in providing e-consumer information and referral through the Web. IntelliHealth, one of the most popular consumer Web sites for health information, is a joint venture of Aetna with Johns Hopkins, which provides much of the site's medical content. These insurer Web sites simulate health care portals but offer less functionality such as restrictive links to other valuable health-related sites. Health insurers and HMOs are targeting the Web as a future channel for e-consumer registration, eligibility verification, and transaction processing.

Internet-savvy health insurance customers in the future may shop for a health plan through discount Internet brokers, just as they can currently shop for automobiles, life insurance, and airplane tickets. Consumers like the price savings of "disintermediation" (eliminating the middleman). Vivius (Vivius.com) gives consumers the ability to design their own health plan on-line. Similar ventures include HealtheCare.com, Oxhp.com, AetnausHealth care.com, and HealthMarket.com. This strategy presumes either that consumers can fund their own medical care or that employers will provide a health benefit contribution for employees to spend as they wish (a defined contribution plan). The jury is out as to whether consumers will demand a personalized health delivery system, but consumers' backlash against managed care has made offering discount health plans a plausible business strategy.

Business-to-Business Models and Services

B2B models and services include but are not limited to the following:

- On-line medical suppliers
- Hospital and physician procurement
- Health insurance services
- Automated services

We've discussed how on-line medical suppliers allow e-consumers to buy medical devices directly And how these consumers need not be individual purchasers but could also be retailers or business organizations. Neoforma, which also serves individual consumers, builds multiple custom marketplaces to meet the needs of leading health care organizations and enables users to buy and sell medical supplies and equipment. It provides an auction site for used and refurbished medical equipment, such as computer tomography scanners, to help e-providers minimize unwanted inventories through using the Internet.

As explained earlier, hospital procurement processes are often tedious, inefficient, and paperwork-intensive. E-commerce technology allows efficient B2B relationships to fulfill health care system supply needs. This strategy provides current and targeted industry information on very specific topics, including access to the multitude of industry journals. Vendor aggregators such as Medpool.com offer hospitals and health care providers one-stop shopping for their supply needs. Other examples include MDLinx.com, and medlinepro.com.

Health insurance companies that provide services on the Web are positioned to become nationwide enterprises, leapfrogging state and local markets. The biggest health plans and HMOs, which are already licensed in multiple states, could jump most quickly to national marketing. Companies such as United Health Care, Aetna U.S. Health Care, CIGNA, and the Blue Cross–Blue Shield Associations have the multimarket presence and local networks to service customers on a national basis. National health plans have moved quickly to adopt the Internet as an integral component of their sales and marketing plans. eBenX (eBenX.com) provides a service that links employers and health plans for the procurement of group health insurance. The company's group health insurance exchange provides an end-to-end solution for all aspects of the procurement process, from request for proposal through premium payment. eBenX independently assesses health plans on behalf of employers and acts as an employer's agent for procurement decisions. The company also facilitates employer and health plan exchanges of eligibility information throughout the benefit year and provides employees with the ability to select and enroll in a health plan on-line.

Finally, the automated services strategy focuses on providing physicians, hospitals, and health care insurance companies with on-line software applications and computerized document management services. GlobalTelemedix (globaltelemedix. com), for instance, has a host of applications that deal with imaging, test results, reports, and referrals. The company helps medical groups with claims processing and insurance eligibility verification. eHealthEngines (ehealthengines.com) builds Web sites for hospitals and medical groups. Other examples include softwatch.com, athenahealth.com, healthit.com, and medscape.com. It should be noted that these e-health applications could be hybrids of B2B and B2C models.

Hybrids and Other E-Health Models and Services

An emerging set of applications has been characterized by efforts to connecting e-consumers (consumer-to-consumer, or C2C) or e-providers (provider-to-provider, or P2P). The P2P model is a subset of the B2B models. Hybrids (for example, combinations of B2B and B2C; C2C and P2P; or B2C and C2C) and other models are used in the following applications and services:

- Electronic medical records (EMRs)
- Connecting e-stakeholders
- E-directories
- Medical digital libraries
- On-line auctions
- Stakeholder health portals
- Communities of e-health learners

EMRs keep details of patient medical history on-line. In compliance with legislated regulations, any data stored on-line are provided on a purely voluntary basis (Chen, 2001). Typical data include information on immunizations, doctor visits, test results, physical appointments, allergies, and diagnoses. Internet connectivity offers a low-cost architecture of intranets and extranets to link internal and external e-provider sites, including physicians' offices, nursing homes, and homes of chronically ill persons. Medical information is universally accessible to participating providers and is stored in data warehouses with huge electronic storage capacities. Patient information can be immediately accessed whenever it is needed for diagnosis and treatment. Health plans and provider-sponsored integrated delivery networks can use data mining to assess and predict risks as well as to measure their own medical care performance against clinical and economic benchmarks.

EMRs can be useful to e-consumers as well as e-providers. Internet-based patient records can allow e-consumers to feel a sense of ownership of their electronic medical records. Internet health information providers such as drkoop.com encourage e-consumers to register their health history and to build a record of their health status over time. Universal patient identifiers (for example, Social Security numbers or other unique identifiers) can be used to allow medical data from future providers to be electronically compiled via the Internet. The goal is to develop informed consumers who are empowered to monitor and manage their own health.

Abaton.com provides EMR data entry and an Internet analysis tool. It allows e-providers to access, update, or analyze health data through the Internet, irrespective of computer platform. E-providers can examine laboratory and imaging results, direct or support an e-clinical care team, make e-referrals, perform e-prescription orders, and analyze outcomes at any time. Abaton.com has built an innovative flexibility into its EMRs, allowing e-providers to gradually adopt software features rather than attempting an instant transition from a paper to a paperless system. Other sites that support EMRs include WebMD.com, Medscape.com, and PersonalMD.com.

Another e-health strategy is to connect all related e-providers and their information systems seamlessly, which is essentially a combination of P2P and B2C applications. Travelocity.com, which links different airline systems, car rental services, and hotel systems for the consumer's convenience and collects a transaction fee from the consumer may be contrasted with e-health connectivity firms, which connect different provider networks for the provider's convenience (not the consumer's) and collects a transaction fee from the provider. These e-health connectivity initiatives can also include EMRs that are accessible through the Internet, assessment of providers' quality or clinical outcomes, and use of quality data in physician selection. A number of e-health connectivity firms have emerged in the past few years. These companies generally collect their revenue from transaction fees, just as Travelocity.com charges a small fee for handling a reservation, just as a travel agent would. Firms running connectivity sites have personnel costs as well as expenses for the hardware needed to create a smooth multiple-user transaction system. One aspect of this strategy is to secure as many revenue-generating links as possible—in other words, increase transaction-based activities. E-health connectivity companies can derive transaction fees from the principals involved when data are moved over the Internet to health plans, physicians, hospitals, clinical laboratories, pharmacies, consumers, and other participants involved in health care financing, marketing, or delivery.

Healtheon/WebMD is one of the largest e-health firms. Healtheon's goal is to become the premier transaction conduit for health data on the Internet. Specifically, the company seeks to provide an on-line route for all provider and insurer data transactions for claims payment, referrals, medical record attachments, benefit eligibility status, and other clinical or administrative payment processes. The appeal of its service is that all a provider needs is a simple Internet connection rather than a proprietary software and hardware package that requires on-site installation, maintenance, and upgrading. To date, Healtheon's primary limitation has been providers' reluctance to adopt its technology. Healtheon's most recent response has been to buy other firms with market share in electronic physician offices. While this strategy has the merit of speed, industry analysts consider the firm to be in a critical phase, during which it must successfully integrate its acquisitions into a seamless enterprise. Other connectivity providers include Cyberdocs.com, Healinx.com, VirtualMedicalGroup.com, eSalveo.com (based in Canada), usmddirect.com, and ehealthcaresymposium.com.

E-directories of providers, specialists, and even information about pharmaceuticals represent another hybrid application. E-directories can be characterized as a hybrid of B2B and B2C models, creating connectivity among multiple shared e-providers and various e-consumers. The Merck Web site (www.Merck.com) features the full searchable text of *The Merck Manual, The Merck Manual of Geriatrics,* and *The Merck Manual of Diagnosis and Therapy.* These manuals provide extensive medical information and resources on medical treatment directed mostly to providers, but these may also be consulted by e-consumers. The site also includes extensive information on a variety of health topics and pharmaceuticals in addition to the standard company information.

Merck has also greatly expanded its consumer-direct (B2C) business with Merck-Medco (www.Merck-Medco.com), a health management and on-line pharmacy offering. This site serves some 65 million HMO and managed care participants with prescription drug care and health management services. The information systems allow participants to maintain health information such as allergies, family history, and other pertinent information in personalized profiles on the Web site. The systems also facilitate communications among patients, pharmacists, and physicians and help to coordinate appropriate drug therapy based on patient health profiles, best clinical practices, and guidelines linked to the patient insurance plan. The provider and physician directories offer patients the ability to search for doctors, specialist groups, or HMOs on-line.

Many directories offer specific searches for dentists, surgeons, ophthalmologists, and many other types of specialists. Some directory sites also offer background information about the listed doctors, including their years in practice, medical schools where they studied, and research specialties.

Hospitals and health plans are employing the Internet to match patients with providers. A growing number of HMOs and health plans offer physician directories that can be searched by zip code as well as clinical specialty. Most Web-browsing health care consumers will ultimately choose a local provider, but some will seek out medical organizations affiliated with world-class experts and active researchers. The Internet allows highly acclaimed hospitals to advertise both nationally and internationally.

Other health care services, such as SeniorPlace.com, offer provider directories for e-consumers seeking information on long-term care providers. SeniorPlace offers a patient referral network (information resource on specialists), listings of providers, and service profiles, with links to Web sites of long-term care providers.

iEnhance.com offers 136 surgical procedures performed by their 1,300 physician subscribers. The site lists costs by region so that e-consumers can find a local specialist. While some physicians and surgeons have expressed ethical and professional objections to this way of doing business due to lack of having face-to-face consultations and associated legal issues, this strategy does empower the e-consumer or e-patient with more information and choice than has ever been available. Other directory sites include healthstreet.com, and physicians-background.com.

Medical digital libraries are a key information resource that preserves knowledge of tested and proven clinical and therapeutic procedures. These Web-based resources act as B2B and B2C hybrids since these can be shared among multiple providers as well as among different groups of e-consumers. Medical digital libraries comprise organized and appropriately indexed knowledge compiled from authoritative sources, integrating definitive medical expertise and knowledge captured from academics and researchers worldwide. In addition, the knowledge captured can be from many cultures and languages, integrating accepted Western medical practices and proven Eastern alternative and complementary approaches. Today, integrative medicine is playing an increasing role in the education of physicians and other health care professionals. This accumulation of knowledge opens the door to linking curative and preventive medicine.

Medical digital libraries can be enhanced with decision support technology to provide expert medical consultation and advice on-line. The e-libraries can be made conveniently available and accessible to both e-providers and e-consumers. E-providers can rely on these digital resources in their practice of evidence-based medicine, while e-consumers can be empowered by expert knowledge that draws on high-quality research. Also, information can be stored and organized for e-providers in a quick-search format that allows the equivalent of thumbing through a reference source, while the same knowledge can be presented to e-consumers in a multimedia form that is easy to read and easy to understand. Research into digital libraries has provided innovative strategies for representing knowledge and displaying the information in a multimedia and integrative or linked fashion. Medical digital libraries promise to preserve expert knowledge for future generations through the use of advancing technologies.

On-line auctions are an emerging hybrid application, combining B2C, B2B, and C2C applications. As discussed previously, e-medical suppliers like Neoforma build multiple custom marketplaces to meet the needs of leading health care organizations and enable both business and consumer users to buy and sell medical supplies and equipment. Eventually, e-consumers will be able to trade among themselves (C2C) via on-line auctions.

Applying this concept to the doctor-patient e-health marketplace, Medicine Online of Huntington Beach, California (www.medicineonline.com) offers consumers the ability to post thirty-six different surgical procedures on-line. Subscribing surgeons have seventy-two hours to bid for the opportunity to do the procedure. Once the potential patient has reviewed all of the posted bids, he or she can then select a surgeon and set up a face-to-face consultation for the surgery. During its first three months in business, Medicine Online successfully arranged for over one thousand procedures. The site currently averages about three hundred patient bid requests per day (Herrmann, 2001). In this model, both the providers (surgeons and specialists) and the patients can be considered e-consumers of on-line auctions. Some physicians and surgeons have expressed reservations about these applications such as ethical and legal aspects of bidding on procedures that must protect the privacy of the e-patients, but they nonetheless foreshadow a form of empowerment of e-patients.

The portal is the face of the Internet that the consumer most commonly sees, the launch point for various on-line activities. Portals can be considered hybrids of B2C, B2B, and even C2C models. Examples of portals include Netscape, Yahoo! and AOL. The portal strategy is to seek to be the first source an e-consumer consults when searching the Internet. Portals derive revenues primarily through advertising, unless they also provide subscription services. The costs of running a portal include personnel, computer hardware to maintain the site, and advertising. Anyone can visit a portal for free, just as anyone can window-shop for free. The critical goal of each portal is to establish a brand name, generating frequent return visits. E-health portals serve as gateways for both e-consumers and e-providers seeking medical guidance and information on new developments. Many portals also provide access to interesting articles, doctor directories, nutrition information, fitness tips, and much more. E-consumers may also use portals to seek out opinions expressed by other e-consumers through support and feedback groups.

Like other portals, health care portals are financed primarily through advertising revenues. Medscape (Medscape.com) provides links on health topics for e-consumers and e-providers and encourages development of support and feedback groups. Medscape was recently purchased by MedicaLogic, an Internet connectivity firm, and refashioned into a combination portal-connectivity enterprise. This illustrates the growth in e-commerce mergers necessitated by weak revenue streams from firms' original strategies. MedicaLogic hopes to attract providers familiar with Medscape to use the firm as a platform for handling electronic medical records and paying claims. Other examples of e-health portals include Achoo.com, doctor.com, doctorslink. com, drkoop.com, helioshealth.com, healthanswers.com, americasdoctor.com, cbs. healthwatch.com, intelihealth.com, doctorpage.com, and healthmall.com.

Communities of e-health learners are appearing in a variety of organized forms and arrangements all over the United States and Canada. Learning communities are characterized mostly by a C2C strategy, providing tools for e-consumers who are eager to learn from one another as well as from the experts, usually free of charge. Of course, many experts and academics provide professional knowledge to these e-health communities. The Maria-Madeline Project, Inc. (www.mariamadeline.com), discussed in the case in Chapter Three, is an example of a learning community for seniors that focuses on senior health and health promotion services.

Mobile Services

By meeting location-sensitive needs for health care information, mobile solutions such as use of PDAs and BlackBerries provide e-health with a unique value stream. Mobile devices can provide professionals, regardless of where they are, with patients' records; a medical alert device; a portable drug reference; or links to articles, journals, and conferences. Mobile devices can also offer remote billing, wireless prescription filling, real-time access to drug references, and convenient patient care management.

Real-time wireless e-health information services provide patients with "just-in-case" mobile applications that permit them to stay in touch with their e-providers via PDAs or low-cost videoconferencing (for example, use of "isight" with Apple desktops). Important medical readings and alerts on patients' physical changes can be delivered to physicians anytime, anywhere through use of wireless or wired technologies. On-site policyholder data can be captured to complete information needed for a health insurance policy. During a screening physical, a medical practitioner can immediately enter all the findings into the insurer database, decreasing the time before acceptance of the policy and billing. Examples of wireless information services include ePhysician.com and e-MedSoft.com.

Conclusion

E-health provides enormous potential for collaboration among e-stakeholders in terms of understanding business structures, testing business models and specifying value propositions. Virtual doctor visits, for example, could be structured on the basis of medical history provided by the patient on-line. Patient records could be made globally accessible so that treatment could be effected regardless of geographical location. The multiplicity of sources contributing to secure medical records could also be streamlined. Patient monitoring systems like Health Buddy could feed into the medical record system, constantly updating patient medical records. Patient medications could come from an on-line pharmacy, where electronically stored medical records automatically generate refill orders, eliminating the need for patients to track prescription refills. Consumers could pre-order medical supplies as needed and have them automatically delivered to their door on a just-in-time basis. Doctors might never be more then an e-mail away. Incorporate some wireless solutions and e-health could be accessible around the clock anywhere that Internet services are available.

To make this vision a reality, major challenges and barriers still need to be overcome. First, a national standard for electronic interface or presentation of information in the United States must be championed and created. Considerable progress on this front has been made and shared among members of the Western European and Canadian informatics communities. One possible solution is to create a Pan-American Standards Council, involving e-health informatics academics and practitioners. Alternatively, a U.S.-based multinational such as IBM or Microsoft or a consortium could host a common Web service infrastructure that could transport electronically stored data files in XML and share them among authorized e-stakeholders.

Making e-health care information available on the Internet also presents a unique set of problems and risks. Quality assurance, a key measure in face-to-face health care education and information therapy, is difficult if not impossible to enforce on the Internet. Alongside numerous reputable and trustworthy sources, many other sites dispense questionable and sometimes dangerous health and medical advice. As with so many other kinds of information on the Internet, the e-consumer must exercise caution and stick with trusted and reputable sites such as www.MayoClinic.com and www.PennHealth.com.

Unfortunately, plenty of sites are more dedicated to generating quick profits and selling useless "cures" than providing accurate patient information. The large volume and continuing proliferation of health Web sites makes regulation and monitoring difficult. The rapid growth and relative convenience of the Internet have left government regulatory agencies in the dust. The U.S. government, for example, has yet to formulate a plan to address taxes for Internet commerce, let alone devise a reasonable strategy to monitor the validity or quality of information provided on the Internet. E-consumers need to act cautiously and exercise good judgment when opting to seek information therapy via the Internet.

Medical ethics has been and will remain a significant issue in regard to patients' e-interactions. Since the inception of the medical profession, interpersonal interaction and personalized, face-to-face patient education and information therapy have been core tenets of the doctor-patient relationship. Managed care has already taken a considerable toll on these relationships by demanding that physicians see more patients in less time and for less money (Stein, 2001; Evenhaim, 2001; Kronhaus, 2001). E-health can further depersonalize these relationships and remove much of the physicality and compassion from the healing arts. Admittedly, e-health has the potential to remove much of the "care" from health care. It is one thing to be able to look up the signs, symptoms, and expected outcomes for one's disease and quite another to be able to discuss and understand the impact of a disease process with a caring, compassionate, and experienced professional.

Today, about 60 percent of physicians still do not use the Internet in their practice (Kerwin and Madison, 2002). Obviously, this is a key obstacle to the success of e-health. Physicians and other health care professionals must be convinced of the benefits of participating in on-line initiatives. Companies building software tools for physicians must create interfaces that are user-friendly enough to induce physicians to adopt e-technologies. Similarly, financial incentives may be needed to convince physicians to buy equipment and enter records electronically (Sweet, 2001). More important, a reimbursement scheme for Internet consultations must be widely adopted. While there are good opportunities for physicians to generate revenues by using the Web, issues of insurance coverage of on-line visits must be resolved.

So far, no clear rules have been generally established for control of and access to on-line patient records (Lumpkin, 2000). This obstacle, perhaps more than any other, may impede e-health growth and development in the coming years. Major concerns over the security, privacy, and confidentiality of patient and other records captured on-line have delayed e-health development by undermining consumer confidence in e-health systems. If customers are not convinced that their personal health data are protected and secure, e-health will not be widely adopted. Recent polls (for example, on medscape.com) indicate that patients are not ready to keep their medical records on-line due to fears of data misuse, overuse, and abuse. Web users are not comfortable with having their medical data "out there" because they perceive that trustworthy security and privacy mechanisms are lacking. Much more research is needed on data privacy, confidentiality, and security in order to move the field of e-health forward.

Chapter Questions

1. Describe the click-and-mortar and virtual e-health models and services. What are their characteristics, competitive strategies, and merits?

2. What strategic opportunities and challenges do you see in e-health today? What is the significance of a strategic e-health framework in helping us to think about the design of e-health business models? Can you think of another way to frame the development and growth of strategic e-health businesses?

3. What can we learn from e-business experience—in particular, from successes and failures in applying B2B, B2C, and hybrid models and services? What major challenges does e-business face today? How can we encourage traditional health care practitioners to move on-line? How can we reassure e-consumers and other e-stakeholders who do not feel comfortable using the Internet for business transactions and services?

4. Why are standards such an issue in regard to e-health success? What about privacy, confidentiality, and security concerns? Why do you think these concerns have not prevented e-business from moving ahead? Why would these issues affect e-health more than e-business initiatives?

5. Imagine that you have been hired to consult with a large investor group to build an e-health business strategy for a profitable e-learning community. Discuss the steps you would take, and justify your proposal. Why do you think the strategy you have suggested would be profitable when most e-learning communities are presently run by volunteers or funded by charity groups?

References

Adams, M. (2000). Forecast 2001: An e-healthcare odyssey. *Pharmaceutical Executive eHealth Supplement*, pp. 12–20. (ISSN 0279–6570)

Allsop, J., & Taket, A. (2003). Evaluating user involvement in primary health care. *International Journal of Health Care Technology and Management, 5*, 34–44.

Baldwin, G. (2001). Consumers ready to point, click, and pay. *Internet Health Care, 2*(1), 12.

Band, W. (2000). Creating value for your customer. *Sales and Marketing Management in Canada, 31*, 4–6.

Bernard, S. (2000). Evolution of the ehealth space. *Pharmaceutical Executive*, pp. 8–14.

Bogen, J. (1999). Imagine this: Future of e-health care. *Health Care Review*, pp. 33–41.

Chen, K. L. (2001). Web-based electronic medical record (EMR) systems: Challenges and solutions. *International Journal of Health Care Technology and Management, 3*, 15–23.

Chin, T. (2000). The e-impact. *American Medical News, 43*(48), 18–19.

Clarke, I. (2001). Emerging value propositions for m-commerce. *Journal of Business Strategies, 18*, 133–148.

Coile, R. C. (2000). E-health: Reinventing health care in the information age. *Journal of Health Care Management, 45*, 206–210.

Evenhaim, A. (2001). Taking e-health relationship management into the next millennium. *Medical Marketing and Media, 36*(2), 104–110.

Fisher, S. (2001). Biometrics is closing on the enterprise. *E-Week, 18*(12), 11–14.

Fonseca, B. (2001). *Pfizer, IBM, Microsoft plan outsourced IT services for doctors.* Retrieved from http://www.infoworld.com/articles/hn/xml/01/03/29/010329hndoc.xml?0330fram

Fotsch, E. (2002). The truth about e-health. *Pharmaceutical Executive*, pp. 112–116.

Goldstein, D. (2000). *Ehealth care: Harness the power of the Internet.* Aspen.

Haugh, R. (2001). Give 'em what they want. *Hospitals and Health Networks, 75*(2), 16–20.

Herrmann, S. (2001). Low bid for surgery? *Healthcare Informatics, 18*(1), 18–20.

Hill, C. (2001). Health online: Should your company purchase a corporate health web? *Compensation and Benefits Management, 17*(1), 52–55.

Kerwin, K. E., & Madison, J. (2002). The role of the Internet in improving health care quality. *Journal of Health Care Management, 47*, 225–236.

Kronhaus, L. (2001). Linking affiliates electronically. *Health Care Informatics, 18*(3), 73–74.

Lazarus, I. (2001). Departmental consensus opens the door to e-health. *Managed Healthcare Executive, 11*(1), 31–33.

Lumpkin, J. R. (2000). E-health, HIPAA, and beyond. *Health Affairs, 19*, 149–151.

Parente, S. T. (2000). Beyond the hype: A taxonomy of e-health business models. *Health Affairs, 19*, 89–102.

Perkins, E. (2001). Pharmaceutical decisions and the Net: More healthcare resources on the Internet. *Searcher, 9*(2), 59–66.

Porter, M. (1998). *Competitive advantage: Techniques for analyzing industries and competitors.* New York: Free Press.

Sedkowski, J. (2001). New 'report card' evaluates healthcare e-commerce marketplace. *Summit, 4*(1), 7.

Siau, K., Southard, P. B., & Hong, S. (2002). E-health care strategies and implementation. *International Journal of Health Care Technology and Management, 4,* 72–80.

Stein, M. (2001). Medical education and the Internet: This changes everything. *Journal of the American Medical Association, 285*(6), 809.

Sweet, P. (2001). Strategic value configuration logics and the 'new' economy: A service economy revolution? *International Journal of Service Industry Management, 12,* 70–88.

Terry, N. (2001). Access vs. quality assurance: The e-health conundrum. *Journal of the American Medical Association, 285*(6), 807–808.

Trevor Rohm, B. (2002). A vision of the e-health care era. *International Journal of Health Care Technology and Management, 4,* 53–62.

Wilcox, D. (2001). Why hospitals aren't rushing into e-commerce. *Hospital Materials Management, 26*(1), 2–12.

E-Health Technology Strategies and Impacts Case

Jung P. Shim, William E. Sorrells

"The illiterate of the 21st century will not be those who cannot read or write, but those who cannot learn, unlearn, and relearn."—Alvin Toffler

Many new information systems and emerging technologies promise significant social benefit and value, but none are more promising than that of the marriage of information technology (IT) with the delivery of health care. Balancing ever-increasing technology demands with the delivery of high-quality patient care is one of today's significant health care organizational challenges. IT offers the potential to expand the access to health care significantly, to improve its quality and delivery, to change the approach to biomedical research such as the use of online drug trial networks, and to reduce the costs of health care. When appropriately deployed, IT can support health care organizations in achieving competitive leverage, market position, quality patient care and efficient operations. These factors will become increasingly important in the future as the costs of health care continue to rise, insurance reimbursements spiral downward, and competition for health care revenues becomes fierce.

Over the past decade, numerous researchers have completed studies in health care and information systems. Among these, Chau and others examined physicians' acceptance of information technology (Chau, Hu, Sheng, and Tam, 1999; Chau and Hu, 2001, 2002). Siau, Southard, and Hong (2002) provided a model for to the use of information systems technologies in health care organizations. Devaraj and Kohli (2000) presented information technology payoffs in the health care industry.

Successful planning for implementation and use of organizationwide IT requires leadership support and organizational commitment. Leaders who fail to leverage IT in the provision of health care will ultimately fail to provide the best information-based health care possible. The case presented here provides an overview of the impact of new and emerging technologies in health care and maps out strategies that health care organizations can use to leverage information systems and technology successfully.

Impact of Information Technology in the Health Care Industry

With medical technologies quickly emerging and forming in tight harmony with computer networks, medical information systems, and decision support systems, information technology is having a tremendous impact on the delivery of health care. Appropriate IT architecture can support organizations in achieving effective and efficient operations, a strong market position, and, most important, improved patient care. Numerous examples demonstrate the successful extension and creation of health care capabilities with the application of IT. It is important to note that while IT does not replace health care, it can provide the ability to deliver quality health care in optimal ways and with optimal outcomes.

Using Information Technology to Improve Health Care at Sea

One of the best examples of the marriage of IT and health care has been undertaken in the U.S. armed forces, and one successful component of this union is the United States Navy's virtual hospital. The Virtual Naval Hospital (VNH) is a digital health sciences library designed to deliver expert medical information to providers and patients at the point of care, helping providers take better care of naval and marine personnel deployed at sea (Ashley, 1999). The floating forces at sea are an extremely isolated group. For the U.S. Navy to deliver high-quality medical care, naval health care providers and their patients need to have convenient access to current and useful medical information. The VNH lowers barriers to accessing information for disease diagnosis, decision support, treatment, and follow-up, as well as for patient education (Ashley, 1999). These barriers are further reduced via a dedicated high-bandwidth, Internet-based network.

By delivering medical information quickly and securely to the point of care, the VNH helps improve clinical outcomes (Ashley, 1999). By moving expert medical information and not people (either clinicians or patients), the VNH uses the Internet as an e-business solution to help provide care, minimizing time, distance, and other obstacles to the physical delivery of care (Ashley, 1999). By reducing naval health care providers' and patients' isolation from information, the VNH contributes to the delivery of enhanced medical care, thus helping to maximize wartime readiness and allowing the navy to fulfill its missions abroad.

Using Information Technology to Reduce Medical Errors

Although the U.S. armed forces use cutting-edge technology for many of their health care missions, many civilian health care organizations have yet to embrace IT, even at a small level, as a tool for the provision of health care. Consider the following figures:

- Estimates indicate that between 44,000 and 98,000 Americans die in hospitals each year as a result of medical errors. A report from the Institute of Medicine (IOM) reveals that approximately 7,000 people per year die from medication errors alone. This figure is about 16 percent greater than the number of people who die from work-related injuries. In addition, medical error–related deaths are rising faster than any other cause of death except AIDS.
- Inadequate availability of patient information, such as timely laboratory results, was directly associated with nearly 18 percent of events involving adverse drug effects (Leape and others, 1995).
- Each year an estimated 770,000 Americans are injured due to adverse drug effects, and up to 70 percent of those injuries could have been avoided by following safety procedures (Classen, Pestonik, and Evans, 1997).
- The IOM report estimates that medical error costs the United States approximately $37.6 billion each year and that nearly half of those costs are associated with medication errors (Ash, Gorman, and Hersh, 1998).

How can IT be used to reduce medical errors? A recent study by the Center for Information Technology Leadership illustrated that nationwide adoption of advanced interconnected computer systems for physician drug ordering in the outpatient setting alone could significantly reduce medical errors. According to the study, more than 2 million adverse drug events and 190,000 hospitalizations per year could be prevented by leveraging and integrating IT into health care business models, simultaneously saving up to $44 billion annually in reduced radiology, laboratory, medication, and hospital expenditures (Center for Information Technology Leadership, 2003). Compared with paper-based methods of clinical information management, electronic medical records could save primary care providers an estimated $86,000 or more over a five-year period (Wang and others, 2003). Cost savings include but are not limited to decreased billing errors, reductions in radiology, reduced drug spending, and improved charge capture for billing purposes.

One hospital on the cutting edge of IT is Cincinnati Children's Hospital Medical Center (CCHMC), a 324-bed tertiary care hospital staffed by over a thousand physicians. CCHMC is deeply concerned with medication safety and patient safety in general. These factors were the driving force behind the development of the hospital's Integrated Clinical Information System (ICIS).

Based on national literature and their own experience, CCHMC believed that most of the errors that ended up in potential or actual patient harm occurred in the medication-prescribing process. They felt the best investment toward minimizing the problem would be implementation of electronic health records, including electronic order entry (also known as *electronic prescribing*). ICIS began in the summer of 2000 as a Web-based portal that physicians and nurse practitioners could use to retrieve laboratory, X-ray, and other results. Next, the designers implemented a radiology order entry system in order to condition physicians to the computer culture.

CCHMC already had physicians getting lab results from computers, but computers were not used to enact or order care. Adding these elements was a key step toward the new system's success, because CCHMC moved culturally from the illegible written order or verbal order to getting clinicians to use the computer, log in, and order something electronically, with a complete, legible, and accurate requisition. The X-ray ordering system evolved from optional to mandatory after about nine months. CCHMC then took an available order entry and clinical documentation system and customized it to fit the specific needs of a children's hospital—for example, accommodating prescribing patterns based on weight and other key parameters (such as size).

A key driver for CCHMC was to bring abundant clinical decision support to the ordering process; decision support was integrated into the work flow so that clinicians could access it without stepping away from the computer or even moving into another application. Now that the ICIS system is available to all physicians within the CCHMC service region, physicians can view the care being provided to their patients, as well as lab results and X-rays. The system also includes an on-line discharge summary to help facilitate the handoff to primary care. Each nurse saves approximately forty minutes per shift by using electronic charts, allowing the nurse to spend more time delivering care than performing health-related documentation.

Using Information Technology for Home Monitoring and Telediagnosis

Connecting physicians and patients electronically by leveraging IT removes barriers to timely health care delivery. The computer technology industry's interest in meeting users' needs has risen to new heights; tools and methods are being created to enhance patient care, and telemedicine is an area that has benefited greatly from improved IT. One of today's fastest-growing areas of telemedicine is health care delivered to consumers' homes via the Internet. The push for this growth has come from the development of home-based information-gathering devices that can routinely deliver information on a patient's vital signs, which is then used by health care providers to assess and improve clinical decisions. Patients with clinically appropriate conditions can be provided with home-based monitoring (telemonitoring) devices, including heart rate and blood pressure monitors, glucometers, and others.

With wireless technologies, patients no longer need cables and cords to connect them to cumbersome information-transmitting equipment; instead, they can move freely about their residence. For example, Philips Medical Systems' home monitoring system uses wireless communications to gather a patient's weight. The patient stands on the scale, and his or her weight is automatically collected and sent wirelessly to a server (National Library of Medicine, 2001).

Another example of telemonitoring is the Telestation from Philips Medical Systems. This system allows efficient two-way communication between care providers and patients with congestive heart failure who are living at home. The system permits care managers to make better-informed, faster patient care management decisions, which lead to reduced emergency room visits, reduced hospital readmissions, and improved quality of life (National Library of Medicine, 2001).

Another initiative that combines IT and health care is the on-line examination, which has been described in some detail in this chapter. This e-health strategy is referred to as telediagnosis, another subset of telemedicine. In telediagnosis, a physician can use remote equipment (with assistance from the patient or the patient's caregiver) to quickly evaluate a patient's condition or prognosis. For example, an ophthalmologist in Santa Fe could perform a retinal exam on a patient in a rural Native American community in northwest New Mexico. This example demands a quality of service that can almost but not quite be achieved with today's Internet. The quality of service limitations in this example involve the probability of the necessary raw bandwidth being available and the guaranteed delivery and security of data (Huang, 1996).

Technology in direct patient care will continue to evolve as new and improved technologies emerge. Patients will wear, ingest, or have implanted medical devices to help provide real-time patient data that will be used to make quick clinical decisions, possibly with the assistance of decision support systems. Such medical devices will include intelligent inhalers that physicians can use to track daily medication usage, disposable electronic wristbands that code all relevant patient information using infrared signals, and embedded glucose monitors that automatically check a patient's blood sugar level, eliminating the need for periodic blood samples. These devices will improve not only the quality and quantity of patient information but also the ability to use time-sensitive information to make knowledge-based clinical decisions that lead to favorable and predictable medical outcomes.

Strategies for Success in E-Health Technology

Health care has evolved into a trillion-dollar industry with a growing variety of participants, including service providers, insurers, and government and regulatory agencies. The landscape of the health care industry will be affected by many forces, including pressures from society, advances in technology, nearly ubiquitous information access in some situations, educated consumers, economic pressures, and medical ethics, to name a few. These forces helped reshape the traditional patient care setting from the fee-for-service physician office and community-based hospital to today's integrated patient service networks and e-health portals. Contemporary service organizations offering integrated patient and family services across the spectrum of health care can provide vast informational and transactional resources. Consider the model of Web-based e-health information systems depicted in Exhibit 12.1.

The success of health care organizations will be measured by their ability to provide a broad range of services along the health care spectrum in a cost-effective and

EXHIBIT 12.1. INFORMATION SYSTEMS AND HEALTH CARE RESEARCH WORKS

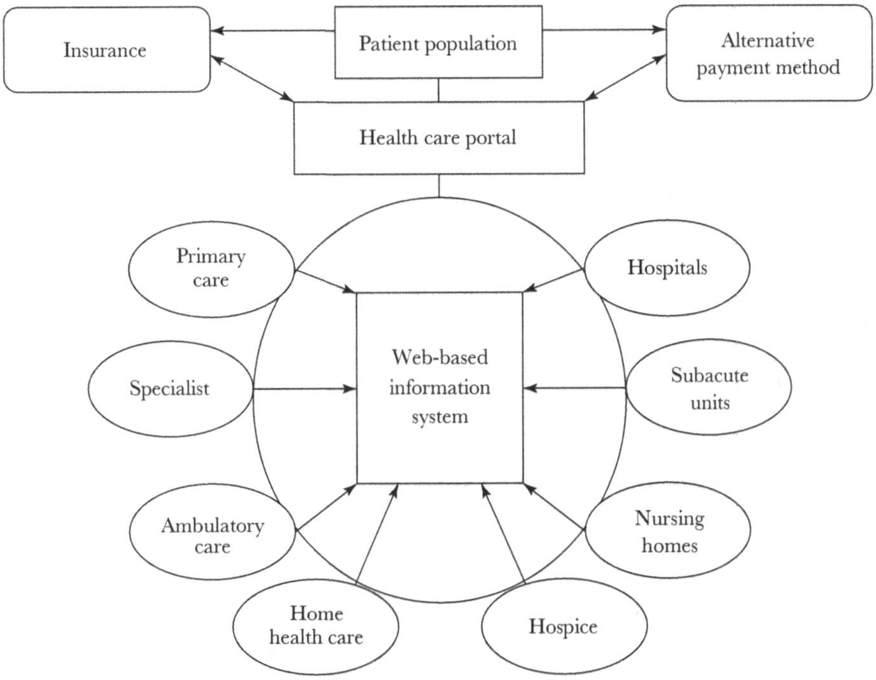

efficient manner, with high-quality clinical outcomes. In order to achieve this level of service, health care organizations are seeking new tools and technology to support their service offerings and define their informational needs.

While emerging IT can provide new opportunities to improve health care and its delivery, numerous challenges limit the potential benefits that IT-enhanced health care can offer. Fiscal restraints appear to be hindering the health care industry's ability to transform isolated departmental and stand-alone systems into enterprisewide, integrated health care solutions. Other challenges include standardizing terminology, incorporating new data types (for example, digital images and patient genotypes) into existing data repositories, developing and implementing decision support system guidelines for use at the point of care, and minimizing the difficulty of integrating applications that reside in heterogeneous technologies.

Bill Gates has describes future businesses as a "digital nervous system" and says that in order to optimize the delivery of health care, critical success factors must be identified (Gates, 1999). His list of factors includes a flexible organizational structure and service delivery mechanism, instant access to business data and information, and a complete understanding of the current health care environment. Organizations must be stronger than ever to successfully provide direction from the present to the future and to map as smooth a course as possible, knowing there will be unforeseeable pressures and roadblocks. Information systems and the corresponding computer-based technologies are tools that can be leveraged to achieve organizational goals. The marriage of health care and IT will be defined by critical criteria such as the following:

- Speed—for example, a response time of less than one second for each information transaction
- Less than 5 percent typing for all input
- Customization for user, place, time, and circumstance
- Consistent enterprise-based, personalized user interface
- 100 percent paperless medical records that can also store images and voice
- E-care systems as extensions of caregivers
- Trusted e-health portals
- Used by 100 percent of physicians because it saves time, improves accuracy, and supports decision making
- Elimination of significant opportunities for error in caregiver environment
- Anytime, anywhere access for authorized users
- Remote care
- Substantial return in labor savings and reduction of medical errors

E-health has already had an impact on the general public. Health care portals and e-health initiatives are experiencing explosive growth. Early adopters of IT in health care stand a good chance of capitalizing on the competitive advantage of information superiority.

Future Trends in E-Health Information Technology

Internet usage in the future will change access to health care and health care information more dramatically than can be foreseen, but it is likely that in the near term, Internet-based e-health technologies will result, at a minimum, in the following:

- Continued expansion of information access for providers and consumers
- Increased public reporting
- Proliferation of patient support groups
- Creation and maintenance of personal electronic medical records
- Risk assessments and health-monitoring tools for use by nonphysicians
- Expansion of current e-commerce links from health care providers to retail pharmacies and medical supply outlets

The Internet is enabling consumers to obtain detailed information regarding health care practices and services. With convenient access to reliable information, patients are becoming better-informed consumers and more active participants in maintaining their own health and well-being. According to a new study by the Pew Internet and American Life Project, a research organization in Washington, the ranks of Americans over 65 who use the Internet have jumped by 47 percent since 2000, making them the fastest-growing group to embrace the on-line world.

Beyond providing reference information, the Internet has enabled health care organizations to offer patients additional access points into their system. Some support on-line chat rooms for patients with similar diagnoses, providing them convenient access to support group therapy and networking. Other health care providers use their Internet site for limited patient access to processes, such as appointment scheduling or completing assessment forms and questionnaires prior to patient visits. Health care providers who have moved ahead in this area have noticed positive by-products of electronic access: patients share a more comprehensive level of information and ensure that their information is accurate, which allows clinical decisions to be made on the basis of accurate information. The bottom line is that patients pay more attention to their health information today than in previous years, possibly because they now have access to more information than ever before.

As stated earlier, the next generation of medical devices will affect the flow, quality, and quantity of patient information. Some of these devices will provide patient-monitoring information that has not been available in the past, whereas others may provide direct integration of their data into third-party clinical documentation applications. These efforts will promote further development and use of information technology, leading to the integration of technology and the clinical practice. In addition, conducting timely and efficient management research on patient outcomes will be critical in order to establish the feasibility and effectiveness of technologically advanced solutions as cost-effective treatments.

The Next Generation Internet (NGI) is an initiative for the integration of higher-speed backbone communication networks to replace the current Internet for many high-bandwidth applications, including medical imaging and other e-health technologies. When the NGI becomes a reality, the virtual house call may become an important and far-reaching means of improving patient care. The idea of the family doctor stopping by a house for an exam or visit was highly valued in large and small communities. In a NGI e-health environment, a physician and patient will be able to engage in a clinical encounter, bringing back the traditions of home health visits. The bond that was developed between physicians and patients often improved clinical outcomes and relieved stress on families with terminally ill family members. In other words, the NGI may offer a way to virtually restore the neglected doctor-patient bond. When voice, images, and data all can travel over the Internet, doctors and patients will be able to use videoconferences to discuss clinical concerns. The real trick is providing this type of service cheaply for both doctors and patient. One strategy is to invest the cost savings realized from preventing hospital visits or admissions in equipping doctors and patients with NGI technology. This would be particularly advantageous for patients who need a large number of clinical visits. The cost savings to the patient in reduced medical care billing, not to mention the fuel savings associated with trips to distant municipalities, could be substantial. In addition, the burden of over-crowded and understaffed hospitals could be significantly reduced, improving the quality of care at brick-and-mortar sites. Here is a hypothetical case in point:

> Mr. Smith is a sixty-three-year-old white male with a complex medical history including hypertension, coronary artery disease, and chronic obstructive pulmonary disease, along with a lifelong diabetic condition. The patient's condition has been determined to be terminal. By using virtual clinical visits, a doctor can possibly prevent an unnecessary clinical admission by identifying a respiratory condition such as pneumonia in its early stages. Assuming an average hospital stay of six days, based on admission history for pneumonia and Mr. Smith's physical condition, a cost savings of over $20,000 would be realized by avoiding this admission.

As you can see, the effects can be astounding. As health care becomes more consumer-driven, clinicians can leverage newer technologies and systems for better health care services and higher operational efficiency within a cost-cutting environment.

Conclusion

One of the most valuable direct benefits of IT's emergence on a global scale is the impact it will have on health care. As medical technologies and processes emerge in conjunction with computer networks, medical information systems, and decision support systems, the Internet and other computer-based technologies will provide, support, and extend health care delivery.

A few short years ago, ubiquitous health care would have been unthinkable. But improvements in information technology have allowed health care to take a great leap forward, providing a bright outlook for the future. With an IT-driven culture shift, health-related information and services can be available anytime and anywhere. Medical researchers will be better equipped to synthesize data into meaningful and sometimes revealing information while collaborating across cultural and business lines, which will ultimately lead to more beneficial treatments. Tomorrow's technology will provide new tools and avenues for health care organizations to provide high-quality and reduced-cost patient care services that are unthinkable today.

Case Questions

1. What are the key barriers to implementing a national health data repository?
2. How can teleradiology and digital medical imaging reduce health care costs?
3. Although information technology can enhance the delivery of health care, does it also create new threats in regard to the protection and security of patient information? If so, what are some such threats?

4. Besides computerized pharmacy refill systems, what other information technologies can be used to minimize or eliminate medical errors in a clinical setting?
5. Who benefits the most from the health care industry integrating health information systems on an industrywide basis? Why?

References

Ash, J., Gorman, P., & Hersh, W. (1998). Physician order entry in U.S. hospitals. *Proceedings of the AMIA Annual Symposium* (pp. 235–239), Portland, OR.

Ashley, D. (1999). U.S. Naval Reserve, the Virtual Naval Hospital: Lessons learned in creating and operating a digital health sciences library for nomadic patrons. *D-Lib Magazine,* Volume 5 Number 5, May 1999.

Center for Information Technology Leadership. (2003). *The value of computerized provider order entry in ambulatory settings.* Retrieved December 2003 from http://www.citl.org/research/ACPOE.htm

Chau, P., & Hu, P. J.-H. (2001). Information technology acceptance by professionals: A model comparison approach. *Decision Sciences, 32*(4), 699–719.

Chau, P., & Hu, P. J.-H. (2002). Examining a model of information technology acceptance by individual professionals: An exploratory study. *Journal of Management Information Systems, 18*(4), 191–229.

Chau, P., Hu, P., Sheng, O., & Tam, K. (1999). Examining the technology acceptance model using physician acceptance of telemedicine technology. *Journal of Management Information Systems, 16*(2), 91–112.

Classen D., Pestonik, S., & Evans, R. (1997). Adverse drug events in hospitalized patients. *Journal of the American Medical Association, 277*(4), 301–306.

Devaraj, S., & Kohli, R. (2000). Information technology payoff in the healthcare industry: A longitudinal study. *Journal of Management Information Systems, 16*(4), 41–67.

Gates, B. (1999). *Business @ the speed of thought: Using a digital nervous system.* New York: Warner Books.

Huang, H. (1996). Teleradiology technologies and some service models. *Computer Medicine Imaging and Graphics, 20,* 59–68.

Leape, L., Bates, D., Cullen, D., Cooper, J., Demonaco H., & Gallivan, T. (1995). Systems analysis of adverse drug events, ADE Prevention Study Group. *Journal of the American Medical Association, 274,* 34–43.

Menduno, M. (1999). Apothecary now. *Hospitals and Health Networks,* 35–36.

National Library of Medicine. (2001). Next generation Internet projects. Retrieved December 30, 2003, from http://www.nlm.lib.gov/research/telefront.htm

Siau, K., Southard, P. B., & Hong, S. (2002). E-health care strategies and implementation. *International Journal of Health Care Technology and Management, 4,* 72–80.

Wang, S., Middleton, B., Prosser, L., Bardon, C., Spurr, C., Carchidi, P., Kittler, A., Goldszer, R., Fairchild, D., Sussman, A., Kuperman, G., & Bates, D. (2003). A cost-benefit analysis of electronic medical records in primary care. *American Journal of Medicine,* 1:114(5), 397–403.

CHAPTER THIRTEEN

E-HEALTH CARE TECHNOLOGY MANAGEMENT

A Multifactorial Model for Harnessing E-Technologies

George Eisler, Sam Sheps, Joseph Tan

Three individuals need to be acknowledged for their invaluable support and cooperation. Jim Flett was one of Canada's most senior hospital administrators. As executive director of the Association of Canadian Academic Health Organisations (ACAHO) at the time of this study, he was instrumental in gaining the support of teaching hospital CEOs across the country for this project. Murray Martin, CEO of the Hamilton Health Sciences Corporation, orchestrated our first audience with the board of ACAHO, which led to their enthusiastic support. Shan Satoglu, program head for health technology management at British Columbia Institute of Technology, provided assistance and objective analysis during the literature content analysis, which was the critical phase of the project.

Learning Objectives

1. Conceptualize e-health care technology management
2. Recognize the benefits and challenges of e-surveying health administrators and executive team members
3. Identify the perceptions of senior health care executives on technology management issues and interpretations of expert opinions and ratings
4. Understand the relationships of HCTM research findings to the results of the Hay Group Study
5. Associate HCTM research findings with an e-HCTM context

Introduction

Human history and development have always been linked dynamically to the technology inherent in tools and means of production. The survival of individuals, clans, tribes, organizations, societies, and empires depends on the power of their technology to harness nature and their environment. The evolution of human civilization from the hunter-gatherer stage to the industrial stage took almost two million years. Amazingly, the evolution of computing and automated information processing technology has taken no more than a few decades, following the Industrial Revolution, two World Wars, the Cold War, and the race to the moon. In the last decade, this trend of accelerating change has been further fueled by instant access to worldwide information, global competition, and the pervasive power of converging advances in computing, information and telecommunication technology, and biotechnology.

The e-health paradigm shift, the topic of this text, is another revolution in the human history of technological developments. The view that e-technology is just an implementation issue or just another operational requirement vying for resources may be one of the key reasons for the current poor coupling of e-technology and e-health care. This view sees e-technology merely as a tool to implement e-health care strategies. It assesses e-technology in terms of return on investment or in terms of satisfying current e-market needs, covering such aspects as identification, selection, acquisition, exploitation, and protection of e-health product or process technologies. Although such tactical e-technology plans are useful (Gregory, Probert, and Cowell, 1996), more compelling is the potential and power of e-technology to radically change clinical and business strategies in health care, not just support e-health systems that mimic traditional systems. Indeed, e-technological innovation has already shifted the competitive balance within the health care industry and is creating more new opportunities for growth, as previous chapters of this text have discussed.

Economists such as Tapscott and Caston (1993) have pointed to technology as an important change agent in the structure of industries and competition. Andersen, Belardo, and Dawes (1994) confirm that the issues are similar in the public service sector arena: "Public expectations for the level and quality of government services were formed in better economic times. Those expectations have grown while satisfaction with their fulfillment has steadily declined. In the past few years, it has become evident that cutting fat, eliminating waste, and preventing abuse is not nearly enough. Government needs to rethink its methods and restructure its approach to public services." Around the world, countries are recognizing that the competitiveness of their health care products and services in the global marketplace depends on their focus on e-technology management. In the e-health environment, the task of managing applications and services is particularly complex. It requires that health care executives master many different skills, including government relations, community liaison, employment of human resources in e-work, financing of e-health business initiatives, e-patient care, research on e-technologies (for example, research based on linked databases), and on-line education. E-health care technology management (e-HCTM), therefore, adds one more dimension to the challenge of harnessing IT for health care in the new economy.

In recent years, e-HCTM and mainstream health care technology management (HCTM) have been receiving attention in developed countries (for example, Japan and countries in Europe and North America) as well as in developing nations (for example, Southeast Asian countries). The World Health Organization (WHO), for example, proclaimed that there were serious shortcomings in the performance of health systems in virtually all countries (World Health Organization, 2000). In the late 1980s, the WHO admitted that its attempts to introduce components of an HCTM system around the world had not been very successful (World Health Organization, 2000). The lack of a working HCTM model or framework and a shortage of technology management skills, expertise, and knowledge among workers in those countries were identified as serious limitations. Without a functioning HCTM or e-HCTM system (incorporating, for example, technology planning, technology life cycle management, and technology assessment and evaluation), long-term support for technology applications and health initiatives is unsustainable. These deficiencies with respect to the management of technology point to the crucial need to align technology strategy and e-business strategy. In other words, the strengthening, linking, and aligning of technology planning and e-business planning in the e-health care context is the essential purpose of e-HCTM. In light of this development, the discussion of this chapter will focus on drawing lessons for e-HCTM from previous research on health care technology management in traditional health care organizations—specifically, large teaching hospitals (Eisler, Sheps, Satuglu, and Tan, 2002).

Multidimensionality of the E-HCTM Concept

Transferring lessons we have gathered from technology management in other industry sectors—particularly the concept of strategic HCTM and the importance of innovation—to health care and e-health care is the beginning step in exploring the concept of e-HCTM.

The complexity of the e-health care environment, the multitude of forces that shape technology decisions, and the uniqueness of the e-health care environment are all justifications for applying e-HCTM to overcome challenges of sustainability, cost, and quality of care. Compared with other industry sectors, such as banking and transportation, the e-health care environment is not only more complex but also more turbulent. The environment is challenging not only because of the complexities inherent in the development and maintenance of a seamless system spanning the continuum of e-health care delivery but also because of the complexity of relationships among stakeholders, including providers, vendors, payers, investors, insurers, patients, the general public (consumers), policymakers, regulators, researchers, and educators.

The Strategic Role of E-Technology

The health care industry is in transition, driven by such changing factors as economic trends, technology products and services, and population demographics. These pressures have resulted in changes in the structure and process of care, financing, and human resource management. The challenge in health care can be summarized as ensuring timely access to high-quality and cost-effective health care services. Health care systems in Canada, the United States, and other developed countries are expected to continue on the road of cost reduction and quality improvement through the growth and diffusion of e-health business models and services (see Chapter Twelve). Reforms in health care have been intended to increase efficiency, flexibility, and integration, as well as to improve health outcomes, community participation, and cost control. Given these sometimes conflicting pressures, a debate about the role of technology as the problem or as an important part of the solution is taking shape. Indeed, e-technology can play a vital strategic role in health care, as it does in other knowledge-based service industries, including banking and entertainment. This is particularly true for information and communication technologies and e-technologies, which can contribute significantly to improved management, cost-effectiveness, customer service, and support. These applications can create opportunities for new e-health services or for new delivery methods for existing services. For these reasons, some governments (for example, the government of British Columbia) have maintained information and communication technologies and e-health applications on their list of priorities even during a period of severe cost reduction (British Columbia Ministry of Health Planning, 2002). Only after a thorough economic evaluation will questions about comparative costs and benefits of various e-technologies, including the status quo, be answerable.

The emergence of e-technology as a lever of economic competitive advantage has created a demand for personnel who can help enterprises take advantage of such technological innovation (Raghupathi and Tan, 2002). In the past, many industries have seen technologies such as computer and telecommunication networks as playing a supportive role, contributing to overhead costs. In other words, these technologies are not seen as central to corporate objectives. Today, e-technologies are beginning to be recognized as significant core enabling assets with major strategic implications for an organization's survival and success. In addition, the power of converging e-technologies is blurring the boundaries between administrative and core technology tools. Many CEOs now believe that such enabling technologies, if managed appropriately, can contribute significantly to the achievement of e-business strategy and new organizational objectives. At the same time, these e-technologies may fundamentally change the way an organization functions as well as the way it relates to its industry sector, sponsors, suppliers, and, most important, its customers or clients. For example, the availability of e-health care through the Internet and related Web services is transforming mainstream health care.

From a marketing perspective, creative and rapid technological evolution generates a volatile technology push on the input side of organizations. Many companies, including giant retailers like Sears and CVS Pharmacy are going on-line to prevent their chain stores from losing customers to a growing list of on-line competitors. On the output side, customers expect reliable, consistent, safe, effective, and efficient service. The convenience of on-line shopping means that they can change their loyalties easily and quickly. They are looking for seamless technology and applications. The challenge, then, is for executives, including health executives, to enable their organization to continually transform the turbulent technology input into a customer-focused and appropriate output in the face of increasingly difficult internal and external constraints (Tapscott, 1996).

"Where change used to occur periodically, it's a way of life now," said Charles Webb Edwards, executive vice president of the Technology and Operations Group at

Wells Fargo and executive vice president and chief technology officer at Norwest Corporation prior to its merger with Wells Fargo. "There is real value in being able to manage . . . change." Strategic planning horizons for most companies are shortening from ten or twenty years to five and, more recently, to three years. "The new approach to strategic planning recognizes that the New World is not predictable, linear, or deterministic. Rather, it is unpredictable, nonlinear, and full of surprises." Rapid technological change is partly responsible for this nonlinearity (McCallum, 1996). Technology strategy is an integral strand in the strategic management fabric of an organization (Badawy, 1998; Husain and Sushil, 1997).

According to McGee and Thomas (1989), what has been missing "is a comprehensive view of how technological change can affect the rules of competition, and the ways in which technology can be the foundation of creating defensible strategies for firms." Restructuring programs, takeover campaigns, and the unprecedented trend toward joint ventures are indications of the new way of doing business, "driven by the need to compete more aggressively and efficiently in world scale markets" (Perrino and Tipping, 1989). Studies have shown that levels of companies' investments in technology explain international differences in productivity and in shares of world markets.

Geisler and Heller (1996) argue that because of economic pressures, our health care system is in crisis. What's more, technology, especially medical technology, has played an increasing role in creating the crisis. They claim that proper and better management of medical technology provides some hope for dealing with the forthcoming challenges.

The World Health Organization defines *health* as a state of total physical, mental, and social well-being, not merely the absence of disease and infirmity. It is now recognized that population and individual health has many determinants not traditionally associated directly with the health care system—for example, air quality and socioeconomic status. Accordingly, e-HCTM includes managing applications of technology that influence the environment, information dissemination, health protection, and disease prevention. It goes beyond just applications of medical technology found in modern acute care systems or for direct medical care. In this context, the term *e-health care technology* applies, in the broadest sense, to more than just e-health information. It includes hardware and firmware devices, software and business processes, health products such as drugs and home care health products marketed on-line, as well as e-prescription and e-home care services. E-technologies that may contribute to quality or sustainability of health care systems (see Chapters One and Two) could be associated with virtual communities (see Chapter Three), e-clinical care (see Chapter Four), e-public health systems (see Chapter Five), e-network infrastructure (see Chapter Six), various e-health domains and applications (see Chapters Seven through Eleven) or other e-health business processes (see Chapter Twelve).

E-Health Care Technology Management Strategy

In this chapter, we review the literature across several industry sectors and combine the results of that review with the findings of our research on technology management in traditional health care organizations. This approach yields general agreement about the basis for e-HCTM strategy; the characteristics of an e-HCTM-focused business; and the responsibilities and capabilities of the e-technology officer, who is equivalent to the chief technology officer (CTO) in traditional corporate settings.

E-HCTM strategy is based on the competitive and turbulent e-health environment, the nature of the e-health business, and the state of e-technology development. Other factors in e-HCTM strategy include considerations of business-specific factors, environmental factors, and customer preferences; creation of strategic advantage and differentiation; development of e-technological expertise, e-business decision-making and problem-solving skills, and human resource capabilities; and readiness for a comprehensive rethinking and readjustment of job descriptions, information systems, governance structure, incentives, and decision-making processes. One of the most important issues is e-health business structure and its value propositions, as has been noted throughout this text. E-health policies hold together a decentralized, virtual workplace with rapid access to global information. In addition to flexible governance structures, management of e-health systems must emphasize seamless information flow, appropriate incentives (for example, for focusing on customers), and innovative performance assessment schemes.

E-HCTM strategy needs to be characterized by managerial vision, foresight, and entrepreneurial spirit. Strong leadership is one of the most critical aspects of success. This entails commitment to knowledge acquisition rather than just product development. Management personnel must know what they want, given the difficult-to-quantify costs and benefits of newer e-technologies and the need for flexibility. Managers must set realistic goals, match the supply of products and services to market demands, and be clearly aware of resources, constraints, and risks. Decisions and attitudes of management must be based on an analysis of competitive position, market intelligence, technical preferences of e-consumers (customers), and internal capabilities. The e-HCTM strategy focuses on the customer, replacing organization-centered approaches with an emphasis on market pull rather than e-technology push.

Management systems must focus on an internally integrated enterprise. These systems must coordinate across functional boundaries; in other words, cross-functional approaches must facilitate convergence of the historically divergent views of technically oriented and market-oriented individuals. Full and meaningful worker and customer participation in the production and delivery process is key to e-health success. Moreover, process management has to replace product management; this shift in focus to flexibility, adaptability, responsiveness, and effectiveness rather than efficiency and costs is necessary mainly because competitive advantage comes from achieving greater customer satisfaction and enterprise knowledge integration by deploying the appropriate e-HCTM strategy, not just from labor cost savings. Above all, the ability of the management team to change, adapt, and avail itself of new opportunities is critical in an environment as turbulent as the e-health marketplace.

E-consumers', e-providers' and the government's expectations have increased because of advances in technological capabilities. For the e-technology officer to move e-HCTM strategy forward, he or she must demonstrate thinking and visionary leadership, the ability to create new ways of funding, and a commitment to the alignment of e-technology with clinical objectives. Thus, the e-technology officer must bridge gaps between virtual team members and engage in continual planning, active resource allocation, development of standards, rapid reorganization when necessary, and adoption and implementation of fundamental changes in the e-business system. He or she must also be a steward of networked leadership, be close to the front line, and build an invisible enabling infrastructure.

The e-technology officer must ensure that promises made on behalf of e-technology applications are kept. He or she must build a viable, productive, and flexible e-technology asset base that can deliver goods and services on time and with a competitive pricing scheme. Moreover, he or she needs to take responsibility for managing technology-driven change and act as a change champion. Overall, this individual must be able to manage in an environment of decentralized decision making with a high level of interfunctional coordination; be conversant in e-business issues and challenges; have a focused commitment, empowered with applicable technical information; and have the skills to effect and manage change. Such an individual will also need relevant technical competence and an understanding of the importance of e-technologies and systems that provide a competitive edge, as well as the need for e-technologies and systems that support the goals of the virtual enterprise.

E-Surveying Health Executives

In this research, we electronically surveyed (e-surveyed) executive team members of the forty largest Canadian teaching hospitals on the topic of HCTM. Our target sample was representative of senior administrators across the Canadian health care system. Selected individuals from this group responded to a newly developed instrument. Factor analysis and cluster analysis were applied to the resulting data set. The research methodology involved the development of a new measurement structure or abstraction ladder (Geisler, 2000) that addresses criticisms of past technology management (TM) research.

Defining Health Care Technology Management

A rigorous content analysis was conducted to develop an acceptable definition of *technology management* and to identify related critical TM capabilities and attributes. A database of 255 articles was searched and 47 related dissertations were read for the sampling unit "defin*" (for "definition") in the abstract or full text, to locate discussions of the definition of technology management. Scanning and integrating the information found in related articles and dissertations and eliminating those that were not relevant to our purpose, we generated the following comprehensive definition of the *technology management* construct:

> *Technology management* (TM) may be defined as a holistic and integrated application of engineering, science, and management capabilities to strategic life cycle management of new and relevant product and process technologies in order to shape, as well as accomplish, the goals and objectives necessary for business success.

From this definition, a schematic diagram for the technology management framework emerges, as shown in Figure 13.1. The final step in the framework, organizational success, can be defined differently in each organization. Business success in health care could, for example, be expressed as improved patient care within given resources. Alternatively, the performance goal may be, for example, the protection of the five health care principles of the 1984 Canada Health Act: comprehensiveness, universality, portability, accessibility, and public administration.

HCTM is a complex, multifaceted process with interlinked activities that clearly encompass more than a single indicator of successful performance. Guided by the notion of an abstraction ladder approach to metric development (Geisler, 2000), the goal was to create a hierarchy of major dimensions, including constructs, dimensions, and variables that describe these dimensions and their measurable indicators. The instrument was constructed from the exhaustive list of individual attributes that resulted from the literature content analysis. The attributes were grouped and regrouped to form indicators in such a way until an intuitively sensible and comprehensible list of indicators emerged. The list of indicators was far more detailed than similar attempts reported in the literature, although it soon became apparent that the indicators could be grouped into variables comparable to those referred to in the literature.

Our study did not develop a new definition for the *technology* construct. Rather, the perspective of technology as an extension of human and organizational ability was adopted from the literature. But based on an extensive literature content analysis, we have proposed a more complete definition of *technology management* to use in studying the concept in a health care setting as well as in generating a model of health care technology management. The proposed definition acknowledges the

FIGURE 13.1. TECHNOLOGY MANAGEMENT FRAMEWORK

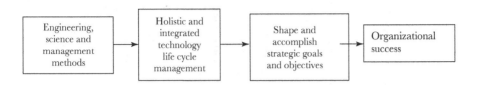

multidisciplinary and integrative nature of the TM construct. It captures the need to manage technology throughout its life cycle, from conception to replacement. Inherent in the definition of TM given earlier is the broadest view of technology. The two most critical aspects of the proposed definition of TM are (1) that technology both shapes and supports organizational strategy and (2) that its objective is to contribute to organizational success, however success is defined for a particular organization.

As we have discussed, the literature content analysis yielded a list of critical attributes for HCTM practice. These attributes, which are summarized in Table 13.1, formed the basis of a metric and thus of a testable HCTM model.

The model consists of three dimensions, which are subdivided into variables and indicators. The collective package constitutes the proposed HCTM model that is to be empirically validated. The individual building blocks are not new to engineering, business, or social science. A body of literature, research, and empirical evidence informs each dimension, variable, and indicator.

Pilot Test and Field Test, Using a Delphi Approach

Using a modified Delphi approach (consultation of experts), a pilot group of senior health care administrators and management consultants were asked to rank and validate the attributes of the HCTM model from the perspective of large-scale health care systems—that is, Canadian teaching hospitals. The focus was on responsibilities at the corporate or executive level. In order to qualify as an expert, an individual had to have been involved in health care management at senior levels for more than ten years. Positions held by these experts during their careers included deputy and assistant deputy minister; CEO, vice president, and chief information officer of a health organization; and director and executive director of a health industry organization. These experts were shown a draft survey and asked to critique the instrument with respect to clarity, comprehension, and ability to complete it. The fifteen pilot participants were also asked to recommend unambiguous descriptors for the state of implementation of each statement category that appeared in the survey.

TABLE 13.1. CRITICAL ATTRIBUTES FOR HEALTH CARE TECHNOLOGY MANAGEMENT FROM CONTENT ANALYSIS

Index	Attribute	Description
1	Core competencies and technologies	The organization defines its core competence and builds an intellectual and technical infrastructure around its core technologies. This infrastructure relates and contributes to all internal and external competitive business aspects, which may include price, quality, flexibility, rapid response, customer service, and reputation.
2	Corporationwide technology strategy	The organization has a *strategic intent*, a focus that drives technology management. The organization develops both a corporationwide technology strategy and an overall business strategy, which are interrelated and aligned with each other.
3	Understands and monitors change	The organization understands how technology and technological change affect market and competitive position, considering the industry, competitors, competitors' strategies, and the organization's position in the industry. This understanding leads the organization to continual questioning of markets and missions and continual development of skills to exploit technological opportunities.
4	Global perspective on innovation	The organization realizes that the global market is increasingly driven by continual technological innovation in which specialization is essential for competitiveness.
5	Local context	The organization considers the local context and infrastructure, including culture of innovation and technological, geographical, social, governmental, and legal factors.
6	Senior technological leadership	The organization believes that innovation can become endemic only with leadership and support from top management and senior executives.
7	Leads organizational change	During all stages of organizational change (exploration, strategic planning, initiation, and implementation), senior management communicates and promotes the vision of the organization with reactive, proactive, preventive, and motivational leadership.
8	Two-way communication, vision, buy-in	Senior management communicates and promotes a vision and helps a shared vision to evolve among organizational leaders, including the CEO and governing boards as well as the company-at-large. Senior management develops effective and timely two-way communication by soliciting input, advice, and feedback and by implementing mechanisms for consensus building. These efforts help to formulate and communicate strategic objectives, to generate support and team spirit for chosen strategies, and to encourage participation and buy-in at all levels.

Index	Attribute	Description
9	Senior management skills	Senior management has commitment, technological competence (stays abreast of developments in present and potential future technologies), strategic competence (knows when to abandon old technologies, support existing ones, or adopt new ones), objectivity when considering new information (maintains effective two-way communication, solicits and considers opinions, decides in a timely manner, generates support), and understanding of the organization's ability to attempt large or difficult projects.
10	All-inclusive technology	The organization promotes technology as part of the organization's thinking at all levels. Technology is not some kind of alien ritual serviced only by the high priests of technology.
11	Long-term experimentation	The organization takes a long-term view toward innovative activities. This perspective is shown through a long-term commitment to experimentation, technological accumulation, and innovation. It is also reflected in a willingness to take risks and in human resource management's predisposition toward constant learning, teamwork, autonomy, initiative, creativity, and freedom to innovate.
12	Rapid response to technological change	The organization has the ability to initiate and respond to technological change swiftly and flexibly, in order to maintain its competitive position. The organization stays abreast of technological developments. R&D exhibits appropriate time-consciousness. Management decisions are made in a timely manner.
13	Learning culture	The organization provides and develops a learning culture that leverages the effectiveness of technological professionals and supports innovation. This culture is indicated by a mutual trust and sharing of ideas; personal commitment; team and entrepreneurial spirit; creativity; calculated risk taking; education and training; the prevalence of systematic thinking over fragmented, sporadic thinking; and synergy. This strong learning culture bonds human assets, senior leadership, and resources to promote core competence and capabilities.
14	Systematic change process	Senior management recognizes change as an opportunity and advocates change through a systematic change process. This includes business process reengineering, continuous improvement, and organizational design. Senior management can manage equilibrium, analyze aspects of the change process (desire and resistance, scope, stakeholder commitment, organizational response), implement change reviews, and act as a change process champion.
15	Incentives to promote innovation	The organization institutes an award, reward, incentive, and celebration system to recognize individual and team accomplishments; to promote creativity, entrepreneurial thinking, innovation, and scanning for innovative opportunities; to encourage education about quality assessment; and to encourage key technological personnel to remain with the organization.

TABLE 13.1. *(continued)*

Index	Attribute	Description
16	Human resource development	The organization recognizes human resource development as the key to building technological capability. The organization builds capability through training (for example, continual development and upgrading of skills, increasing emphasis on know-how); recruitment of innovative individuals; effective two-way communications; and multiskilling (active sharing of expertise within and throughout the organization). The organization has a proactive program to track pockets of high expertise, technical excellence, and leading-edge talent.
17	Internal knowledge	The organization develops and exploits its internal knowledge base by sponsoring opportunities for knowledge sharing and organizational learning; by implementing a system to maintain knowledge and skills independent of personnel leaving the firm; by extensive sharing of information for effective decision making; by promoting communication across product lines; and by establishing an advisory committee that includes users, technologists, and senior management. At the national level, the country establishes a direct formal link between science and technology producers and users.
18	Performance management	The organization develops a performance management system that targets internal and external customer satisfaction, that includes key performance measures, and that sets high performance goals.
19	Integration of the innovation chain	The organization links R&D, manufacturing, and marketing through formal multifunctional teams with top management support and through multidisciplinary R&D cores in each market, each with its own mission to be managed in terms of network, vertical, and horizontal integration with suppliers, customers, and external sources of expertise.
20	Internal R&D	The organization establishes and strengthens in-house R&D activity by increasing financial allocations and committing resources to understanding the technological future. Research leaders have sufficient years of experience and technical maturity.
21	Integrates R&D with organization	The R&D department has the following proficiencies: ability to convert an initial innovative concept to a marketable product; ability to inform and involve other parts of the organization in decisions and developments that affect them; and ability to accept and incorporate the direction of research chosen by senior management with the needs and wants of the market and the capabilities of the organization.

Index	Attribute	Description
22	External knowledge	The organization keeps up on relevant technical developments through various external sources by gaining and exchanging information and ideas through suppliers, customers, professional networks, user groups, global interorganizational networks with public agencies, academic organizations, competitors, and clients; by scanning for, spotting, and tracking trends and opportunities in the world market environment; by using competitors to benchmark, examining the adaptability of their best practices; and by understanding how the organization is perceived in the market.
23	Organizational flexibility	The organization creates flexibility through employee empowerment (job and role flexibility that allows employees to initiate and seek innovative opportunities), virtual organization and horizontal organization (decentralized multidisciplinary teams, multifunctional managers and generalists, well-educated and highly skilled employees, and continual and intensive collaboration and integration among functional and specialist groups).
24	Resources	The CTO develops access to sustained and sufficient external and internal resources (physical, financial, venture capital, and so on) to explore potential technologies in the chosen area, to support ongoing operations, and to take the research effort all the way to the intended conclusion.
25	Comprehensive CTO responsibilities	The organization has a chief technology officer to act as technological gatekeeper (manages, retrieves, and disseminates corporationwide technological knowledge through distributed knowledge systems); spokesperson and technology strategist (fosters recognition of innovation needs and matches these needs to core technologies, ensures sponsorship of needs research, and ensures cooperation among key organizational elements); supervisor and coordinator of technology efforts; manager of corporationwide technology, technology policy, and technology adoption, acquisition, and implementation; participant in corporate business planning; and galvanizer of a vision of product lines that go beyond current customer needs. The CTO is also responsible for selecting a committed product champion for each technological product.
26	Technology scanning	The organization identifies and monitors emerging strategic technologies through systematic technology scanning of internal product groups, internal R&D, professional literature, professional bodies, university research, collaborative partners, seminars, suppliers and potential suppliers, customers, and competitors.
27	Product champions	The organization assigns a committed product champion to each project.

TABLE 13.1. *(continued)*

Index	Attribute	Description
28	Customer focus	The organization focuses on the end user by understanding user needs and anticipating future needs, linking technology to the market, and responding to needs quickly. This focus on user needs is achieved by making line managers ultimately responsible for customer service, developing efficient customer linkages, involving users in the development process, enhancing customer service levels, analyzing the company's role in the value chain, identifying potential needs and opportunities for innovation, respecting customers' values (ethics), changing products and markets through relative diversification, emphasizing market pull rather than technology push, creating a corporate vision based on market realities, and incrementally developing products or processes to meet consumer needs.
29	Effective technology selection	The organization strategically selects technologies by reviewing past selection processes; identifying the appropriate decision maker; assessing potential for synergistic integration (with existing technologies, structure, operational procedures, and skills); assessing production criteria (managing production economies of scope and economies of scale, production automation decisions, and make or buy strategies); and assessing potential for competitive advantage (ability to meet short-term and long-term product development needs, potential for growth of market and market share, and ability to equal or surpass competing technologies in quality, cost, or reliability).
30	Life cycle management	The organization manages technology across the technology life cycle, focusing on costs and critical success factors
31	Strategies for acquisition of technology	The organization acquires technology by transferring technology, deciding to make or buy, producing it under license, developing it through in-house R&D, contracting for external R&D, outsourcing, negotiating joint venture agreements, acquiring a company, attracting key personnel, making alliances, adapting useful foreign technologies, and acting on information from technology scanning or early warning systems such as failures of existing technologies.

Index	Attribute	Description
32	Equipment control and maintenance	The organization formalizes aspects of equipment development (formal design methods and automated tools for technology development), implementation, and operations (enforcing standards and quality control, requiring product certification, monitoring and planning obsolescence and replacement).
33	Diverse knowledge base to reduce product development time	The organization maintains a diverse level of technological knowledge (including past, present, and potential technologies) and reviews these technologies for radical or incremental innovation, to reduce new product development time and shorten innovation cycles.
34	Assessment	The organization critically evaluates its technological performance and decisions by making reviews of benchmarking and of technological and organizational change part of the management process. The organization establishes and maintains technology standards, to ensure quality.
35	Protection of knowledge	The organization understands that it must protect its information in order to maintain its uniqueness. The organization minimizes the risk of unplanned technology transfer by monitoring its communication with other companies; creating patents and licensing agreements, confidentiality clauses, and designs that prevent copying or reverse engineering; implementing knowledge security and ownership; and spreading knowledge of particular processes or technologies across several people.

Note: Detailed citations for each of the thirty-five attributes are provided in Eisler (2002).

Source: Eisler (2002).

It was envisaged that the outcomes of this e-survey would lead to a new research agenda for HCTM and e-HCTM. It was also hoped that the outcomes would influence curriculum development in health care technology management training in Canada and other countries. Therefore, the Canadian College for Health Service Executives, based on its own survey on desirable attributes of future health service leaders, published this statement: "Health care leaders carefully and successfully adapt some features of the private sector model for use within the public sector infrastructure. Technology conscious leaders are increasingly able to guide its infusion to their best advantage" (Canadian College for Health Service Executives, 2000). The statement was used to motivate respondents to fill out the questionnaire. Pilot participants were informed about the national character and the expected target audience of the study. They were presented with the prototype questionnaire, which included forty-two indicators, and asked to do the following:

- Complete the survey, keeping any large health care organizations with which they were familiar in mind
- Identify whether and how specific statements should be altered
- Add any missing statements that they thought were important
- Express concerns they might have about the appropriateness of the indicators being grouped into the identified domains and the categories within each domain
- Identify examples of additional real and practical evidence or indicators that could be used to support statements about the extent of implementation in the various categories (for example, strategic plans, job descriptions, budgets)
- Comment on the comprehensiveness and comprehensibility of the instrument

In the follow-up field test, senior managers of four regional referral organizations, representing a variety of administrative responsibilities, participated; specifically, the CEOs of four medium-sized health service organizations in British Columbia provided e-mail addresses of their executive teams (vice presidents, CEOs) and individuals reporting to the executive team members (senior managers). These sixty-four executives and senior managers represented eight different areas of responsibility. With thirty-three responses from sixty-four individuals on the e-mail list, overall response rate was 52 percent and ranged between 43 percent and 64 percent for the four participating institutions. As in the pilot test, respondents were asked to comment on content, wording, and structure of the instrument; however, no changes to the instrument were suggested. The importance of the topic of technology management was confirmed by a consistently high average rating from each organization. On the six-point Likert scale in which 1 meant "of least importance" and 6 meant "of greatest importance," average ratings from each organization ranged from 5.6 to 5.9.

Feedback from the pilot study as well as from the follow-up field test was used to further refine the questionnaire. Following the pilot test and the field test, the survey instrument was reshaped and reformatted before it was used in the national survey.

Validity and Reliability Issues and the Gap Score

The literature supports our approach to the evaluation of validity and reliability concerns about our research instrument (Lewis, 1993). Content validity was optimized through the iterative process by which the instrument was developed. Content analysis informed the instrument, and expert opinions from the pilot test and field test stages refined the instrument.

The following steps were used to establish different types of validity with respect to the instrument:

- Face validity and content validity of the instrument development process was supported by existing literature (see Table 13.1).
- Refinements were made based on initial expert suggestions from academic researchers and on comments and suggestions received from experts in the field in the pilot test and field test to achieve significant content validity.
- The field test stage further tackled content as well as structure, clarity, and comprehensibility of the survey instrument.
- Construct validity was addressed through a factor analysis of all responses.
- Concurrent validity was eventually addressed through a comparison of our research findings with a performance review of the same institutions that was completely independent of our research; this review, conducted by the Hay Group Study, uses a completely different metric.

The internal consistency coefficient, Cronbach's alpha, was computed with SPSS statistical software and applied to each of the three major dimensions (factors) resulting from the factor analysis of the field test data. An alpha of .8 is desirable. Reliability of the instrument was assessed by calculating this coefficient for each of the indicators according to the factors established by the factor analysis. For all indicators, Cronbach's alpha was found to range from .79 to .94.

In addition to generating Likert ratings for each indicator, a single measure was established to capture each respondent's perception of the gap between the ideal extent of implementation (as reflected in a rating of 6 on the Likert scale) and the perceived extent of implementation (which could be represented by a score from 1 to 6 on the Likert scale) for twenty-six HCTM indicators. Gap scores were weighted by using the respondent's assessment of the importance of the respective indicator. This resulted in a gap score, a composite variable given by the following formulation:

$GS = (6 - E) \times B$, where

GS = gap between ideal and perceived implementation

6 = ideal implementation rating

E = rating of perceived extent of implementation

B = rating of perceived benefit or importance of implementation

A gap score (GS) was derived for each respondent. The term $(6 - E)$ can be interpreted as an indication of room for improvement, because an E score of 6 would indicate full implementation. The factor B is a weighting factor based on the perceived importance of the item. For example, perceived full implementation of an indicator would yield a gap score of 0—that is, $GS = (6 - 6) \times B = 0$, whereas deeply perceived need for an indicator to be implemented in the responding organization would yield a very high gap score—for instance, $GS = (6 - 1) \times 6 = 30$. Here, an implementation rating of 1 (meaning "not at all") would yield the highest gap score if the indicator's importance was also rated as 6 (meaning "very great"). Gap scores, therefore, range from 0 to 30.

An average gap score (the average of responses from a particular organization) of, say, less than 8 for an indicator can then be interpreted as "This indicator has been implemented to a high level and would not require additional attention for improvement." This could be either because the indicator has been well implemented (rating of 5 or 6) or because the importance was rated lower than other indicators (4 or less). Field test results indicated that the instrument and the gap score meaningfully and consistently capture differences in perception among senior managers from different organizations with regard to known HCTM factors.

Altogether, responses from the organizations that participated in the field test can be grouped into major clusters. Our analysis of the field results uncovered three primary dimensions, or clusters. Cluster A, the low gap cluster, represented responses from executives in organizations achieving average gap scores of between 6 and 10. Cluster B, the moderate gap cluster, comprised organizations with an average gap score of more than 10 and less than 15, while Cluster C, the high gap cluster, consisted of organizations receiving average gap scores of 15–19.

One could interpret this finding as an indication of poorer-performing clusters (Clusters B and C) versus better-performing ones (Cluster A) in the eyes of their senior managers. Moreover, some respondents whose responses generally fell into Clusters A or C appear to have a more consistent view of their organization's performance than those whose answers generally fell into Cluster B. Finally, Cluster A organizations seem to have reached a high level of HCTM performance. Consistent with this finding, the organizations found in Cluster A are among those nationally recognized for their quality management systems. Our next step was to verify results of this field test in a wider national survey.

Web-Based Survey Design

The survey instrument was designed on the basis of the list of attributes and administered via a Web-based delivery system. This strategy was adopted because our target audience comprised very busy executives. The questions posed in the survey were ordered in a logical sequence that was based on the overall model, which was laid out for participants in a cover letter. Given that the target audiences for the survey were knowledgeable senior executives, it was deemed unnecessary and probably unhelpful to scramble the sequence of the statements; this was verified by our pilot-testing of the instrument. As in the Lewis study on the information resource management construct (Lewis, 1993), respondents used a Likert scale to rate their perception of the importance of various HCTM factors and the extent of the implementation of these factors in their organization.

Obviously, a survey can only be employed if the intended audience can be assumed to have access to appropriate technology. While our intended participants were believed to have Web access, other major reasons for using e-surveying in our case included the following:

- Senior health administrators are too busy to take the time to answer mail-in questionnaires.
- The speed and convenience of e-surveys would encourage a high response rate and result in faster return of the surveys.
- E-surveys ease data handling and permit convenient data analysis.

Developing and posting the e-survey on the Web involved a number of critical steps. The most time-consuming aspect of the process was determining the correct e-mail addresses of hundreds of potential participants. Repeated exchanges of notes and information to and from representatives of the executive offices of the participating organizations took place. The survey content, including all associated notes and rating scales, was developed as a Microsoft Word document; Web pages with forms for accepting data input were generated with Dreamweaver 4.0 Web design software. Rather than using purchased Web survey software, the Web survey tool was custom-designed in order to achieve a more professional look. A thank-you page was automatically generated and sent to the respondent on receipt of a survey response. The survey was sent electronically to hundreds of senior managers whose e-mail addresses had been identified. Data files of submitted responses could easily be created and exported directly into an Excel database and spreadsheet program.

Anonymity of respondents and their organizations was ensured. Even so, the process allowed reminders and requests for responses to individuals from whom none had been received within the specified time period. Distribution of the e-survey, receipt of responses, and creation of the data set for statistical analysis were all accomplished within a six-week period; in contrast, gathering and correcting compiled e-mail addresses took eight weeks.

The National Survey

In February 2001, the Executive Committee of the Association of Canadian Academic Health Organisations (ACAHO) enthusiastically endorsed the research reported here. The Executive Committee members, the CEOs of some of Canada's largest teaching hopitals, shared the view that HCTM approaches in the Canadian health care system could be and needed to be strengthened. Their support and active promotion of this project presented an invaluable opportunity to attract participation from senior managers across Canada's teaching hopitals. The list of ACAHO member organizations was compared with the list of organizations ranked by number of technology-intensive beds from the Canadian Health Association guide. This list indicated that ACAHO member organizations included most of the major and most technology-intensive health care organizations. It was felt that the senior managers of these organizations were best positioned to assess HCTM practices in Canadian health care agencies.

Following the decision of the ACAHO's Executive Committee, which included the CEOs of six of Canada's largest health care organizations and ACAHO's executive director, to sponsor this national survey, letters were sent to the CEOs of member organizations to ask for their organization's participation. With the aid of ACAHO, requests were issued to the CEOs for the e-mail addresses of their executive teams and their senior management. The collection, validation, and verification of the e-mail addresses were a considerable undertaking that had to be completed prior administration of the e-survey.

Factor analysis was used to explore the data for patterns and to reduce the number of variables to a more manageable size. Survey responses were clustered by individual organizations and further analyzed using analysis of variance (ANOVA) to identify systemic differences in HCTM practices. However, this analysis was inconclusive, suggesting the possibility that senior managers with direct patient care responsibilities were responding differently from those who did not have direct patient care responsibilities because of differences in the pattern of observed responses. Executive team members (vice presidents, CEOs) were responding differently from senior managers reporting to VPs. Cluster analysis was used to investigate the underlying data groups and patterns more thoroughly. In this sense, it was used to optimize the comparison and identification of differing HCTM practices and capabilities.

Research Findings with Relevance for E-Health Care Technology Management

Thirty-three ACAHO member organizations were invited to participate in this national e-survey project. In the end, approximately 850 individuals in twenty-eight organizations received the survey electronically. Of these, 324 responded, representing an average response rate of approximately 38 percent per participating institution (range of 24 percent to 58 percent).

Confidentiality of the respondents and the organizations were protected through the assignment of an organization code between 1 and 33, which will be used for the remainder of this discussion. For example, organization 1 submitted thirty-six acceptable responses, reflecting a 33 percent response rate from the executives and senior managers who received the survey. Of these thirty-six respondents, six executive members had patient care responsibilities (for example, the vice president of nursing and vice president of nursing), while seven did not (for example, the vice president of finance and vice president of support services). Of the responding managers reporting to vice presidents, eight had patient care responsibilities and fifteen did not. The respondents were first asked to rate the importance of the topic of the survey (1 = not at all, 2 = very little, 3 = little, 4 = some, 5 = great, and 6 = very great). The overall result was that 317 of 324, or 98 percent, rated the topic's importance as great or very great. No respondent rated the importance at less than 4.

In addition, when respondents were asked to rate the importance of the individual indicators, every indicator scored an average rating of 5 or greater on the six-point rating scale. This implies that, on average, the 324 respondents agreed on the great importance of each indicator. The results validated both the instrument and the applicability of our HCTM model to the health care setting.

Factor Analysis

Factor analysis was performed to identify the degree of separation and aggregation of underlying variables, or *latent variables,* on which the twenty-six measured indicators loaded (for specific variables, see headings under each dimension such as "Technology Strategy," "Chief Technology Officer," and so on). The resulting model is presented in Table 13.2, which shows the apparent loading of the twenty-six indicators onto three primary dimensions, or factors. Thus, it was no longer necessary to treat the indicators separately for further analysis; these three dimensions, or factor loadings, define the primary units for analysis. For the purpose of our discussion and to ease comparison, the numbering of the revised indicators has been retained in Table 13.2.

TABLE 13.2. REVISED MODEL OF INDICATORS

Strategic Management (Dimension 1)	Management of Change and Innovation (Dimension 2)	Organizational Management (Dimension 3)
Technology Strategy 1. Technology and business strategies are aligned. 8. Technology is linked to customer needs.	*Customer Focus* 9. Line managers are responsible for customer service. 13. Performance management is based on customer satisfaction.	*Effectiveness and Flexibility* 2. Key technology is supported by infrastructure. 16. Technology diffusion and transfer are encouraged.
Chief Technology Officer 3. Executive formulates technology strategy. 4. Executive administers and manages technology strategy.	*Change Management* 10. Senior management participates in change management 11. Corporate learning culture prevails. 12. Senior management promotes an organizational vision and direction. 19. Organization has strategies for responding to change.	*Operations Management* 22. Organization uses sound project and process management. 23. Technology life cycle is systematically managed.
Knowledge Management 5. Vision of technology is monitored through routine scanning. 6. Environmental factors relevant to technology strategy are identified.	*Integration of Innovation Chain* 14. Communication system promotes technology. 15. Innovation system integrates R&D and operations. 20. Organizational design uses multi-functional teams.	*Assessment and Evaluation* 24. Technology-related risks are evaluated. 25. Technology assessment informs technology decisions. 26. Performance due to technology management is evaluated.
	Human Resource Management 17. Human resource development and planning is key to technological capability. 18. Accomplishments are formally recognized. 21. Skilled employees seek innovative opportunities.	

Developing a technology strategy that is aligned with business strategy to meet the highest possible order of customer needs represents dimension 1 of the model. The more sophisticated the organization's ability to become aware of relevant new technologies, the more timely its ability to adapt or adopt emerging technologies will be. If those emerging technologies cannot be supported or sustained because of environmental factors, their usefulness will be limited. Thus, dimension 1 also includes technology and environmental scanning and further suggests that the development, implementation, and administration of the technology strategy needs to be driven and managed from the executive level.

The model further implies that in addition to the development of a technology strategy, the organization has to be nimble in order to make necessary changes in business direction or adapt to new ways of meeting customer needs. Dimension 2 therefore focuses on change management. Key elements of the change management dimension are a customer service attitude that permeates the organization and a change management process driven by the executive team. Celebrating technology as part of the solution, keeping an eye on the future of the organization, and celebrating integrated multifunctional teams are other components of this dimension of the model. A human resource strategy that fosters innovation and creativity in line with strategic technologies is considered another critical aspect of this dimension.

Dimension 3 of the model represents the organizational and operational management component of HCTM. Once strategic direction has been established and the organization has been prepared for change, the success of the implementation and operation depends on organizational and operational management. This continuous and iterative process should encompass every stage of the technology life cycle and should be well supported by ongoing evaluation and assessment of performance and risks at the technological level and the organizational level.

These new dimensions were used to test for significant differences in responses between and among various categories of respondents. This was necessary to establish whether all responses from individual organizations could be treated as coming from the same population for the purpose of response comparisons within and between organizations. The resulting p-values ($p = .25$ for patient care versus non–patient care managers; $p = .5$ for executive versus non-executive managers) indicated no significant differences in gap scores between the categories of respondents within organizations. Thus, all responses from the same organization could be grouped for the purpose of testing for significant differences between organizations.

One key question to be answered in our research was the ability of the instrument to differentiate between organizations in regard to their HCTM approach. The twenty organizations that supplied five or more responses were included in this part of the analysis. Based on ANOVA and the resulting p-values ($p < 0.001$), significant differences were found in the way in which senior managers across the twenty organizations perceived the state of HCTM in their organization.

Cluster Analysis

A cluster analysis approach was used to determine if the organizations grouped around similar mean gap scores for each of the three dimensions. Cluster analysis of the twenty organizations with more than five responses yielded an apparent three-cluster taxonomy:

- Cluster 1: Organizations 1, 2, 3, 5, 6, 7, 9, 11, 13, 14, 17, 18, 19
- Cluster 2: Organizations 4, 8, 10, 12, 16
- Cluster 3: Organizations 15, 20

Testing for significant differences between and among these clusters indicated a statistically significant difference ($p < 0.001$) between the mean gap scores of clusters of health care organizations along each of the three dimensions identified. Since Cluster 3 consisted of only two institutions, with comparatively few responses, further analysis focused primarily on the differences between Cluster 1 and Cluster 2 organizations. The average gap scores for every indicator were lower for Cluster 2 than for Cluster 1 organizations. In addition, the significant differences between the two clusters of organizations, based on the perceptions of their senior managers, are influenced more by some variables than others.

The importance of implementing each indicator was not rated as highly as the importance of the indicator itself. This was consistent for every indicator. The mean scores for implementation range from 3.15 to 4.46, demonstrating greater variability than those for indicators with a standard deviation range of 1.01 to 1.62. The mean gap scores ranged from 8.4 to 14.66, with a standard deviation range of 5.45 to 8.27. This considerable variability raised questions about the factors contributing to the different perceptions. Statistical analysis showed that the key factors contributing to the variability were significantly different responses from senior managers representing different organizations. In fact, the participating organizations fell into two main groups of perceived HCTM performance—that is, Cluster 1 and Cluster 2 organizations.

Table 13.3 lists the twenty-six variables in the survey in the order of the percentage difference between Cluster 1 and Cluster 2 mean gap scores. Percentage differences range from 6.54 to 56.42 percent. On a national basis, the two indicators (indicator 3 and 4) with the highest percentage difference were also the ones with the highest variability.

Based on the analysis, the major differences between the two clusters from the perspective of senior managers could be identified. Cluster 2 managers rated their organizations very highly (low gap score) in the following three areas:

- Indicator 3: Executive member formulates technology strategy.
- Indicator 4: Executive member administers and manages technology strategy.
- Indicator 12: Senior management promotes organizational vision and direction.

TABLE 13.3. GAP SCORE DIFFERENCES BETWEEN CLUSTER 1 AND CLUSTER 2

Indicator	Difference	Percentage Difference	Cluster 1	Cluster 2
7	0.61	6.54	9.33	8.73
22	0.80	7.46	10.73	9.93
10	1.24	13.15	9.43	8.19
9	1.53	13.53	11.31	9.77
25	1.89	14.26	13.25	11.36
17	2.00	15.85	12.62	10.62
8	2.34	16.03	14.60	12.26
2	2.15	16.17	13.30	11.15
21	2.33	17.72	13.15	10.81
20	2.36	18.50	12.76	10.39
23	2.58	18.57	13.89	11.31
15	2.59	18.82	13.76	11.16
24	2.20	19.00	11.58	9.38
6	2.49	20.66	12.05	9.56
19	3.27	21.48	15.22	11.95
11	2.54	21.77	11.67	9.13
18	3.34	24.38	13.70	10.36
14	2.83	24.50	11.55	8.72
16	2.94	25.28	11.63	8.69
1	3.93	28.98	13.56	9.63
13	4.02	28.98	13.87	9.85
12	2.69	29.89	9.00	6.31
5	3.98	31.61	12.59	8.61
26	4.86	31.52	15.42	10.55
4	5.71	48.15	11.87	6.15
3	7.29	56.42	12.92	5.62

In contrast, Cluster 1 managers rated their organizations particularly poorly (high gap scores) in the following areas:

- Indicator 8: Technology is linked to customer needs.
- Indicator 19: Organization has strategies for responding to change.
- Indicator 26: Performance due to technology management is evaluated.

The distribution of indicators in the four quartiles of the gap score range is shown in Table 13.4.

At one end of the spectrum, Cluster 1 managers rated none of the indicators in the lowest quartile of gap scores, compared with Cluster 2 managers, who placed four indicators there, the top two of which were indicators 3 and 4. On the other end, seven indicators were rated in the highest quartile for Cluster 1 as opposed to none for

TABLE 13.4. INDICATOR DISTRIBUTION

Gap Score Quartile	Cluster 1 Indicators	Cluster 2 Indicators
6.0–8.4		3, 4, 12, 10
8.5–11.0	12, 10, 22	16, 14, 11, 24, 6, 1, 9, 13, 22, 18, 20, 26, 17, 21
11.1–13.5	9, 14, 24, 16, 11, 4, 6, 5, 20, 3, 21, 25, 2, 1	2, 15, 23, 25, 19, 8
13.6–16.0	18, 15, 13, 23, 8, 19, 26	

Cluster 2. These seven Cluster 1 indicators were led by indicators 8, 19, and 26, which also were deemed to need the most attention according to the overall national averages.

The largest differences in reported perception based on implementation ratings and gap scores between Cluster 1 and Cluster 2 managers related to indicators 3 and 4 of our HCTM model.

Indicator 3 states: "A designated member of the executive team is responsible for the formulation of the organization's technology strategy."

Indicator 4 states: "A designated member of the executive team is responsible for the administration and management of the organization's technology strategy."

These are the two indicators that focus on the function of a chief technology officer (CTO). This result strongly confirmed the message from the literature about the necessity of executive attention and leadership for HCTM. As a member of the executive team, the CTO typically reports directly to the CEO. Indicators 3 and 4 imply that this individual is responsible for staying abreast of present and potential future technologies and for leading the strategic decision-making process about when to adopt, support, or abandon technologies. Along with providing leadership, coordination, and facilitation, the responsibilities of the CTO include such activities as gatekeeping, advocacy, funding, sponsorship, policy and procedure development, promotion, capacity building, and overseeing the technology management system.

Not all hospitals have a CTO, in which case the responsibilities discussed here are either taken up by the CEO or, more likely, delegated to someone else such as the chief financial officer or chief operations officer. The CTO's job is to understand the strategic business issues, the customers, and the technology. The CTO should be an effective leader and command the respect of his or her employees, managers, and peers. The CTO should demonstrate vital communication skills. This finding implies that a good CTO probably can translate technical issues so that they can be readily understood by nontechnical personnel.

Cluster 1 hospitals were shown to be weakest in the indicators that also presented the highest need for improvement on a national, systemwide basis—namely, indicators 8, 19, and 26.

Indicator 8 states: "Technology is linked to clearly identified customer needs and priorities."

Indicator 19 states: "The organization has strategies to respond flexibly and rapidly to technological change."

Indicator 26 states: "The organization's performance as a function of technology management activities is routinely evaluated and benchmarked."

A high gap score on indicator 8 implies a lack of ongoing access to information about current and future needs and priorities of customers and staff. Indicator 19, similarly, addresses how quickly the organization responds to shifts in technological trends. A high gap score here implies that the organization ignores "market pull" strategies as part of its customer relations policy, essentially going along with "technology push." Product development times, innovation cycles, and overall cycle times for putting ideas and innovations into practice are longer than expected relative to industry norms. Finally, a high gap score for indicator 26 implies a lack of systematic performance reviews for different aspects of HCTM. These might include their impact on overall organizational goals, objectives, and customer service, including, for example, annual performance evaluations of the executive fulfilling the CTO role.

From our analysis, the instrument (the e-survey) is able to distinguish between senior managers' differences in perceptions of their organization's standard of HCTM. Significant differences ($p < 0.001$) between Cluster 1 and Cluster 2 organizations can be consistently identified across all three dimensions of HCTM. In particular, the perceived presence of chief technology officer roles in the organization seems to contribute strongly to the differences in mean gap scores between the clusters. Other strategic management and change management variables are perceived as being implemented to a greater extent in Cluster 2 institutions. Improvements seem to be possible along all three dimensions.

Overall, our results and statistical analysis indicated that there are significant differences in HCTM sophistication among Canadian teaching hospitals. The major differences occur in areas of strategic technology management (dimension 1), followed by change management (dimension 2), and, to a lesser extent, organizational management (dimension 3). The perceptions of senior managers are not significantly influenced by their area of responsibility relative to patient or non–patient care or by their position in the reporting structure. Improvements are generally needed in all areas addressed by the indicators identified in our HCTM model.

The Hay Group Study

As pointed out earlier, the purpose of the entire HCTM exercise is to improve performance in terms of achieving the strategic goals and objectives of the organization. For a private sector organization, this may be expressed as competitive advantage, market share, profitability, return on investment, or other such measures. What would be the performance measures for public sector agencies such as the hospitals that participated in this study? What difference does it make that one cluster of hospitals seems to manage technology better than another cluster?

Fortunately, answers to these questions have been provided independently by ACAHO information about operational efficiency and clinical efficiency that is generated on a confidential basis. The Hay Group in Toronto compiled the data in an annual report entitled *Benchmarking Comparison of Canadian Hospitals*. The Hay study was commissioned by the hospitals in an effort "to improve the efficiency, effectiveness and quality of their care processes." The comparisons were based on Canadian hospital separation data, on accounts and statistics reported to Ministries of Health, and other data provided by the participating hospitals.

We made use of the Hay study to validate the results of our own study. To determine whether there was any association between HCTM performance of the two clusters of hospitals identified in our study and the measures of performance used in the Hay study, we examined the outcomes provided by the Hay study on the following two summary measures:

- The measure for the overall clinical efficiency of a hospital is the percentage of inpatient days that could be reduced if a hospital were to achieve benchmark levels of performance. The smaller the percentage, the more efficient the hospital.
- The measure for the overall operational efficiency of a hospital is the potential reduction in operating cost, including direct care, administrative, and support functions. Subject to some caveats, the hospital with the smaller potential reduction can be considered more efficient with respect to the areas examined by these comparisons.

If an average gap score of 6 (over all responses and all indicators for each organization) was considered the benchmark target, the potential HCTM improvement could be calculated and expressed in terms of potential percentage reduction. We can use this measure to compare our results to those of the Hay study.

Four of the five Cluster 2 hospitals and eleven of the thirteen Cluster 1 hospitals participate in annual benchmark comparison studies. Confidential summary statements provide participating organizations with feedback about the room for improvement if they operated at benchmark levels on specific performance indicators. From the summary statements, it was clear that Cluster 2 hospitals had considerably less room for improvement, suggesting a strong correlation between their high HCTM performance and their clinical and operational efficiency.

Conclusion

Our research generated a technology management conceptualization consisting of a definition, its attributes, and a metric. Development of a validated and reliable instrument amounted subsequently to the formulation of a first-order HCTM model. This model represents both a theoretical perspective that can be further tested empirically and a framework for applying HCTM practice in the real world.

A key question in our research relates to the impact of HCTM sophistication on health care organizational performance and success. Our study was able to explore to some extent the relationship between clinical and operational efficiency and technology management performance, which was discussed in terms of a comparison of our study results with those of the Hay Group study. Unfortunately, our study did not address the more strategic impact of HCTM performance on customer satisfaction and customer service levels relative to customer needs; this is a topic for future HCTM research.

Our purpose in this concluding section is to conceptualize how the findings from our HCTM research challenge us to view the importance of the customer (consumer, patient, or client) in health care more critically. Specifically, the need to understand in detail the various consumer groups and their needs, priorities, and values can be applied meaningfully in an e-health context. We will come back to this topic a bit later in the section, but first we will consider some of the implications of our findings.

We believe that further HCTM and e-HCTM research is clearly needed to test the generalizability of our three-factorial model. Our analysis suggests that this three-dimensional HCTM model can also be used to serve not only as the basis for creating a HCTM training curriculum, but as practical guide for the establishment of a HCTM strategy in a health care organization. It may also be the basis for an e-HCTM curriculum, as well as a practical tool for generating an e-HCTM strategy by providing benchmarks for future research.

In terms of e-HCTM curriculum, we have seen how the e-health paradigm components in this text can be divided into three major themes. First, the e-health foundation (Chapters Three through Six), which corresponds to dimension 3 of the HCTM model (organization management) because of the concentration on how organizational perspectives and infrastructures are to be reshaped through e-health thinking and the management of virtual organizations. Second, e-health domains and applications (Chapters Seven through Eleven) correspond to dimension 2 of the HCTM model (change management) because of the focus on how different sectors of main-stream applications of health services must now be changed and managed into new domains and alternative forms of e-health services. Finally, e-health strategies and impacts (Chapters Twelve through Fifteen) correspond most clearly to dimension 1 (strategic management) because of the need to focus this paradigm shift at a strategic management and policy level, rather than at operational or lower levels in order to achieve organizational success and high system performance.

In terms of generating an e-HCTM strategy, our study recognizes the increasing power of technology (in our case, e-technology) to meet the needs of e-consumers and e-providers in revolutionary and unpredictable ways. In this sense, our focus is on harnessing the power of e-technology through e-health care technology management. Like other potentially strategic resources such as health, human resources, and financial resources, e-technologies should and can become more commonly understood assets that must be managed well if high payoffs are to be expected. Executive-level attention is critical in facilitating the alignment of an organization's overall business strategy and its e-technology strategy in order to achieve high-performing e-health systems. The empirical evidence from our study is clear on this matter: to be successful in the current turbulent and unpredictable technology environment, organizations need to anchor technology management at the vice presidential level. Both traditional health care and e-health care systems have efficiency goals and consider innovation and technology to be tactical tools to accomplish existing services at lower cost or to produce more services at a given cost. The judgment of what constitutes strategic technology needs to be made with full knowledge and information about the customers.

Strategic technology improves the manner in which customer needs are met. It is aimed at the highest order of customer needs achievable under prevailing circumstances. One key research area emerging from our study is the definition and identification of customers, customer groups, and customer needs in health care or in the case of e-health systems, e-consumers, e-consumer groups, and e-consumer needs. Organizations like teaching hospitals are faced with competing customer interests (provincial services, community services, research and education services), not to mention internal "customer" interests, including those of doctors, nurses, and technicians as well as patients. Resource planning of any kind—human, technological, or financial—is difficult unless the primary customers and their needs are well defined.

With the emergence of e-health, a whole new scenario of e-customer and e-consumer relationships is unfolding, with significant implications for providers and agencies of health care services. In e-health, e-consumers and e-patients must take center stage, and their needs must be considered very carefully. Definition of e-consumers, e-stakeholders, and their hierarchy of needs is essential. Everyone in the e-health system must be clear on whose needs are to be met by a particular technology and be prepared to adjust if better ways to meet those needs are discovered.

Groups of e-customers or individual customers may prioritize their needs differently. Most expressed needs are simply a means to another end, intermediate needs that can sometimes be leapfrogged with e-technology. Without a thorough understanding and explicit statement of this hierarchy of customer needs, no effective e-technology strategy can be developed.

While most organizations attempt to tackle various aspects of the e-technology management model, the lack of an integrated framework limits organizations and individuals, preventing them from realizing the full potential and benefit of those attempts. Without an e-technology management focus and framework, there is no basis for relating technology management ideas; thus, the response to those ideas is fragmented. An example might be the often-lamented difficulty of bringing research results to bear on practice environments through a linkage and exchange process (see, for example, Robson, 1993). Using a fragmented approach may lead to only limited success in changing environmental conditions; for example, individuals may be trained in new technologies but then may return to environments that do not have a suitable support framework in place. A cohesive framework would optimize the benefit of individual actions. Applying the HCTM model to e-HCTM would at the very least provide a foundational perspective from which ideas about e-HCTM can be generated and shared.

E-health care systems should not overlook the importance of e-technology management responsibility. There seems to be some opposition to the idea of a central executive coordinator of technology strategy and implementation, primarily due to the breadth of e-technology in health care. It is important to remember that inherent in the HCTM model is the concept of multidisciplinary and multifunctional teams with representation from both research and operations departments. In a similar vein, e-technology management training and research needs to be strengthened from a multidisciplinary and multifunctional perspective. E-technology has made the critical leap from being a tactical resource to also being a strategic resource. While a broad view of potentially strategic e-technology is important, an e-HCTM framework focuses efforts on strengthening the managerial aspects of an organization for e-technology use and application.

Finally, a number of issues relate to the application of the HCTM model and its implications for e-HCTM. The HCTM model consists of a hierarchy of dimensions, variables, and indicators. As mentioned earlier, there is a body of literature dealing with the basic and applied science fundamentals underlying each indicator. While knowledge could undoubtedly be expanded in each of these facets, some examples of priority research areas for HCTM and for e-HCTM are listed here:

- How are the customers in e-health care different from those in traditional health care? What are their differing needs, and what order of priority may be attached to those needs (that is, what is their hierarchy of needs)? What are the implications for HCTM versus e-HCTM?

- Aside from health administrators and executive team leaders, who would be key targets for an e-survey on HCTM and e-HCTM? Are the views of these groups potentially the same or different in traditional and e-health care systems?
- What concretely differentiates clusters of high-performing and low-performing health care organizations in terms of HCTM? How would this information apply to e-HCTM, a system with apparently quite different e-technology management perspectives and performance capabilities?
- How significantly do HCTM and e-HCTM contribute to clinical and operational efficiencies, quality and levels of care, and customer (or e-consumer) satisfaction?

Organizations should be guided by market pull as opposed to technology push considerations. The public's unlimited demand for customized, high-quality, rapidly delivered, and low-cost health care is well documented. E-providers and e-customers today are demanding ready access to global e-health information to achieve the highest level of health care. This, and the rapid rate of e-technological development, require both public and private sector organizations to manage e-technology and innovation strategically, albeit for different combinations of economic and altruistic motives. The perspective of e-technology as a strategic resource implies willingness to change the business fundamentally if the needs of customers can be better met with different technology.

Chapter Questions

1. How is e-HCTM strategy defined on the basis of the extant literature? What emerging dimensions define HCTM and can in turn be applied to e-HCTM?
2. What is the significance of e-surveying health administrators and executive team members on a topic such as health care technology management?
3. What characteristics do you expect to find in well-managed e-health care systems? Why? Who are the best people to manage e-technologies?
4. What are some of the areas for future research in e-HCTM?
5. Imagine that you have been asked to oversee a new e-health initiative on moving a large pharmacy chain store on-line. What steps would you take with respect to e-technology applications and management of these applications in the longer run to ensure sustainability?

References

Andersen, D. F., Belardo, S., & Dawes, S. S. (1994). Strategic information management: Conceptual frameworks for the public sector. *Public Productivity and Management Review, 17*(4), 335–353.

Badawy, M. K. (1998). Technology management education: Alternative models. *California Management Review, 40*(4), 94–116.

British Columbia Ministry of Health Planning. (2002). *A new era for patient centred health care: Building a sustainable, accountable structure for delivery of high-quality patient services.*: Author.

Canadian College of Health Service Executives. (2000). *Survey of leadership skill requirements.*: Author.

Eisler, G. (2002). *Health care technology management (HCTM): An assessment of its application in Canadian teaching hospitals.* Unpublished doctoral dissertation, University of British Columbia, Canada.

Eisler, G., Sheps, S., Satuglu, S., & Tan, J. (2002). *Health technology management in Canadian teaching hospitals: An empirical investigation.* Paper presented at the Hospital of the Future Conference, Chicago, Illinois.

Geisler, E. (2000). *The metrics of science and technology.* Westport, CT: Quorum Books.

Geisler, E., & Heller, O. (1996). *Managing technology in healthcare.* Boston: Kluwer.

Gregory, M. J., Probert, D. R., & Cowell, D. R. (1996). Auditing technology management processes. *International Journal of Technology Management, 12*(3), 306–319.

Husain, Z., & Zafar Husain, S. (1997). Strategic management of technology—A glimpse of literature. *International Journal of Technology Management, 14*(5), 539–578.

Lewis, B. R. (1993). *The information resource management concept: Domain, measurement, and implementation status (Technology planning).* Doctoral dissertation, Auburn University, Auburn, AL. (Available from UMI Dissertation Services)

McCallum, J. S. (1996). Changing at warp speed: Managing technology. *Business Quarterly, 60*(31), 87–89, 92–93.

McGee, J., & Thomas, H. (1989). Technology and strategic management progress and future directions. *R & D Management, 19*(3), 205–213.

Perrino, A. C., & Tipping, J. W. (1989). Global management of technology. *Research Technology Management, 32*(3), 12.

Raghupathi, W., & Tan, J. (2002, December). Strategic IT applications in health care. *Communications of the ACM, 45*(12), 56–61.

Robson, C. (1993). *Real world research: A resource for social scientists and practitioner-researchers.* Cambridge, MA: Blackwell.

Tapscott, D. (1996). *The digital economy: Promise and peril in the age of networked intelligence.* New York: McGraw-Hill.

Tapscott, D. and Caston, A. (1993). *Paradigm shift: The new promise of information technology.* New York: McGraw-Hill Inc.

World Health Organization. (2000). *The World Health Report 2000: Health systems: Improving performance.* Geneva, Switzerland: World Health Organization.

Evidence-Based Medicine Case

Barry P. Markovitz

Professionally our methods of transmitting and receiving the results of research are generations old and now totally inadequate for their purpose. (Vannevar, 1945).

A second-year medical student hears a psychiatry professor lecture about Freud's theories. He asks the professor what evidence there is to support these theories and receives this answer: "I don't think there is any. I certainly don't believe this stuff; I was asked by the department chair to give this lecture." On rotation in internal medicine, a medical student is required to present evidence to support her treatment plans for every new patient she has admitted. She finds this exciting and challenging compared with the usual routine of following the attending physician's preferences without supporting evidence. A student is asked to read an article to help determine the proper course of treatment for a particular patient. The attending physician provides this disclaimer: "No one really does this in real life."

These three experiences are noted as defining moments in the careers of three authors (Brian Haynes, Sharon Straus, and Scott Richardson, respectively) of a very popular handbook called *Evidence-Based Medicine: How to Practice and Teach EBM* (Sackett and others, 2000). First formally introduced in a 1992 article in the *Journal of the American Medical Association,* (Evidence-Based Medicine Working Group, 1992), evidence-based medicine has become known as "the means by which current best evidence from research can be judiciously and conscientiously applied in the prevention, detection, and care of health disorders" (Haynes and Haines, 1998). The term *research* in this context refers almost exclusively to clinical research. So was the concept of using scientifically derived information to guide medical care just invented in 1992? Of course not, but even today, health care is far too heavily influenced by the individual practitioner's beliefs, experiences, and preferences. Indeed, the correlation between the strength of evidence to support a practice and the frequency of its use remains poor (Rich, 2002).

The explicit process known as *evidence-based medicine* or, more generically, *evidence-based health care,* truly represents a paradigm shift, as defined by Thomas Kuhn (1970). Prior to the explosion of research findings available in the past few decades, physicians for generations had little more than their mentors and personal experience to rely on in deciding what was best for their patients. With the advent of the controlled clinical trial, therapeutic interventions could be rigorously tested for efficacy. The principles of clinical epidemiology were developed and applied to interpret patient-oriented research. The old paradigm was based on the assumption that clinical experience and understanding of pathophysiology were sufficient to diagnose and treat most patients. That paradigm has faded away. The new paradigm still calls for clinical experience and mechanistic understanding but also calls for a knowledge of how to use the rules of evidence to properly interpret the medical literature for direct patient care. Although publications on clinical research trials have increased dramatically, many studies have substantial flaws that may limit their application. A critical eye is necessary to evaluate such reports.

Why evidence-based medicine, and why now? With exponentially increasing numbers of outcome-oriented clinical trials, systematic reviews, and evidence-based guidelines being published, clinicians need a consistent approach to search for, appraise, and apply this evidence to the care of their patients. Classic continuing medical education programs do not necessarily improve physicians' skills; pathophysiological treatment often fails; and traditional textbooks are typically out of date with regard to recent innovations by the time they are published.

Evidence-based medicine (EBM) comprises five stages:

- Developing the clinical question relevant to the patient at hand, typically formatted by the PICO acronym: In a given **p**atient population, does a particular **i**ntervention, **c**ompared with controls or standard therapy, result in an improved **o**utcome?
- Searching for the evidence, usually in bibliographic databases such as the National Library of Medicine's MEDLINE
- Critically appraising the evidence for its validity, results, and applicability
- Integration of the appraised evidence with the patient's values and preferences
- Self-evaluation of the process to continually improve its efficiency and effectiveness

It becomes obvious early in this process that many relevant clinical trials may address one's patient's problems. Systematic reviews can be structured and concise summaries of two or more original clinical studies designed to address a focused question; when quantitative analysis is performed, the term *meta-analysis* applies. The methodology and results of a systematic review can be critically appraised in a manner analogous to the appraisal process of a primary clinical investigation. When systematic reviews are analyzed on the basis of individuals or organizations, evidence-based clinical practice guidelines may be published. As one might expect, the guidelines, like the studies, can and should be viewed through the prism of critical analysis.

Each clinical situation requires a unique set of questions to filter the studies and interpret the results. The Users' Guides to the Medical Literature are a series that has appeared in the *Journal of the American Medical Association* since 1992, offering structured methods of critical appraisal of original trials on therapy, prognosis, diagnosis, and harm, as well as guides to interpretation of systematic reviews, clinical practice guidelines, and many other peer-reviewed publications on health care. For example, for trials of a therapeutic intervention, in order to appraise the paper's validity and root out various sources of bias, one might ask the following questions (Guyatt, Sackett, and Cook, 1993):

- Was the assignment of patients to treatment groups randomized?
- Were all patients who entered the trial properly accounted for and attributed at its conclusion?
- Were patients, health workers, and study personnel blind to treatments?
- Were the groups similar at the start of the trial?
- Aside from the experimental intervention, were the groups treated equally?

In assessing a therapy article's results, we ask the following (Guyatt, Sackett, and Cook, 1994):

- How large was the treatment effect?
- How precise was the estimate of the treatment effect?

The terminology of clinical epidemiology can put results in terms that providers and patients can grapple with more appropriately than with a "statistically significant difference" measured by a "*p*-value." For dichotomous outcomes, the concepts of *relative risk, relative risk reduction, absolute risk reduction,* and *number needed to treat* are the relevant markers of effect. The importance of each of these terms is demonstrated in Exhibit 13.1, in which two hypothetical treatments have identical relative effects but very different absolute mortality rates.

Finally, we ask about the applicability of the study's results (Guyatt, Sackett, and Cook, 1994):

• Can the results be applied to my patient's care?
• Were all clinically important outcomes considered?
• Are the likely treatment benefits worth the potential harm and costs?

After following this process, one should have a reasonably sound notion of whether the study in question is valid, what the results are, and whether they are truly applicable to one's patient.

The Users' Guides series has been updated and condensed into a textbook, finally compiling into a single tome the "liturgy" of EBM. While the basic methodology of EBM may be suitable for a textbook (although this itself is debatable, a point that the authors readily concede), the evidence needed to practice EBM cannot be so easily packaged, and that is where the Internet plays a vital role.

The Internet as a Source for Evidence

The original 1992 article that introduced EBM describes a clinical scenario wherein a curious resident conducts a computerized literature search in the library, at a cost of one hour of time and $2.68, including the photocopying charge (Evidence-Based

EXHIBIT 13.1. THE IMPORTANCE OF DICHOTOMOUS MEASURES OF EFFECT

	Treated Mortality Rate (Percentage) A	Control Mortality Rate (Percentage) B	Relative Risk of Death (RR)	Relative Risk Reduction of Death (RRR)	Absolute Risk Reduction of Death (ARR)	Number Needed to Treat to Prevent One Death (NNT)
Formula			A/B	1 – A/B	A – B	1/ARR
Treatment X	10%	40%	0.25	0.75	30%	3.3
Treatment Y	0.1%	0.4%	0.25	0.75	0.3%	333

Medicine Working Group, 1992). Ten years later, the same search would likely be conducted in the hospital ward or clinic, quite possibly at the patient's bedside, at no charge. The article chosen might be printed out on the nursing station's laser printer or simply read on-line or saved in an Adobe portable document format (PDF) file for later printing or e-mail distribution. A version of the article could be available for downloading directly into the resident's portable digital assistant (PDA), never using paper. And the entire process of searching and retrieval might take only a few minutes at most, rather than an hour.

Indeed, it is astounding how far and fast the biomedical information retrieval technology of the Internet has spread in less than a decade. Virtually every bibliographic database in the biomedical sciences is available on-line, and those managed by the U.S. National Center for Biotechnology Information (NCBI) and National Library of Medicine (NLM) are accessible free of charge. The premier such database, MEDLINE, now available at PubMed (http://www.pubmed.gov/), contains over 11 million citations from 4,600 journals from seventy countries. The "Clinical Queries" function provides direct evidence from clinical trials and is particularly useful for clinicians. It incorporates a series of built-in filters that are specific to the type of query. There is a separate button for articles about therapy, prognosis, diagnosis, and etiology, which allows rapid focusing of searches on only the most relevant citations (Haynes and others, 1994). In addition to citations and abstracts, direct links to the full text of the on-line paper are often available, although either an institutional or an individual subscription to the journal in question is usually necessary to actually view the full text. Over 3,500 journals enable this "link out" feature from PubMed.

A separate but related issue, the concept that for-profit private companies (publishers) should control the record of scientific accomplishments, is being called into question. Numerous initiatives are trying to break down the centuries-old concept that scientists, who are usually publicly funded, should turn over copyright of their written analysis to publishers, who then require the authors and their peers to buy back this written record. Although this may be a reasonable model for commercial writers, who seek profit from sales of their work as the publishers do, with the advent of the Internet and the minimal cost of distribution of electronic "papers," scientific authors often seek as wide a distribution as possible of their work with as few barriers as possible. In some cases, the financial firewalls are beginning to crumble. Scientists are joining boycotts of publishers that do not enable free access to their manuscripts on the Internet, at least after a limited period of time. The Public Library of Science (http://www.publiclibraryofscience.org), one organization calling for open access, has received signatures of support from over 30,000 scientists from 180 countries. Some journals now provide access to their archives three to twelve months after initial publication. Other journals have been free on the Web for several years, and new journals with altered business models (author pays instead of reader pays) are being developed. This is a critical issue for the future of EBM and the Internet, for without access to the full text of clinical research on-line, there is insufficient evidence with which to practice evidence-based medicine.

Other companies provide access to MEDLINE with proprietary interfaces, the most popular of which is OVID (http://www.ovid.com). In addition to point-and-click access to sophisticated searching functions, OVID has contracted with numerous publishers to provide their journals' full text from within the application, which is now most commonly accessed over the Internet with a browser. With many institutions paying for OVID access, clinicians and researchers can easily access thousands of publications' full texts either at no cost to the user or for a nominal yearly fee. OVID also provides full access to a number of other resources that are valuable for the evidence-based clinician. MedScape (http://www.medscape.com) also provides a search interface to MEDLINE and has arrangements with a number of journals to display selected full-text articles. Silverplatter (http://www.silverplatter.com), another proprietary service affiliated with OVID, offers access to MEDLINE and other databases.

Not all medical journals are cited in MEDLINE. The Institute of Scientific Information maintains several large scientific bibliographic databases, including the Current Contents series, which is now available by institutional subscription as the Web of Science (http://isiknowledge.com/wos/). CINAHL is a nursing and allied health bibliographic database, and CANCERLIT provides references related to cancer studies. EMBASE, maintained by the publisher Elsevier Science, includes some journals not referenced in MEDLINE. In addition, it provides subsets for more directed searching, such as EMBASE Pediatrics and EMBASE Anesthesiology.

Either with the aid of built-in filters—for example, at PubMed or in OVID—or by learning to manually add screening terms to searches, the evidence-hungry clinician can rapidly focus on relevant clinical trial reports, then continue the process of critical appraisal and application. Tools for learning EBM techniques are widespread on the Internet and will be discussed in the next section. But often there are numerous studies that are relevant to the patient question at hand. In such cases, it is far more appropriate and efficient to look for and appraise systematic reviews or evidence-based guidelines, should they exist. Is there a rapid way to access these secondary evidence sources on-line? In PubMed, a search can be limited to systematic reviews and to meta-analyses in OVID. The Cochrane Collaboration is an international group dedicated to creating, disseminating, and maintaining systematic reviews of virtually every aspect of health care. The Cochrane Library of Systematic Reviews is on-line (http://www.cochranelibrary.com/) and available by individual or institutional subscription. These reviews are rigorously prepared with structured software and are peer-reviewed and regularly updated. The United Kingdom's National Health Service Centre for Reviews and Dissemination at the University of York maintains the Database of Abstracts of Reviews of Effects (DARE) on-line (http://nhscrd.york.ac.uk/darehp.htm). Since DARE represents a regularly updated source of summaries of systematic reviews obtained from a variety of sources, it should be a clinician's first stop in a search for such resources.

Using systematic reviews, original clinical research, and consensus opinion under rigorous and structured rules, many organizations (for example, the American Academy of Pediatrics and the Society of Critical Care Medicine) have developed guidelines that summarize the current best evidence in the diagnosis and management of a variety of disorders. Unlike previous generations of consensus statements, which were often simply the opinion of experts, evidence-based guidelines explicitly present the evidence behind the recommendations and grade the recommendations accordingly (Oxford Centre for Evidence-Based Medicine, 2002). A unique source for such guidelines is the National Guideline Clearinghouse (NGC) (http://www.guideline.gov/), sponsored by the U.S. Agency for Healthcare Research and Quality. Only clinical practice guidelines from professional societies or organizations that have a documented evidence-based approach are included on the NGC site, which makes available nearly a thousand guidelines in either full-text or summary form.

When confronted with a clinical problem, it is usually not immediately clear whether original research, systematic reviews, guidelines, or other focused sources will be most useful in the specific case. What is needed is a metasearch engine that scours numerous other search sites and presents a coherent list of results. SUMSearch at the University of Texas Health Science Center is just such a resource (http://sumsearch.uthscsa.edu/). SUMSearch performs contingency searching—that is, it alters its search based on the number of results obtained, broadening or narrowing the focus as necessary—of PubMed, DARE, NGC, and other quality sites. It provides pull-down menus for filtering, based on the type of clinical question (therapy, prognosis, and so on), age group, and language. Search results are presented in an extremely user-friendly format, based on evidence type and source.

There are additional secondary sources of evidence. Structured critical appraisals and other succinct summaries of original clinical research studies (and of systematic reviews and guidelines) are available as independent journals and on a number of established Web sites. The American College of Physicians and American Society of Internal Medicine (ACP-ASIM) publishes the *ACP Journal Club* (http://www.acpjc.org), and the journal *Evidence-Based Medicine* is from the BMJ Publishing Group (http://ebm.bmjjournals.com/). A long-standing resource, Patient Oriented Evidence that Matters (POEMs) (http://www.infopoems.com/), offers such succinct and structured summaries and is now available by subscription. This resource is integrated with a search engine and a version for PocketPC PDAs. The University of Michigan Department of Pediatrics maintains a collection of Critically Appraised Topics (CATs) (http://www.med.umich.edu/pediatrics/ebm/), concise evidence-based summaries of research that addresses a particular patient issue. The PedsCCM Evidence-Based Journal Club posts peer-reviewed, structured critical appraisals of clinical trials and systematic reviews pertaining to intensive care medicine (http://PedsCCM.wustl.edu/EBJournal_club.html).

The Turning Research into Practice (TRIP) database (http://www.tripdatabase.com/) is a comprehensive resource for evidence sources on the Internet, cataloguing sources from seventy-five sites, including the abstracting and appraisal sites. Search results are grouped according to source—for example, peer-reviewed journals, guidelines, journal clubs. In addition, the TRIP site includes links to relevant chapters in Internet-based textbooks and digital image sources, recognizing that some users also require the type of background information that a textbook can still provide effectively.

For the busy clinician, tracking down and appraising the necessary information still sounds like a lot of work! If there were resources that synthesized validated evidence resources into a user-friendly interface, more physicians might be amenable to practicing evidence-based medicine. *Clinical Evidence* (http://www.clinicalevidence/com/) is a quarterly print and Web publication of the BMJ Publishing Group. Organized by clinical topics (for example, stroke management, myocardial infarction prevention), *Clinical Evidence* discusses focused questions and presents very succinct conclusions. Evidence appraisals are hyperlinked from the conclusions, enabling rapid drill-downs to the primary source material. Exhibit 13.2 shows a sample screen that illustrates the utilitarian user interface of this valuable resource.

Cliniguide, available via OVID, presents disease management information in a stripped-down textbook interface, also taking full advantage of hyperlinking to make more detailed material with source evidence appraisals readily available. EBM Solutions (http://www.ebmsolutions.com/) is a care management application that is available to physicians and patients on the Web; it was developed by six academic medical centers. The site offers succinct evidence-based guidelines on various aspects of management of numerous common conditions. Unique to EBM Solutions, symptom constellations (for example, abdominal pain in children and chronic cough) are also listed, improving the usefulness of this resource.

Although evidence-based medicine decries the pejorative label of "cookbook medicine," in the face of overwhelming evidence from nearly every health care field that consistency of approach is a critical factor in explaining improved outcomes, decision support tools are being developed to steer practitioners to the "proper" diagnostic or management strategy for a patient with a given symptom complex or disease. Interactive calculators on the Web (and downloadable versions for PDAs) can determine everything from free water deficits to a patient's risk of breast cancer. The National Center for Emergency Medicine Informatics (http://www.ncemi.org/) provides a wide range of such calculators and acuity scores. Some could readily be labeled clinical decision support tools. For example, the simple Ottawa rule for ankle fracture, with the answers to three simple questions, can reliably predict the need for a radiograph of the ankle (Stiell and others, 1993). The more complex Goldman acute myocardial infarction probability calculator can also be used as a decision support tool (Goldman and others, 1988). Unique to pediatrics is Isabel, an on-line interactive tool that aids in differential diagnosis and also chronicles unique cases and treatment algorithms (http://www.isabel.org.uk/). A remarkable on-line tool, Evidence-Based On-Call (http://www.eboncall.co.uk/), offers nearly comprehensive evidence for the diagnosis and management of a limited number of common conditions, free of charge.

Resources for Learning Evidence-Based Medicine on the Internet

As many sites exist to learn about or provide tools for EBM as exist to provide evidence with which to practice EBM. With the hyperlinked Internet, it is hard not to find (or stumble on) this vast network of EBM resources. Certainly, a reasonable starting point for someone who wishes to learn about EBM would be one of the "mother ships" for

EXHIBIT 13.2. CHAPTER INTRODUCTION TO *CLINICAL EVIDENCE*

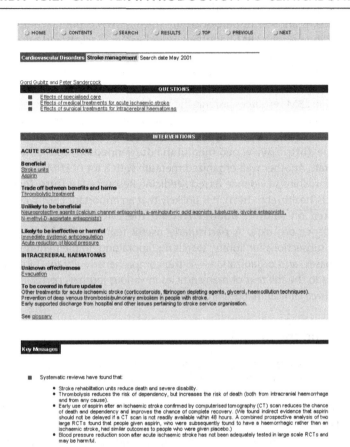

EBM, either McMaster University's Health Information Research Unit in Canada (http://hiru.mcmaster.ca/) or the Oxford Centre for Evidence-Based Medicine in the United Kingdom (http://cebm.jr2.ox.ac.uk/). These two sites offer both internal educational resources and links to the vast array of resources elsewhere on the net. For learning how to practice Evidence Based Medicine, the Clinical Epidemiology for Effective Clinical Practice Online Tutorial at IntensiveCare.com is also an excellent starting point (http://intensivecare.com/Tutorial.html). The Introduction to Evidence-Based Medline tool, a joint effort of Duke University Medical Center Library and the Health Sciences Library at the University of North Carolina–Chapel Hill is another self-paced tutorial (http://www.hsl.unc.edu/lm/ebm/index.htm).

Many consider the Users' Guides to the Medical Literature series (mentioned earlier) to be the defining scripture of EBM, and the full text of the entire series is now freely accessible on-line at the Canadian Centres for Health Evidence (http://www. cche.net/usersguides/main.asp). A version of the guides with more interactive features is also available on-line by individual or institutional subscription (http://www. usersguides.org). The Centre for Evidence-Based Medicine at Mount Sinai Hospital in Toronto, Canada, is another resource-rich site (http://www.cebm.utoronto.ca/). This is the home of the popular EBM handbook noted earlier (Sackett and others, 2000); it offers supplementary materials and updates to the text. Also available at this site is a free EBM calculator for PalmOS and PocketPC PDAs, which enables rapid calculations of risks, odds ratios, and more. The site also maintains an excellent annotated set of links to on-line EBM resources around the world.

The basic science of evidence-based medicine is clinical epidemiology, and the Web has vast resources in this field; many are listed on the Epidemiology and Biostatistics Resources page (http://www.ped.med.utah.edu/genpedscrr/Epibio.htm) at the University of Utah. Another well-organized metasite with a list of EBM links is the University of Hertfordshire's Evidence Based Medicine Resource List (http://www.herts. ac.uk/lis/subjects/health/ebm.htm). It is unlikely that an important EBM Web site exists that is not listed on Andrew Booth's Netting the Evidence page (http://www. nettingtheevidence.org.uk/). A particularly useful feature of this site—which is organized into subsections for library, searching, appraising, implementing, software, journals, databases, and organizations—is the comprehensive library (bibliography), with direct links to the full text of many articles in various journals pertaining to EBM, systematic reviews, clinical trial design, and more.

The Future of EBM and the Internet

It is clear that evidence-based medicine and the Internet are thoroughly intertwined to the extent that it is virtually impossible to practice effective and up-to-date EBM without the use of the Internet. Because new generations of health care providers have grown up with computers and the Internet, teaching them how to use the Web to practice EBM is superfluous. However, they do need training on how to practice based on the best available evidence and where to go to find that evidence. Proper application of the tools of clinical epidemiology also requires a set of skills that must be learned. Above all, young trainees must be shown how to integrate EBM into their clinical routines; in many programs, it remains a separate academic exercise. EBM could never have evolved to its current state without the Internet, but the ongoing development of the on-line world does not guarantee the success of EBM. That will still require thoughtful, caring, and rational health care providers.

Case Questions

1. What is the significance of EBM for e-health care?
2. Why is the Internet an effective means or infrastructure for promoting EBM? What other platforms or infrastructures could be used?
3. Why is access to full-text clinical research critical to practicing EBM? How does one ensure the authoritative nature of the source from which evidence is to be gathered?

4. How can patients assist their caregivers in finding an appropriate evidence-based treatment for their symptoms? Imagine that you are asked to design a Web site to provide EBM support to patients. What features, design elements, or interface elements are needed to ensure that the site can provide this support in a convenient way?
5. How can EBM be integrated into clinical routines? How can the training of new residents help the integration of EBM? What is the impact of EBM on the future of e-health practices?

References

Evidence-Based Medicine Working Group. (1992). A new approach to teaching the practice of medicine: Evidence-Based Medicine Working Group. *Journal of the American Medical Association, 268*(17), 2420–2425.

Goldman, L., Cook, E., Brand, D., Lee, T., Rouan, G., Weisberg, M., Acampora, D., Stasiulewicz, C., Walshon, J., Terranova, G., et al. (1988). A computer protocol to predict myocardial infarction in emergency department patients with chest pain. *New England Journal of Medicine, 318*(13), 797–803.

Guyatt, G., Sackett, D., & Cook, D. (1993). Users' guides to the medical literature. II. How to use an article about therapy or prevention. A. Are the results of the study valid? Evidence-Based Medicine Working Group. *Journal of the American Medical Association, 270*(21), 2598–2601.

Guyatt, G., Sackett, D., & Cook, D. (1994). Users' guides to the medical literature. II. How to use an article about therapy or prevention. B. What were the results and will they help me in caring for my patients? Evidence-Based Medicine Working Group. *Journal of the American Medical Association, 271*(1), 59–63.

Haynes, B., & Haines, A. (1998). Barriers and bridges to evidence based clinical practice. *British Medical Journal, 317*(7153), 273–276.

Haynes, R., Wilczynski, N., McKibbon, K., Walker, C., & Sinclair, J. (1994). Developing optimal search strategies for detecting clinically sound studies in MEDLINE. title to come, *1*(6), 447–458.

Kuhn, T. *The structure of scientific revolutions.* Chicago: University of Chicago Press, 1970.

Oxford Centre for Evidence-Based Medicine. (2002). *Levels of evidence and grades of recommendation.* Retrieved on December 29, 2002, from http://www.indigojazz.co.uk/cebm/levels_of_evidence.asp

Rich, M. (2002). From clinical trials to clinical practice: Bridging the gap. *Journal of the American Medical Association, 287*(10), 1321–1323.

Sackett, D., Straus, S., Richardson, W., Rosenberg, W., & Haynes, R. (2000). *Evidence-based medicine: How to practice and teach EBM.* Edinburgh, Scotland: Churchill Livingstone.

Stiell, I., Greenberg, G., McKnight, R., and others. (1993). Decision rules for the use of radiography in acute ankle injuries: Refinement and prospective validation. *Journal of the American Medical Association, 269*(9), 1127–1132.

Vannevar, B. (1945, July). As we may think. *Atlantic Monthly,* 101–108.

CHAPTER FOURTEEN

E-SECURITY

Frameworks for Privacy and Security in E-Health Data Integration and Aggregation

Joseph Tan, Patrick Hung

The authors would like to acknowledge Kerry Taylor (CSIRO, Australia), Christine O'Keefe (CSIRO, Australia), James Gray III (RSA Security Inc., USA), Dickson K. W. Chiu (The Chinese University of Hong Kong, Hong Kong), and Mike Leung (PNM Solutions, Hong Kong) for their helpful suggestions and comments. In addition, the authors acknowledge the contributions of their past and present students, including those from the University of British Columbia, British Columbia Institute of Technology and Wayne State University, especially those who assisted with the literature review and with general research, including graphing, editing and checking references, and gathering materials presented in these chapters. Any omissions remain the responsibility of the authors. This work was supported by grants from the Office of the President of Wayne State University and other sources.

Learning Objectives

1. Articulate the intent of the security process
2. Understand the purpose of e-health data integration, and understand aggregation issues
3. Know the differences between a security framework and a privacy and consent framework
4. Characterize the security and privacy requirements of e-health data integration services and the dynamic nature of aggregation issues
5. Recognize the e-security implications of using e-health data integration services for policymakers, practitioners, and researchers
6. Generate a formal, rigorous e-security policy for e-health data integration, to prevent unauthorized users from accessing aggregates

Introduction

In today's era of e-health care informatics and telematics, there is a growing need for automated and integrated views of health information to guide rapidly changing health care planning activities and increasingly sophisticated health-related policy-making, as well as fulfill the information requirements of daily e-clinical care and e-patient management. Because e-health care information about individuals, groups, communities, and selected populations is mostly distributed across many different electronic databases, this information needs to be integrated in order to accomplish meaningful and intelligent decision making. This need has led to increased research on digital health data linkages and integrated views or, more formally, the theory and practice of *e-health data integration* (e-HDI).

Applied research in e-HDI services shows that integrated views in e-HDI can be provided in different information formats through the use of intelligent electronic health data access, analysis, and visualization tools (Lacroix, 2002). In particular, data mining and clustering techniques, which are discussed more fully in Chapter Eleven, can be used to unveil hidden patterns and complex knowledge that may have implications for future health research and health services planning, requirements, and recommendations. New developments in bioinformatics and e-diagnostic techniques are opening up enormous potential to screen for early warning signs and symptoms and to identify risk factors through accumulated and linked health data sets. Indeed, through Web interfaces, e-HDI services have already resulted in the creation of virtual communities that fill the needs of e-workers, e-providers, e-vendors, and Internet-savvy e-consumers who are also often geographically dispersed.

However, e-HDI services that link e-patients' health data sets to other sources of patient-specific data pose significant risks to the security, privacy, and confidentiality of stored patient data. These data sets often contain identifiable and sensitive information such as genetic or demographic data about individuals—for example, name, age, sex, address, phone number, employment status, family composition, and DNA profile (Quantin, Allaert, and Dusserre, 2000). Not only will disclosure of sensitive information of particular individuals potentially create personal embarrassment, but it may also, very possibly, lead to social ostracism (France, 1996).

Similarly, as e-HDI services encompass a great number of *aggregates*, or *integrated views*, the use of these aggregates for scientific research and related work will increase threats to security and privacy, especially in a cross-institutional, multiprovider environment (Moehr, 1994). Given that e-HDI services exist to aggregate the data sets in previously isolated databases for different users in a loosely coupled environment, their security must be rigorously guarded in order to ensure patient confidence (Ishikawa, 2000). At the same time, the dynamic nature of e-HDI services makes security issues challenging. Some of the most pressing security issues and privacy concerns that we have observed in e-health information management include (1) acquisition, storage, and processing of health data; (2) consent for processing and disclosure of e-health data; and (3) rights of the data subject (typically a patient about whom the data are being collected) to access and rectify his or her own health data set (France, 1996).

Earlier chapters of this text refer frequently to the need for e-security, which is essentially the design and development of frameworks for security as well as privacy, systems that safeguard against misuse or abuse of emerging e-health care applications and networks. In this chapter, we review the extant literature on security and privacy issues in order to generate appropriate security and privacy frameworks to guide future e-health care systems designers and developers. More significantly, we provide a specific treatment of security issues involved in aggregation of e-health data. In particular, we construct a formal specification for generating an e-security policy within the context of e-health data integration. We conclude the chapter with some suggestions about directions for future research in e-HDI services.

Security and Privacy Frameworks

In the last few years, a significant role of e-HDI initiatives or services has been to provide a technological platform to enable the improvement of e-health care treatment services (Grimson and others, 2001). For example, doctors who use e-HDI services to access patient medical records stored in diverse databases maintained by various health care provider groups and organizations will have a distinct advantage over those not privy to such rich patient information, which will be aggregated from diverse sources such as databases of past treatment data, medication records, and diagnostics, including digital image libraries and laboratory test reports associated with a patient. Moreover, such integrated views might be capable of being configured differently at different locations and thus be usable in varying contexts. However, this convenience does come with the cost of guarding the security, privacy, and confidentiality of the released information.

Recently, health data management that supports policymaking and high-level decisions in e-health services has been shifting its emphasis from treatment to prevention via the use of e-HDI services (Sheng and Chen, 1990). An example is the FluNet system, which aggregates worldwide information on potential threats arising from the spread of influenza-related viruses (see Chapter Five). Along these lines, e-HDI services integrate data sets from disparate health and social databases into integrated views for policymakers, practitioners, and researchers, who often use the results to conduct additional analyses. Partly owing to this development, scientific research has now become an integral part of our understanding of new strategies for management of chronic diseases such as diabetes and of patient treatment planning in specialties such as oncology (Moehr, 1994). As integrated data provide a more complete and comprehensive view of the patient care history and resulting patterns of applied treatment modalities, these can be used to guide future disease management and treatment planning.

While these developments may accelerate our knowledge of interfacing between clinical and medical sciences on the one hand and social and public health strategies on the other, and while they may help us to apply new findings to a host of health care services and treatments, there is always the danger of potential misuse, overuse, and undetected abuse of e-HDI services. Despite the inherent risk of such problems, research in the area of e-HDI security and privacy has been neglected, resulting in a significant gap in our knowledge of the issues in constructing a security policy for use when aggregating e-health data.

Our health care system has evolved on the implicit foundation of security, privacy, and confidentiality of patient records, and the emerging e-health care system and environment is bringing security and privacy issues to the fore. Indeed, the future of e-health depends on our understanding of these issues. The new security and privacy requirements confronting e-health care provider organizations and e-health data custodians are needed because of increasingly complex information technology and integrated e-technology architecture, coupled with widely distributed e-network availability (see Chapter Six).

Unfortunately, even traditional health care information systems have not been adequately audited, inviting fraud and abuse. Health care information technology has focused chiefly on administrative transactions such as laboratory results, patient registries, and traditional hospital financial information systems.

With the evolution of direct-to-digital clinical data systems, e-providers have begun to aggregate and edit data that were captured internally. This has resulted in distributed data entry (data entry from different locations) that is evolving into high-value transactions, thereby generating the "deep" trend in health care informatics. In contrast, the "wide" trend is promulgated by the movement of patient care outside the walls of the traditional inpatient environment. Not only has health care been shifting toward outpatient and ambulatory care settings, but it has also moved toward the provision of e-clinical care within an e-health care system and environment. Mainstream health care organizations are integrating modes of health care delivery in this way, regrouping themselves into highly distributed "integrated delivery networks" and e-delivery networks. These new delivery networks require applications in multiple environments in order to increase the number of access points available to users. The new networks also require a wide variety of access modalities for extracting and aggregating relevant health data sets.

Framework for Security

Before delving into the topic of security, we should first be clear about the intent of the security process. The primary challenge facing e-providers and e-health information custodians is how to handle the ubiquitous access requests from a variety of users over multiple channels who are attempting to get connected to information. Security requires that all access to information be guarded and provided only to authorized users. Thus, the challenge for e-health care managers becomes how to deploy and support increasingly complex applications across diverse environments while maintaining adequate levels of security. The essential question remains: How should the risk of releasing the information be balanced against the legitimacy of needs and the value of the released information to the user? This question is further complicated by the fact that providing some information often fuels user expectations for more information, as well as by generally increasing expectations in regard to convenient access, easy-to-use and easy-to-interpret information displays, and rapid release of information.

Today, privacy legislation in the United States (for example, the Health Insurance Portability and Accountability Act of 1996) and in Canada (for example, Bill C-6) and adoption of strong industry standards (for example, ISO 17799) have led to heightened awareness of security issues. Even so, we do not want to design systems so heavily weighted toward privacy protection requirements that they become very difficult to use, thereby defeating the purpose of making information accessible. In other words, we do not want powerful systems with rich stores of information that eventually have to be abandoned due to lack of use or usability. On the other hand, users should not be granted unrestricted access to more systems, which will only result in more user identifications and passwords to remember, let alone more potential for misuse, overuse, and abuse.

Based on our discussion, then, it seems that in planning any security application, a number of key considerations should be examined, including the following:

- Understanding the relative value of the information to the requester
- Application of available security tools to form a sound security framework
- Construction of a security policy for use when accessing aggregates
- How to evaluate compliance with the security policy and framework

The value of any particular piece of information is contingent on the need of the requester and will differ from one requester to another. Depending on what is already known, a new piece of information may or may not be valuable to a person in any particular situation. Moreover, some requesters hesitate to reveal their true intent when requesting particular information. If, for example, a patient is in need of medication, then it may be important to know the patient's medication allergies and other medications. Hence, knowing the reason why a particular piece of information is requested will go a long way toward specifying whether the requester has a legitimate claim to the information and should therefore be provided with it.

A strategy that simply encourages the implementation of a security technology system application by application is impractical and prohibitively expensive versus one in which security is managed via integrated applications. In the e-health care context, security need to entail calculated diligence in applying available tools to safeguard against potential risks. Many useful tools such as the ISO/IEC 17799 standard are available to formulate a sound security framework. The International Organization for Standardization (ISO) and the International Electrotechnical Commission (IEC) stipulate the characteristics of specialized systems for worldwide standardization. The ISO 17799 standard was published to provide an international framework for information security. The standard was not developed specifically for the health care industry; rather, the scope of the document encompasses cross-sector applications. Ten key areas that encompass a sound security framework are identified in the ISO 17799 standard. Each section provides explicitly detailed protocols that meet the security concerns associated with that area.

Of these ten areas, two stand out as most essential for security planning: (1) the formulation of a sound security policy from which security solutions can be generated and practiced and (2) compliance with the security policy and framework. Compliance monitoring ensures that all the key areas of the security framework are functioning properly. Issues of privacy and confidentiality of health information are closely related to the security of health information use and distribution.

Framework for Privacy and Confidentiality

Privacy is a basic human right, a central tenet of our free and democratic society. It is a measure of respect for personal autonomy and the dignity of the individual, and it forms the foundation of the basic rights outlined in documents such as the U.S. Constitution and the Canadian Charter of Rights and Freedoms, including freedom of speech, of association, and of choice. It is fundamental to both Canadian and U.S. societies. George Radwanski, the privacy commissioner of Canada, defines *privacy* as the right to control information collected about oneself, including its use and disclosure (G. Radwanski, "Patient Privacy in the Information Age," speech given at *E-Health 2001: The Future of Health Care in Canada,* Toronto, 2001). Privacy, therefore, has to do with our decisions on what personal information we want to share and with whom, trusting that it will be used for the purposes for which the information was requested.

While *privacy* relates to one's right to prevent one's health-related information from being shared with anyone and to control what information is revealed, *confidentiality* refers to the responsibility of custodians and recipients of an individual's health information to use or disclose it only as authorized. These concepts differ from *security*—the procedures, techniques, and technology employed to protect information from accidental or malicious destruction, alteration, or access, as discussed in the previous section. In other words, security mechanisms are used to implement privacy and confidentiality policies. As e-health care gives a new dimension to the health care industry, it also brings new threats to the security, privacy, and confidentiality of patients' medical records.

Imagine, for example, that Julie, a hypothetical high-profile political science professor at a state university, has been nominated for governor of her state or province after the resignation of the former governor. Suppose that at first, her nomination is hailed statewide because of her professionally faultless record. Her manifest qualifications clearly supersede questions of partisanship politics. However, an opposition party's nominee secretly hires a hacker to delve into her medical history. Soon, information about her past medical misadventures leaks to the press. Many years ago, she had an abortion, and she has also undergone treatment for depression at some point in her life. These facts anger many of her strong supporters, who are also strong anti-abortion activists. The fallout from the information leak drives Julie back into therapy for depression, raising further doubts as to her mental stability. Results of a recent uterine biopsy raise further doubts about her overall health. Julie is eventually forced to withdraw from the governor's race.

This illustration shows how lack of proper management and security in regard to health information, particularly e-health information, can be a significant factor in the violation of an individual's rights and privacy. Legislation such as the Health Insurance Portability and Accountability Act of 1996 (HIPAA) standards play an important role in creating security solutions to prevent such security breaches; one of the primary objectives of these standards is to "guarantee security and privacy of health information."

Obviously, Julie's case shows that personal health information is a critical area in which privacy should be enforced. Nothing is more intimate and deeply personal than one's health information. A massive amount of data has been collected over the years by trusted caregivers, and with e-health care systems, all of the data pertaining to one's physical and mental health can be conveniently housed in electronic health records. In some instances, the information will include sensitive medical information, such as the presence of a genetic predisposition to disease (for example, the breast cancer gene) or risk factors for a particular disease; history of depression or other mental illness; surgical interventions; treatment for sexually transmitted diseases; fertility status; or history of alcohol or drug abuse. Definitely, the amount of data that should be treated as strictly confidential is huge. The case of Professor Julie demonstrates how the release of this type of information can lead to significant negative personal consequences. If appropriate health information privacy is not guaranteed, the care provider–patient relationship will also be affected, possibly complicating the ethical and medical dimensions of a complex situation.

Given that it is not unusual to hear about privacy violations, particularly the inappropriate release of health information to third parties, it is easy to understand why privacy advocates have been intensely concerned about potential abuses and resulting discrimination. Dire consequences of inappropriate revelation of health information have included denial of insurance coverage, loss of job opportunities, refusal of mortgage financing, and more. Imagine how quickly these consequences would multiply in a completely wired society. The protection of e-health information privacy should therefore be of even greater concern to society than to individuals. If there were no legislated obligation for e-care providers to maintain confidentiality of health information, how frequently would fear of exposure prevent people from seeking medical attention? What would the implications be for public health issues such as HIV/AIDS and other sexually transmitted and infectious diseases?

It can be argued that individuals should have ownership of their own health information. However, once a caregiver collects the information, the organization to which the caregiver belongs almost always wants to assert some rights over the information.

Consequently, privacy rules and legislation must be enforced on the premise that privacy is a right that is essential to the integrity of an individual. E-health care providers must be considered merely information custodians, not owners. Custodianship gives these providers access privileges but also a responsibility to maintain the individuals' trust. In this sense, confidentiality is the obligation of caregivers to protect personal information that is entrusted to them and includes an implicit understanding that information will not be disclosed except in limited situations. Custodians are also responsible for ensuring that the information is not misused or used for purposes other than those for which it was originally intended. This moral, ethical, and legal duty is articulated in most professional codes of conduct for example, HIPAA Information Privacy Policy and the Canadian Standards Association (CSA) Model Privacy Code. The CSA code is an adaptation of the privacy standards originally developed by the OECD. The list of fair information practices it delineates are accountability; identifying purpose; consent; limiting collection; limiting use; disclosure and retention; accuracy; safeguards; openness; individual access; and challenging compliance—that is, an individual should be able to challenge the care provider's compliance with privacy requirements.

Privacy Legislation and Consent

The importance of privacy is clear when one reviews the regulatory frameworks covering the subject on both sides of the U.S.-Canada border. The province of British Columbia, for example, has a health privacy law, the Freedom of Information and Protection of Privacy Act, which applies only to public sector organizations. In Canada, Bill C-6, or the Personal Information Protection and Electronic Documents Act, includes privacy regulations for both the public and private sectors at the national level. This legislation further mandates provinces to formulate legislation to deal with personal privacy within the private sector.

Canada's privacy commissioner sounded the alarm bell when his office discovered that a federal government department, Human Resources Development Canada (HRDC), had a linked database with information from four other departments. Even though individual health care information was not being collected, HRDC was eventually forced to inactivate and dismantle the linked database due to public pressure and increased scrutiny by the privacy commissioner. This case clearly underscores the importance that Canadians place on privacy.

In the United States, HIPAA consists of two titles: (1) HIPAA Health Insurance Reform, which protects health insurance coverage for workers and their families whenever they change or lose their jobs, and (2) HIPAA Administrative Simplification, which requires the Department of Health and Human Services (DHHS) to establish national standards for electronic health care transactions and national identifiers for providers, health plans, and employers, as well as provisions for security and privacy of health data. The Centers for Medicare and Medicaid Services were entrusted by the DHHS with the responsibility of enforcing the transaction and code set standards as part of the administrative simplification provisions.

The issue of what constitutes *informed consent* has been debated for years in the health care arena, but never so vigorously as in today's emerging e-health environment. When individuals enter the e-health care system, are they truly aware of how their data may be used, with or without their express or implied consent? Just what uses of the data are considered ethical or unethical? E-health care managers are challenged with these concerns on a daily basis because various stakeholders find it very tempting to access personal data for purposes other than those originally intended. Seaton (2001) states, "Consent is proving to be the greatest challenge for health informatics professionals in the whole realm of privacy. . . . [It] is tough to define, tough to collect, tough to track, and tough to prove" (p. 28). This challenge is further complicated by the fact that many professionals are still not fully aware of the differences between security of the health information system and privacy and consent issues.

Firewalls and data encryption help to ensure the security of the system but do not offer any protection against inappropriate or malicious uses of stored information by those with access privileges. Security is more tangible than the notion of consent, which can encompass many subtle ethical dimensions; for example, a person may have a moral objection to the research for which his or her medical data were submitted, even if his or her identity is protected. Given the public's increased sensitivity about human rights and privacy, should the use of e-health information be restricted to only those purposes expressly consented to? Clearly, if the answer is yes, health care organizations will face major challenges in gathering enough data to plan and evaluate e-health care services appropriately. This rhetorical question, however, does point to operational difficulties in managing consent to disclosure of information. How can we satisfy ethical concerns about consent but also ensure that information is used for the greater good of society? An important element of any health organization's consent policy is internal education. Unfortunately, when it comes to multiple internal uses of health information, the health care system in general has not paid much attention to the issue of consent (Gostin and Hodge, 2001).

Accordingly, education on privacy and security must begin internally. Most organizations require staff to sign oaths or letters of confidentiality but do little in the way of educating employees with regard to confidentiality, privacy legislation, and consent. In fact, most employees are probably unaware of exactly where patient information resides after data have been entered into the electronic health records or on the Internet or elsewhere. Even though it may not be practical to explain every detail of the data trail to employees or e-caregivers, e-health organizations still need to ensure that their employees fully understand the issues of consent and confidentiality and how to deal with them at all stages of data collection, analysis, and release.

E-Health Data Integration

In conducting our literature survey on security, privacy, and confidentiality of health information, we found that most health informatics research focuses either on the ethical and legal dimensions or the appropriate methodological approach for guarding the security, privacy, and confidentiality of patient information, especially in services involving shared data. Little research has been conducted specifically on data aggregation with respect to issues of data confidentiality, data integrity, identity authentication, and access authorization in health informatics, particularly in the context of e-HDI services.

Security and Privacy Requirements of e-HDI Services

The literature on e-health data integration services proposes data standardization policies and both hardware and software solutions that focus on security and privacy issues in health data processing, storage, and collection, particularly for the electronic medical records (Toyoda, 1998). Consent to process and use integrated data sets would include, for example, a clear definition and a right to accept the purpose of the e-HDI service by the data subject or the patient (Moehr, 1994). In addition, there have been many discussions about the ethical right of the data subject to access and modify his or her personal medical records. For instance, a group designated "WG4" in the International Medical Informatics Association is working on the security and privacy issues of health informatics (International Medical Informatics Association, 2001). The focus of this group, while not specifically on the issues of achieving security for aggregated data in the context of e-HDI services, has been on the ethical use and distribution of electronic health and medical records among e-health practitioners and health services provider organizations.

In our discussion, the concept of *aggregation issues* refers to matters of security, confidentiality, and privacy that arise in the context of e-HDI services when two or more data sets are considered more sensitive together than each is separately. Take the example of an aggregate view of patient medical records at hospitals (with the data sets representing a group of employees from a particular organization) and their claims at a Medicare center which in the Australian context refers to a medical insurance organization or any other claim center. Here, the integrated view is deemed to be more sensitive than if the data sets were viewed separately because the combined data set allows the employer to know where or under what specific illnesses the majority of the claims fall and thus possibly which specific individuals or clusters of employees are most likely to be included in these claim groups. Such knowledge discovery resulting from the higher-level aggregation might allow and perhaps encourage the employer to adopt new policies to support hiring of workers falling outside certain categories or to begin outsourcing certain types of work (thereby retrenching certain categories of workers) because the aggregate data reveal a particular trend in increased medical costs for the employer.

On the basis of the preceding example and of more detailed level analyses of data aggregates, we can therefore state that it would only be ethical and acceptable to limit integration. For example, if one of the integrated data sets were to be given to a user (viewer) who is not authorized to see the sensitive data or were to be stored in a place (for example, a computer) not considered appropriate for sensitive health data, then no part of the data sets that would allow a sensitive aggregate to be formed should be included. (Data already available for the integration in question would remain available.) Otherwise, key aspects of security requirements in e-HDI services could be breached, including but not limited to data confidentiality, data integrity, identity authentication, and access authorization.

Modeling security enforcement is of paramount importance in many public, industrial, and commercial application domains, especially e-health care. Applications that require security enforcement include on-line office automation, e-government planning, e-medical diagnosis, e-mail communications, and e-networks and e-commerce systems that involve interactions between e-consumers and e-business entities (B2C applications) or between e-businesses (B2B applications). E-health data integration involves a set of heterogeneous and distributed hardware and software systems (that is, databases and networks) open to frequent sharing and exchange of e-health information and transactions. It is not surprising, then, that such data sharing activities could lead to conflicting interests or potential breaches of security measures and requirements. In any event, illegal violation of security and privacy through access of data has to be monitored, controlled, and reported meticulously. A violation is an access of systems by unauthorized users or processes. An authorized user or process circumvents or defeats the access controls of a system to obtain unauthorized access to classified information or data. The violation breaches the security policy and procedures of a system in a manner that could result in the loss or compromise of classified information or data. Thus, an e-HDI service has a set of distinct administrative domains (that is, networks and database management systems) and responsibilities that demands a complex and rigorous security policy.

If we look at e-HDI services in terms of confidentiality (Bakker, 1998), we find that first, confidentiality means that all data interchange and communications must and should only be restricted to authorized parties so that the information being entrusted to the users will not be shared with unauthorized personnel. Confidentiality focuses on preventing unauthorized disclosure of e-health data, especially identifiable and sensitive information. In other words, all access must be restricted to parties that are legally and fully authorized to have it. Prior researchers (Louwerse, 1998) have introduced the ethical need-to-know principle for restricting the accessibility of health data (Clark and

Wilson, 1987). Similarly, Bobis (1994) proposes a right-to-know concept to describe levels of access that e-health practitioners should have to e-patients' medical records, which correspond to the services the e-health practitioners are providing to individual patients. In regard to methodological approach, Tsujii (1998) describes a public-key cryptosystem for e-medicine and related e-medical records that will help maintain data confidentiality and integrity in the context of secure communications.

Data Integrity in e-HDI Communications

In the context of e-health, *data integrity* focuses on preventing unauthorized modification of e-health data sets. In other words, data integrity is nothing more than ensuring that the data sent as part of a larger exchange are not modifiable in transit. If the data are modified or forged, those alterations or modifications should be readily identified and discarded. Obviously, the motivation for maintaining data integrity is to prevent inappropriate e-health treatment caused by corrupted e-health data. Imagine what the consequences might be if an e-physician were to view diagnostic data that have been altered. The distributed infant and maternity care system in Finland, for example, adopts a combination of secure socket layer (SSL) and Internet protocol security (IPSec) procedures to maintain data confidentiality (Kouri and Kemppainen, 2001). SSL is a protocol for transmitting information by using a private key to encrypt data that is transferred over the Internet. As both Netscape Navigator and Internet Explorer support SSL, many Web sites use SSL to obtain confidential information such as credit card numbers. IPSec is a framework of open standards for supporting network-level data confidentiality over Internet Protocol (IP) networks by using cryptographic security services as well.

Tan, Wen, and Gyires (2003) also discuss the application of public-key cryptography infrastructure (PKI) and certificates to ensure confidentiality and to verify the authenticity of mobile users in the context of e-business and e-health information exchanges and transactions (see also Chapter Six). Another interesting variation on the theme of secured data transmission is the use of "invisible" watermarks or other data hiding techniques. Chao, Hsu, and Miaou (2002), for example, discuss a data hiding technique to secure an electronic medical record transmitted over the Internet and to ensure data confidentiality, integration, and authentication. We will now consider the issue of authentication in e-HDI services, keeping in mind that many of the security properties we are discussing overlap one another.

Authentication and Authorization in e-HDI Services

Essentially, *authentication* in e-HDI services has to do with ensuring that the identity of a user cannot be forged or altered. Hence, authentication focuses on the verification of the identity of users of e-health data. Put simply, the identities of users of e-health data must be true and verifiable. Barber (1998) advocates the use of digital signatures in e-health services by using the RSA encryption algorithm along with the password management of traditional health information systems. In another case, a commercial clinic information system, CliniCare, uses a secure asynchronous message exchange service called Health Link to maintain confidentiality and obtain user authentication (Moehr and McDaniel, 1998).

Authorization in the e-health care context means ensuring that e-health data can be accessed only by authorized users. This is especially important for aggregated data. Kaihara (1998) describes the security issues of authorization for computerized medical records from the perspectives of intrahospital use, interhospital use, and storage. Smith and Eloff (1999) discuss a set of authorization issues that apply in the context of e-health care information systems. Malamateniou, Vassilacopoulos, and Tsanakas (1998) propose an authorization infrastructure based on a work flow system for handling virtual medical records in a loosely coupled database environment. The proposed architecture implements an automated interorganizational treatment process with a security policy for granting and revoking access privileges for e-health practitioners. The authorization architecture considers the time interval in which the operation can be performed and the location from where the operation can be performed. It means that the architecture only authorizes data access at specific locations and times that depend on what service is being rendered. For example, the data access is only authorized if the request is from the office's computer during the working hours at a company. Community health information networks (Williams, Venters, and Marwick, 2001) build access control into the design of the e-network security architecture (Please refer to Chapter Six for further details.) Sadan (2001) discusses the authorization and integrity problems that apply to sharing information between e-patients and e-health providers in the context of co-documentation and co-ownership of medical records. Although various authorization models have been proposed, aggregation issues have not been covered or considered, despite the fact that aggregation issues should have a direct impact on how authorization of users and integrated views are conceived.

Past health informatics research on communications architecture has focused on secure communication protocols. For example, Mea (2001) describes the security issues of communications in a multi-agent paradigm for e-medicine systems. Blobel (2000) proposes a security infrastructure for e-medical record systems that adopts the technologies of PKI and smart cards. In addition, Ishida and Sakamoto (1998) propose a secure communications model that consists of subdividing e-health data into fragments and forwarding encrypted fragments through multiple secure paths. However, it is not clear that this is more secure than the traditional approach of sending the medical record as a whole. Blobel and Roger-France (2001) propose a set of tools that uses unified modeling language for analysis and design of secure e-health information systems. The tools provide a layered security model with security services and mechanisms but do not consider aggregation issues.

Very little health informatics research has studied aggregation issues in order to offer a formal specification for generating a security policy for e-HDI services. The aggregation issues discussed in Lunt (1989) are based in the context of a multilevel database in which the sensitivity level of each data set is preclassified. Further, Lunt mainly focuses on the issue of quantity-based aggregation without a formal specification. A quantity-based aggregation is a collection of up to N data objects of a given type is not sensitive, but a collection of greater than N data objects is sensitive. As we have emphasized, e-HDI has to aggregate data sets from previously isolated databases without a central classification scheme. Because of this, a security policy that addresses the specific issues involved in e-HDI services is critical in order for e-HDI services to be widely accepted.

In light of the discussions we have found in the literature, we present, in the next section, some important aggregation issues in the context of a formal specification.

E-Health Data Aggregation Issues

For administrative and clinical purposes, e-medical records may often contain a combination of textual and numerical information that is similar to the data that are typically captured in relational databases. For diagnostic and other practical purposes, e-health databases should also provide graphic or pictorial information such as X-ray or endoscopy images and histopathology pictures. Typically, specific e-health data sets used in e-HDI services include not only electronic medical records but also other patient-specific data such as medical insurance claims. The implication is that an enormous range of data sets can be exposed to security threats through e-HDI services. To restrict the scope of our discussion, however, we will focus primarily on electronic medical records stored in the form of relational e-health data sets (Louwerse, 1998), which are used in most e-health databases employed within a shared network environment.

The principle of information privacy and disposition (International Medical Informatics Association, 2001) states that "All persons have a fundamental right to privacy, and hence to control over the collection, storage, access, use, communication, manipulation and disposition of data about themselves." In an e-health system, data access should be restricted to e-health professionals only and should be based on the need-to-know principle. In other words, in principle, e-providers working with e-patients can only have access to data about the patients whom they treat. Moreover, e-health data relating to psychiatry care may be separated from those relating to home care. These separate data regarding the same patients may not be accessible to other providers in the same system—that is, different views of the patient data may be permitted based only on providers' need to know. E-health data are primarily transferred among authorized users, and the use of e-health data for research requires the consent of the individual patients concerned.

Traditional health data sets housed within hospitals are mainly governed by a set of privacy regulations that determine the aim and scope of the input of the data registration, the type of data included, the rights of data subjects, and access rights (Louwerse, 1998). Access to e-health data should be just as securely protected. Yet recent developments in e-HDI will only deepen the conflict between individual privacy concerns and the pressure for health information from nonmedical institutions (for example, insurance companies), unless a rigorous security policy framework is developed for e-HDI services (Anderson, 2000).

Architecture of e-HDI Services

Figure 14.1 shows the architecture of e-HDI services, which consists of a set of databases at N locations (for example, a hospital and a Medicare center); e-HDI middleware (typically, a powerful server that accepts the stream of requests from the e-HDI services, connects the databases from different locations, combines the requested data sets from the databases into integrated views, and makes the integrated views available to the e-HDI services); and the e-HDI services (which interface with the users' requests, send the requests to the e-HDI middleware, and send the integrated results to the users).

FIGURE 14.1. ARCHITECTURE OF E-HEALTH DATA INTEGRATION

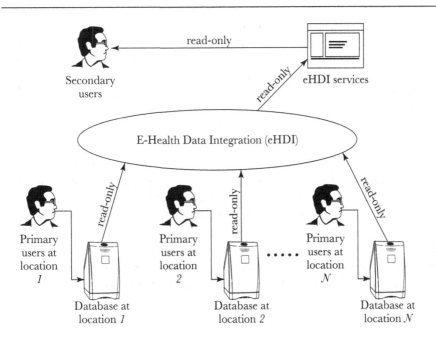

In this scenario, the e-health data access channels are all read-only because most of the cases only involve read-only operations. An example is the Ohio cancer-related research project, which is structured as an e-HDI service to support different users in accessing specific cancer information as well as extracting integrated views on accumulated cancer data (Koroukian, Cooper, and Rimm, 2001). With this arrangement, we can see that there are two types of e-HDI users. The primary users are the e-patients and e-health service providers such as doctors and nurses. E-patients can access their own health data, communicate with e-health service providers, and even manage health insurance claims. E-health service providers use health data for a variety of purposes. For example, e-physicians may want to review an e-patient's medical records to evaluate the appropriateness of the e-consultation provided. The secondary users include policymakers, practitioners, and researchers who use the data for research, social services, public health, regulation, litigation, and commercial purposes (such as marketing and the development of new medical technology) (Anderson, 2000).

Aside from the many reasons we have discussed, another reason that security issues need to be studied and tackled seriously in e-HDI services is that the systemic use of patient-identifiable health information poses additional potential threats to the security, privacy, and confidentiality of e-patient information. For example, one published survey (Anderson, 2000) reported that in the United States, some people do not file insurance claims or see health service providers for fear that disclosure of their health information may hurt their job prospects or ability to obtain insurance coverage. Note that a user can also belong to both the primary and the secondary user groups, which may cause conflicts; for instance, a doctor can be a health service provider and an e-HDI health informatics researcher. Of course, a doctor may also be a patient. Because this section of the discussion focuses primarily on secondary e-HDI users, the term *users* will refer to secondary users unless otherwise specified.

Figure 14.2 shows a sample schema for e-health data integration, including the attributes of the data for each data set in the schema. Tables 14.1 to 14.4 show sample data for each data set.

In e-health data integration, each database consists of a collection of data sets. From a relational database perspective, a data set may be conceptualized as a view composed of a set of relations. Each data set represents an entity (for example, a patient) with a set of attributes (for example, the patient's name, Medicare number, and diagnosis). In addition, these data sets (such as those provided in Tables 14.1 through 14.4) can be joined to form many different sets or views of data sets, with different categories of data integrated in each view. As an illustration, the medical records with identities (that is, patient-id) "298495," "298496," and "298497" that are shown in Table 14.1 can be treated as a data set. An integrated view in e-health data integration is composed of a set of data sets (for example, patients and Medicare claims).

FIGURE 14.2. SAMPLE SCHEMA FOR E-HEALTH DATA INTEGRATION

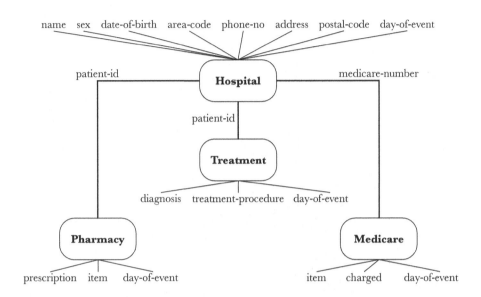

Associations between data sets are represented by *join-attributes* (common attributes)—for example, medicare-number or patient-id—which allow the data sets to be joined to obtain an integrated view (Lunt, 1989). Table 14.5, for example, is an integrated view of the data sets from Hospital, Treatment, Pharmacy, and Medicare through the association of the major keys, namely, patient-id and medicare-number.

It has been suggested that to guard against possible infringement of privacy and confidentiality of patient information, the integrated view should not disclose the identity of the patients involved (Moehr, 1994). Thus identifying information (that is, medicare-number and patient-id) in Table 14.5 is hidden, to ensure anonymity. In e-health data management, *anonymity* means that users provided with aggregate data will not be able to access the subject's identity unless they have separately been authorized to do so (for example, because they are primary users).

Anonymity is related to security, privacy, and confidentiality; it is an important principle in e-health informatics, especially when disseminating information to secondary users. One commonly cited case example in the literature is that of the adopted child (Heinlein, 1996). The adopting parents, who are responsible for the child's medical care, have a right and a need to know the birth parents' medical histories but not

TABLE 14.1. SAMPLE DATA FOR HOSPITAL

patient-id	name	sex	date-of-birth	medicare-number	area-code	phone-no	address	postal-code	day-of-event
298495	John Smith	male	06/04/1969	2506351429	02	62167031	. . .	6201	10/8/2002
298496	Ken Ackland	male	07/09/1976	3506371168	02	62298032	. . .	6201	10/8/2002
298497	Jason Mcfee	male	15/03/1980	5766311472	02	63237089	. . .	6201	11/8/2002

TABLE 14.2. SAMPLE DATA FOR TREATMENT

patient-id	diagnosis	treatment-procedure	day-of-event
298495	lung problem	X-ray	10/8/2002
298495	tuberculosis	injection	11/8/2002
298495	tuberculosis	injection	12/8/2002
298495	tuberculosis	injection	13/8/2002

TABLE 14.3. SAMPLE DATA FOR PHARMACY

patient-id	prescription	item	day-of-event
298495	Myambutol® 100mg tablets	30	11/8/2002
298495	Myambutol® 100mg tablets	30	12/8/2002
298495	Myambutol® 100mg tablets	30	13/8/2002

TABLE 14.4. SAMPLE DATA FOR MEDICARE

medicare-number	item	charged	day-of-event
2506351429	55808	$154.85	10/8/2002
2506351429	104	$25.50	11/8/2002
2506351429	104	$25.50	12/8/2002
2506351429	104	$25.50	13/8/2002

their identities. When the adopted child comes of age, he or she also has those same rights and needs, but the anonymity of the birth parents may and should still be preserved in many circumstances. However, the problem of preserving patient anonymity is outside the scope of this discussion.

An aggregation problem arises whenever some collection of data sets (that is, integrated views) is more sensitive than the individual data sets forming the aggregate. Most likely, the relations "Hospital," "Treatment," and "Pharmacy" would be stored on a hospital intranet. It is reasonable to assume that all these databases would be protected appropriately and robustly from most security threats. The integrated view in Table 14.5 should not cause any harm to the individual patients because their identities are hidden. However, this may not always be the case. Although the data contained in Table 14.5 are not direct identifiers, a combination of those data may somehow allow individual patients to be identified.

Generally speaking, protecting the identities of patients just by including only the nondemographic portion of the e-health data is inadequate. To appreciate how data

TABLE 14.5. AN INTEGRATED VIEW OF HOSPITAL, TREATMENT, PHARMACY, AND MEDICARE

item	diagnosis	treatment-procedure	prescription	charged
1	lung problem	X-ray	none	$154.85
2	tuberculosis	injection	Myambutol® 100mg tablets	$25.50
3	tuberculosis	injection	Myambutol® 100mg tablets	$25.50
4	tuberculosis	injection	Myambutol® 100mg tablets	$25.50

are to be protected in the context of e-HDI security, one must understand the three layers of secrecy that are traditionally considered in e-health informatics—namely, the content layer, the description layer, and the existence layer (Smith, 1988). The *content* layer focuses on protecting both the actual e-health data and the association formed in e-HDI from the users. In Table 14.5, both the identities of the data subjects (that is, the individual patients) and the associations between the different data sets (that is, the join-attributes such as medicare-number and patient-id) should be hidden from the users. The *description* layer emphasizes hiding the e-HDI security policy from the users. This layer is more restrictive because the users do not even know which security rules are enforced in the e-HDI services. Finally and most restrictively, the *existence* layer concentrates on hiding the existence of any e-health data that the users have not been permitted or authorized to view. This is the most restrictive layer. Its primary purpose is to reduce security threats by keeping users completely unaware of the e-health data that have been hidden from them.

Owing to the lack of research in the e-HDI domain and the need to build a first-level formalization of an e-HDI security policy, our goal here is to construct a first-cut yet rigorous e-security policy for e-HDI by observing different types of aggregation rules that can be formulated at the level of the content layer.

E-Security Policy for E-Health Data Integration

An e-security model for e-health data integration must support protocol-independent, declarative e-security policies. An *e-security policy* is a set of rules and practices that specify or regulate how a system or organization provides security services to protected electronic health resources. Accordingly, a security assertion is typically scrutinized in the context of an e-security policy.

Briefly, engineering an e-security policy begins with risk analysis and ends with a set of security assertions that is ready for integration into the e-security policy framework. In the context of e-HDI services, risk analysis identifies security threats in a particular scenario and a set of security assertions is designed in conjunction with rules and practices to regulate how sensitive information is managed and protected within such a loosely coupled execution environment. An e-security policy is often formalized or semiformalized within the context of an e-security model that provides a basis for formal analysis of security properties. In this section, our goal is to generate a set of specifications for constructing an e-security framework for e-HDI services.

Because e-health data integration involves many participants, widely diverging group interests can potentially clash (Moehr, 1994). Sheng and Chen (1990) consider the issue of conflicts in e-HDI in the context of schema integration. Aggregation problems can be avoided if conflicts of interest between users and data sets can be identified and accounted for in the e-security policy framework before the integrated view is delivered (Hung, 2002). Attempting to hide subjects' identities and related sensitive information from users of aggregate information is related to the concept of sanitization. *Sanitization* (Brewer and Nash, 1989) means disguising a subject's information, particularly to prevent the discovery of that subject's identity as a measure of privacy.

A first-level e-HDI security framework can be understood in terms of four types of aggregation:

- Context-dependent aggregation
- Quantity-dependent aggregation
- Time-dependent aggregation
- Functionality-dependent aggregation

We propose that *users* = $\left\{u_1, \ldots, u_n\right\}$ be a set of *n* users and *views* = $\left\{v_1, \ldots, v_m\right\}$ be a set of *m* views. The value of *m* is then determined by $|P(\text{data sets})|$ or the power set of data sets from all databases in the e-health data integration (for example, at locations $1, \ldots, N$ as shown in Figure 14.1).

Context-dependent aggregation is based on an actual value of an attribute, the association of an attribute with a specific value or a range of values, or the associations among several attributes and their values (Lunt, 1989). Further, these attributes may be associated with different data sets. In this type of aggregation, the need for conflict of interest regulation (CIR) can be represented as a binary relation in the format of first-order predicate calculus as follows:

$$\exists \, \mathrm{CIR}\,(v, u) \rightarrow \left\{ \exists \, u.e \mid (u.e \cap v \neq \emptyset) \wedge s \subseteq u.e \right\} \tag{1}$$

where $v \in$ *views*, $u \in$ *users*, *u.e* refers to existing data sets at *u*'s disposal, and *s* refers to sensitive information.

Simply, the statement asserted here is that if there exists CIR between the integrated view *(v)* and the user *(u)*, then there may also exist an intersection between the existing data sets at the user's disposal *(u.e)* and the integrated view *(v)* and the fact that the user's existing data sets *(u.e)* contain sensitive information. For example, neither the users who can access the databases at the hospital (that is, "Hospital," "Treatment," and "Pharmacy" in Figure 14.2) nor the users who can access the databases at the Medicare center (that is, "Medicare" in Figure 14.2) should be permitted to access the integrated view shown in Table 14.5. This should not be allowed because the information available to each of the user groups on the subjects' identities may make it possible for them to use data mining techniques to infer the identities of the subjects in the integrated view (Glymour, Madigan, Pregibon, and Smyth, 1996). Although the integrated view (Table 14.5) does not contain identifying information, both user groups could identify the patients' identities with very little difficulty.

Quantity-dependent aggregation means that a collection of up to t e-health data of a given type is sensitive. In other words, if the size of the integrated view (that is, the number of records) is lower than a specific threshold (t) (Quantin, Allaert, and Dusserre, 2000), the users may also be able to identify the subjects' identities, even though the sensitive information is hidden in the integrated view. In this type of aggregation, the CIR can be represented as a binary relation in the format of first-order predicate calculus as follows:

$$\exists \, \text{CIR}\,(v, u) \rightarrow |v| < t \tag{2}$$

where $v \in$ *views*, $u \in$ *users*, and t refers to the threshold level.

In this case, we have the assertion that if there exists CIR between the integrated view *(v)* and the user *(u)*, then the number of records in the integrated view *(v)* may be less than a specific threshold *(t)*. For example, users may be able to identify a particular patent's identity if there are less than ten patients with a specific diagnosis (for example, AIDS) in a hospital (that is, $t = 10$) . The risk of identifying a patient decreases when the value of t increases (Quantin, Allaert, and Dusserre, 2000).

Time-dependent aggregation means that the sensitive level of an integrated view may vary with time. Certain e-health data may have a different sensitivity level during a normal period than during a crisis. For example, if a serious infectious disease such as tuberculosis is spreading in a region, the integrated view may have to include the subjects' identities in order for the policymakers and researchers to take further action. In this type of aggregation, the CIR can be extended into a binary relation with a time factor in the format of first-order predicate calculus as follows:

$$\exists \, \text{CIR}\,(v, u) \rightarrow ext - \text{CIR}\,(v, u, p) \tag{3}$$

where $v \in$ *views*, $u \in$ *users*, p equals a period of time, and *ext*-CIR refers to a binary function to determine whether CIR exists with the time factor.

Here, the statement provides that if CIR exists between the integrated view *(v)* and the user *(u)*, then it might also imply that there exists CIR between a user *(u)* and a view *(v)* within a particular period of time *(p)*. Furthermore, time factors should also be considered sensitive information. The integrated view in Table 14.5 hides the day-of-event information because this information may be a clue to the subject's identity; for example, an employer might be able to infer an employee's identity if the employee was on sick leave at the time the information was collected.

Functionality-dependent aggregation means that some sensitive information can be inferred via information provided by other attributes and vice versa. In this type of aggregation, the CIR can be represented as a binary relation in the format of first-order predicate calculus as follows:

$$\exists CIR(v, u) \rightarrow \exists v.a_1 \vee v.a_2 \vee \ldots \vee v.a_h \Rightarrow s \tag{4}$$

where $v \in views$, $u \in users \Rightarrow$ is *implies*, $(1) \vee (2) \vee (3) \vee (4)$, $v.a_1, v.a_2, \ldots, v.a_h$ refers to the set of h attributes in the integrated view, and s refers to sensitive information.

Briefly, the assertion goes like this: If there exists CIR between the integrated view *(v)* and the user *(u)*, then there may exist one or more attributes in the integrated view *(v)* that can imply sensitive information *(s)*. For example, users can narrow the possibilities of where a patient might live if the patient's telephone area code is presented and can narrow them even further if the postal code is also presented, even though the address may not be shown.

At this point, it is important to note that there are disjunctive relationships among the CIR rules discussed above such that $(1) \vee (2) \vee (3) \vee (4)$, meaning that more than one of the four types of aggregation can apply at the same time. These CIR rules can be used as security assertions in an e-security policy. Based on these security assertions, the e-security policy must be able to check whether there exists CIR between the users and the integrated views. Once the e-security policy, whether in part or as a whole, is violated (that is, CIR exists), the simple solution is to abort the request. However, this may not be as easy as it sounds because such an action may in turn cause other concerns, including denial of services and availability that could require a further investigation.

Availability focuses on preventing unauthorized withholding of e-health data or resources. Availability is especially important in e-health services because often the care provided either has to be continued or is ongoing.

In this sense, it is also necessary to control the ability of an authorized user to copy e-health data by means of implemented policies. Once a user has read e-health data of a certain sensitive level, the e-security policy must ensure that any data item written by that user in regard to that case or patient has a sensitive level at least as high as the level of the e-health data previously read because the user's knowledge of sensitive data may permeate anything he or she subsequently writes.

Conclusion

Health care information might be considered the most intimate and personal information that is systematically collected and maintained about an individual. In most countries, e-health information is classified as sensitive information. This is because electronically stored data containing sensitive information can be easily and conveniently released, and disclosing sensitive information to outsiders can cause direct or indirect damage to an individual. Although security breaches have occurred in the era of paper records, the potential harm has been multiplied by electronic databases because information can now be transferred to a large number of people within extended boundaries. Imagine now that these various databases containing sensitive information are to be integrated and the aggregate data provided to a wide variety of users, including e-health practitioners, researchers, lawyers, and business and government policymakers. How should the security, privacy, and confidentiality of patient information be protected?

The e-health paradigm shift from a traditional care model toward a shared care (multi-provider care) model is also reflected in the security framework of e-HDI services. The establishment of continuous e-care chains in covering the continuum of care will also mean sharing information by means of e-HDI services. Systems designed to support shared care will be used by many independent organizations, some of which will be virtual, and each organization's security must therefore be systematically taken into consideration and examined in great detail.

It has been demonstrated that the use of an e-security framework for e-HDI services will provide the foundation for secure yet easy-to-access shared care systems. For example, information about e-patient medication is crucial for e-medical practice. Properly implemented medication e-registry systems are rare today, and information is fragmented into several systems and organizations. E-HDI services will be invaluable both for planning e-patient treatment and for research. E-HDI services are therefore a good example of the next generation of client-centered e-health information services that will be shared among e-provider organizations. But how can we ensure adequate security so that e-HDI services can flourish for the legitimate purpose of enhancing e-patient care and treatment?

Traditionally, secrecy provisions have protected privacy in health care. In our mainstream organization-centered health care model, organizational security together with password-based access control has been considered sufficient to protect patient data in medical information systems. In e-HDI services, security issues are much more complex because they involve aggregation of data and how conflicts of interest between users and the integrated views can be reconciled. We have looked at different types of aggregation and the secrecy provisions that need to be enforced at the level of the content layer. Much more research is still needed to fully understand the potential for e-security violations in the use of e-HDI services.

We see three research directions that can build on and expand the current work. First, an e-security policy for e-health data integration is needed in order to resist both intentional and accidental security threats (Clark and Wilson, 1987). One of the classic security policies for dealing with conflict of interest regulation is "Chinese wall" security policy (Brewer and Nash, 1989). *Chinese wall security policy* contains a set of access control rules such that no person can ever access data (objects) on the wrong side of the security "wall." It provides freedom of choice in the subject's initial access rights. The major objective of the Chinese wall security policy is to prevent information flows that cause conflict of interest for individual consultants in financial institutions. Webster's Dictionary defines "conflict of interest" as a conflict between the private interests and the official responsibilities of a person in a position of trust. The original application of Chinese wall security policy is illustrated as follows. Organization information is stored in datasets. Initially, each consultant has the potential to access any dataset. Once a consultant has access to a dataset of a particular organization, that consultant is not allowed access to datasets of any other competing organization. However, Chinese wall security policy is not directly applicable to e-HDI services because the policy was mainly designed for financial companies. For example, Chinese wall security policy does not involve any data integration activity. In addition, e-HDI users have different roles (for example, researchers and practitioners) that are not supported by Chinese wall security policy. Several revised Chinese wall security policies have been approved for different applications such as financial data analysis (Lin, 1990, 2000; Meadows, 1990); however, a specific version of Chinese wall security policy for e-health data integration needs to be investigated.

Second, countermeasures for e-HDI services have to be selected, implemented, and supervised in order to reduce the risks of security violations. Risk analysis is an examination of the components of risk of a particular system within a particular environment in a particular location (Smith and Eloff, 1999). Risk analysis identifies how a breach of security could affect a system and determines the seriousness of potential consequences to the health services unit (for example, a hospital or a Medicare center) (Bakker, 1998). An on-the-spot security risk factor (Hung, Karlapalem, and Gray, 1999) can be used to assess the level of risk associated with a set of subjects (users) retrieving a set of objects (integrated views). Thus, a security risk factor mechanism can be an appropriate approach for e-health data integration.

Finally, security enforcement may lead to execution failure. Availability is also an important property of security for e-HDI services. Thus, an escape mechanism may be required, by means of which emergency access could be granted, provided the user (1) has a special authorization and (2) specifies the reason for needing emergency access (Louwerse, 1998). In particular, the study of trade-offs such as breaking the access control rules (for example, conflict of interest regulation) versus resilience to execution failure is a challenge for future research to explore. Furthermore, resilience to subject (for example, data set) failures (Hung, Karlapalem, and Gray, 1999) implies the ability to complete the execution of activities even when some subjects are unavailable or have failed or when some access control rules are violated. Thus, an escape mechanism is required for e-HDI services to maintain reliable services for different users.

In real life, an e-health institution may not easily grant privileges to external users to access its e-health data unless the external users are authorized for some specific purposes such as academic studies. Referring to the privacy act in many countries, the aggregation problem has to be solved any time a user is authorized to access the e-health data with the subject's (the patient's) prior consent. In conclusion, e-security policy is an important topic in e-HDI services.

Chapter Questions

1. Differentiate *privacy, security,* and *confidentiality.* Why are these terms easily confused?
2. What is an e-security policy framework? What is its significance to e-health care?
3. Why is it important to study data aggregation issues? Why has prior research in health informatics not focused on these important issues?
4. Differentiate the security approaches used in the U.S. and Canadian health care systems. Are you aware of the approach used in any other country? How are privacy and confidentiality of patient data guarded on the basis of legislation in those countries?
5. Imagine that you are a physician who has been asked to oversee John, who is unconscious and has just been admitted into the hospital after fainting in the street after his face turned red. After checking his pulse and other related symptoms, you feel very strongly that you need his medical records in order to treat John properly. John carries a smart card, and fortunately, your hospital has a smart card reader. However, the only information you can find about John or his family is a code written on a small piece of paper, which appears to be the password needed to unlock the information contained on the smart card. As a medical professional, do you check John's records (which may be encoded on his smart card, along with other private information about him) without his consent? Or do you treat him as best you can without having the essential information? Why?

References

Anderson, J. (2000). Security of the distributed electronic patient record: A case-based approach to identifying policy issues. *International Journal of Medical Informatics, 60*(2), 111–118.

Bakker, A. (1998). Security in perspective: Luxury or must? *International Journal of Medical Informatics, 49*(1), 31–37.

Barber, B. (1998). Patient data and security: An overview. *International Journal of Medical Informatics, 49*(1), 19–30.

Blobel, B. (2000). The European TrustHealth Project experiences with implementing a security infrastructure. *International Journal of Medical Informatics, 60*(2), 193–201.

Blobel, B., & Roger-France, F. (2001). A systematic approach for analysis and design of secure health information systems. *International Journal of Medical Informatics, 62*(1), 51–78.

Bobis, K. (1994). Implementing right to know security in the computer-based patient record. In, *Proceedings of the International Phoenix Conference on Computers and Communications* (pp. 156–160), Phoenix, AZ, USA.

Brewer, D., & Nash, M. (1989). The Chinese wall security policy. In *Proceedings of 1990 IEEE Computer Society Symposium on Security and Privacy* (pp. 206–214), Gamma Secure Systems Ltd., Camberley, Surrey, United Kingdom.

Chao, H., Hsu, C., & Miaou, S. (2002). A data-hiding technique with authentication, integration, and confidentiality for electronic patient records. *IEEE Transactions on Information Technology in Biomedicine, 6*(1), 46–53.

Clark, D., & Wilson, D. (1987). A comparison of commercial and military computer security policies. In, *Proceedings of 1987 IEEE Symposium on Security and Privacy* (pp. 184–194).

France, F. (1996). Control and use of health information: A doctor's perspective. *International Journal of Biomedical Computing, 43*(1–2), 19–25.

Glymour, C., Madigan, D., Pregibon, D., & Smyth, P. (1996). Statistical inference and data mining. *Communications of the ACM, 39*(11), 35–41.

Gostin, L., & Hodge, J. (2001). *The National Centre for Health Statistics white paper: Balancing individual privacy and communal uses of health information.* Retrieved from Model State Public Health Privacy Web site at www.critpath.org/msphpa/ncshdoc.htm

Grimson, J., Stephens, G., Jung, B., Grimson, W., Berry, D., & Pardon, S. (2001). Sharing health-care records over the Internet. *IEEE Internet Computing, 5*(3), 49–58.

Heinlein, E. (1996). Medical records security. *Computers and Security, 15*, 100–102.

Hung, P. (2002). Specifying conflict of interest in Web Services Endpoint Language (WSEL). *ACM SIGecom Exchanges, 3.3*, 1–8. Retrieved from http://www.acm.org/sigs/sigecom/exchanges/

Hung, P., Karlapalem, K., & Gray, J., III. (1999). Least privilege security in CapBasED-AMS. *International Journal of Cooperative Information Systems, 8*(2–3), 139–168.

International Medical Informatics Association. (2001, March). *A code of ethics for health informatics professionals (HIPs).* Retrieved from International Medical Informatics Association Web site at http://www.imia.org/pubdocs/Code_of_ethics.pdf

Ishida, Y., & Sakamoto, N. (1998). A secure model for communication of health care information by sub-division of information and multiplication of communication paths. *International Journal of Medical Informatics, 49*(1), 75–80.

Ishikawa, K. (2000, November). Health data use and protection policy; based on differences by cultural and social environment. *International Journal of Medical Informatics, 60*(2), 119–125.

Kaihara, S. (1998). Realisation of the computerized patient record: Relevance and unsolved problems. *International Journal of Medical Informatics, 49*(1), 1–8.

Koroukian, S., Cooper, G., & Rimm, A. (2001, December). *The linked Ohio cancer incidence surveillance system and Medicaid files: An example of health data integration.* Retrieved from the National Association of Health Data Organizations Web site at http://www.nahdo.org/meetings/16meeting/meetpres/koroukian NAHDO—Dec 2001.pdf

Kouri, P., & Kemppainen, E. (2001). The implementation of security in distributed infant and maternity care. *International Journal of Medical Informatics, 60*(2), 211–218.

Lacroix, Z. (2002). Biological data integration: Wrapping data and tools. *IEEE Transactions on Information Technology in Biomedicine, 6*(2), 123–128.

Lin, T. (1990). Chinese wall security policy: An aggressive model. In, *Proceedings of the Fifth Annual Computer Security Applications Conference* (pp. 282–289).

Lin, T. (2000). Chinese wall security model and conflict analysis. In, *Proceedings of the 24th Annual International of Computer Software and Applications Conference (COMPSAC 2000)* (pp. 122–127).

Louwerse, K. (1998). The electronic patient record: The management of access. Case study: Leiden University Hospital. *International Journal of Medical Informatics, 49*(1), 39–44.

Lunt, T. (1989). Aggregation and inference: Facts and fallacies. In, *Proceedings of the 1989 IEEE Symposium on Security and Privacy* (pp. 102–109).

Malamateniou, F., Vassilacopoulos, G., & Tsanakas, P. (1998). A workflow-based approach to virtual patient record security. *IEEE Transactions on Information Technology in Biomedicine, 2*(3), 139–145.

Mea, V. (2001). Agents acting and moving in health care scenarios: A paradigm for telemedical collaboration. *IEEE Transactions on Information Technology in Biomedicine, 5*(1), 10–13.

Meadows, C. (1990). US Naval Res. Lab., Washington, DC. Extending the Brewer-Nash model to a multilevel context. In, *Proceedings of 1990 IEEE Computer Society Symposium on Research in Security and Privacy* (pp. 95–102). Oakland, CA, USA.

Moehr, J. (1994). Privacy and security requirements of distributed computer based patient records. *International Journal of Bio-Medical Computing, 35*(1), 57–64.

Moehr, J., & McDaniel, J. (1998). Adoption of security and confidentiality features in an operational community health information network: The Comox Valley experience—Case example. *International Journal of Medical Informatics, 49*(1), 81–87.

Quantin, C., Allaert, F., & Dusserre, L. (2000). Anonymous statistical methods versus cryptographic methods in epidemiology. *International Journal of Medical Informatics, 60*(2), 177–183.

Sadan, B. (2001). Patient data confidentiality and patient rights. *International Journal of Medical Informatics, 62*(1), 41–49.

Seaton, B. (2001). The chief privacy officer: Coming soon to a management team near you! *Healthcare Information Management and Communications Canada, 15*(5), 58–59.

Sheng, O., & Chen, G. (1990). Information management in hospitals: An integrating approach. In, *Proceedings of Annual Phoenix Conference* (pp. 296–303), Scottsdale, AZ, USA.

Smith, E., & Eloff, J. (1999). Security in health-care information systems: Current trends. *International Journal of Medical Informatics, 54*(1), 39–54.

Smith, G. (1988). Identifying and representing the security semantics of an application. In, *Proceedings of Aerospace Computer Security Applications Conference* (pp. 125–130).

Tan, J., Wen, H. J., & Gyires, T. (2003). M-commerce security: The impact of wireless application protocol (WAP) security services on e-business and e-health solutions. *International Journal of M-Commerce, 1*(4), 409–424.

Toyoda, K. (1998). Standardization and security for the EMR. *International Journal of Medical Informatics, 48*(1–3), 57–60.

Tsujii, S. (1998). Revolution of civilization and information security. *International Journal of Medical Informatics, 49*(1), 9–18.

Williams, M., Venters, G., & Marwick, D. (2001). Developing a regional health care information network. *IEEE Transactions on Information Technology in Biomedicine, 5*(2), 177–180.

Integrated Selective Encryption and Data Embedding for Medical Images Case

Qiang Cheng, Yingge Wang, Joseph Tan

This case proposes a new scheme for transmission of medical images that uses selective encryption integrated with functional data embedding. Selective encryption can speed up computation in comparison with full encryption methods using classical cryptosystems, yet it often has insufficient security or other drawbacks. The proposed new scheme embeds functional data into the image seamlessly, losslessly, and in a standards-compliant way. The selected parts of the image are encrypted efficiently. Information integration of medical images and functional data is achieved, with high levels of security and privacy. New functions may be enabled within the proposed framework. The new method has proven to yield high security and will result in significantly less computation. Experimental results demonstrate the effectiveness of the proposed scheme.

Background

The development of imaging technologies has made medical images a key component of electronic patient records. These images are often transmitted between image producers, such as radiology and pathology departments, and image requesters, such as health professionals and medical departments. With increased computing capability and broadband communications, transmission of medical images across networks will become commonplace in e-medicine and mobile medicine.

There are stringent requirements for the quality of medical images in transmission and storage. Oftentimes, especially for primary diagnosis, the medical images are not permitted to have any single-bit modification after acquisition. In e-medicine or mobile health applications, in which electronic patient and medical records are transmitted through open networks such as the Internet, insecure transmission environments expose these records to interception, impersonation, and other attacks (Schneier, 2000; Stajano, 2002). To protect the security of patient data, cryptographic methods must be applied. In general, a typical medical image is huge, which makes encryption computationally expensive or even prohibitive for small or mobile devices.

Standard cryptosystems are designed for the simplest multimedia data, plain text. For images (including image sequences), the computational complexity of these standard ciphers is high. To reduce the computational load, selective encryption methods have been proposed for multimedia data. Selective encryption enciphers only the important parts of multimedia data. The existing selective encryption methods often

The authors thank X. Luo for his help in programming the rate and distortion curves.

suffer from some drawbacks, such as insufficient security level, insignificant reduction of computational complexity, and incompatibility with existing industrial standards. Here, we propose a new scheme, *integrated selective encryption and data embedding* (I-SEE), to protect the security of medical images.

Data embedding methods have been proposed for multimedia copyright protection, traitor tracing, and covert data transmission. New functions can be enabled in an innocuous, seamless, and standards-compliant way. Existing data embedding methods, however, have several potential weaknesses; for example, the security of embedded data is not high, and the amount of information that can be reliably embedded usually is quite limited.

I-SEE—which integrates data embedding with selective encryption for high security, large amounts of embedded information, and moderate computational overhead—addresses these challenges. Selected parts of the image data are combined with functional data such as the patient's name, identification number, and even diagnosis. Then the composite data are encrypted. In this process, both partial image data and functional data are reversibly compressed for embedding purposes. At the receiving end, the encrypted data are first deciphered with proper cryptographic keys, and then the embedded textual data and the image parts are decompressed. The embedded data transmit important information reliably along with the images. Compared with existing selective encryption methods, our scheme achieves high levels of security with significantly reduced computational complexity and is capable of embedding a significantly high volume of textual information. I-SEE makes possible new functions such as partial availability of image contents for previewing or content-based retrieval purposes, and seamless integration of medical images with relevant associated medical data.

Rationale for I-SEE

Secure communications and storage often make use of cryptographic techniques, including standard encryption algorithms such as triple Data Encryption Standard (DES), International Data Encryption Algorithm (IDEA), Rijndael Advanced Encryption Standard (AES), and Rivest-Shamir-Adleman (RSA), which were originally designed for text (Qiao and Nahrstedt, 1998). Recently, selective encryption methods have been proposed to reduce computational requirements (Qiao and Nahrstedt, 1997; Shi, Wang, and Bhargava, 1999; Zeng and Lei, 2002; Wu and Guo, 2001). These methods apply encryption or scrambling methods (such as DES, IDEA, XOR) or permutation to parts of multimedia data in the frequency domain or spatial domain or by modifying entropy codec, a term used in image compression. Note that the entropy codec is used for image compression and decompression in the system.

The existing selective encryption methods, however, have several known weaknesses that may be potentially exploited by an attacker. For video selective ciphering, the zigzag permutation algorithm (Tang, 1996) can be cryptoanalyzed by known-plaintext or ciphertext-only attacks (Qiao and Nahrstedt, 1998). The video encryption algorithm (Qiao and Nahrstedt, 1997) encrypts every other bit of the MPEG stream and the required computation is 50 percent of full encryption, without considering the selection overhead (Wu and Guo, 2001). The real-time video encryption algorithm selects the sign bits of each macroblock and encrypts them using DES or IDEA (Shi, Wang, and Bhargava, 1999). It has been argued that encryption of sign bits and also more significant bits may still lead to information leakage (Wu and Guo, 2001). In the entropy codec design (Wu and Guo, 2001), video or image data are encrypted, using multiple Huffman coding tables and multiple state indices in the QM coder. The coding tables and state indices are known only to the encoder and decoder and thus are part of secret keys. This gives rise to inflated key size, however.

In general, these methods suffer from one or more drawbacks such as insufficient security, increase in key size, decrease in compression efficiency, or insignificant reduction of computation compared to full encryption (Qiao and Nahrstedt, 1997, 1998; Shi, Wang, and Bhargava, 1999; Zeng and Lei, 2002; Wu and Guo, 2001). Because a medical image is of little value without relevant associated data (Van de Velde and Degoulet, 2003), we propose a new scheme that seamlessly integrates the associated data into medical images and selectively encrypts the combined image data. The drawbacks of existing selective encryption are effectively addressed with the proposed algorithm; it has low computational complexity yet high levels of security. Without proper cryptographic keys, the resulting medical images are of little value due to degradation of image quality as well as the lack of relevant associated functional data. With the keys, the original medical images and associated data can be exactly reconstructed and made readily available. Compared with the original image or original textual data, the size of the data storage space resultant image decreases.

The proposed scheme exploits a reversible data embedding method (Luo, Cheng, and Tan, 2003). Data embedding, including watermarking, steganography, and fingerprinting, is an emerging technique for multimedia copyright protection, authentication, traitor tracing, and covert communication (Cox, Kilian, Leighton, and Shamoon, 1997; Cheng and Huang, 2001, 2003; Fridrich, Goljan, and Du, 2001; Cheng, Wang, and Huang, 2004). By embedding invisible secondary data into multimedia data, including images, the secondary, secret-bearing data are associated with the multimedia in a seamless and standards-compliant way.

Data embedding techniques can be roughly classified into two categories according to the characteristics of the embedding: nonreversible (lossy) or reversible (lossless). *Nonreversible,* or *lossy,* methods result in degradation in image quality that cannot be eliminated at the receiving end; in contrast, *reversible,* or *lossless,* methods yield only degradation that is removable at the receiving end. Existing reversible data embedding methods can only embed a small number of message bits, but I-SEE reversible embedding imprints a large volume of associated functional data into images.

Medical images and relevant medical data are usually separated in existing medical information systems (Van de Velde and Degoulet, 2003). Correct links or indices must be established between images and their associated data. Any incorrect or lost links lead to mistakes in medical practice. Thus, the integration of medical images with associated functional data is desirable, if it can be done securely. A large volume of data embedding can fulfill the need for medical information integration. Data embedding techniques alone, however, cannot guarantee the security of multimedia data. The embedded data must be protected with cryptographic methods.

Our novel I-SEE scheme incorporates reversible data embedding and selective encryption in order to enhance the security of images as well as integrate images with functional data. Our reversible data embedding method modifies both image data and header files. At the transmission end, functional or textual data are embedded into the medical images. The embedded, composite images are transmitted through the channel; at the receiving end, both the embedded data and the original medical images are recovered perfectly. The reversible property guarantees that the medical images have no loss in quality, and the functional data are transmitted in a covert and reliable fashion. This proposed scheme is different from both existing selective encryption and existing data embedding methods. High security and seamless association of functional data with images are achieved with moderate computational complexity. Partial availability or total obfuscation of image contents can be chosen flexibly, depending on the application or user preference.

System Framework of I-SEE

Our I-SEE system requires processing at the transmitting and receiving ends. To send the image and associated functional data, the transmitter selects some parts of an image for data embedding and encryption. These parts are reversibly compressed and padded with proper functional data, which may also be reversibly compressed. The compressed image parts together with the (compressed) functional data have the same size as the original image parts. Then, the modified parts, consisting of compressed data and embedded data, are partially encrypted. Finally, the encrypted data are put back into the original positions in the image. This modified image will be transmitted through the communication channels.

Exhibit 14.1 shows the transmission and recovery cycle of the whole process.

EXHIBIT 14.1. PROCESSING AT THE TRANSMISSION END (TOP) AND THE RECEIVING END (BOTTOM), USING THE I-SEE FRAMEWORK

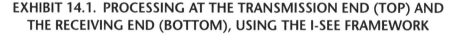
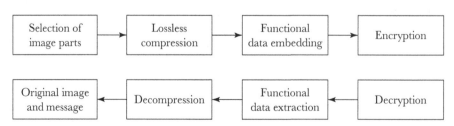

At the receiving end, the encrypted parts are first deciphered with proper cryptographic keys. Then, the embedded data are extracted to obtain the associated information. The compressed image parts are reconstructed perfectly, and consequently, the original image is recovered without any modification. This recovery process is also shown in Exhibit 14.1.

System Transmitter Processing

First, the transmitter needs to select the proper parts of an image for further data embedding and encryption. The framework considered above can be easily extended to compressed images by selecting some parts of the compressed bitstream resulting from a specific codec like JPEG or JPEG2000. Considering the stringent requirement of high image quality for diagnosis purposes, we mainly focus on uncompressed medical images in this discussion. We use the effective bitplanes (those consisting of at least one nonzero bit) of the medical image as the basic parts for data embedding and encryption. Other parts of the image can be defined in other ways and similarly employed within the framework of I-SEE.

There are two different modes for using the bitplanes: selecting the most significant bitplanes (MSBs) or selecting the least significant bitplanes (LSBs) for I-SEE. Different modes can be adopted for different purposes. Because the MSBs are more significant for human perception than the LSBs, and the MSBs have similarities to the original image, while the LSBs are mostly random in appearance, different selections have different effects on the visual quality and data embedding rate. Essentially, if partial visibility of the medical images is required in content-based image retrieval applications or for preview, peer review, or research purposes, the LSBs can be employed. If the image contents need be hidden, the MSBs should be selected. The LSBs cannot be compressed much compared with the MSBs. Thus, MSBs are preferred if a higher data embedding rate is desired. One bitplane or several bitplanes together can be used, depending on the volume of the data to be embedded. The more bitplanes used, the higher the volume of functional data that can be embedded.

Next, the selected image parts are losslessly compressed. Several methods can be used for the lossless compression: JPEG-LS, JPEG, JBIG2, entropy coding such as static Huffman coding or dynamic or adaptive Lempel-Ziv (LZ) and its variants like Lempel-Ziv-Welch (LZW) (Cover and Thomas, 1991). In this case, we employ the LZW algorithm. In the LZ algorithm or its variants (Ziv and Lempel, 1978), the source sequence is sequentially parsed into strings by searching for the shortest string that has not appeared so far. Each string consists of a prefix that has occurred earlier and a last bit that is new. The string is coded by the location of the prefix and the value of the last bit. The decoding reverses the steps and recovers the source sequence without error. LZ or LZW coding is universal in the sense that it is independent of the distribution of the source—that is, given an arbitrary source, it achieves an average code word length which is asymptotically equal to the entropy rate of the source. The LZ or LZW algorithm is adaptive–that is, it does not need to learn the exact probability distribution of the source, in contrast to static algorithms like Huffman coding.

The medical images must be indexed in order to keep track of their locations and characteristics. Existing standards such as DICOM usually provide header files to collect and organize relevant patient and study demographic data. However, more electronic health record (EHR) data should be considered—for example, personal information of patients, (such as name and identification number), lab results, observations, diagnosis, and so on. These data may not always be physically associated with the images, due to the limitations of the header files or for security or privacy reasons. Merging these EPR data with corresponding medical images will facilitate information management and information integration. In doing so, the security of both the medical images and the EPR will be enhanced, and the privacy of the EPR will be better preserved; once the EPRs are directly embedded into the images, they remain unavailable even after the selective encryption is deciphered, unless the correct authorizations are provided. With the associated functional data, the performance of content-based image retrieval can be augmented, taking into account information in both image and textual modes.

Our I-SEE framework incorporates a data embedding scheme to achieve the information integration. We apply LZW coding to functional information, usually in the form of plain text, to compress it losslessly into a binary stream, then merge it into the compressed image parts. The merging can be simple concatenation or more sophisticated deterministic mixing—for example, interleaving techniques used in wireless communications to combat bursty errors or fast fading. Here, we chose a block interleaving method (Proakis, 2001). The two compressed data streams are merged such that the combined size is exactly the same as the original size of the selected image parts or multiples of the bitplane size. To this end, we pad with zeros when necessary. The method of merging and the positions of the extra zeroes will be contained in the header file—for example, using the FileMetaInformationVersion or StudyDescription field. If the number of bitplanes is changed, the corresponding fields in the header file will have to be changed correspondingly—for example, BitDepth and FileSize fields in the DICOM format. Our method of functional data embedding maintains compliance with standards because the merging of image with textual data and the modification of the header file adhere to rules or options of the standards.

After the integration of functional text and image, we encrypt the combined data. Only the modified data are encrypted, while unchanged parts are not. Standard ciphers such as triple DES, IDEA, or Rijndael AES, can be used for this purpose. To reduce complexity, we propose to employ the XOR operation for enciphering. A cryptographically secure random sequence controlled by a secret key can be generated efficiently (Stinson, 2000; Stajano, 2002), and the sequence, used as a one-time keypad, is XORed with the combined textual and image data. Since XOR sequence is generated using a seed, as long as the receiver has the same seed, by performing XOR again, the message can be recovered. In this case, we make use of a separate private key owned by the receiver to encrypt the secret key to the random sequence. The

encrypted key to the random sequence is provided in the header file. More sophisticated off-line distributed or group key management will be designed for better security control and will be discussed in our future work. The computational complexity is
proportional to the size of the selected image parts and only a fraction of what would
be required for full encryption. After encryption, we put the combined data back into
their original positions in the selected image parts.

It can be observed that modification of the MSBs has significant impact on the
visual quality of the image, while modification of the LSBs has insignificant impact. At
the same time, the volumes of data that can be embedded by using MSBs and LSBs
are different. If the MSBs are used, the volume is large; if the LSBs are used, it is small.
As mentioned earlier, the visual impact and volume of data embedding are important
factors in selecting image parts for encryption in various applications. To quantify
the volume of embedded data and visual degradation of the medical image, we
define *rate* and *distortion* as follows:

The rate R of the I-SEE is defined as the average number of functional bits that can
be embedded into the image per pixel; thus, its unit is bits per pixel (bpp). The rate R
depends on how well the image parts can be compressed. The fundamental limit of the
reversible compression is the *entropy rate* of the selected image parts (Cover and Thomas,
1991). If we consider bitplane or bitplanes X, the rate R has an upper bound of $r - H(X)$,
where $H(X)$ denotes the entropy rate of the source X, and r is the number of bits per
pixel for original parts X. The value of r, for example, is 1 if X is the MSB, 2 if X is the first
two MSBs, and so on. If the lossless compression coder is asymptotically optimal, such
as the LZ coding for an ergodic source, then the larger the size of X, the closer the rate
R is to the upper bound. The MSBs are usually less random-like than the LSBs and have
a smaller entropy rate than the LSBs. Thus, the MSBs yield a larger rate R than the LSBs.
The distortion D of the I-SEE is measured using the peak signal-to-noise ratio. It is simply a measure of the *mean squared error,* which is defined as the average squared difference between the modified and the original images. The rate-distortion curve can be
obtained empirically.

We conducted experiments using sixty medical images that range in size from 128
x 128 to 1024 x 1024 and in modality from computed tomography, ultrasound, and
magnetic resonance imaging (MRI) to digital X-ray, digital subtraction angiography
(DSA), and nuclear medicine. A range of organs were shown in these images. Because
different imaging modalities have different gray scales (for example, most MRI images have 12–16 bits, while DSA images have 8–12 bits), we selected the LSBs for encryption. The motivation to select the LSBs is to obtain partial observations of medical
images. The LSBs were considered consecutively. In our experiment, we considered only
8 LSBs at most. Exhibit 14.2 plots the empirically obtained rate-distortion curves using
the sixty images. We plot the rate and distortion against the number of LSBs.

Note that the rate-distortion curve can also be plotted with the rate R as a function of the distortion D. Our plot clearly demonstrates an increasing trend in rate
and a decreasing trend in distortion as consecutive LSBs selected for encryption are

EXHIBIT 14.2. RATE AND DISTORTION CURVES FOR IMAGES, BY NUMBER OF CONSECUTIVE LSBs SELECTED FOR ENCODING

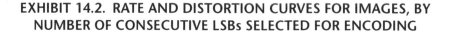

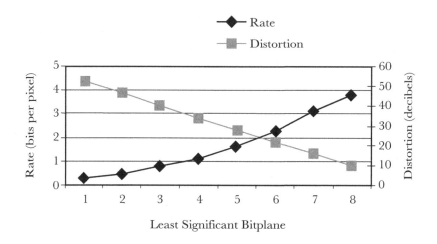

increased. If some significant bitplanes are used (or the lowest LSBs are excluded), the rate R becomes significantly higher, and the distortion D becomes lower, as explained before. Users can use the rate-distortion curve to choose a proper operational point for their I-SEE system.

System Receiver Processing

At the receiving end, the processing that was performed at the transmitting end is reversed. The receiver must possess the private key to decrypt the key that is used to generate the pseudorandom sequence. Since all processing at the transmitter is reversible, both the original image and the embedded functional data can be reconstructed simultaneously without error. The computational complexity is proportional to the size of the selected image parts.

Conclusion

We propose the integrated selective encryption and data embedding system for transmission of medical images. Functional patient and medical data are seamlessly embedded into the medical image and compressed losslessly in a way that complies with industry standards. Selected parts of the image are efficiently encrypted. Integration of medical images and functional data is achieved, and high security and privacy of data are maintained. New functions may be possible within the proposed I-SEE framework—for example, multimodal content-based image retrieval. Our future work will consider the issues in managing distributed and group keys in an I-SEE system.

Case Questions

1. In what circumstances is a random-like encrypted image preferred? In what situations is partial availability of a medical image useful?

2. What are the potential benefits of the integration of images with electronic patient record data?

3. Application of I-SEE to medical image communications is considered in this case. Can you envision applications of I-SEE to the storage of medical images in a database? Please explain your answer.

References

Cheng, Q., & Huang, T. S. (2001, September). An additive approach to transform-domain information hiding and optimum detection structure. *IEEE Transactions on Multimedia, 3*(3), 273–284.

Cheng, Q., & Huang, T. S. (2003, April). Robust optimum detection of transform-domain multiplicative watermarks. *IEEE Transactions on Signal Processing, 51*(4), 906–924. (Special issue on signal processing for data hiding in digital media and secure content delivery).

Cheng, Q., Wang, Y., & Huang, T.S. (2004, August) Performance analysis and error exponents of asymmetric watermarking systems. *Signal Processing, 84*(8), 1429–1445.

Cover, T., & Thomas, J. (1991). *Elements of information theory.* New York: Wiley.

Cox, I. J., Kilian, J., Leighton, F. T., & Shamoon, T. (1997). Secure spread spectrum watermarking for multimedia. *IEEE Transactions Image Processing, 6*(12), 1673–1687.

Fridrich, J., Goljan, M., & Du, R. (2001). Invertible authentication. In, *Proceedings of The International Society for Optical Engineering Photonics West Security and Watermarking of Multimedia Contents III,* San Jose, California, USA,, January 22–25, 2001 (Vol. 3971, pp. 197–208).

Luo, X., Cheng, Q., & Tan, J. (2003). A lossless data embedding scheme for medical images in application of e-diagnosis. In, *Proceedings of the International Conference of IEEE Engineering in Medicine and Biology Society (EMBS '03),* Cancun, Mexico, September 2003.

Proakis, J. G. *Digital communications* (4th ed.). New York: McGraw-Hill, 2001.

Qiao, L., & Nahrstedt, K. (1997). A new algorithm for MPEG video encryption. In, *Proceedings of the International Conference of Imaging Science, Systems, and Technology (CISS'97),* pages 21–29, Las Vegas, NV, July 1997.

Qiao, L., & Nahrstedt, K. (1998). Comparison of MPEG encryption algorithms. *International Journal on Computer and Graphics, 22*(3). (Special issue on data security in image communication and network.), Urbana, IL, U.S.A.

Schneier, B. (2000). *Secrets and lies: Digital security in a networked world.* New York: Wiley.

Shi, C., Wang, S.-Y., & Bhargava, B. (1999). MPEG video encryption in real-time using secret key cryptography, West Lafayette, IN In, *Proceedings of the International Conference of Parallel and Distributed Processing Techniques and Application,* Las Vegas, NV, June 1999.

Stajano, F. (2002). *Security for ubiquitous computing.* New York: Wiley.

Stinson, D. R. (2000). *Cryptography: Theory and practice.* Boca Raton, FL: CRC Press.

Tang, L. (1996). Methods for encrypting and decrypting MPEG video data efficiently. In, *Proc. ACM Multimedia,* Boston, November 1996 (pp. 219–230), Boston, MA.

Van de Velde, R., & Degoulet P. (2003). *Clinical information systems.* New York: Springer.

Wu, C.-P., & Guo, C.-C. J. (2001). Efficient multimedia encryption via entropy codec design. In, *Proc. SPIE Security and Watermarking of Multimedia Content,* San Jose, CA, January 2001 (Vol. 4314), San Jose, CA, USA.

Zeng, W., & Lei, L. (2002). Efficient frequency domain selective scrambling of digital video. *IEEE Transactions, Multimedi*a.

Ziv, J., & Lempel, A. (1978). Compression of individual sequences by variable rate coding. *IEEE Transactions On Information Theory,* IT-24, 530–536.

CHAPTER FIFTEEN

E-HEALTH IMPACTS ON THE HEALTH CARE AND HEALTH SERVICES INDUSTRY

Surfing the Powerful Waves of E-Technologies

Joseph Tan, David C. Yen, Sharline Martin, Binshan Lin

Learning Objectives

1. Characterize the functions and business processes of various sectors of the health care and health services industry
2. Realize the positive impacts of applying e-technologies in various health care and health services sectors
3. Recognize the risks associated with applying e-technologies in health care
4. Articulate the various stages of e-health evolution
5. Chart the future of e-technologies in health care

Introduction

A vision of better population health and human well-being has continually motivated those in the health care field to innovate and invent new ways of applying technology. E-technologies promise to revolutionize our society, and it is this trend that has brought about the e-health care era and has contributed to the e-health paradigm shift. E-technologies have already begun to enhance various aspects of health care—for example, the ability to communicate with individuals, groups, and communities through the use of e-health records, e-public health information systems, e-networks, and Web services (see Parts One and Two of this text); our access to media-rich e-health information and knowledge through the use of complex e-consultation and e-monitoring technologies and e-health intelligence software (see Part Three); and our ability to interconnect e-consumers, e-vendors, e-providers, and other e-business entities through e-health commerce applications (see Chapters Twelve through Fourteen). Put simply, e-technologies have already significantly affected many industries, ushering in the next generation of health care—that is, the e-health marketplace.

In the past, health care providers and consumers have been slow, even reluctant to embrace e-health care applications, primarily because of the limited power and newness of e-technologies. Many stakeholders have feared that e-health could not ensure the security of health care data in general and the privacy and confidentiality of sensitive patient information in particular (see Chapter Fourteen). With new advances in cryptography and firewalls, digital signatures and certificates, and wireless security protocols, security concerns faced by the health care industry have eased significantly, and an increasing number of mainstream health care business sectors are now considering moving into e-health care. E-consumers are adopting emerging e-health applications for their many potential benefits, including increased speed and accuracy of health information exchange, lower cost of services, convenient access to media-rich e-health information and knowledge, and more efficient and effective health care decision making. Many e-consumers, for example, are demanding increasingly rapid and ready access to multimedia information and in-depth knowledge of health care in order to help them make better choices and informed decisions.

Similarly, e-providers and e-health managers are looking toward e-technologies to bring about significant reductions in costs while preserving and maintaining high-quality health care. The proliferation of electronic mail systems, the Internet, the World Wide Web, and the emergence of organizational intranets and extranets as innovative extensions of local area networks and wide area networks, as well as the introduction of various forms of e-diagnostic systems, including linked and distributed databases, e-clinical decision support systems, e-medicine, e-home care services, and e-prescription systems, have resulted in a need to understand the impacts of emerging e-technologies and applications on various sectors of health care and health services, particularly among health administrators, practitioners, and patients (Tan, 2001; Tan with Sheps, 1998). Eoffering Corp, for example, has conducted a survey that indicates that the market for e-health care services is about to explode (Fell and Shepherd, 1998). While there are no predictable statistics available for the e-health care market, the indication has been that the e-health care marketplace, when combined with mainstream health care services, has now exceeded 14 percent of the gross national product (GNP) in the United States; in addition, the possibilities of extending services to a global marketplace are also expanding (see Chapters One and Two and Chapter Twelve).

In this chapter, we explore characteristics of various traditional health care and health services sectors and examine how emerging e-technologies are affecting them. Some benefits and risks created by e-technologies are also highlighted. To accomplish this, we first present an overview of the health care and health services industry, followed by a general discussion of the impacts of emerging e-technologies on various sectors. The major characteristics, tasks, functions, traditional approaches, and potential applications of e-technologies will be factors in the discussion. Next, we focus on some potential impacts and challenges of using e-technologies to evolve new e-health businesses. We explore the growth and development of e-technologies and the managerial strategies, directions, and implications of employing these technologies in health care and health services sectors. Finally, we conclude the chapter with a brief look at potential future innovations and trends in e-technologies.

E-Technologies in Various Health Care and Health Services Sectors

The mainstream health care and health services industry encompasses various sectors, including hospitals, physicians' offices, medical insurance companies, nursing homes, and home health care agencies, as well as pharmaceutical and health care product companies. Although the characteristics, tasks, and functions of each sector differ, all the sectors share the common goal of providing consumers with health care goods and services. Each of these sectors has also evolved to its own stage of the e-health revolution. In this section, we take a look at how emerging e-technologies gradually but surely affect each sector.

E-consumers' expectations of e-businesses, including health care businesses, are continually increasing. E-health consumers are demanding the same privileges they receive from other e-businesses. With the advent of e-technologies, e-consumers have access not only to media-rich e-health information and high-speed communications but also to direct purchase of e-health goods and services. In light of increased competition among e-health care providers and heightened awareness among e-consumers, many sectors of the health care and health services industry are now anxious to use emerging technologies to meet the challenges and needs of a new generation of e-consumers, e-providers, e-insurers, e-vendors, and other e-stakeholders.

For some traditional health care organizations, harnessing e-technologies may be the only way to solve their looming financial troubles; for others, it represents new and exciting opportunities to regroup, restructure, and even expand their share of the growing global market. Either scenario provides good reasons for examining the different sectors to determine how e-technologies will change the ways they conduct their businesses.

Hospitals and Physicians' Offices

Traditionally, hospitals provide acute and, in some cases, intermediate and longer-term health care services for the ill. Most hospitals have numerous departments, including admission and discharge, emergency and acute patient care units, laboratories, radiology, pharmacy, medical record archives, and ancillary departments. Seamless networking, collaboration, data exchange, and communication among departments are important to maintaining efficient and effective managerial and operational activities.

Typically, a patient is admitted either through the hospital emergency room or directly from a referring physician's office. Except for emergencies, every admission requires pre-certification from an insurance company. Traditional pre-certification involves multiple phone calls as well as detailed preparation of insurance company paperwork. Delays are often caused by the time required for physicians, nurses, pharmacists, and social workers to record and properly code the required information. Such medical records are also confidential and as such should be retrievable only by the health professionals directly responsible for patient care. Once discharged, a patient may need continuing therapy and prescription drugs for home treatment. Often, a physician prescribes medication either by supplying a written prescription or by calling a pharmacy of the patient's choice. Either of these procedures can be very time-consuming for both health care professionals and patients.

Unlike hospitals, which are often heavily subsidized by government funding, physicians' offices are private business units whose ultimate goal is to make profits. With the emergence of managed care and new restrictions on insurance reimbursements, patients with minor needs are now seen more and more in doctors' offices rather than in hospitals. Simple medical and surgical procedures once performed in hospitals, such as the administration of chemotherapy and minor biopsies, are now frequently performed in physicians' offices. The rising demand for these services is creating an increased need for medical products and equipment at physicians' offices.

Faced with increasing pressure to reduce expenses, along with changing health care consumer expectations for greater accountability and higher-quality care and services, hospitals as well as physicians' offices nowadays are trying to cut costs while maintaining quality of services. To manage their day-to-day business activities more efficiently and effectively, both groups are turning to emerging technologies for new and innovative ways of doing business. Strategic uses of e-technologies can help achieve the goals of reduced costs and more time for patient care. To this end, e-technologies such as intranets and extranets can prove to be effective. For example, e-technologies can be used for marketing, for providing on-line scheduling information to patients, and for the exchange of information between e-caregivers and e-patients and between users and insurance companies.

An increasing number of hospitals and physicians are using the Internet as a marketing tool. According to Fell and Shepherd, use of the Internet in hospital marketing has grown from 16.5 percent in 1995 to 32.2 percent in 1998 (Fell and Shepherd, 1998; Moynihan, 1999). Web access, external e-mail, physician referral services, research, employee recruitment, and education were the main Internet-related functions or tasks used by hospitals. In addition, the study points out that 56 percent of the surveyed hospitals not currently using Internet technologies plan to do so very soon (Fell and Shepherd, 1998; Meszaros, 1996).

In addition, the study argues that e-technologies such as the Internet can be applied to provide pre-admission and postdischarge information to patients. Providing pre-admission information such as instructions on preparation for surgery over the Internet could reduce the paperwork and the number of telephone calls between health providers and patients. It could also alleviate patients' anxiety and help patients make informed decisions. Similarly, discharge instructions and prescriptions can also be made available through the Internet in cases where the physician is not immediately available to write the prescriptions. This could lead to reduced costs, less paperwork, and fewer phone calls between the physician and the pharmacist or between the physician and the patient.

E-technologies can also be employed as networking tools to facilitate collaboration in e-consultation and for e-clinical follow-up services. In addition to supporting quicker and more effective decisions, these tools can provide e-health care providers with rapid access to rich and appropriate e-patient medical information. Provided that information exchange and transmission activities can be kept secure, Web services and e-health data integration services (see Chapter Fourteen) can support health care professionals in coordinating activities among providers and in exchanging critical e-patient information in a cost-effective and user-friendly fashion.

Dr. Joseph Catalano, an orthopedic surgeon at Baptist Hospital East in Louisville, Kentucky, surmises that use of the Internet to access patient information not only reduces expenses but also saves time and eliminates paperwork. He likes being able to use the Internet to check laboratory results for his patients (Benmour, 1999). With this technology available, physicians and health care providers can make quick and at times life-saving decisions because they have direct and convenient on-line access to critical patient medical information. To safeguard the confidentiality of patient information, Dr. Catalano's hospital uses encryption software that scrambles data before transmitting them. Users (physicians and other health care professionals such as nurses and laboratory technicians) are required to enter user identification information and secret passwords before any medical data can be retrieved. As reported elsewhere, encryption software has proven effective in keeping patient medical information secure and confidential.

Other uses of e-technologies include rapid access to e-patient information from referral sources, e-prescription services, e-procurement of supplies, and e-registry of new patients. For example, many products used in hospitals and physicians' offices can be purchased directly over the Internet rather than dealing with salespeople. More competitive pricing and direct connection to suppliers are strong reasons for e-purchasing, which can also result in substantially greater control over expenses and long-term time savings. Extensive ordering paperwork, valuable time spent with sales agents, and lengthy shipment delays can be minimized or, in some cases, eliminated.

Nursing Homes and Home Health Care Agencies

Nursing homes are health care institutions for the elderly as well as for those who are debilitated and need longer-term health care services than hospitals can provide. As a result of new advances and breakthroughs in medical and other life-prolonging therapeutic technologies, these institutions have gained popularity in the latter part of the twentieth century, especially among those elderly people who want to maintain a more independent form of living. Home health care agencies also provide continuing health care services to patients who have been discharged from a hospital or hospice and who prefer to be cared for at home. The introduction of managed care systems and diagnostic related groups in the pursuit of decreasing health care costs from shorter hospital stays have created a booming industry for home health care. Chapter Nine of this text is devoted to the topic of e-home care services.

Owing to the extended length of stays at nursing homes as well as the extended time that patients spend in home health care, a large number of medical records have to be maintained by nursing homes and home health care agencies to support the collaboration between the nurses, pharmacists, physical therapists, and doctors who are providing patient care. Traditional means of communication among these health providers are telephone calls, faxes, or hard-copy memos. These types of communication often cannot be completed in a timely fashion, prohibiting quick decisions. These methods may also involve extensive amounts of paperwork.

Like other health care and health services sector businesses, both nursing homes and home health care services can make good use of e-technologies to increase efficiency and effectiveness. For example, the Internet or other e-technologies can be used to send e-mail messages and to directly link computer systems in order to transfer e-patient data. Nonetheless, use of e-technologies by these operations needs to be well planned, controlled, and monitored. A nursing home or a home health care agency operating under contract with the U.S. government is subject to the Privacy Act of 1974, which imposes limitations on the disclosure of medical information collected by government agencies. In addition, the Health Insurance Portability and Accessibility Act of 1996 places further restrictions on the disclosure of patient information (see Chapter Fourteen). Many Canadian provinces and U.S. states have additional laws regarding the distribution and disclosure of medical records and other health care information. Hence, nursing homes and home health care agencies not only face the challenges of complying with medical record security, privacy, and confidentiality requirements but risk losing federal and managed care revenues and may also incur fines if their e-security measures prove improper or inadequate.

The trend toward quality home health care is on the rise as a result of the increased cost of traditional health care and the higher life expectancy rate associated with medical and technological advances. Home health care professionals travel to patients' home settings to provide health care services. Removed from the traditional corporate infrastructure, a home health care provider faces unique challenges. In order to provide quality care, home health care providers must be able to conveniently access patient information when needed, capture admission assessments, and collaborate with other health care team professionals in a timely and effective manner. They must also be able to stay in touch with their supervisors or managers in order to ensure that appropriate actions are taken and the appropriate people are kept informed.

E-technologies can provide effective solutions. According to Nugent (1999), "Internet-based technology will provide the necessary infrastructure for health care professionals to access data warehouses, data marts, HEDIS, reporting tools, and data mining systems." In other words, home health care workers can take advantage of e-technologies to access critical patient data when needed, transmit patient information, and connect with supervisors or managers to identify best actions and practices for complex situations requiring immediate action.

Pharmaceutical and Health Care Product Companies

Pharmaceutical and health care product companies provide health care products to hospitals, physicians, and patients. The primary role of these companies involves new product research and product sales. Traditional business-to-business (B2B) and business-to-consumer (B2C) sales in the health care industry are done with telephones, paper, and faxes or in drugstores and through personal sales. Product advertisement and education of potential customers in regard to products is typically done through television, newspapers, and magazines.

E-technologies provide new sales solutions for pharmaceutical and medical product companies, many of which are detailed in Chapter Twelve. For instance, with a simple mouse click, patients and health care providers can obtain product information and purchase products on-line. Within the health care industry, B2B and B2C revenues due to on-line marketing and e-operations are predicted to rise significantly over the next several years due to revenues from e-operations.

While using e-technologies has distinct advantages for pharmaceutical companies, some disadvantages and unsafe practices are also associated with these applications. For example, Pill Box Pharmacy, a popular Internet pharmacy, allows visitors to order medications such as Viagra, Propecia, and homeopathic drugs on-line. Visitors connected to the Pill Box Pharmacy Web site can seek an on-line prescription by linking to Medical Center Net; a doctor employed by that Web site approves or declines a prescription based on the customer's answers to a preset questionnaire (Weber, 1999). This practice provides potent medication prescriptions without physically evaluating patients. Pamela Gemmel, a spokesperson for Pfizer, the manufacturer of Viagra, has stated that the company does not support such on-line prescription of medication (West, 1998).

Medical Insurance Companies

Medical insurance companies, which provide insurance coverage for health care consumers, are major stakeholders in the health care and health services industry. Insurance companies pre-certify a patient's eligibility for medical and clinical procedures.

For example, they determine the length of stay that hospitals will be compensated for, compute payments to different parties, and dictate which health services particular patients are entitled to receive under their insurance plan. Because the major functions of medical insurance companies are to provide insurance coverage, decide on the length of stay for a given diagnosis, and compute reimbursement according to specific coverage plans, the medical claims filing and claims reimbursement process require a considerable amount of attention and validation. Traditional communications among the medical insurance company, the patient, and the health care provider involve phone calls, faxed information, and mailed correspondence. Manual paperwork can be very time-consuming, so these approaches usually result in longer response times than a direct electronic data interchange connection. E-technologies can provide on-line information about eligibility, benefit status, out-of-pocket expenses required, and procedure pre-certification. These resulting increased operational efficiencies will in turn translate into greater clinical effectiveness. Thus, use of these e-technologies can not only can significantly reduce costs and processing time but also simultaneously improve the quality of health care delivery.

Until recently, on-line transmission of Medicare claims was not legally permitted. In 1998, however, the Health Care Financing Administration provided directions to providers on how to maintain and transmit medical data electronically (Moynihan, 1999).

◆ ◆ ◆

Table 15.1 details the major characteristics and stakeholders involved in the different health care and services sectors and outlines how e-technologies will affect these sectors.

Our discussion on the task characteristics and uses of Internet technologies across the various health care and health services sectors brings us to two key questions: (1) What impact will e-technologies have on traditional health care? (2) What are the challenges in applying e-technologies to health care? We begin with the impacts of e-technologies on health care.

The Power of E-Technologies

Strategic use of e-technologies creates a competitive advantage for health care organizations and providers by offering the potential to lower costs, improve consumer satisfaction, increase quality of care, and strengthen consumer-provider relationships. In addition, employers that apply e-technologies successfully can expect to improve efficiency, create new opportunities, and provide more effective programs for employees in terms of decreased absenteeism and increased productivity (Wilkins, 1999). Other advantages include faster and more convenient access to health care services for the

TABLE 15.1. E-TECHNOLOGIES IN VARIOUS SECTORS OF THE HEALTH CARE INDUSTRY

Sector	Characteristics	Parties Involved	Impact of E-Technologies
Physicians' offices and hospitals	Large amount of paperwork related to medical records, payment, and (for hospitals) admission	Patients, doctors, pharmacists, suppliers, nurses, and (for hospitals) social workers and other health professionals	• Marketing tool • Access information • Get information about medical products • Exchange information
Nursing homes and home health care agencies	Reasonable amount of paperwork	Health care providers, physicians, nurses, pharmacists	• Share information • Provide fast and accurate link to other systems • Provide more flexibility for remote patients (for home health care)
Pharmaceutical and health care product companies	Some paperwork	Hospitals, patients, physicians, suppliers and retailers	• Accomplish B2B and B2C e-commerce activities
Medical insurance companies	Transformation of information and paperwork	Patients, health care providers, and insurance companies	• Provide on-line information about policies and procedures • Share information about medical claims

disabled, for remote and isolated patients, for the elderly, and for underserved rural, urban, and inner-city populations.

We have seen that e-technologies such as e-medicine (Chapter Eight), e-home care services (Chapter Nine), e-diagnostic decision support (Chapter Ten) and e-health intelligence (Chapter Eleven) will enable e-health care consumers to participate much more in managing their own medical records and health needs. E-patients, regardless of their mobility status, will be able to access the finest health care systems and the best e-care providers in the world simply by traveling either physically or virtually to an e-medicine-enabled hospital or health research center.

The e-health paradigm shift is changing the concept of health care. Whereas in the past, patients had to travel and wait to see a care provider before health care services could be rendered, with the help of e-technologies, expert clinical information and knowledge from many sources can now be transferred to the patient either directly or through an intermediary (such as an on-line physician). For instance, emergency services can be rendered to a traveling patient in a different country with data captured in smart cards carried by the patient or extracted real-time from a relevant database stored in the patient's home country. This powerful concept promises to revolutionize the business functions and characteristics of the mainstream health care and health services industry. Already, e-consumers are providing their physicians with research information on their diagnosed illnesses, as well as alternative therapeutic solutions that they have learned about via the Internet and other e-technologies. Moreover, e-patients are shifting attention to preventive care and lifestyle changes rather than concentrating on curative treatments. Coile and Trusko (1999) predict that "Internet-accessible information may reduce the potential demand for health services by the baby boomers in decades ahead. It could also result in a dramatic decline in demand for acute care services, as a healthier lifestyle kicks in and life expectancy jumps unexpectedly."

A number of generally positive apparent impacts of e-technologies on current health care services and business processes have been reported:

- Reengineered business processes and reduced administrative and clinical costs
- Increased customer empowerment and satisfaction
- Strengthening of patient-provider-insurer relationships
- Enhanced quality of care services and clinical outcomes

All sectors of the health care industry, including profit and nonprofit health care stakeholders, providers (for example, hospitals), payers (for example, insurance companies), employers, practitioners, public health officials, educators, system developers, consumers, and others must be prepared to face significant changes. Both health care and computer professionals, for example, must be aware of how changes in the use of e-technologies will affect them both as facilitators of the development of these applications and as health care consumers. As a facilitator, one must examine the design and development of applications in order to capture, organize, store, rationalize, and present health information in new ways; facilitate the replacement or integration of existing processes and systems with emerging technologies; and the manage new technologies and integrated systems. As a consumer, one must keep confidentiality, ethics, privacy, and security; usability; and political and societal impacts in mind. We will explore some of the more beneficial impacts of e-technology in the following sections.

Reengineered Business Processes and Reduced Administrative and Clinical Costs

At the very least, health care providers and other stakeholders can begin to reduce administrative and medical costs by improving work flows and significantly reengineering inefficient and costly business and administrative processes. This is an inexpensive and low-risk way to make good use of emerging e-technologies. For instance, the World Wide Web can be used to coordinate otherwise time-consuming and complex communications between e-consumers and e-providers in place of fragmented paper trails and time-consuming chains of phone messages. Many health care organizations are also allowing patients to do their own scheduling and appointments on the Internet. Intranets and extranets provide significant enterprisewide communications, including prior announcement and dissemination of intended changes in policies and processes that require substantive input and participation from employees. This method efficiently and effectively tests reactions and feedback without direct confrontation. Costs associated with postage, paper, long-distance telephone bills, meetings, personnel, and unnecessary processes can all be eliminated through the use of e-technologies to streamline administrative operations.

According to Healtheon CEO Steve Curd, time wasted on the phone in the health care system costs $200 to $300 billion annually (Delevett, 1999). Curd further estimates that a telephone call with a simple question costs an insurer $4 when overhead costs such as salary and rent are added, whereas the Internet can handle the same transaction for a small fraction of these costs. In a case example reported by Raghupathi and Tan (2002), an Internet-enabled patient record system installed by a practice with 26,000 patients in four clinics (Cabarrus Family Medicine in Concord, North Carolina) frees up time for the patients, residents, physicians, and their secretaries. Cabarrus doctors were spending about 40 percent of their time sifting through paper-based patient records. With the e-technology in place, physicians and residents can access medical records quickly, using standard browser technologies. Although we do not know how much storage space is being axed, the paperless system probably also resulted in a substantial cost savings on annual rental of physical space for storage of paper-based records.

On the medical side, e-medicine, videoconferencing and Web services can decrease the number of nurses' and nurse's aides' visits required in home health care settings, thus effectively reducing labor costs. Virtual visits can be prescheduled on a regular basis, for example, to ensure that the patient suffering from a chronic illness such as lower back pain will follow-up on instructions pertaining to pain medication and other therapeutic procedures (for example, regular stretching exercises and healthy lifestyle behaviors).

Medical cost savings can also be obtained by educating consumers about prevention and self-management of chronic diseases. Health care Web sites on the Internet and kiosks installed in public places can provide useful information and can educate patients about early symptoms, thus encouraging e-consumers to seek early medical attention and to use appropriate health care resources. The same technologies can also be applied to e-health promotional programming (see the case in Chapter Three). Some have pointed out that prevention and "early detection [are equivalent to] . . . less intensive, more appropriate treatment, [and which, in turn] . . . translates into lower costs" (Deckmyn, 1999; Wilkins, 1999).

Health care consumers can take an active role in the treatment process by making use of Internet-based self-care treatment plans. In this sense, patients can conveniently co-manage their own diseases on-line with health care professionals. It has been noted that through use of early and frequent e-mail communications, automated treatment reminders, and shared on-line resources patients can co-manage their own diseases on-line with health care professionals through early and frequent communication via e-mail, through automated treatment reminders and through sharing of online information (Shaffer, 1999; Wilkins, 1999). E-patients who have difficulty in using e-technologies can work with an intermediary. Today, many elderly patients have grandsons and granddaughters who will show them how they can learn to use the Internet and experience intergenerational programming (where the younger generations are working alongside the older generations in the use of Internet software), and through this, a better social link between these generations has emerged, as demonstrated in the case discussed in Chapter Three.

The use of new technologies often promises to increase the efficiency and productivity of workers. Although workers may feel stressed by the compressed time frames that result from electronic work techniques before they have a chance to adapt, many of them have been willing to learn the new trade with the understanding that the Internet is here to stay and computing skill is an essential for daily living. In other words, people are expected to do the same or more work as workers refuse to do more than they expect and ask for more money, with technologies serving as "substitute workers." It is believed that over time, as people adapt to new technologies, new ways of doing things will further increase the limits of growth of e-technological applications. New procedures and new capabilities may also combine to evolve completely different forms of business. Chapter Twelve illustrates how many traditional brick-and-mortar organizations are moving into e-businesses and how this move creates hybrid models of e-commercialization in health care.

Increased Customer Empowerment and Satisfaction

Apart from affecting professional e-health care providers, e-technologies can empower e-consumers to access information about their illnesses and ways to treat themselves. In a related area, e-consumers can also obtain support from other non–health care professionals—for instance, others with the same illness. Patients with chronic diseases such as cancer, diabetes, and AIDS can draw support from other patients with similar illnesses through Web chats, on-line support groups, and newsgroups. Ultimately, this will enable and empower these e-patients to understand their illness, the associated symptoms, and the treatment alternatives. It will also allow the patients to view the physical and emotional effects of the disorder through the eyes of someone else going through a similar experience. It has been claimed that "among the most powerfully supportive experiences for patients and caretakers is the sharing with others who have already 'been there'" (Wilkins, 1999).

Educating and empowering e-health care consumers through on-line information enable them to become active participants in their own health care, thus potentially resulting in higher satisfaction. Making information and networking tools available and conveniently accessible allows health care consumers to participate in planning their treatment regimen and to compare notes with others. This may further enhance their trust in e-health providers, perhaps enough to allow them to share previously hidden concerns with their practitioners. Moreover, reduction of emergency care, acute care admissions, and unnecessary visits to the doctor will save the health care system a significant amount of money.

Wilkins observes that "[i]t is becoming more common for patients to supply for their physicians with the latest disease research and treatment gathered over the Internet" (Wilkins, 1999). A new generation of educated consumers feels it is not only their right to discuss their health conditions with their physicians but also their responsibility to challenge their physicians to stay current regarding of new treatments and procedures. Thus, knowledge gained through proper use of e-technologies is enabling an evolving open dialogue between providers and patients. Over time, if such a dialogue results in positive interactions, not only will a stronger provider-patient relationship evolve, but both the patient and the provider will be able to feel comfortable that the patient is in control of his or her own health management. Again, this will result in higher patient satisfaction.

In addition, patients will be more satisfied when they can get answers to general health questions with a mouse click rather than having to travel, wait in line, and spend a copayment fee. Many e-consumers are already using on-line banking and e-bill payment and thus have mastered the skills they need to fill out e-claims for medical expenses and to e-schedule physician appointments. When patients can manage claim forms for themselves, not only are they empowered, but providers and insurers also realize huge cost savings.

Strengthened Patient-Provider-Insurer Relationships

Many examples that were previously mentioned will combine to promote and strengthen patient-provider, provider-insurer, and patient-insurer relationships. Hence, in this section we need only to briefly lay out a few typical examples. When a patient walks into a physician's office, the clerical or nursing personnel typically have to call the insurer to determine the patient's eligibility and which treatments are covered. Healtheon Corporation, a company based in Santa Clara, California, is marketing an Internet-enabled system that gives physician's offices immediate access to such information (Delevett, 1999), allowing verification procedures to be simpler and more efficient.

Once the physician has rendered a service, it usually takes weeks or even months to get insurance reimbursement because claim forms and procedures are designed for manual processing, which often takes a significant amount of time. By processing e-claims through secured e-technologies, e-providers will eventually speed up the payment process. The same applies to e-consumers who claim medical expenses incurred during travels or other emergency situations. The resulting efficiencies will enhance and strengthen patient-provider-insurer relationships. Indeed, the rapport among these stakeholders is key to the success of health care service providers. A key reason why consumers switch providers or health insurers is the lack of efficient and effective service on the part of the provider or insurer. The costs for the insurer or provider when a patient moves are enormous in the long term.

Providers, insurers, and patients can all be kept in close contact with one another through the use of e-technologies. For example, if a new screening procedure for colon cancer or a new treatment for hair loss is approved by an insurer, both providers and patients can be alerted and services quickly made available for appropriate patients. Posting these announcements and alerting the respective providers and patients effectively serves as a marketing effort for the insurer.

An insurer can use e-technologies to match patients with providers and encourage e-patients to provide feedback on their experience with those providers, allowing the insurer to develop data to help decide whether to renew a particular provider's contract when it comes due. Not only would such on-line evaluation enhance the patient-insurer relationship, but employers (who often pay a significant portion of the health care costs of their employees) would also benefit from a more productive and less dissatisfied workforce and fewer days lost to illness. E-technologies that can be used to strengthen patient-provider-insurer relationships include e-mail, on-line chats, postings on bulletin boards, organizational extranets, community networks, and mobile health care technologies such as wireless bedside PDAs.

Enhanced Quality of Care Services and Clinical Outcomes

Historically, information related to the development of a disease, as well as the risks and benefits of treatment, was not easily available or accessible to health care consumers. With advances in e-technologies, however, today's e-consumers can educate themselves about risks and benefits of alternative treatment options for particular illnesses.

An informed and educated consumer is likely to participate actively in his or her own treatment plan. As we have noted, this tends to create higher consumer satisfaction with regard to treatment outcomes. E-technologies also allow e-consumers and e-patients to choose their own physician or hospital and to check on the status of their insurance coverage on-line. Given what we know about the mind-body connection, autonomy in consumer decision making is likely to aid in achieving favorable medical outcomes for patients.

While any e-technology by itself cannot turn water into wine in terms of providing cures for sick patients, e-technology is a significant tool in the health care process. High-performing health organizations generally are managing these technologies better than other organizations (see Chapter Thirteen). This is why some patients prefer to be treated in one facility rather than another. Patients also seek physicians who use technologies appropriately and intelligently. Indeed, many chiropractors, physical and occupational therapists, and even acupuncturists are turning to the use of e-technologies to differentiate themselves from their competitors. How best to use e-technologies to achieve improved quality of care services and enhanced clinical outcomes is still a matter for further research and gaining further expertise, but at the very least, patients are impressed by the image of competence, efficiency, and responsiveness projected by e-health care providers and are spreading the word about their positive experiences.

Risks in Applying E-Technologies

Risks associated with applying e-technologies in health care and health services include the following:

- Organizational, cultural, and societal impacts
- Security, privacy, standards, and legal issues
- Mismanagement of e-technologies

Organizational, Cultural, and Societal Impacts

Some organizational, cultural, and societal impacts relate to potential job losses in traditional health services fields as a result of the changes needed to integrate e-technologies, including structural changes in the industry leading to closures of hospital beds and traditional health care organizations, changes in roles and responsibilities, redesign of mainstream health care systems leading to changes in funding and investment directions, and redesign of traditional work definitions.

Individuals, groups, organizations, communities, and society in general will respond differently to the introduction of new e-technologies, depending on their underlying culture and belief systems. For example, when hospital administrators are forced to cut their budgets, they most often believe that clerical personnel and middle managers should be laid off because clerical and administrative workload can better be reduced with the use of computers than can physician and specialist workload.

If a corporate intranet is to be installed, nurses and nurses' aides will have to be trained to use it, but physician training may have to wait, although physician training is often a more sensitive issue than that of implementing a nursing training program. If physicians refuse to use the networks, it is often assumed that the interface provided for them is not good enough and that some other specialized technologies may have to be put in place. Hence, the social and cultural dimensions of professional acceptance or resistance are key factors in any e-health technology project.

Similarly, when a health care organization attempts to install an e-prescription system, pharmacists may fear that having physicians e-prescribe the appropriate drugs for their own patients may diminish the pharmacists' role, which may not be acceptable to the organization or to both the physician and pharmacist groups. Such changes touch on the social and cultural fabric of the organization because when physicians order manually, the organization can hold the pharmacists responsible for checking the appropriateness of the medication and ensuring that the correct dosage or medication is being ordered. Furthermore, even if such a change takes place, resistance may surface later, perhaps in the form of concerns over patient safety and quality of care, so that the change becomes difficult or impossible to implement. In contrast, it is easier to create a direct link between a pharmacy chain and a doctor's office, because the role of the pharmacist will not be affected.

The same notion of the cultural context for acceptance of e-technology applies in major corporations. For example, if a corporation wanted to make ordering prescriptions on-line mandatory for a group of retirees, major resistance and political lobbying might be encountered because some retirees would not be ready to go on-line. They would prefer to visit their local pharmacies, gaining assurance from those whom they have trusted for years and discussing dosages and alternative prescriptions face to face. Many elderly patients also do not like having to remember a series of passwords and policy identification numbers and fear being kicked out of the system for not doing it correctly. They are also fearful of security and privacy violations, because of the many horror stories that they have heard over the years. Conversely, if the system were to be presented to newly hired school teachers, the reaction might well be different, given the group's likely experience with the Internet and also their intense time management issues.

In general, the experiences of traditional business during the evolution of e-commerce and e-business initiatives are expected to repeat themselves in traditional health care services as they evolve into the e-health care era. Some suggestions on how to avoid the cultural pitfalls such as those that have been described include running parallel systems rather than an outright automation, having an evaluation component to study and guide the e-technology implementation process, and generous use of multiple consultants in the beginning stage to better managed the transition process. Some organizations will outsource many of the technologically advanced functions until the organization has built enough in-house expertise. However, barriers involving security, privacy, standards, and legal issues are expected to keep the e-health revolution from accelerating at this time.

Security, Privacy, Standards, and Legal Issues

As discussed previously, the many positive changes brought about by e-technologies have been accompanied in some cases by user resistance, fear, and anxiety; violations of security, confidentiality, and consent; issues regarding the legality of e-health practices; concerns about privacy and ethics; issues brought on by a lack of standards and standardization; issues of data validity and identity authentication; and concerns about potential misuse, misinterpretation, and mismanagement of electronic information sources.

Data security and patient information confidentiality, two of the most important concerns about applications of e-technologies in the health care and health services industry, are discussed in detail in Chapter Fourteen. According to the American Medical Association (AMA), individuals or agencies can legitimately access confidential medical data only with bona fide intent. To enhance digital and electronic data exchange for health care services, the AMA has developed guidelines for imposing stringent security procedures to prevent unauthorized access to computer-based patient records (Meszaros, 1996). Chapter Four also discusses these issues in regard to how they affect electronic health records. In this section, we briefly review some of the security requirements and solutions.

Electronic access is typically controlled through the use of passwords, software encryption of information, or other means such as scannable bar-coded badges. To use e-technologies for health care and health services effectively, it is important to define who will be granted access and what level of data the patients will be allowed to access. Although data security and confidentiality of patient information are the biggest challenges, software solutions have emerged to tackle these challenges. Encryption software uses complex mathematical algorithms, or keys, to encode a message, thereby ensuring that only a computer using the same keys will be able to read the message. An encrypted patient record sent via e-mail, for example, would appear to be gibberish to an unauthorized user who opens the e-mail. This safeguards the confidentiality of patient information and helps to ensure data security. In another approach, firewalls combine hardware and software to separate an internal computer system from the outside world. Firewalls usually require passwords or codes embedded in specific computers to grant access to the protected system.

Lack of standards also fuels user resistance to e-technologies. While the Health Insurance Portability and Accountability Act, passed in 1996 (see Chapter Fourteen), made some progress in establishing standards, the difficulty of implementing common software without compatibility standards and the tedious process of achieving standardization among major stakeholders are obstacles to the effective adoption of e-technologies in health care.

Mismanagement of E-Technologies

Another major risk category in implementing e-health technologies has to do with mismanagement of e-technologies. According to a survey by the Northeast Chapter of the AMA, "only 14 percent of physicians would recommend the Internet as a medical information resource for patients" (West, 1998). This attitude is attributed to the fact that physicians believe that consumers will be unable to distinguish high-quality information from poor-quality information on the Internet. Since virtually anyone can post information on the Internet, it is sometimes difficult to separate scientific medical information from not-so-scientific claims. Further, the potential for misuse of information (such as that in patient records) that is collected and then made available via the WEB is another major concern.

In Chapter Thirteen, we discussed the management of e-technologies as a key to organizational success in harnessing the power of these technologies. Among the difficulties encountered by organizations are lack of leadership to oversee the growth and development of appropriate e-technological applications within health organizations. Unfortunately, many traditional health care administrators are hesitant to invest in e-technologies because a number of major hospitals and corporations have suffered major implementation failures and losses in trying to move on-line (see Tan with Sheps, 1998). In addition, health care organizations often lack technological expertise because it is difficult to find people with the appropriate technical skills who are also familiar with health care systems. The history of health care computing in Chapter One testifies to the risks associated with new technologies.

Surfing the Waves of E-Technology

Despite all the risks of potential mismanagement of e-technologies, expected consequences in terms of moving toward new business models, a more efficient and productive workforce and greater consumer empowerment and satisfaction warrant our continuing attention to the growth and development of e-technologies in health care. Two important questions arise from our foregoing discussion about e-technologies:

- What key functions need to be computerized or transformed in order to best capitalize on the power of e-technologies?
- What stages must such a transformation undergo before it can be considered complete?

With respect to the first question, we feel that e-technologies can contribute most significantly to two major domains and applications: (1) organizational management functions and internal operations, and (2) e-consumer needs and e-provider roles and responsibilities.

The crucial functions to be automated for organizational management functions and internal operations include patient care management, patient records management, administrative and practice management, insurance claims processing, supply chain relationship improvement, medical applications and services integration, and better matching of service with marketing demands. A simple example is the use of electronic health records (see Chapter Four) in which clinical and financial information can be integrated via e-networks and other e-technologies (see Chapter Six) to help make strategic and operations planning and resource allocation decisions as well as to facilitate patient care management and insurance claims processing.

The market for health care services is generally determined by the participation of health care providers and consumers. With e-technologies, e-consumers (that is, customers) will become more aware of trends in health care and ways to evaluate the state of their health. They will have better means of preventing illness and will experience greater personal empowerment because they will have access to medical information and knowledge. E-technologies also promote many other possibilities, for example, self-care, sharing of remedial actions among e-communities, better use of available on-line resources, and greater competition in the health care marketplace.

In addition to educating e-health consumers, the aggregation of professional content will be on-line as a resource used to educate medical professionals such as doctors, nurses, and hospital administrators and will provide greater accountability among these practitioners in achieving the goals of evidence-based medicine. Ultimately, evidence-based medicine will improve the primary purpose of the on-line educational component and help delineate measures for benchmarking best practices, thereby leading to a more credible performance evaluation of e-providers. Thus, adopting e-technologies can enhance professional career development and development of new competencies through continuing education, job redesign (by working and collaborating on-line), new hiring opportunities as a result of new skill development, credential renewal and audit, and professional certification. E-technologies change the roles and responsibilities of the e-providers beyond just on-line or continuing education as a new system of health care services is being engendered.

With respect to the second question we raised, we believe that three stages of e-technology development occur during its implementation in health care: (1) the information-focused stage, (2) professional services–focused stage; and (3) marketing integration–focused stage.

The earliest form of e-health care, the information-focused stage, typically begins with automating such tasks as acquiring, regrouping, and consolidating relevant medical information based on the ability of e-technology to interconnect different communities of consumers and professionals who intend to share, obtain, access, and use the information. In this stage, health care sectors attempt to make use of the virtual information flow, aggregate similar information, redistribute the information in a different form, and construct a substantial infrastructure for the information. One goal is to generate revenues so that these applications can become self-sustaining or even become profitable. We call this stage of e-health evolution informating e-health care.

In the professional services–focused stage, the health care sectors leverage their existing base of customers, consumers, and skills through the use of e-technologies in order to offer a broader portfolio of e-medical services by integrating their products and services with other partnering e-health care providers. Experience with e-technologies in the first stage can evolve new strategies for engaging in partnerships with other e-businesses. This represents an expansion of traditional isolated services into a more comprehensive and aggregated health care management or service delivery mechanism. We call this stage of e-health evolution e-servicing e-health care.

In the final stage of evolution, the marketing integration–focused stage, we envision a number of health care sectors forming a market-oriented strategic alliance to gain a significant competitive advantage. Several sectors are improving insurance claims processing, on-line patient management, electronic patient record management, automated facility management, and hardware and software integration and development by linking private clinics, research centers, nursing homes, pharmaceutical companies, and hospitals together via e-technologies. E-technology allows the network of e-stakeholders to share resources and information. The Internet and the World Wide Web are ideal platforms for the communication and dissemination of useful and accurate information. These technologies can provide cost-effective, timely, and specific e-health information to users on a global scale. In this way, e-health services can become global and ubiquitous. We call this stage of e-health evolution globalizing e-health care.

Given the gradual evolution of e-health and the pervasive power of e-technologies, there is a need to understand managerial e-health delivery strategies and supporting technologies further in order to link e-technologies for isolated rural and inner-city users into the global electronic health village, despite learning, language, geographical, and cultural barriers.

E-Health Delivery Strategies and Supporting Technologies

A key e-health delivery strategy is to place greater emphasis on on-line health information education and training. We believe that the new generation of e-consumers will be more educated, aware, and interested in charting their own course of health. This trend reflects many factors, including dissatisfaction with the current medical system, advances in health computing technology, and a shift in emphasis from the traditional view of the health care provider as the authority on treatment decisions to the empowerment of the e-consumer as the informed decision maker.

This shift in authority from provider to consumer calls for a new type of partnership, one in which e-providers and e-patients learn to make mutually agreeable decisions. To ensure success, convenient access to relevant and high-quality e-health care information via e-learning is critical. Indeed, for e-consumers, greater access to high-quality e-health information is itself a form of medicine (sometimes referred to as information therapy). The goals of information therapy include increasing the health knowledge of e-consumers, providing assistance with self-care, and giving e-consumers the ability to manage their own health care. Each of the communication components of the Internet—including bulletin boards, e-mail, Internet chat groups, Web security and Web data aggregation services, and the World Wide Web—provides a solution for better delivery of e-health care information to e-consumers. The bottom line is that these technologies offer access to a wealth of media-rich e-health information in an affordable, accessible, private, and convenient manner.

E-commerce is also a major force in changing the e-health care system (see Chapter Twelve). For example, IBM, as a leader in electronic commerce and computing technology, is developing an Internet-based health network known as HealthVillage. HealthVillage is an on-line community composed of patients, clinicians, health management professionals, and health organizations. It uses Internet technology such as e-mail, moderated electronic chats and forums, and Web browser tools. HealthVillage aims to offer high-quality health information and services in a personalized, comfortable, and manageable way. Its appeal will be based on several virtual Internet applications, including the HealthVillage Library, the Time-Life Medical Center, the Village Square, the Mall, and Member Services.

The HealthVillage Library is a user-friendly virtual library where the consumer can access current health information news through periodicals, journals, and references. This Internet-based library will have the capacity to run global searches and link the consumer to existing public information databases around the world. The Time-Life Medical Center provides consumer-oriented information designed to educate the user on health issues ranging from childhood asthma to coronary artery disease, diabetes, and depression. As a part of HealthVillage, the center will offer comprehensive diagnostic information for new patients and family members.

The Village Square works like a newsgroup in that key events and village news can be posted, and the square provides a virtual meeting place for health consumers to engage in informal dialogues on topics of mutual interest. More formal discussions coordinated by a health professional can also take place. At the Mall, consumers can purchase health-related products, such as books, fitness equipment, health food, home health nursing, and nonprescription pharmacy products. Finally, Member Services offers consumers customized "offices" within HealthVillage that allow access to personal information such as their benefit plans and health status information. Physicians and health care organizations can communicate with individual health consumers via these virtual offices and introduce specific programs or services (solutions.ibm.com/healthcare).

Other e-technologies can include hybrid strategies (see Chapter Twelve); complete on-line courses on particular health-related topics, either run independently or as part of a total degree program; virtual meetings; and on-line seminars, workshops, and conferences. Virtual reality is also a particularly interesting means of letting users participate in e-health evolution and solutions. This topic is the subject of Chapter Sixteen.

Managerial Challenges and Implications

The evolution of e-technologies as part of the health solution for the future also faces some challenges. For example, these technologies have been shown to be more readily accessible to those in better social and economic conditions and thus may work against the concept of equitable and universal health care by further dividing the population into those who have access and those who do not (see Chapter Eight). A further concern is the quality of the e-health information being disseminated via some of these technologies, particularly the Internet, and the difficulties of regulating or validating information quality. Ultimately, the user (typically, the e-consumer) has the responsibility of separating high-quality and credible information from inaccurate and unreliable information.

Given the likely changes in future e-technologies in health care, one important question is how these changes will affect management challenges, the definition of new roles and responsibilities, and the overall implications for all of the targeted users, from clinicians and technical operators to technical executives, administrators, and managers to policymakers and consumers (patients). The clinicians and technicians will be concerned about changes in their workplaces and work responsibilities that may be brought about by the introduction and use of e-technologies. As a group, they are more inclined to adopt a technological perspective on information and communications technology (ICT) and change. Health executives, administrators, and managers will generally see e-technologies as a change agent for improving the effectiveness of decision making and organizational problem solving. Since they are more interested in fitting the technology to organizational needs, they tend to adopt an organizational perspective on ICT and change. Finally, policymakers and patients are more concerned with how e-technologies in general will be adopted and will evolve over time; these people will be motivated toward a sociotechnological perspective of ICT and change.

Although different terminology has been used, these three perspectives are clearly recognized in both health computing and information technology management literature. The impact of these differing perspectives on future managerial implications and challenges will be highlighted by again using the example of IBM's HealthVillage.

From a technological perspective, the application and use of HealthVillage technology could drastically change the way that health professionals and clinicians practice health care. By becoming a paid subscriber to this on-line service, a professional would be able to reach new clients and perform services without being impeded by geographical distance and time zone differences. In theory, a clinician could even do away with costly physical offices, a regular schedule, and much paperwork. Groups of professionals could form partnerships via a virtual referral network. All they would need would be a virtual storefront, from which they could provide efficient and coordinated services that would distinguish them from their local competitors.

From an organizational perspective, HealthVillage technology would allow organizational needs to be met in new ways via the use of e-technologies. Health executives and managers, to make this new form of health technology work for them, would need to make a paradigm shift to allow e-work, e-management routines, virtual meetings, and a new generation of e-workers who would behave very differently and have very different expectations from traditional workers. New means of partnership formation and collaborative ventures would also define new roles for e-health managers and e-health executives. Meeting organizational needs in such an environment would require a flexible, adaptable, and revolutionary management style that would go beyond traditional ways of negotiation, policymaking, casting of votes in person, analytical problem solving, individual attention to details, and decision making.

From a sociotechnological perspective, the application and use of HealthVillage technology would mean a movement toward an integrated, virtual, community-based e-health care. Maintaining the ideals of equitable and universal health care has been a particular challenge for policymakers, especially in a multi-tiered health care system such as the United States and HealthVillage technology promises to ease that challenge. Medical information and knowledge would proliferate and become accessible at a fraction of the cost of accessing the same information traditionally. Empowered consumers would be expected to play new roles in making decisions regarding their own health and well-being. Those who still had not learned to use the new information technology would feel pressure to do so, and those who had learned it would find enormous growth in the amounts of information, knowledge and expertise that could be gained or accessed.

Given the preceding analysis of the different perspectives on the use of e-technologies for different stakeholders in the health care system, it is important to recognize the emergence of the self-learning and intelligent organization to meet future challenges in health care (see Chapter Three). According to Burn and Caldwell (1990), an intelligent organization has the following characteristics: (1) it centers on learning, (2) it promotes advanced technologies for decision support, (3) it encourages collaborative efforts among individuals and groups, and (4) it is information literate. These characteristics effectively integrate the three perspectives, providing a balanced approach to the managerial challenges that are likely to be posed by future e-technologies.

Conclusion

E-technologies have transformed many lives in today's society. With a simple mouse click, many e-consumers and e-providers are now able to enjoy the efficiencies these technological breakthroughs can provide—for instance, the ability to obtain a wealth of information or facilitate easier and faster individual-to-individual contacts, individual-to-group or individual-to-organization communications, group-to-group networking, or even B2B and B2C information exchange through e-mails, listservs, and other on-line and e-commerce applications.

Today's e-health care consumer demands quality care at a low cost. As a result, various sectors of the health care and health services industry are embracing e-technologies to provide more efficient work flows and reduce time lags in services and administrative processes. Using paper, telephones, faxes, and mail to transfer patient medical data from one facility to another, make diagnostic information available to patients, and organize collaborative activities among various stakeholders such as hospitals, insurance companies, physicians' offices, and nursing homes normally results in time lags. In contrast, e-technologies efficiently and effectively support these tasks, eliminating many of the time lags. As we have seen, coordinating activities among e-health care professionals via e-mail, ordering medical products through e-procurement software, providing on-line prescriptions through e-prescription applications, and accessing patient data instantly via mobile handhelds are some of the ways that e-technologies can be used to change the landscape of health care and to benefit the various health care and health services sectors.

As a result of using e-technologies, many health care and health services sectors are beginning to acquire a competitive advantage. Recent developments in data security have provided an impetus for traditional health care to gradually embrace new technologies and for e-health care to flourish. The increasing benefits of adopting e-technologies opened the eyes of an increasing number of traditional brick-and-mortar health care institutions at the end of the last century, and further innovative applications of these technologies can be expected in the current century. The trend appears to be toward e-health, e-consumers, e-physicians, e-insurers, e-vendors, and e-clinical care services.

Chapter Questions

1. Why is the power of e-technologies so pervasive? Give concrete examples of applications of e-technologies throughout the various sectors of the health care and health services industry.

2. How do e-technologies affect traditional health care providers, including physicians, nurses, health administrators, and patients?

3. What is meant by patient empowerment? Can the use of textbook knowledge rather than Internet knowledge empower patients? If so, why should patients use the Internet?

4. Differentiate informating e-health care and globalizing e-health care, and articulate your vision of future developments of e-technologies in health care.

5. Imagine you are asked to evaluate HealthVillage as a next-generation e-health system. What steps would you take? Create a list of criteria you would use to conduct this evaluation, and discuss what you expect to find.

References

Benmour, E. (1999). Hospital technology speeds information delivery. *Business First–Louisville, 15*(46), 38.

Burn J., & Caldwell, E. (1990). *Management information systems technology.* Oxford, England: Alfred Waller, 1990.

Coile, R., & Trusko, B. (1999). Healthcare 2020: The new rules of society. *Health Management Technology, 20*(8), 44–48.

Deckmyn, D. (1999, August 2). Internet health care to grow. *Computerworld, 33*(31), 25.

Delevett, P. (1999). Tech Rx. *Business Journal Serving San Jose and Silicon Valley, 17*(12), 29–31.

Fell, D., & Shepherd, D. (1998). Hospital marketing and the Internet Revisited. *Marketing Health Services, 18*(4), 44.

Meszaros, L. (1996). Patient confidentiality a big concern with Web access. *Physician's Management, 36*(7), 15.

Moynihan, J. (1999). New security guidelines will foster EDI use. *Healthcare Financial Management, 53*(1), 57.

Nugent, D. (1999). Providing solutions for the growing trend toward home healthcare. *Health Management Technology, 20*(8), 28.

Raghupathi, W., & Tan, J. (2002, December). Strategic IT applications in health care. *Communications of the ACM, 45*(12), 56–61.

Shaffer, R. A. (1999, September 27). The Internet may finally cure what ails America's health care system. *Fortune, 140*(6), 274.

Tan, J. (2001). *Health management information systems: Methods and practical applications* (2nd ed.). Sudbury, MA: Jones & Bartlett.

Tan, J., with Sheps, S. (1998). *Health decision support systems.* Sudbury, MA: Jones & Bartlett.

Weber, D. (1999). Web sites of tomorrow: How the Internet will transform healthcare. *Health Forum Journal, 42*(3), 40–45.

West, D. (1998). On-line prescriptions have adverse reactions. *Pharmaceutical Executive, 18*(11), 28.

Wilkins, A. S. (1999). Expanding Internet access for health care consumers. *Healthcare Management Review, 24*(3), 30–41.

E-Communities Case: Scalability Challenges in Information Management

Harris Wu, Joseph Tan, Weiguo Fan

A dramatic number of e-health communities (or e-communities) have emerged to provide e-health information and allow patients and health care professionals to share their knowledge and experience. In 1998, 60 million adults sought health care information on the Web (Taylor, 1999). A Harris poll in August of 2000 showed that 98 million adults had used the Web to find health information or contribute their experiences (Harris Poll, 2000). E-communities have more benefits than just the ones experienced by patients. Internet technology can facilitate the distribution of important medical information and knowledge to the medical community (Detmer and Shortliffe, 1997). Web-based dissemination of medical evidence has helped evidence-based medicine, a new medical paradigm based on meta-analysis of medical evidence, to replace the traditional authority-based paradigm (Brownson, Baker, Leet, and Gillespie, 2003).

Federal and state agencies, health care organizations, local communities, and individuals have set up thousands of e-communities. Yahoo alone provides forty-three health subcategories linking to 19,000 sites (Rice and Katz, 2001). On-line health communities range from small groups of people who face similar medical problems to large professional and commercial sites that provide many services, including the opportunity to interact with other people.

Recently, there appears to be a tendency toward consolidation of such e-communities (E-Health Initiative, 2004). Smaller organizations have found that they do better by investing in intranet systems and extranet systems rather than content-intensive Web portals because of the expenses to create, monitor and maintain such e-communities which, in turn, requires a critical mass of participation in order to survive for the long run. Many Web communities have failed simply because not enough people participated in them (Preece, 2000). From the larger perspective of the field of e-health, consolidation of e-communities helps avoid duplicate investment in providing general medical information to the public and reduces costs in integrating heterogeneous information systems. Moreover, a large e-community can obtain a critical mass of participants, which produces network benefits and enables tasks such as statistical knowledge mining. Besides cost savings, large-scale e-communities present new opportunities for evidence-based medicine and medical knowledge discovery. Small e-communities will still exist, but most of them will center on specific diseases or specific regions.

Large e-communities such as drkoop.com and WebMD.com have millions of users and documents. In this case, we discuss some scalability challenges and promising directions for information management in large e-communities. We have placed these challenges and directions in three broad categories: information delivery, information organization, and knowledge mining.

Information Delivery

Information overload presents a formidable challenge to e-community users. In a large e-community, the problem usually is not insufficient information; rather, the problem is how to get the specific information needed. Decades of information retrieval research have dealt with information overload and medical information retrieval, yet e-communities present some new unique challenges, including information quality, handicapped information users, and personalized information delivery.

The quality of information is extremely critical in e-communities. Inaccurate information can cost lives. Traditional information retrieval research has focused mainly on two measures: precision rate (the percentage of results that are relevant) and recall rate (the percentage of relevant information that is retrieved). Accuracy and other quality measures have rarely been the focus of any studies.

One idea for addressing the quality of information in a huge repository is collaborative filtering. An e-community contains a huge amount of information, much of which is contributed by individual users; thus, it is impractical to examine each piece of information. Collaborative filtering is a technique that harnesses the power of multitude. Information can be filtered by collaborative efforts of e-community users, through mechanisms such as voting, ratings, and relevance feedback. Users in an e-community, as well as documents, can be evaluated according to the information they contribute. For example, the Hub/Authority approach (Kleinberg, 1998) builds on the premise that "good" people (people who are considered to be an "authority") should contribute "good" information and identifies high-quality information (linked to source) in a system.

Another challenge in an e-community is that users may not be information workers in their daily lives. Traditional information retrieval research has tended to serve information workers, who are skilled in processing information. In an e-community, the users, including those traditionally trained health care professionals and alternative medical providers (for example, physiotherapists, chiropractors, acupuncturists), may be unfamiliar with information processing tasks such as searching and browsing on-line and providing clients with on-line transactional processing. With the recent trend toward mobile health care, many users have started to access health information through handheld mobile devices, which have stringent input and output limitations. Further, some patients are handicapped either physically (for example, by poor eyesight) or mentally. In short, many e-community users are not ideally suited for information tasks. To serve these users, the workload of using an e-health information repository has to be minimal. More focus must be placed on delivering concise, solution-oriented information rather than intermediate results such as clusters or lists of possible answers.

Question answering is a promising technique that may serve the needs of e-community users. Question answering combines information retrieval and natural language processing (Radev, Libner, and Fan, 2002). Users who have difficulty performing typical information processing tasks can use information from the community through a natural language question interface, which can be speech-based or text-based. Recent research has examined the application of question answering to the medical field. For example, Leroy and Chen (2001) developed an ontology-enhanced medical concept mapper, which transforms natural language questions to efficient database queries containing proper medical terminology. Wu, Radev, and Fan (2004) suggest a combination of question answering and summarization to support information retrieval through handheld devices.

Personalized information delivery is another challenge for an e-community. In typical information retrieval, users need to initiate information requests. In an e-community, however, both patients and health care professionals can benefit from proactive information push—that is, providing information before it is requested. For example, doctors can benefit from newsletters on medical breakthroughs or availability of new drugs related to their field. Patients can benefit from articles that pertain to their current health situation; using such information may effectively prevent them from developing certain health problems or lead them to new disease management approaches. Thus, information push is just as critical as information pull in e-communities.

Recommender systems (Resnick and Varian, 1997) are one way to approach personalized information delivery. By profiling users either through explicit questionnaires or passive observation of their behavior, e-communities can provide personalized information both on demand and before it is requested. Fan, Gordon, and Pathak (in press) have compared various profiling techniques and proposed a unified framework for profiling consumer information retrieval needs.

Information Organization

One major challenge for e-communities is how to organize heterogeneous information from various sources. Individual users contribute a large amount of information to an e-community. Lack of a common format for data from various sources makes it difficult to organize them. Furthermore, e-communities need to exchange information with one another, so that users can use information from multiple communities. In this section, we describe several promising directions for information organization: Semantic Web, XML, and Web services.

One encouraging research area encompasses recent extensive work on Semantic Web (an approach in database modeling that provides more emphasis to data semantics aside from syntax) and development of appropriate classification of ideas and ontologies by medical research communities. Resources in e-communities tend to be rich in human-readable and human-understandable annotation, but each resource uses its own terminology. An e-community not only needs semantically consistent and precise definitions of the data within the community but also needs ways to transfer or exchange the information with other communities. Successful integration and exchange of information hence depends on both a shared language for communication (a *terminology*) and a shared understanding of what the data mean (an *ontology*). Examples of ontologies include the Unified Medical Language System (UMLS) and WordNet. UMLS contains over 730,000 concepts in its thesaurus. Recently some research has applied Semantic Web solutions to generate context-specific ontologies that use knowledge representation languages (Stevens, Goble, Horrocks, and Bechhofer, 2002). Once an ontology is in place, documents in an e-community can be organized according to the ontology, based on a traditional lexical-statistical approach (Hersh, 2003).

XML (eXtensible Markup Language) provides another promising way to package information in e-communities. For example, Lacroix (2002) used object Web wrappers (software) to provide XML-based access to the data and map the query results back to a semantically consistent representation. The view published by the wrapper includes information about not only the content available from the associated source but also the query capabilities supported by that source. From an object-oriented perspective, the view contains information on both attributes and methods of data objects. These views allow the query engine to process complex queries on heterogeneous information.

Web services provide a layered architecture for information organization across different e-communities or different sources within an e-community. For example, Kemp (2002) presents a mediator-based multilayered architecture that defines three views of the data: the internal schema, the conceptual schema, and the external schema. The *internal schema* is the format that the mediator obtains the data in; the *conceptual schema* is the mediator's internal view of these data; and the *external schema* is the representation that the mediator publishes. The mediator performs the required data transformation between input and output layers (see Neural Networks in Chapter Eleven). The external schema (output) of one mediator may be used as the internal schema (input) of others, permitting a series of mediators to be used to define the federated schema. This layered approach supports multiple alternative views of the data while promoting significant mediator reuse, thereby yielding a more efficient neural net.

Knowledge Mining

Data mining and clustering techniques are discussed in Chapter Eleven. In this section, we stress one unique challenge that also represents an opportunity for e-communities: mining of user actions.

In an e-community, the user actions, in addition to the content of their postings, provide an excellent source of knowledge. For example, associations between symptoms can be inferred from users' sequential visits to different documents in a Web site. In another case, extensive requests for information regarding flu and fever from users in a certain region can provide an early warning to the region's medical authorities. Mining user actions has additional benefits in content-based knowledge discovery (see, for instance, Swanson, 1989). For example, user actions can be analyzed (and hence knowledge can be extracted) for specific periods of time, regions, or groups of people. In addition, passive observation of user actions is not as intrusive as soliciting user input through questionnaires or user registrations. However, harnessing user actions is not an easy task. Popular e-communities such as drkoop.com have millions of visitors every day (Preece, 2000), who take tens of millions of actions (for example, Web page navigation decisions).

Some emergent research in navigation mining has obtained encouraging results in making use of the information contained in user actions. Using a truncated technique based on singular value decomposition (an algebraic technique), Wu, Gordon, DeMaagd, and Fan (in press) analyzed 13 million navigations collected from a Web community. The analysis showed trends in user actions over different periods of time. Both data collection and analysis techniques were shown to be scalable to large e-communities. Their research also points out some security and privacy challenges that occur in observing user actions.

Conclusion

The preceding discussion of some of the scalability challenges and some of the most promising directions for information management in large e-communities is not meant to be comprehensive. However, the discussion should provide some insights into the challenges and opportunities involved in building large e-communities.

Case Questions

1. How might scalability challenges in information management affect future e-health community endeavors?
2. How do the ideas of data mining in this case differ from traditional data mining in other businesses? What are the challenges in applying data mining to e-communities?
3. Do you think scalability is an important issue in information management? Support your argument.
4. Delineate a scenario in which you want to use knowledge mining to improve the functions of e-communities. What are the drawbacks and advantages?

References

Brownson, R., Baker, E., Leet, T., & Gillespie, K. (2003). *Evidence-based public health.* Oxford, England: Oxford University Press.

Deerwester, S., Dumais, S., Landauer, T., Furnas, G., & Harshman, R. (1990). Indexing by latent semantic analysis. *Journal of the American Society for Information Science. 41,* 391–407.

Detmer, W., & Shortliffe, E. (1997). Using the Internet to improve knowledge diffusion in medicine. *Communications of the ACM, 40,* 101–108.

E.-Health Initiative. (2004). *Connecting communities for better health.* Retrieved from http://ehealthinitiative.org

Fan, W., Gordon, M., & Pathak, P. (in press). Effective profiling of consumer information retrieval needs. *Decision Support Systems.*

Harris Poll. (2000). Retrieved from www.ada.org/adapco/daily/archives/0008/0811.html

Hersh, W. (2003). *Information retrieval: A health and biomedical perspective.* New York: Springer.

Kemp, G., Angelopoulos, N., & Gray, P. (2002). Architecture of a mediator for a bioinformatics database federation. *IEEE Transactions on Information Technology in Biomedicine, 6,* 116–122.

Kleinberg, J. (1998). Authoritative sources in a hyperlinked environment. In *Proceedings of the Association for Computing Machinery—Society for Industrial and Applied Mathematics Symposium on Discrete Algorithms, Journal of the Association for Computing Machinery, 46*(5), September 1999, pp. 604–632.

Lacroix, Z. (2002). Biological data integration: Wrapping data and tools. *IEEE Transactions on Information Technology in Biomedicine, 6,* 123–128.

Leroy, G., & Chen, H. (2001). Meeting medical terminology needs: The ontology-enhanced medical concept paper. *IEEE Transactions on Information Technology in Medicine, 5,* 261–270.

Preece, J. (2000). *Online communities.* New York: Wiley.

Radev, D., Libner, K., & Fan, W. (2002). Getting answers to natural language queries on the Web. *Journal of the American Society for Information Science and Technology, 53,* 359–364.

Resnick, P., & Varian, H. (1997). Recommender systems. *Communications of the ACM, 40,* 56–58.

Rice, R., & Katz, J. (2001). *The Internet and health communication: Experience and expectations.* Thousand Oaks, CA: Sage.

Stevens, R., Goble, C., Horrocks, I., & Bechhofer, S. (2002). OILing the way to machine understandable bioinformatics resources. *IEEE Transactions on Information Technology in Biomedicine, 22,* 135–141.

Swanson, D. (1989). A second example of mutually-isolated medical literatures related by implicit, unnoticed connections. *Journal of the American Society for Information Science and Technology, 40,* 432–435.

Taylor, H. (1999). Explosive growth of a new breed of cyberchondriacs. *Harris Poll,* 11.

Wu, H., Gordon, M., DeMaagd, K., & Fan, W. (in press). Mining Web navigations for intelligence. *Decision Support Systems.*

Wu, H., Radev, D., & Fan, W. (2004). Toward answer-focused summaries. In M. Maybury (Ed.), *New directions in question answering.* Cambridge, MA: MIT Press.

PART FIVE

E-HEALTH PROSPECTS

An overview and a vision of e-health were provided in Part One of this book, followed by a discussion of the foundations of e-health in Part Two. Part Three explored e-health domains and applications. Part Four discussed the management of e-health and how it affects the health care and health services industry. Part Five, the final part of this book, deals with the development of trends leading to the evolution of the e-health paradigm shift. Chapter Sixteen recognizes the emergence of virtual reality as another frontier of e-health systems and environments. Chapter Sixteen also analyzes the concept of consumer-driven e-health systems and links this concept with the fundamentals of e-health that have been stressed throughout this book. Finally, the chapter attempts to chart the future of e-health technologies and what humans can make of these technologies.

CHAPTER SIXTEEN

E-HEALTH PROSPECTS

Mobile Health, Virtual Reality, and Consumer-Driven E-Health Systems

Joseph Tan

Learning Objectives

1. Understand the development of trends leading to the evolution of the e-health paradigm shift
2. Recognize the emergence of mobile health care as a frontier of e-health systems and environments
3. Recognize the emergence of virtual reality as another frontier of e-health systems and environments
4. Articulate the concept of consumer-driven e-health systems
5. Specify the steps involved in generating performance-based, future-oriented e-health applications
6. Chart the future of e-health technologies and what humans can make of these technologies

Introduction

During the turn of this century, we have been and still are witnessing an electronic information and knowledge revolution that parallels and, in many respects, clearly surpasses the industrial revolution of the past millennium. Just as the industrial revolution and its social implications changed the way of life not only for workers but also for families, organizations, and communities, so will this knowledge diffusion affect workers, families, organizations, and communities. Where once railroads, motorways, and machinery contributed to building industrialized communities and brought great economic benefits to corporations situated on or linked to busy crossroads and prepared and willing to jump on the bandwagon, now growing electronic and wireless networks are providing similar competitive advantages to new forms of organizations, a new breed of knowledge workers, and a new generation of cross-disciplinary thinkers. All of these stakeholders are learning about the power of emerging e-technology and discovering new ways to harness the power of this awesome technology (see Chapter Fifteen).

Accordingly, the proliferation of electronic mail systems, the Internet, and the World Wide Web and the emergence of intranets and extranets, e-communities, e-medical and remote patient monitoring devices, and Web services, as well as the introduction of mobile technologies have generated new computing and network applications in health care. As discussed in Parts Two and Three of this text, e-health records and databases (Chapter Four), e-public health information systems (Chapter Five), e-networks (Chapter Six), e-rehabilitation (Chapter Seven), e-medicine (Chapter Eight), e-home care (Chapter Nine), e-diagnostic decision support (Chapter Ten) and e-health intelligent systems (Chapter Eleven) together have called for a significant expansion of knowledge and training among analysts, managers, practitioners, and researchers. Most critically, stakeholders need to understand the prospects of e-health care technologies for future growth and development amid emerging frontiers and applications and evolving health care systems and environments.

The traditional role of health management information systems is to provide administrators with automated solutions for routine transaction processing problems (Tan, 2001). Health management information systems were built to resolve generally isolated, well-structured departmental information processing needs. These systems diffused and proliferated in the late 1970s and the early 1980s. Their acceptance among health administrators and clinicians (for example, physicians and nurses) has now been widely and clearly documented in mainstream health informatics literature. In Tan with Sheps (1998), the focus shifted to health decision support systems as the next paradigm for computerized applications, with the concept of using computer models and knowledge-based systems to support managerial and clinical decision making. In this context, a health decision support system may be defined as "any computer-based intellectual mechanisms useful for supporting and augmenting organizational or system users' cognitive abilities and skills in making complex decisions via the application of a mix of data, models, and knowledge elements through interacting with a convenient (typically, graphical) interface" (Tan with Sheps, 1998, p. xvii).

The key feature that distinguishes health decision support systems from traditional health management information systems is the combined use of data, models, and knowledge elements to enhance and extend the perceptual and cognitive effectiveness of health administrators and clinical decision makers. This enhanced effectiveness is normally accomplished by extending the range and capability of managerial thinking and clinical problem-solving processes rather than merely providing a system for automating routine, programmable, and repetitive tasks or functions (Keen and Scott-Morton, 1978). Although this more advanced concept of automation was proposed as early as 1978 by Keen and Scott-Morton, its application to solving semi-structured and higher-order health care decision problems was never fully appreciated until the late 1980s and the 1990s.

Today, as this text has emphasized, we are experiencing a further shift in the e-health care paradigm, in which information and communications technology is applied not only to assist individuals and organizations in solving routine and semi-structured problems but also to network, educate, and even transform the health and well-being of individuals, groups, communities, and entire populations. Indeed, it now appears that transformation is now virtually the only constant in the evolving health care system.

This chapter focuses on the prospects and transformational role of e-health systems and how to go about designing and growing future-oriented applications of e-health technologies. I will first survey some emerging frontiers of e-health technologies and applications—namely, mobile health care and virtual reality. Both offer natural extensions of the concepts, domains, methodologies, and cases discussed throughout this text. These topics, along with areas such as nanotechnology in health care, are expected to be the subject of future textbooks in health computing.

To complete this chapter, I take a closer look at consumer-driven e-health systems from the perspective of generating future-oriented e-health applications. I discuss the analysis of end user information requirements to aid the reader in understanding traditional health care technology planning and design. I then argue that this traditional perspective is inadequate for prospecting and building consumer-driven, future-oriented e-health care information systems. Accordingly, I discuss a new accountability expectations framework in detail, to provide an understanding of the rationale and underlying process for evolving strategically relevant, performance-based, and consumer-oriented e-health systems. The goal is systems that will satisfy consumer requirements, both by developing successful interventions for change and by promoting the health and well-being of individuals, families, groups, organizations, communities, and populations.

Mobile Health Care

Mobile computing has been touted by many industries as the next frontier. Apparently, this trend will include health care, although the development of mobile health is expected take longer than developments in other fields because of familiar concerns about standards, security, privacy, and confidentiality of e-patient data (see Part Four, particularly Chapter Fourteen; Tan, Wen, and Gyires, 2003).

Nonetheless, the transition and transformation from traditional computing technology and methodology to a wireless platform is already happening in many of our routine work and leisure activities. Hence, it is only a matter of time before this transformation moves into the realm of health care. The benefits for mobile health will be significant, given that immediate data capture and retrieval will become convenient when specialists, physicians, dentists, pharmacists, nurses, nurses' aides, public health professionals, and home health care workers all begin using wireless-enabled personal data assistants (PDAs).

Many executives today have converted to a mobile platform, making schedules, writing memos, engaging in complex analysis, listening to music, creating alerts and alarms, and e-mailing via BlackBerries, Palm Pilots, iPods, advanced pagers, cell phones, and other handheld devices. These handhelds provide a very convenient platform for generating future-oriented applications in health care. For example, both Pocket PCs and Palm Pilots are currently being tested and used for e-prescribing, capturing charges (e-billing), on-line research, e-book resources and references, e-patient education, e-clinical tools, and real-time retrieval of daily scheduling information.

Mobile Health Clinical Applications

Not only is wireless computing changing the lives of e-health stakeholders, but its effects are also becoming evident on a global and extraterrestrial scale. News articles about medical breakthroughs describe how e-medicine can be transmitted to the North and South Poles and even to outer space, providing e-care services to astronauts on the space shuttle. When one begins to fathom the countless possibilities that mobile computing technology opens up, the result is a growing stream of future applications and opportunities for scientific advances in almost every imaginable occupation. With regard to future-oriented e-patient care, the following list of ideas is only a sampling of the ways in which handheld technology can transform patient-caregiver interactions and provide instantaneous improvements.

- *Automated alerts:* using cell phones, pagers, and handheld devices to alert patients about doctor's appointments, or remind patients of scheduled medication, vitamins or supplements, self-administered blood sugar tests, walking and stretching exercises, or e-mail prompts for messages from e-providers or home health care personnel.
- *E-diagnosis:* using e-diagnostic decision support software to input patient symptoms and verify diagnoses using a clinical protocol reference database; obtaining information to support the practice of evidence-based medicine.
- *E-patient safety and error reduction:* using automated functions to calculate correct dosages and reduce the possibility of dosage errors; to graph and chart medication consumption for e-care monitoring; to flag errors in e-health records due to captured inputs that do not make sense, for example, spelling errors and missing information; and to ease the transmission of patient self-reports by beaming patient input on drug reactions from one device to another, thereby offering immediate alerts in case of errors.
- *E-patient monitoring and tracking:* recording information such as vital signs, medical history, prescriptions, allergies, and patient laboratory data at the point of care and updating patient records as care is administered or as soon as possible; immediately after patient information has been updated, the information can be transmitted between devices and synchronized with network computers for review by caregivers and e-providers.
- *E-referencing:* providing reference-based information to e-consumers on various aspects of health care and services and to e-providers, including evidence-based medicine and clinical care protocols as well as information resources such as e-directories of prescription drugs, referrals, and experts.
- *E-prescriptions:* transmitting prescription orders directly to pharmacies and using specialized software programs to reduce error by automatically checking drug interactions and eliminating errors due to misreading of physical handwriting.

In order for a wireless personal computer (PC) or Palm to be used for medical purposes, a nurse or physician must register the handheld with some support services such as ePhysician, an e-information service model in support of physician's office daily workflow and problems founded by Dr. Stuart Weisman. Registration is accomplished on the first synchronization with ePhysician, which is compatible with over fifty practice management system (PMS) software. Following registration, data stored in the PMS database, which include items such as provider information, patient demographics, insurance information, and appointments, are imported on a scheduled basis into the ePhysician remote database by way of the Patient Data Exchange program.

One application of this kind of wireless technology is an e-prescription system. With the elimination of handwriting, a physician can send an e-prescription order directly to the pharmacy, where encryption programs allow fast and inexpensive verification of the credentials of the prescribing physician. A prescription software package such as ePad requires the provider to customize the drugs, pharmacies, and formulary information that appear on both the handheld and the communicating PC. The selected medications, pharmacies, and formulary information, in tandem with the patient identification information (name, appointment, and demographic information) are then transferred to the handheld unit each time the PC is synchronized with the handheld where data is also transferred from the handheld to the PC. The key benefit of an e-prescription system is therefore the elimination of potential medication errors due to human transcription and increased efficiency and accuracy in the dispensing of medication and refills.

Besides clinical applications, mobile health encompasses health administration applications.

Mobile Health Administration Applications

Wireless technology can also be used to lighten the load for health administration processes and procedures. Again, the following list is just a sample of the many possibilities:

- *E-billing and e-charge capture:* a direct method of efficient, accurate, and concise billing, including automatic billing and electronic capture of charges. This increases the reliability and accuracy of data transfer from the point of care to the official records, speeding up business transactions.
- *E-messaging:* giving doctors, nurses, aides, and other caregivers continual access to remotely located e-patients and e-provider colleagues through wireless technology.
- *E-credentialing:* securely verifying the integrity of caregivers' credentials by means of encryption programs.

- *E-recording:* capturing treatment records and other measurements electronically at the point of care, for automatic updating of network computers in a timely fashion, thus drastically reducing the possibility of error and increasing patient safety.

- *E-tasking:* taking advantage of the portability of handhelds to monitor personal information such as appointments and prescheduled meetings. Reminders and other documentation can be dispatched automatically via e-mail.

Mobile Health Delivery Systems

EPocrates Rx Pro, a popular PDA program for e-prescription services, is an example of a mobile health delivery system. Information is available for each drug, including dosage recommendations, administration routes, cautions, typical patient reactions, drug interactions, metabolism information, retail costs, manufacturer, safety data, and recalls. EPocrates Rx Pro will also recommend alternative and substitute drugs, particularly when a patient's formulary does not cover the initial option; this is known as *e-prescription referencing.* Multicheck, another useful feature of the Rx module, evaluates two or more drugs and compiles a list of drug interactions.

The SUNY Upstate Medical University, located in Syracuse, New York, has been educating students to become qualified physicians for over 160 years. The university comprises the medical center with a teaching hospital, a Level 1 trauma center, a burn unit, the Center for Evidence-Based Practice, many specialty clinics, and an expanding biomedical research facility. Dr. R. Eugene Bailey of the SUNY Medical University, uses his PDA an average of two dozen times per day for a "variety of reasons. . . . [Uses include] teaching students, diagnosing illnesses, determining treatment, prescribing medication, determining drug interactions, calculating dosages, and performing all necessary steps that are involved with quality patient care without the concern restraints on physical location and proximity to the subjects." Bailey goes on to point out that his PDA allows him to conveniently review various articles and current events in the medical field through publications such as *Drug News Weekly* and *DrugLink,* a monthly newsletter that provides abstracts of drug-related articles from a good selection of journals. Like Dr. Bailey, many physicians are shifting to wireless computing applications, a trend that is especially appealing to the younger generation of trained doctors and nurses.

In addition to the wireless devices of mobile health care, other new technologies are being applied in the medical sciences—for example, virtual reality, sound waves, voice recognition and other advanced interface technologies, gene therapy, and nanotechnology. Due to the newness of some of the other technologies, the focus in the next section will be on virtual reality, a future-oriented e-health application that is already making a difference in fear therapy, among other uses.

Virtual Reality in Health Care

Virtual reality (VR) has been employed for years, particularly in entertainment and design modeling, but it has only recently been applied to health care. According to Strickland, Hodges, North, and Weghorst (1997), VR uses one of several modeling languages to create imaginary environments, or *virtual environments* (VEs), which permit real-time, user-controlled actions. VEs are computer-presented visions that give the feeling of another place. The user is given a head-mounted device, which projects a VE and eliminates any background noise (interference from "real reality"), effectively fooling the mind into believing the images are real. The user's hands may be free to move around or may have a remote control that allows redirection of movements through the VE. The user's actions are tracked, so that the environment can constantly readjust in order to interact as the real world would. For example, in its bid for the 2008 Olympics, the city of Toronto, Canada, used VR software to create the sight and feel of a new city landscape. The judges could be ushered into a VE to see different parts of the city from the sky as if they were flying over the city.

Virtual reality technology offers new and promising opportunities in every field, not just health care. However, it is especially suitable for enhancing the teaching and delivery of health care because of its ability to realistically simulate real-life situations and environments. Users are able to perform or practice complex tasks and challenging procedures without taking a lot of risk. In the Toronto VR example, city redesigns can be tested before the city is actually rebuilt to welcome the Olympics. In health care, the stakes are even higher than they are in an Olympic bid, because care providers are dealing with human lives and well-being. In such a field, the risk-free practice available through VR technology is invaluable.

Many VR applications are in the early stages of experimentation. VR has been carving out niches in particular health care areas, especially those that have not been adequately addressed by traditional medical science, including medical education, surgery, mental health, and rehabilitation.

Virtual Reality in Medical Education and Surgical Intervention

Telerobotic and telepresence surgery are examples of VR applications. Whereas the former entails the virtual control and use of remote surgical instruments, someone else other than the surgeon, who is not physically present, may manipulate the surgical instruments locally in the latter. In any case, these surgical interventions are performed with the aid of satellite communications where surgeons in a remote location perform procedures on a virtual image of the patient. A telerobotic prostatic biopsy on a human patient has been accurately performed. Although past results have been satisfactory, it is believed that further improvement in the technological architecture can reduce overall time delays while improving the time consistency between and within sched-uled surgeries, thus greatly enhancing the technique.

Surgical Simulator, a stylized replica of a human abdomen with several essen-tial organs, allows surgeons and residents to practice surgeries in a VE and predicts outcomes far more accurately and with very reduced risk compared with real-life prac-tice. For example, the use of the virtual scalpel, clamps, and staples on these visualized organs can be varied, and the short-term or long-term consequences for various sur-gical interventions can then be assessed. This is a particularly safe environment for training new surgeons.

Three-dimensional (3-D) visualization of anatomy is yet another VR application. With 3-D visualization, not only is the surgeon able to visualize the intended proce-dure more accurately, but the technology is able to scale, rotate, reposition, overlap, and reconstruct images that have been previously scanned and stored digitally into specialized equipment such as a Picture Archiving Communication System (PACS). Oyama and others (1997) report that 3-D visualization offers new breakthroughs for cancer research, diagnosis, and treatment. For example, VR software enables estimates of cancer invasion to surrounding organs based on virtual cancer images of individ-ual patients. The software can be used to help explain procedures and findings to can-cer patients in order to obtain their informed consent. 3-D visualization can also be combined with other VR techniques to simulate complicated surgeries. Satava (1995a) notes that in difficult brain tumor operations, for example, MRI scans of the patient's tumor can be fused with video images of the patient's actual brain, allowing a previ-ously impossible level of precision in X-ray vision, especially when the tumor is im-planted in the brain tissue. With 3-D visualization, the next generation of medical students will be able to learn anatomy, not from a textbook with overlapping trans-parencies, but by exploring organs inside and out through manipulation of 3-D im-ages (Satava, 1995b). Use of 3-D visualization tools coupled with interactive modeling (which allow the users to participate actively) allows dentists to better understand jaw articulation, while simulation of jaw movements helps dentists to deal with com-plex contact points and observe the actual functioning of the human jaws, thereby learning how to better treat their patients.

VR offers special needs educators a novel means of interacting with some of their hardest-to-reach students—for example, those with Down's syndrome and autism. The Learning in Virtual Environments (LIVE) program is the product of a network of re-searchers working together to develop tools for severely learning-disabled people. In this instance, users are exposed to virtual activities that simulate real life scenarios such as riding on a plane or shopping at a market to give them a feel of what can happen in real life activities. LIVE has been used to teach Makaton symbols, a language system used by children with a wide range of learning disabilities. VR provides new hope for success in an area in which traditional educational strategies and tools have generally failed.

Finally, VR can be used in hazard simulations—for example, in a simulation of a terrorist attack. In the real world, we cannot summon hazardous events at will, yet there is a need to prepare and plan effective mitigating steps (Mitchell, 1997). VR software can be combined with geographical information systems to simulate rescue operations for terrorist attacks (see Chapter Five). A VE allows first responders to practice novel and creative mitigation steps that might otherwise remain untried. Imagine too how VR can be applied to prepare military personnel for warfare against terrorists and for rescue missions to recover injured soldiers. All of these can be performed safely in a VE, and the skills learned have been found to translate well into real life (Inman, Loge, and Leavens, 1997).

Virtual Reality in Phobia Therapy

Acrophobia (fear of heights) can be a debilitating phobia. People with acrophobia avoid heights whenever possible, and this can interfere with their daily activities and routines. Therapy often takes the form of exposing these victims to varying heights in order to decrease their level of anxiety. Traditional therapy entails placing the victims in increasingly threatening real-life situations (in vivo exposure), controlling the exposure periods. VR effectiveness studies conducted on acrophobia treatment show that besides being safer and less embarrassing, exposure therapy in a VR environment had better outcomes than the traditional approach (Strickland, Hodges, North, and Weghorst, 1997).

Similarly, VR treatment for fear of flying offers many advantages compared to the traditional approach. Virtual flights taken by patients can achieve the same clinical outcome as actual flights. In a virtual flight passenger simulation, the patient can look out the window and see the changing ground and sky scenes. Such VR therapy has been shown to be as effective as in vivo exposure, at a significantly reduced cost (Rothbaum and others, 1996). Whereas the cost of actual airline tickets for patients and therapists are quite prohibitive, initial investment in VR hardware and software can be spread over many patients for years, making VR therapy possible for many more people.

Treatment for fear of spiders and other insects has also been attempted via VR exposure. Victims can expose themselves to increasingly frightening situations in the VE until their anxiety gradually decreases. Realistic virtual exposure can be achieved not only with virtual spiders but also with the tactile enhancement of large fuzzy plastic spiders (Carlin, Hoffman, and Weghorst, 1997). Other phobias treatable with VR therapy include fear of driving, fear of public speaking, and agoraphobia, which is the fear of being helpless in an inescapable situation—such as being trapped inside a burning building or being caught in rising floods. Agoraphobia often causes a person to avoid spaces or situations associated with anxiety. Many studies in VR therapy for phobias such as fear of public speaking and agoraphobia have produced remarkable results. More studies are being done, but VR therapy for phobias will likely become a growth industry.

Body image disturbances, which are believed to lead to eating disorders, have also been very difficult to treat with traditional therapies. A virtual environment offers a novel way for users to receive therapy, because it requires the user to pass tests and to perform tasks. These tasks must be completed in order for the patient to advance to the next level or to get into the next room. For example, they may have to eat something, weigh themselves, or choose which body image among many simulated versions best represents their true body size. Other symptoms—such as pain, insomnia, fatigue syndrome, and feelings of hate and anger—can all be treated in innovative ways with VR applications that use VE scenarios. Imagine taking a virtual cable car up a virtual mountain to ski; such an experience might teach you how to ski, help overcome your fear of heights and skiing, or even relieve the stress of your daily work and activities. It may also provide opportunity to those who will never have the possibility of performing the same activities physically due to impairments or other reasons. This brings us to the next topic on virtual reality in rehabilitation.

Virtual Reality in Rehabilitation

Rehabilitation may be the area in which VR will have the most impact and bring about the greatest transformation in human living. Not only do VR technology promise to make the blind "see" and help the paraplegic "walk," but we have yet to fathom the limits of this technology in related areas (Max and Burke, 1997). In a simulated VE, disabled people can safely engage in all kinds of activities and be relatively free of the limitations imposed by their disabilities. Moreover, there is evidence that skills learned in a VE are transferable to the real world. For example, disabled people can practice navigating their wheelchairs in dangerous situations. Owing to the limitations of current technologies, there is, of course, a trade-off between performance observed within the simulated system and in real life. Even so, research has shown that driving skills of those who may have impairments or are learners and are being trained increase as a function of time spent in VR (Inman, Loge, and Leavens, 1997). Moreover, VR therapy promotes compliance by making the entire rehabilitative process more enjoyable, motivational, and appealing (Bowman, 1997).

DataGlove and WristSystem technologies, which measure human movements, have been discussed and illustrated in Greenleaf (1997). These technologies are being used by occupational and rehabilitation medicine specialists, ergonomists, industrial safety managers, biomechanical researchers, and risk management consultants to study physical movements of patients undergoing rehabilitation. When worn during normal daily tasks, for example, these gloves (and wrist systems attached at the end of the gloves) measure how long the wrist, hand, and arm are positioned at specific angles; they also measure maximum, minimum, and mean wrist angles. Such information can then be usefully applied to study and help patient overcome poor ergonomics such as challenges faced with Carpal Tunnel Syndrome. VR-based rehabilitative workstations simulate occupational tasks as well as tasks of daily living. VR technologies can also help people with vocal impairments communicate. Computer mapping of hand movements in the GloveTalker, for example, can permit one who previously would have been locked inside oneself to convey more complex ideas.

Physical rehabilitation has obvious VR applications, but VR can also reach people with specific attention and movement disorders. Paradoxical walking or the diminished ability to walk voluntarily is a condition suffered by patients with Parkinson's disease. The difficulty of walking can be overcome if only stationary objects can be placed along the walk paths. VEs can be used in presenting the virtual images to the nondominant eye and scrolling the objects toward the subject along a virtual ground plane. Perception of the objects stabilizes appropriately as the subject walks over them. The VE can create images of such stationary objects with the use of special glasses and can superimpose these images onto the real environment, enabling people with paradoxical walking disorder to walk again (Weghorst, 1997). Attention deficit disorder and visual impairments are other domains in which VR rehabilitation is believed to be effective as the VR provides users with visual cues of objects in the surrounding space (Wann, Rushton, Smyth, and Jones, 1997).

Recovery from a stroke is often rapid during the first few weeks but normally plateaus before full functionality is reached. Traditional therapy often helps to prevent an early plateau, but it is hoped that VR therapy can help patients achieve a higher level of functionality as a result of gradual exposure and safe training experimental treatments. VR systems can either be used alone or as a complementary treatment modality alongside traditional treatment. The criteria, of course, should be whether value is added to the rehabilitation process, therefore justifying the required capital investment and technical expertise needed to set up VR therapy.

Trade-Offs in Virtual Reality Therapies

Although VR offers many opportunities in the treatment of otherwise difficult-to-treat conditions, some possible risks to patient health and safety must be considered. For example, people who suffer from migraines are believed to be susceptible to adverse physiological effects from VR. VR machines may be prone to errors such as creating visual distortions, which may induce hallucinations or exacerbate symptoms of existing mental illness. Such possible adverse effects need to be monitored and evaluated when applying VR therapies. Because patients are unaware of their real physical environment during VR therapy, attention should also be paid to physical environments so as to avoid possible trauma caused by accidents.

Owing to the effects of VR on the vestibular system or the body's sensors for movement, some patients experience motion sickness ("cybersickness"), while others suffer from a small epileptic event ("flicker vertigo") following their VR exposure. Stanney and Kennedy (1997) suggest that cybersickness may be reduced by providing the user with an optimal level of user-initiated control over their movements in the virtual world. Results from their VR studies indicated that VEs tend to produce fewer oculomotor-related (O) disturbances, such as eyestrain and more disorientation (D) than neuronegative (N) symptoms, such as nausea (Stanney and Kennedy, 1997). Hence, in order to ensure safety, VR patients and users should allow for recovery time before engaging in risky psychomotor activities such as operating motor vehicles.

The exact causes of cybersickness and other VR aftereffects such as flicker vertigo are not fully understood. While there are standards for binocular image alignment, there are no tolerance standards for the amount of dynamic mismatch the visual system can tolerate in terms of either convergence or focus. Eyestrain caused by a poor quality head-mounted device (HMD) or ocular alignment is better understood. Design of the HMD may result in a dynamic mismatch with the user's visual system. Enforcing specific standards to limit the amount of dynamic mismatch may reduce the eyestrain. Viire (1997) suggests that the standards established for eyeglass prescriptions would be a practical place to begin specifying HMD design standards.

Light source and noise levels are other considerations in ensuring the safety of VR therapies. Because lighting from many VR systems shines directly at the user's eyes, the light levels must be safe. Moreover, some VR systems use potentially dangerous sources of light such as lasers, which can damage eyes. VEs can produce loud noises at close range, which can also pose risks to users. Fortunately, existing standards for safe sound levels can be applied, and the effects of sound exposure at various decibels can be controlled and managed properly.

The next section covers a critical topic that can pave the way for the future success of e-health systems—that is, what must happen to generate future-oriented, performance-based e-health systems that satisfy consumer and user requirements and expectations.

Consumer-Driven E-Health Systems

With active and increasing grassroots participation from consumers and community groups, e-health may soon become a household word. Whether health organizations like it or not, and regardless of what the major insurers may try in order to stop health care reform, consumers and payers such as employers and third parties (for example, the government) will continue to play major roles in determining the future of health care, particularly e-health care. Advocates of consumer-driven health care systems argue for a transformation in the current system that will ultimately allow consumers to decide for themselves how they are going to pay for health care. Employers, on the other hand, are also taking the initiative in order to get the most out of the money they spend on employee health care. Major manufacturing firms such as General Motors, Ford, and Chrysler need to ensure that health care costs are sufficiently contained in order to stay profitable. Similarly, the government is always trying to find the best formulas to help keep a lid on the escalating costs of health care.

With these trends, we will be seeing some drastic changes in the way health care will be financed in the future. Many consumers are already turning to alternative modalities such as integrative medicine, preventive medicine and therapies, and e-health. One financing suggestion is that the premiums paid for health care go into a savings account until health services are rendered. Other schemes include ensuring that the services meet the requirements and expectations of the consumers and the employers based on needs and priorities. Some employers are even demanding that cost-saving services such as e-prescriptions be instituted as the norm, regardless of employee preference. The U.S. government and government-funded research agencies have been studying the financing of health care costs, legislation on security and privacy of patient records, health care technology assessment issues, challenges to the quality and safety of health care services, and managed care schemes.

Hence, we are beginning to see some real changes emerging in health care and e-health care. Put simply, if insurers and other traditional health organizations continue to turn a blind eye to changing trends in health care and a deaf ear to the new generation of informed and Internet-savvy consumers, these organizations may soon be replaced by emerging competitors who are responsive to the demands and requirements of consumers and employers.

Analyzing User Information Requirements

In light of changing trends and paradigm shifts in our health care system, we close this chapter with a discussion of how to understand user information requirements (IRs), which is basic to any systems development. Information requirements affect how a system designer or developer elicits and specifies the relevant, useful information that is expected to be available from an information system (IS).

In health systems development, the problem of having data without useful or meaningful information is usually the result of having too much rather than too little information. This problem is especially pervasive in e-health applications because massive amounts of data are often collected, accumulated, and then presented to serve many different purposes. Moreover, the data are often gathered from a variety of sources without a good rationale or adequate planning. Instead, data gathering can be motivated by reporting needs or sometimes by fear of potential requests for more information from diverse e-stakeholders (for example, the government, e-health providers, e-payers, e-patient advocacy groups, and users, who include e-consumers, managers, directors, and referring clinicians).

Data collected for a particular use may not be transferable or even relevant for other uses. Informational needs vary in focus and volume according to the type and level of planning and decision making that is to be undertaken (Tan, 1995). For example, strategic planning typically requires the integration of external and internal data sources, whereas routine operations concentrate mainly on internal data sources. There often is a lack of clarity as to the relevance of the data collected to meet user IRs. Even so, it is obvious that when inadequate planning or attention is given to user IRs at the beginning of the system development cycle, the resulting information system will likely be irrelevant, leading rapidly to its disuse and obsolescence. This happens because users or decision makers who interface with the system will not benefit if the system cannot deliver the information they need or want.

Notwithstanding, the process of analyzing user IRs is complex and poorly understood or enforced in everyday practice. As a result, many systems provide poor or inadequate support to users. Conceptually, the traditional process for analyzing user IRs can be configured as a three-stage framework, as shown in Figure 16.1.

At the *conceptualization* stage, which is closest to the real-world representation, the context for modeling is the actual environment in which empirical problems and needs are observed and interpreted. Conceptualization is the point where empirical reality is gradually translated into mental models and concepts, which are then articulated as key system design ideas and elements. The representation of these elements (or entities) and their interrelationships is necessarily complex because these are often the by-products of the interplay of many poorly defined variables, including legal, cultural, socioeconomic, political, environmental, technological, and epidemiological variables. These variables are frequently difficult, if not impossible, to define operationally. In fact, their meanings and interrelationships are often the subject of multiple interpretations that depend on a manager's or an analyst's view of the world. Yet in this beginning step of IR analysis, elements of real-world objects and their interrelations have to be reduced from highly dynamic environments in which economic, political, legal,

FIGURE 16.1. TRADITIONAL PROCESS FOR ANALYSIS OF USERS' INFORMATION REQUIREMENTS

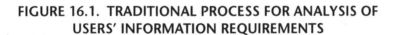

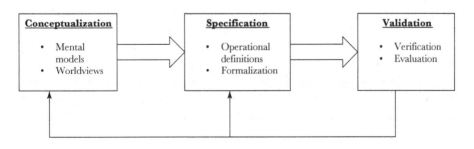

social, and technological variables are constantly evolving to more concrete and tangible measures (see Chapter Thirteen for more on defining e-health care technology management and strategy).

Next, the process of *specification* involves moving from a mental representation of abstract ideas and concepts to a more logically defined and formalized model. This is the stage in which key stakeholders, particularly users, attempt to move toward an information processing model of the real-world situation. Typically, the chief analyst is responsible for providing the specification in a form that is readable for both the end users and the programmers. In this regard, concepts and variables of the conceptual phase now have to be operationally defined as constructs, and the complex but observable phenomena in question must now be reduced to a manageable model that depicts the information flow. In short, conceptual elements and their relationships are translated into corresponding data objects (entities) and linkages (relationships). Many transitional models are formed during this transformational stage, each of which may be relatively abstract compared with the physical models that will follow in the final stage. Specification is the part of the IR analysis process that brings about a consensus of perspectives and concerns among key stakeholders; the analyst and system developer notes these perspectives and concerns.

Finally, the *validation* stage is an attempt to determine whether a valid set of user IRs has actually been created. During this phase, the earlier specification is refined, to provide an accepted and measurable reflection of the perceived system performance gaps and accepted solutions, both of which are now limited to the information system context. Thus, the objective is to achieve a working prototype. This intermediate product is a computer-based prototype that adequately captures the specified design model. In fact, the design model produced during validation is analogous to an architectural blueprint of a building, waiting for construction. This blueprint is the method for communicating between users and analysts, and it spells out the details of the proposed structure and contents of the information flow system. It is also a document for the contractor (programmer) to use in verifying, evaluating and building the system.

The journey from conceptualization to validation involves a series of mental transformations. Different analysts will choose different routes of mental transformation, which explains, in part, why different e-health solutions may be proposed to achieve the same purpose. The possibility of multiple solutions implies that there can be as many e-health applications as there are conceptualizations and interpretations of real-world phenomena. This is also one of the reasons why effective communication between analysts and end users at all three stages determines whether the resulting information system solution will meet the ends of all stakeholders.

A key limitation of the user IR analysis process just described is the lack of emphasis on bridging the user's IRs with the overall system's information needs and values. In short, the traditional view limits the conceptualization of user IRs to mostly operational and tactical levels of thinking. Thus, the resulting information system design concepts or ideas depend greatly on somewhat biased and subjective communications of particular user needs to the analysts. Owing to the complexity and potential frustration for an analyst in interacting with a group of end users who may well be unable or unwilling to communicate what they need or want from a shared perspective, most analysts find it convenient to focus the conceptualization process toward the views of a particular user. Thus, to meet the needs of a multiplicity of users with different or even conflicting needs and wants, analysts develop a network of isolated and fragmented systems, each of which satisfies the needs of a different set of individual users. In other words, the traditional IR analysis process supports the development of individualized or compartmentalized systems, not integrated user-oriented networks or systems.

A related limitation of the traditional approach is users' lack of an agreed-on basis for defining constructs and validating user needs and requirements. In other words, the validation process in the traditional IR analysis approach assumes that the design concepts and elements can be verified through a series of structured analyst-user interactions. What is missing is the notion that the constructs and variables to be verified should be linked to accepted standards that are shared among key stakeholders. In short, there is no explicit sense of what the constructs or variables might be for different users. The problem is aggravated in e-health applications designed to support multiple-level users with conflicting needs and wants. Thus, a new perspective for understanding strategic e-health system planning and design is needed—that is, a perspective that will not only align users' IRs with the general system mandate and purpose but ensure that all e-health users share the same views about needs and priorities.

Finally, the traditional approach emphasizes formalization of information system solutions for well-defined, structured, and isolated systems rather than integrated, dynamic e-health decision problems. The traditional specification process requires that analysts map user IRs onto a formalized model, using the systems approach, defining outputs via a backward chain of reasoning to the inputs (and validating inputs to outputs via a forward chain of reasoning). Because this level of reasoning and formalization is possible only if the decision systems are somewhat well-structured, the potentially high benefits of developing e-health applications using more qualitative and consumer-oriented data for semistructured and complex decision systems cannot be easily accommodated.

Many key e-health problems occur at the high levels of intraorganizational and interorganizational problems—for example, difficulties with the integration of health care services or the sharing of information among strategic partners and users. Thus, there is a need to develop more integrated perspectives that would effectively guide and accommodate the development of mixed applications to support well-structured, semistructured and ill-structured decision problems. Therefore, an accountability expectations framework, developed on the basis of a consumer-driven problem-solving model, is proposed to guide future e-health system planning and design.

The Accountability Expectations Framework

The *accountability expectations framework* (Modrow and Mathias, 1998; Tan and Modrow, 1999, 2003) refers generally to identifying a set of expected performance measures or indicators through which management can be held accountable for particular decisions or actions vis-à-vis clearly defined requirements and expectations from the consumer's end. As presented in Figure 16.2, the accountability expectations framework begins with specifying the ideal e-health model, followed by the identification of specific problems evolving within dynamic mandates and environments for which adequate information to make decisions must be captured. In other words, the information available must be sufficient for users to make the decisions and judgments for which they will be held accountable. Various e-health alternative solutions must be evaluated in an attempt to bridge problem gaps—that is, when the difference between the desired and observed performance is deemed unacceptable, new efforts should be made to ensure that a wide variety of innovative e-health solutions are examined. Indeed, solutions generated in this manner are likely to be adaptive and dynamic.

For e-health systems to be strategically and dynamically relevant, then, these systems should link users throughout the network system and set desired performance criteria. This linkage provides the basis to ensure that users achieve their performance goals within the bounds of the e-health system mandate and purpose. One necessary condition for this linkage is the existence of consumer-driven, albeit explicit and clearly defined measures of performance or standards for benchmarking performance. In other words, consumers must be surveyed in order to generate the measures.

Since users' characteristics differ (for example, e-providers differ from e-consumers in their roles and needs), users' standards for benchmarking and monitoring performance will also differ. For instance, e-providers may have explicit performance standards for determining success, defined in terms of market share, return on investment, net profit, and other clearly articulated and measurable indicators. All user decisions in such an environment would be clearly linked to the performance measures, and the quality of decisions made could be judged in relation to these measures.

As another example, imagine that a physician or an employer wants a mobile system to reduce expensive and often extraneous physician consultation costs related to manual prescription services. On this basis, one requirement for an effective mobile e-prescription application would be the ability to provide relevant and precise e-prescription information directly to pharmacists without the need for further consultation with a physician. If the pharmacists still have questions after receiving

FIGURE 16.2. ACCOUNTABILITY EXPECTATIONS
FRAMEWORK FOR E-HEALTH INNOVATIONS

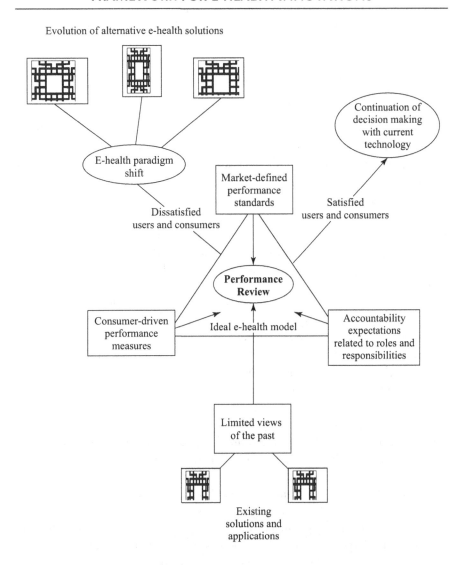

the information or if patients have complaints about their prescriptions, these problems should be tracked to provide a basis for evaluating the effectiveness of the mobile e-prescription solutions. In this sense, the mobile e-prescription system will not only reduce opportunity costs and increase productivity but also add value by assessing the effectiveness of medication intervention for the patients.

The analysis of existing prescription solutions compared with mobile or other potential solutions can also yield insights for evolving future prescription systems (for example, virtual prescription applications). Closing-the-gap analysis and continual benchmarking via evidence based medical practices, therefore, require analysts and users (in our case, the employer, the physician, and the pharmacist) to focus on identifiable and measurable differences between expected and observed performance and between newly designed solutions and existing solutions. The ideal e-health model should focus on measurable performance standards and indicators at the competitive level and system performance measures at the user accountability level. Based on an understanding of ideal versus current solutions, we can then evolve an e-health application that will adequately support the user information and decision-making roles and responsibilities. Such a system will generate the information needed or wanted, not just provide massive databases that may overload users with irrelevant and unwanted data.

Strategic thinking in the e-health context moves toward understanding performance measures and adding value to the health care process. The critical questions are "How is performance to be determined?" and "What value has been added by the introduction of the e-health solution?" For instance, if overprescription or patient safety becomes a concern, it would be important to add a verification function in the system to set limits on prescriptions so as to make pharmacists aware of these concerns. Viewing clinical performance in terms of traditional process outcomes such as adequate supplies and scheduling of order fillings and refills versus our proposed performance outcomes such as quality assurance and resulting health outcomes is analogous to making products available without being concerned about their quality. Nonetheless, in the competitive e-market system, profitability is an important criterion. Hence, the strategic relevance of e-health solutions must be linked to both the system's environment and performance outcomes.

As discussed at the beginning of this text, five basic strategies govern the outcomes of e-health systems and guide the development of future e-health systems: (1) specifying e-health core value propositions; (2) understanding the characteristics of the e-health service model; (3) involving the community of e-stakeholders; (4) strengthening the potential for a critical mass of transactions, to ensure sustainability and eventual profitability; and (5) examining e-health potential to accommodate future features such as product or service expansion, population growth, and global development.

E-health applications that are strategically relevant, consumer-driven, and performance-based will include applications that track user satisfaction data, systems that perform accounting and budgeting analysis, solutions that capture information on quality assurance and on public perception, systems that track complaints and facilitate their resolution, and applications that monitor competitive funding sources and the success with which developers of innovative e-health solutions can compete for these funds. In the end, regardless of whether the e-health applications are intended for e-providers or e-consumers, effective e-health solutions are those planned and designed to determine what users want and need, and those that can be used to monitor particular interventions in an attempt to reduce performance gaps and evaluate the effectiveness of the interventions. Because change is an essential characteristic of e-health, these solutions will be evolutionary in nature.

Conclusion

The future of e-health relates to the expansion of perspectives, the continuing growth of the Internet and other e-networks (Parts One and Two), the emergence of new domains and applications (Part Three), and the implementation of new strategies, management approaches, and impacts (Part Four) as well as the application of new and emerging mobile health networks and technologies, virtual reality, and other advancing technologies (Part Five). All of these developments will ultimately amount to the blurring of corporate communities on one hand and the blurring of user communities on the other. The defined roles of e-suppliers, e-providers, and e-customers are becoming less distinct. Therefore, it is still critical to come back, as I have in the final part of this chapter, to ask, "What is it that the consumers or the customers want? How do we go about designing something that is precisely what the market wants? What performance measures determine success?"

Today, companies are reaching outside their walls to encourage growth and development that incorporate many collaborative partners. This is already happening in the U.S. e-health marketplace. Under this model, many stakeholders hope that the health care industry will become more globalized in a positive, inclusive sense and less centralized. Understanding how to nurture organizations through the transition from a command-and-control focus to a virtual model while keeping them integrated will be a challenge for the government, the health insurance companies, provider groups, and many e-health venture capitalists and entrepreneurs in this century.

The most important message to be relayed in this text is that e-health systems should focus not on creating profit but on providing a competitive advantage, encouraging further innovations and more significant change for the improvement of human health and well-being. This is what distinguishes e-health from e-business. While new business functions must be created and competitive advantages can be realized, the goal is to reach out to the underserved and to those who have limited access. The need for effective universal access to health services has changed how the health care industry values health care goods and services. In the past, making health care goods and services available to individuals was the primary goal. Later, the focus became the quality of health care goods and services that can be provided to all patients within a region. With the globalization of markets and the shift in emphasis to ubiquitous computing, the focus is now on what benefits can be derived from the provision of health care goods and services. In other words, can preventive care and preparedness for potential public health hazards be achieved with new ways of performing health care? The change in the industry is also a movement from structured to unstructured processes. Being able to capitalize on complex processes will enable e-stakeholders, including e-vendors, e-payers, e-providers, and, most important, e-consumers to use the latest e-health technologies in new ways.

As we have noted throughout this text, a new paradigm in health care, the e-health paradigm shift, has emerged. This has led to new expectations among e-consumers of health care. Virtual reality, with its great promise for medical training and education, is one example of how e-health technology can help to achieve these increasingly higher expectations. From information management to surgical simulations and 3-D anatomy, new generations of medical students will learn how to meet these raised expectations by embracing the new paradigm. With this learning will come substantial advances that will revolutionize the way we think about current practices and methods. Already, some experts believe that if we can use nanotechnology to cure cancer, cancer patients will no longer need to endure harmful treatments such as radiation or laser surgery. Instead, molecular-level healing elements (nanotechnology) might destroy only targeted cancer cells without affecting neighboring cells. How successfully we combine our knowledge of these new technologies with health care services will be the determining factor in our future health and well-being.

The next breakthroughs in strategic e-health care applications are expected in the areas of integrated e-systems, intelligent e-networks, and e-robotics (Raghupathi and Tan, 2002). Indeed, the ability to integrate e-clinical and e-administrative information about e-patients means that doctors can provide better care at lower cost. For example, integrated e-clinical support systems can provide e-health professionals in a distributed clinical setting with on-line, real-time history of e-patients accessed from a master patient database. These systems will also allow e-physicians and other e-providers to track and analyze e-patient care history, e-test results, and e-billing and cost information. Typically, such applications combine data warehouses, electronic data entry, messaging, networks, and graphical user interface tools. The most enlightened health care organizations are now discovering that higher-quality care can in fact lead to lower costs.

Future research in e-health strategic planning and design should focus on a basic understanding of the different competitive environments in which health care services can operate and the strategic role and relevance of e-health applications in the different environments. In this regard, an important area to investigate is the appropriate mix of e-health investments in order to maximize strategic expertise and competitive advantage for private nonprofit systems and public sector health organizations. For example, senior management and chief information officers in these environments could be surveyed to find out where or in what areas they perceive that investments in e-health solutions would yield the greatest strategic benefits, and why.

Similarly, a critical question to study is how the process of e-health strategic planning and design should be managed as it moves from isolated intraorganizational concerns to integrated intraorganizational and interorganizational systems and from single-user to multi-user applications. In this context, research on issues related to differences in the strategic thinking, planning, and management of e-health thinking in private sector versus public sector health environments is particularly warranted. I have also noted the importance of understanding how consumer-driven e-health will eventually affect the financing of e-health.

In summary, we stand at a crossroads. The technology we know today has the potential to be applied for the great good of millions of people, even entire populations. At the same time, the ongoing suffering in this world, fighting over limited resources, torturing of human beings, and killings not only of animals but also of large numbers of human beings must be reversed. Technology is only as good as its appropriate use to better the lives of others. Having that power in our hands, we must go about using it well. This, in essence, is the future of e-health care. The ideal and most significant paradigm shift will be the shift in human thinking—that is, applying new and emerging technologies not to destroy the human race but to create a peaceful and healthy world.

Chapter Questions

1. Provide a framework for understanding mobile health. How is mobile health different from and similar to e-health? What other domain or area might be the next frontier?
2. Give an example of a virtual reality application. Why might VR therapies be considered or expected to be superior to conventional therapies? What are the potential side effects of VR for phobia therapies?
3. Why is it important to understand the accountability expectations framework? What significance does this understanding have for our design of future-oriented e-health applications and solutions?
4. What is meant by an adaptive solution?
5. Imagine that you have the power to install an e-health application that would reverse the aging process. Describe the potential characteristics of such a solution, and indicate how it would actually be useful. How might such an innovation be evaluated?

References

Bowman T. (1997, August). VR meets physical therapy. *Communications of the ACM, 40*(8), 59–60.

Carlin, A. S., Hoffman, H. G., & Weghorst, S. (1997). Virtual reality and tactile augmentation in the treatment of spider phobia: A case report. *Behaviour Research and Therapy, 35*(2), 153–158.

Greenleaf, W. (1997, August). Applying VR to physical medicine and rehabilitation. *Communications of the ACM, 40*(8), 43–46.

Inman D. P., Loge, K., & Leavens, J. (1997, August). VR education and rehabilitation. *Communications of the ACM,* 40(8), 53–58.

Keen, P., & Scott-Morton, M. (1978). *Decision support systems: An organizational perspective.* Reading, MA: Addison-Wesley.

Max, M., & Burke, J. (1997). Virtual reality for autism communication and education, with lessons for medical training simulators. *Studies in Health Technology and Informatics, 39,* 46–53.

Mitchell, J. T. (1997). Can hazard risk be communicated through a virtual experience? *Disasters, 21*(3), 258–266.

Modrow, R., & Mathias, R. (1998). Universality: Moving beyond access to outcome [Editorial]. *Canadian Journal of Public Health, 89*(2), 77–78.

Oyama, H., Wakao, F., Mishina, T., Lu, Y., & Honjo, A. (1997). Virtual cancer image data warehouse. *Studies in Health Technology and Informatics, 39,* 151–154.

Raghupathi, W., and Tan, J. (2002, December). Strategic IT applications in health care. *Communications of the ACM, 45*(12), 56–61.

Rothbaum, B. O. Hodges, L., Watson, B. A., Kessler, C. D., & Opdyke, D. (1996). Virtual reality exposure therapy in the treatment of fear of flying: A case report. *Behaviour Research and Therapy, 34*(5–6), 477–481.

Satava, R. M. (1995a). Medical applications of virtual reality. *Journal of Medical Systems, 19*(3), 275–280.

Satava, R. M. (1995b). Virtual reality, telesurgery, and the new world order of medicine. *Journal of Image Guided Surgery, 1*(1), 12–16.

Stanney, K., & Kennedy, R. (1997). The psychometrics of cybersickness. *Communications of the ACM, 40*(8), 67–68.

Strickland, D., Hodges, L., North, M., & Weghorst, S. (1997). Overcoming phobias by virtual exposure. *Communications of the ACM, 40*(8), 34–39.

Tan, J. (1995). *Health management information systems: Theories, methods and applications* (1st ed.). Gaithersburg, MD: Aspen.

Tan, J. (2001). *Health management information systems: Methods and practical applications* (2nd ed.). Sudbury, MA: Jones & Bartlett.

Tan, J., & Modrow, R. (1999). Strategic relevance and accountability expectations: New perspectives for health care information technology design. *Topics in Health Information Management, 19*(4), 84–97.

Tan, J., & Modrow, R. (2003). *Strategic health management IS: Focusing on performance-based indicators.* Paper presented at the 13th American Chinese Management Educators International Conference on Pacific Rim Management, Seattle, July 13-August 2.

Tan, J., with Sheps, S. (1998). *Health decision support systems.* Sudbury, MA: Jones & Bartlett.

Tan, J., Wen, H. J., & Gyires, T. (2003). M-commerce security: The impact of wireless application protocol (WAP) security services on e-business and e-health solutions. *International Journal of M-Commerce, 1*(4), 409–424.

Viire, E. (1997). Health and safety issues for VR. *Communications of the ACM, 40*(8), 40–41.

Wann, J., Rushton, S., Smyth, M., & Jones, D. (1997). Rehabilitative environments for attention and movement disorders. *Communications of the ACM, 40*(8), 49–52.

Weghorst, S. (1997). Augmented reality and Parkinson's disease. *Communications of the ACM, 40*(8), 47–48.

Virtual Reality Case

Joseph Tan, Pency Tsai

Originally conceived by the founder of VPL Research, Jaron Lanier, to refer to immersive virtual reality, in which users are thrown into an artificial computer-generated three-dimensional environment, the term *virtual reality* (VR) refers to a computer-generated interactive multimedia environment into which the user is assimilated, so that he or she becomes an active participant in a virtual world (Pantelidis, 1995; Passig and Eden, 2000). Other closely related terms include *cyberspace, artificial reality, virtual worlds,* and *virtual environments.*

Over the decades, the best-known VR applications have been in the entertainment industry. In fact, VR hype is now almost ubiquitous in that sector, in video games, movies, and more. VR simulations are found in many environments that range from education to military and pilot training and even practice for space shuttle missions. Architects, for example, use VR to envision a building before it is built, to minimize potentially costly mistakes. Molecular biologists use VR to explore the microscopic world of molecules and to "experience" intermolecular forces. The same immersive technology is used to assist people in exploring their phobias (Dunkley, 1994). VR applications are becoming progressively more compelling in many aspects of our lives.

Generally speaking, there are two types of VR technologies. *Immersive virtual reality,* the more advanced technology, fully surrounds users with a computer-generated environment. Users typically wear helmets, data gloves, and a body suit with visual display units and speakers. Thus, the system is able to track users' responses to the simulations. *Non-immersive virtual reality,* which is used primarily for academic purposes such as distance learning, permits users to interact primarily with a three-dimensional (3-D), computer-generated display. The following case focuses on immersive VR technology.

Entering Immersive Virtual Reality Environments

To enter immersive virtual environments (VEs), one must wear special equipment such as data gloves, goggles, and earphones, which receive inputs from the computer. A head-mounted display created by Evans and Sutherland in 1965 was the first device that provided immersive virtual experience. A *head-mounted display* (HMD) is a helmet that covers the user's full face and that contains an optical system and two miniature display screens that continually send images to the eyes. At all times, a motion tracker recognizes and measures the position and movement of the user's head. The

HMD allows the image-generating computer to adjust the scene representation to the appropriate view. Thus, the viewer can "look around" and "walk through" the surrounding VE (Beier, 2004). Several types of HMDs (LCD-display HMD, projected HMD, small-CRT HMD, and single-column-LED HMD) may be used. However, with all HMDs, VR is often quite intrusive, uncomfortable enough to give rise to alternative types of VEs, such as BOOM and CAVE.

The BOOM (*binocular omni-orientation monitor*) is a device mounted on a mechanical arm that has tracking sensors located at the joints. Users must secure the monitor and hold their face up to it. The computer then generates appropriate scenes based on the positions and orientation of the joints on the mechanical arm (Aukstakalnis and Blatner, 1992). Through the use of projected stereo images on the floor and walls of a room-sized cube, the CAVE (cave automatic virtual environment) provides users with the illusion of immersion. Several persons wearing lightweight stereo glasses, for example, can enter and move freely inside the CAVE. Head tracking systems continuously adjust the stereo projection to the current position of the leading viewer.

A *data glove* is an input device equipped with a fiber-optic bend sensor, which helps users sense and generate their finger movements. The sensor also transmits the data to the VR computer. Some sophisticated data gloves can even record movements from wrists and elbows. In the virtual world, users can point to, grip, and push objects, so the use of the data gloves sensually enriches the immersive experience.

Virtual Reality Cases in Health Care

We now move to VR cases in Health Care, including training and education applications, psychology and psychiatry, and phobia therapies.

Training and Education. Computer graphics have been adapted in the Animated Dissection of Anatomy for Medicine (ADAM). With an extensive collection of two-dimensional anatomy drawings, ADAM creates a 3-D effect by cutting away tissue layers and sections.

Another form of VR-like training simulation is electronic laparoscopic simulation. Dunkley (1994) notes that electronic laparoscopic simulations may act like VR. For instance, trainees (students) can insert simulated instruments into an electronic mockup of a body and perform surgeries. Internal organs are displayed on monitors, and the surgeon's virtual movements can be sensed through the use of immersive VR technology. Thus, VR simulation can effectively increase the medical students' skills without risking patients' lives. Using advances in medical knowledge and the evolution of computerized training models, VR provides an alternative medium for medical students to practice medicine.

Many nursing schools continue to add more theoretical courses while shortening the length of practical training so that nurses can enter the workforce sooner. This practice results in deficiencies in clinical experience. With the aid of VR simulations, students can now practice their skills without adverse impacts on patients. Moreover,

VR can also assist students in gaining critical thinking skills by giving them opportunities to take risks and make correct decisions. With VEs, students also have the opportunity to experience care settings similar to those they will face in real life. For example, VR allows nursing students to practice inserting an intravenous line. Students can also practice conducting patient assessments on the desktop, using virtual anatomical 3-D models, while tracking simulated electronic patient records.

Rehabilitation. Virtual reality has been proven effective as a treatment tool in rehabilitation. VR allows disabled individuals to practice tasks they wish to accomplish in real life without fear of pain or further injury. VR can be used in occupational therapy to improve balance and dynamic standing tolerance, especially in geriatric patients. It can also help patients with spinal cord injuries to overcome some of the physical limitations that affect their mobility and to increase their level of independence as well as the quality of their daily life.

It is often difficult to conduct accurate and controlled assessments of stroke patients' memories. There is scanty empirical evidence about how to address problems related to loss of prospective memory (Brooks, 2004). Prospective memory is the type of memory that is needed to complete future tasks, such as remembering to give a note to someone when you next see them, to pick up milk on the way home, or to keep an appointment. By testing prospective memory through simulations in VEs, a better assessment of the memory loss can be achieved. This will also help overcome some of the difficulties such as designing real world tasks for effective rehabilitation programs on stroke patients.

Surgical Applications. VR can provide 3-D anatomical views of internal organs as well as bones for simulations of surgical operations. This kind of practice enables surgeons to visualize the intended procedure more accurately, which improves their perception in the operative field. In addition to helping surgeons prepare for surgery through simulations, VR technology can circumvents many problems in actual surgery. For example, during a brain operation, VR technology can be used to fuse an MRI scan of the patient's tumor with a video image of the actual brain, which can obscure much of the X-ray image and result in loss of surgical precision if the tumor is deeply embedded in the brain tissues (Satava, 1995).

The most extreme use of VR in surgery is telepresence surgery, in which the surgeons in a remote location perform procedures on a virtual image of the patient. Their movements are electronically transmitted to a medical telerobot that performs the procedure on the actual patient (Iovine, 1995).

Psychology and Psychiatry. The use of VR in medicine is not new; various VEs for health care have been developed for surgical procedures, preventive medicine and patient education, medical education and training, visualization of massive medical databases, and architectural design for health care facilities. However, there is a growing recognition that VR can play an important role in clinical psychology as well. VR applications can provide a range of services from diagnostic tests to therapeutic improvements. VR is an effective medium of treatment for a variety of disorders. One example is the use of VR in the treatment of phobias. Patients are helped to overcome their irrational fears and apprehensions through virtual exposure to phobogenic stimuli. A controlled study by Hodges and Rothbaum showed VR to be effective in remedying acrophobic subjects' anxiety and avoidance of heights (Kooper, 1995). Besides being time-efficient and cost-effective, VR defines a very controlled environment for phobia treatment. In other words, VR phobia treatment eliminates the variables that might prevent treatment receivers from successfully identifying and addressing the stimuli of interest. It is also worth mentioning that most people with phobias prefer to undergo virtual exposure rather than being exposed to a feared situation or object in vivo. We will now examine the use of VR for treatment of phobias in more detail.

Types of Phobias

Phobias can be divided into three categories: social phobias, specific phobias, and panic disorders. Social phobias, also known as social anxiety disorders, occur when individuals have excessive anxieties in social situations; such as, parties, meetings, interviews, restaurants, making complaints, writing in public, eating in restaurants, and interacting with the opposite sex, strangers, and aggressive individuals. Specific phobias, also known as simple phobia, is a persistent, irrational fear of, and compelling desire to avoid, specific objects or situations. Panic disorder is marked by recurrent, spontaneous fear and panic attacks. A panic attack is an intense period of fear or discomfort.

The National Institute of Mental Health estimates that at least 5.3 million Americans have a social phobia. Furthermore, the Surgeon General's *Report on Mental Health,* issued at the end of 1999, indicates that approximately 7 percent of Americans are disturbed to some extent by social phobias in their daily life (Smith, 2004a). Unfortunately, social phobias are only one type of fear. The NIMH further indicates that more than one out of ten Americans has had one or more specific phobias. A telephone study of one thousand adults done by Penn, Schoen, & Berland Associates, Inc., for Discovery Health shows that 7 percent of Americans report themselves as suffering from a phobia. Shockingly, about 40 percent admit that they have a great fear of a specific object or a specific situation. For example, Americans have fears of snakes (40 percent), rats (58 percent), and cockroaches (23 percent). Moreover, 24 percent of American women and 17 percent of men acknowledge the fear of being in crowded or open spaces. It is estimated that roughly a third of all Americans admit to having had panic attacks. Despite these high indices of fear, only about 11 percent of all people with phobias seek professional help.

According to Dr. Roger Burket, associate professor and director of residency training at the University of Florida's Division of Child and Adolescent Psychiatry, children often suffer from the same phobias and anxieties as their parents do (Smith, 2004a). His research indicates that many people learn phobias by hearing about their parent's fears or witnessing their parents' reaction when feared situations or objects are presented. According to Dr. Cary Savage, director of the Cognitive Neuroscience Group in the Department of Psychiatry at Massachusetts General Hospital and Harvard Medical School, it is not clear whether phobic reactions of children of parents with phobias are biologically inherited or attributable to early learning.

People with specific phobias are usually aware of their abnormal fears. Only when the fear interferes with their lives, however, do they seek professional help. Common phobias include fear of animals, insects, heights, elevators, flying, automobile driving, water, storms, and blood or injections.

Phobic disorders rarely develop after the age of twenty-five, according to the National Mental Health Association. Studies funded by the National Institute of Mental Health show that a specific phobia may be inherited or may result from damage to the amygdala, a small structure in the brain that may be responsible for fear responses (Smith, 2004c). However, serious social phobias may develop later in life or can be transformed into panic disorders, which are characterized by chest pains, heart palpitations, shortness of breath, dizziness, or abdominal distress. People who suffer from social phobias also have a 50 percent chance of simultaneously suffering from other psychiatric problems, such as depression, substance abuse, or panic disorder.

Traditional Versus Virtual Reality Therapy (VRT)

Medicine and other cognitive-behavioral therapies have traditionally provided remedies for phobias. The most effective and well-recognized phobia therapy is exposure therapy; that is, gradually exposing people with phobias to the stimuli that cause fear. For example, repeated exposure to footbridges, outdoor balconies, and glass elevators, virtual or otherwise, has been proven to successfully decrease patients' fear of heights and, furthermore, to change their previous outlook on heights as they become accustomed to heights (Hodges and others, 2001).

During VR exposure treatment, when patients are put into VR environments, their fears get activated; patients begin to experience physical reactions when in feared situations, such as sweating, "butterflies" in the stomach, and weak knees. Although the reactions are initially rather strong, with the help of the virtual reality therapy, most patients usually recover from their fears quite quickly. Progressively, they are also more able to face their fears in real life. Virtual reality exposure therapy places the client in a computer-generated world where they "experience" the various stimuli related to their phobia. The patient wears a head-mounted display with small TV monitors and stereo earphones to receive both visual and auditory cues. VR Therapy tends to cost less than vivo exposure. The "phobic" experience is in total control without leaving the therapist's office and the segments of any phobia can be repeated, allowing the patient to gradually reduce fear and anxiety. People once resistant to traditional treatment may find Virtual Reality Therapy acceptable.

A test of VR therapy's efficiency has been the treatment of combat-related posttraumatic stress disorders (PTSD) among Vietnam veterans (Hodges and others, 2001). Patients may develop PTSD after a traumatic change in their lives, such as a severe car accident or a sexual assault. High avoidance of retrieving past traumatic memories, sleep difficulties, nightmares, and flashbacks are some symptoms of PTSD.

Combat-related PTSD affected approximately 830,000 Vietnam War veterans (Hodges and others, 2001). VR therapy can provide much needed help in facilitating retrieval of past traumatic memories. For patients suffering from PTSD, the virtual world is a place they could go to confront their fear or to confront a traumatic experience. Studies have shown that retrieval of past traumatic memories can help cure PTSD symptoms.

Conclusion

Virtual reality technology has many potential applications in medicine, including surgical training; tele-operated robotic surgery; assessment and rehabilitation of phobias and other social, behavioral, and neurological disorders; and diagnosis and rehabilitation of physical disabilities. Virtual reality today offers a new paradigm for human-computer interaction, in which users are no longer simply external observers of images on a computer screen, but active participants within a computer-generated three-dimensional world. Most of the psychological therapies carried out with the help of virtual reality rely on the principle of exposure. Possibilities offered by VR in the field of the cognitive-behavioral therapies are numerous. VRT has not replaced the role played by therapist. Indeed, his/her presence near to the patient remains essential. It seems that VR reinforces the therapeutic relation between patient and therapist on a collaborative mode.

Case Questions

1. Define virtual reality. Name the different types of virtual reality.
2. What are the major areas in which VR can be applied to health care?
3. What effective is VRT in treating phobic disorders?

References

Abrams, R. (2002, April 10). A nurse's viewpoint: A new beginning. *HealthLeaders.com,*

Aukstakalnis, S., & Blatner, D. (1992). *Silicon, mirage, the art and science of virtual reality.* Berkeley, CA: Peachpit Press.

Beier, K. (2004, February 10). *Virtual reality: A short introduction.* Retrieved on March 4, 2004, from http://www-vrl.umich.edu/intro/index.html#Applications

Brooks, B. M., Rose, F. D., Potter, J., Jayawardena, S., & Morling, A. (2004). Assessing stroke patients' prospective memory using virtual reality. *Brain Injury, 18*(4), 391–401.

Cunningham, D., & Krishack, M. (1999). Virtual reality: A holistic approach to rehabilitation. *Study Health Technology and Informatics, 62,* 90–93.

Dunkley, P. (1994). Virtual reality in medical training. *Lancet, 343*(14), 1218.

Hodges, L. F., Anderson, P., Burdea, G., Hoffman, H. G., & Rothbaum, B. O. (2001, November/December). Treating psychological and physical disorders with VR. *IEEE Computer Graphics and Applications,* 25–33.

Iovine, J. (1995). *Step into virtual reality.* Windcrest/McGraw-Hill.

Kooper, R. (1995). Virtual reality exposure therapy. Retrieved from http://www.cc.gatech.edu/gvu/virtual/Phobia/phobia.html

Pantelidis, V. (1995). Reasons to use VR in education. *VR in Schools, 1*(1), 9.

Passig, D., & Eden, S. (2000). Improving flexible thinking in deaf and hard of learning children with virtual reality technology. *American Annals of the Deaf, 145,* 286–291.

Riva, G. (1998). Virtual reality in paraplegia: A VR-enhanced orthopedic appliance for walking and rehabilitation. *Study Health Technology and Informatics*

Rothbaum, B. O., Hodges, L. F., Kooper, R., Opdyke, D., Williford, J., & North, M. M. (1995). Effectiveness of computer-generated (virtual reality) graded exposure in the treatment of acrophobia. *American Journal of Psychiatry, 152*(4), 626–628.

Roy, L. S. (2002). The virtual reality revolution: Technology changes nursing education. *Nursing Management, 33*(9), 14–15.

Satava, R. M. (1995). Medical applications of virtual reality. *Journal of Medical Systems, 19*(3), 275–280.

Smith, A. (2004a). *Facts about phobia.* Retrieved from http://health.discovery.com/centers/mental/phobias/facts.html

Smith, A. (2004b). *Phobias A to Z.* Retrieved from http://health.discovery.com/centers/mental/phobias/phobialist.html

Smith, A. (2004c). *Treatment of phobia.* Retrieved from http://health.discovery.com/centers/mental/phobias/treatment.html

Smith, A. (2004d). *Virtual treatments.* Retrieved from http://health.discovery.com/centers/mental/phobias/virtual.html

Weiss, P., & Jessel, A. (1998). Virtual reality applications to work. *Work, 11*(3), 277–293.

NAME INDEX

Viire, E., 535, 547
Voigt, B., 283, 290

W

Wachter, G., 51, 52, 175, 189
Waddell, G., 296, 297, 314, 320, 321
Wahr, J., 279, 290
Waites, K. B., 154
Wakao, F., 277, 289, 546
Walczak, S., 310, 321
Walker, C., 449
Walshon, J., 449
Walter, S., 169, 180, 189
Wang, C., 187, 189
Wang, Q., 36
Wang, S., 398, 405
Wang, S.-Y., 480, 481, 487
Wang, Y., 190, 479, 481, 487
Wann, J., 534, 547
Ward, R. E., 287
Warner, P., 126
Watanabe, M., 240, 241, 260
Watson, B. A., 546
Weber, D., 496, 514
Weghorst, S., 530, 532, 534, 546, 547
Wei, C., 260, 266, 330, 331, 352, 353, 354, 355, 356, 360, 361

Weisberg, M., 449
Weisman, S., 528
Weiss, P., 553
Welsh, T. M., 209, 210, 223
Wen, H. J., 168, 189, 365, 462, 478, 526, 546
West, D., 496, 507, 514
Wheatley, M., 71, 82
Wheeler, L., 274, 282, 288
White, J., 224
Whitehouse, F., 287
Whitten, P., 141, 154
Wilcox, D., 380, 396
Wilczynski, N., 449
Wilkins, A. S., 497, 501, 502, 514
Williams, M., 463, 478
Williamson, J., 271, 287
Williford, J., 553
Wilson, D., 462, 475, 477
Winker, M. A., 211, 224
Witteman, C.L.M., 321
Wnek, J., 332, 352
Wolfson, H. G., 289
Wondrow, M., 189
Wong, T. K., 214, 222
Woods, D., 205, 224
Woodward, B., 175, 186, 189, 190, 191, 194, 200
Woollet, A., 28, 36
Wouden, J., 126

Wright, D., 240, 243, 260
Wu, C.-P., 480, 481, 488
Wu, H., 515, 517, 519, 520
Wu, J., 274, 290

X

Xydis, T. G., 191, 192, 197, 200

Y

Yap, C. S., 259
Yasnoff, W., 41, 52, 129, 130, 131, 132, 155
Yen, D. C., 489
Yu, P., 331, 351

Z

Zadeh, L. A., 314, 321
Zafar Husain, S., 411, 439
Zait, M., 332, 352
Zanasi, A., 351
Zeller, R. L., 252, 260
Zeng, W., 480, 481, 488
Zhang, J., 170, 181, 189
Zhang, Y. T., 190, 191, 194, 200
Zhou, X., 189
Ziv, J., 483, 488
Zmud, R. W., 248, 252, 259

SUBJECT INDEX

A

Abaton, 388

Absolute risk reduction, 442

Acceptance: of e-home care, 284–285; of EHRs, factor critical to, 103, 106; ensuring, 24, 33; obtaining, 33; as requisite for e-medicine implementation, 253; social and cultural context of, 505; unresolved issues of, 241

Access network, 168

Access to care, addressing issue of, 5, 11, 38, 39, 543–544

Access to information. *See* Information access

Accessibility requirements, 172, 173, 174–177

Accordant, 385

Accountability: privacy principle of, *110*; public, emphasis on, 40, 96

Accountability expectations: framework for, 540–543; increasing pressure to adapt to, 4

Accuracy: of e-DSS, 311, 312,

313; of EHRs, issue of, 123; privacy principle of, *111*; of public health data, 135

ACP Journal Club (ACP-ASIM), 445

Active surveillance, 135

Actual visit, meaning of, 272

Acute care needs, driven by, issue of, 45

Ad hoc wireless network, defining, 192

Adaptation, over time, to new technology, 501

Addis Ababa University, 248

Administrative and clinical cost reduction. *See* Cost reduction

Administrative and policy diagnosis, 84

Administrative and support applications, 214–219

Administrative benefits, 100–101

Administrative concerns, 240

Administrative data warehouse (ADW), 139, 140, *141*

Administrative Simplification, 458–459

Administrative training, 213

Admission-discharge-transfer

(ADT) system, 61

Advance appointments, issue of, 118–119

Advanced Informatics Distributed Medical Access Network (AIDMAN), 183–184

Adverse drug effects, 398

Advisory Council on Health Infostructure (ACHI), 94–95, 96, 109, 115

AenausHealthcare, 385

Aetna, 385, 386

Affordable care, 44

African continent, 236

African Human Development Indicators, *246*, 260

Age and experience, general practitioner awareness levels influenced by, 117

Agency for Healthcare Research and Quality, 445

Agglomerative clustering, 335

Aggregates, service encompassing, 452. *See also* E-health data integration (e-HDI)

Aging population trend, 269–270, 272, 281